Navigating Pediatric Brain Tumors

Angela Mastronuzzi • Andrea Carai
Editors

Navigating Pediatric Brain Tumors

Springer

Editors
Angela Mastronuzzi
Area of Hematology-Oncology,
Cell Therapy, Gene Therapies, and
Hematopoietic Transplantation Bambino
Gesù Children's Hospital, IRCCS
Rome, Italy

Department of Life Sciences and
Public Health
Università Cattolica del Sacro Cuore
Rome, Italy

Andrea Carai
Neurosurgery Unit
IRCCS Bambino Gesù Children's
Hospital
Rome, Italy

ISBN 978-3-032-18991-2 ISBN 978-3-032-18992-9 (eBook)
https://doi.org/10.1007/978-3-032-18992-9

This Springer imprint is published by the registered company Springer Nature Switzerland AG
The registered company address is: Gewerbestrasse 11, 6330 Cham, Switzerland

Preface

Pediatric brain tumors occupy a unique and humbling place in medicine. They are the most common solid malignancy of childhood and among the most heterogeneous and complex diseases in medicine. A single diagnostic category can encompass more than a hundred molecularly distinct entities, each with its own natural history, therapeutic vulnerability, and impact on the developing child. To care for these children is to navigate uncertainty with precision, and compassion with scientific rigor.
This textbook was born from that duality.

Over the last decade, our understanding of pediatric central nervous system tumors has undergone a profound transformation. The era in which classification rested solely on histology has given way to an integrated molecular era, defined by the WHO Classification of CNS Tumors, 5th edition, DNA methylation profiling, and next-generation sequencing. Entities once grouped together are now recognized as fundamentally different diseases. These discoveries have transformed not only tumor classification but also therapeutic decision-making and our vision for the future of pediatric neuro-oncology.

A critical part of this molecular revolution is the growing recognition of Cancer Predisposition Syndromes (CPS). A significant proportion of pediatric brain tumors—far higher than previously appreciated—arises in the context of an underlying germline predisposition. From Neurofibromatosis Type 1 and Type 2, Tuberous Sclerosis Complex and Gorlin Syndrome, to Li-Fraumeni Syndrome, Constitutional Mismatch Repair Deficiency, and other newly described entities, these syndromes reshape our clinical approach. Identifying a predisposition syndrome influences tumor surveillance strategies, informs therapeutic choices and radiation avoidance, guides genetic counseling for the family, and has profound implications for siblings and future generations. For this reason, this textbook integrates germline predisposition not as a separate topic, but as an essential perspective through which every tumor type should be considered.

Yet, for all our molecular advances, the core challenge remains unchanged: a brain tumor in a child is never just a tumor. It exists within a developing brain, within a child who must continue to grow and develop, and within a family whose life has been profoundly altered. Surgical decisions must be weighed against functional preservation. Oncological efficacy must be weighed against long-term neurocognitive outcomes. Survival must be weighed against quality of survival. No single discipline can address these challenges alone.

For this reason, *Navigating Pediatric Brain Tumors* is intentionally multidisciplinary. It is designed as a comprehensive resource for all professionals who care for children with CNS tumors—pediatric and adult neuro-oncologists, neurosurgeons, radiation oncologists, neuroradiologists, neuropathologists, clinical geneticists, neurologists, endocrinologists, rehabilitation specialists, neuropsychologists, nurses, and trainees across these fields.

A central principle guiding this work is that palliative care is not an alternative to disease-directed therapy, but an essential and concurrent component of it.

In pediatric neuro-oncology, palliative care is not synonymous with end-of-life care. From the time of diagnosis, children experience a substantial symptom burden together with profound emotional and psychosocial challenges affecting the entire family. Therefore, early integration of palliative care is essential. In this textbook, principles of palliative care are integrated throughout the clinical continuum, from state-of-the-art symptom management and psychosocial support, to compassionate communication about goals of care, and to competent and dignified end-of-life care focused on minimizing suffering.

Our ultimate goal is to provide a clear, evidence-based, and humanistic guide to clinical practice—whether the intent is cure, disease control, or comfort.

This book is dedicated to our patients and their families. Their courage and resilience in the face of extraordinary adversity inspire our work and remind us that while we navigate tumors, they are navigating childhood itself. Our greatest measure of success lies not only in survival but in lives lived with the least possible suffering and the greatest possible quality of life.

We hope this textbook will serve as a trusted companion in that endeavor.

Rome, Italy — Angela Mastronuzzi
2026 — Andrea Carai

Contents

Epidemiology

1

Teresa Perillo

1.1 Incidence

Brain tumors are the most common type of solid childhood tumors, as well as the leading cause of cancer-related death among children. Based on Global Cancer Observatory (GLOBOCAN) 2020 estimates, there were 30.766 new cases and 15,337 deaths due to primary brain and Central Nervous System (CNS) cancer tumors in children and adolescents (age 0–19 years) in 2020, 24,388 of which were children 0–14 years old [1]. Nevertheless, incidence differs among countries, thus reflecting the impact of the accessibility of the community to health care. It ranges from approximately 0.3 to 5.14 cases per 100,000 children in different parts of the world, with the highest rates reported in the United States, where incidence of all primary brain and other CNS tumors in children and adolescents <20 years of age was 6.06 per 100,000 children from 2012 to 2016 [2]. The incidence was reported to be higher in non-Hispanics compared to Hispanics (6.35 vs 5.14 per 100,000) as well as in Whites compared to Blacks (6.29 vs 4.71 per 100,000). Additionally, the incidence of all CNS tumors was higher in girls compared to boys (6.13 vs 5.98 per 100,000). The observed elevated incidence in girls might be driven by meningioma in 15–19-year-old females [2].

T. Perillo (✉)
Pediatric Oncology and Haemathology, Bari, Italy

1.2 Distribution

The fifth edition of the World Health Organization (WHO) Classification of Tumors of the Central Nervous System, published in 2021, introduced major changes in brain tumor classification due to new molecular diagnostic features [3].

Twenty-two tumor types were introduced, based on specific molecular alterations. Low-grade gliomas (LGGs) are the most frequent brain tumors of childhood, accounting for a third of all cases [4]. Pilocytic astrocytomas are the most common pediatric low-grade tumors, and they have a very favorable prognosis. Most of them are located in the cerebellum and suprasellar region, but they can appear elsewhere. Embryonal tumors are a heterogeneous group of malignant CNS tumors and they are the second most common brain tumors of childhood. Embryonal tumors account for approximately 20% of childhood brain tumors [5]. The old term "PNET" has been replaced by the term "CNS embryonal tumor," based on molecular profiling. Medulloblastomas (MBs) and other CNS embryonal tumors are the two main types of embryonal tumors. MBs account for more than 60% of childhood embryonal tumors, and 70% occur in children under the age of 10 years; one third of cases arise in children under the age of 3 years. Ependymomas are the third most common brain tumors of childhood, accounting for 5–10% of CNS neoplasms in children; 90% arise in the posterior fossa, and the

A. Mastronuzzi, A. Carai (eds.), *Navigating Pediatric Brain Tumors*,
https://doi.org/10.1007/978-3-032-18992-9_1

remainder are spinal. Ependymomas are still classified as grades 1, 2, or 3 according to the degree of anaplasia. The rare subependymoma is grade 1, while grade 2 and 3 ependymomas are supratentorial or infratentorial in location. Posterior fossa ependymomas are subdivided into PFA, occurring predominantly in infants, and PFB ependymomas, occurring in older children. Pediatric-type high-grade gliomas (HGGs) account for 10% of brain tumors in children and have a poor prognosis. Among them, the diffuse midline glioma is a still a lethal tumor that affects young children, and H3K27-altered tumors are associated with worse survival than wild-type counterparts [6]. As for overall age distribution, according to the CBTRUS report, among children aged 0–14, gliomas and embryonal tumors accounted for 49.7% and 12.3% of brain and other CNS tumors, respectively. The most common glioma histopathology was pilocytic astrocytoma (20.4%). Medulloblastomas, atypical teratoid/ rhabdoid tumor (ATRT), and all other embryonal tumors accounted for 67.3%, 16.9%, and 12.1%, respectively, of embryonal tumors in children. Regarding distribution of tumors by site and histopathology in adolescents (ages 15–19 years), the most common histopathology in adolescents was tumors of the pituitary (35.6%). Gliomas accounted for 28.5% of brain tumors, and the most common glioma histopathology in adolescents was pilocytic astrocytoma (7.7%) [7].

1.3 Prognosis

Recent diagnostic and therapeutic advances have led to improvement in survival and quality of life for many children with CNS cancers. However, the prognosis for many children with brain tumors remains poor, and treatments have long-term sequelae. Prognosis of pediatric brain tumors (PBTs) varies greatly and depends on various factors, including tumor histology, tumor location, age at diagnosis, race, ethnicity, and sex. The 10-year survival for children aged 0–19 diagnosed with malignant brain and other CNS tumors was estimated at 72% with lowest (17%) and highest (96%) survival rates being attributable to high-grade gliomas and pilocytic astrocytomas, respectively [2]. Overall, tumors located in the brain stem show the poorest survival compared to tumors located at any other site; survival is better for older children compared to very young children that cannot be treated intensively. As for race, survival was reported to be poorer among non-Hispanic Blacks and Hispanic children compared with non-Hispanic Whites in the United States for the period of 2001–2008; 5-year relative survival was reported as 77.6% for non-Hispanic White patients, 69.8% for non-Hispanic Black children, and 72.9% for Hispanic ones [2].

1.4 Risk Factors

No direct cause for brain tumors has been identified; genetic and environmental factors play a combined role in the pathogenesis of brain tumors [8].

1.5 Cancer Predisposition Syndromes and Family Risk

The application of sequencing approaches has demonstrated that 8–19% of pediatric CNS tumor patients harbor a germline alteration in a classical tumor predisposition gene [9]. Neurofibromatosis type 1 (NF1) and type 2 (NF2), tuberous sclerosis complex, Li-Fraumeni syndrome (LFS), Gorlin syndrome, familial adenomatous polyposis (FAP), and constitutional mismatch repair deficiency (CMMRD) are the most common genetic syndromes predisposing to nervous system tumors. Optic pathway gliomas and brainstem low-grade gliomas are the most common intracranial neoplasms found in NF1, and an increased incidence of high-grade gliomas has been noted as well (50-fold higher when compared to the general population) [9]. The most common tumors seen in NF2 are vestibular and non-vestibular cranial and spinal nerve schwannomas, peripheral nerve schwannomas, meningiomatosis, intracranial or spinal meningiomas, and ependymomas. In the pediatric age group, the most frequent symptoms and signs of NF2 are related to underlying skin or spinal tumors [10]. SEGA is the only CNS tumor seen in TS [11]. Children with CMMRD are usually affected within the first two decades of life. HGGs are the most common brain tumors; however, medulloblastoma and supratentorial primitive embryonal tumors have also been reported and usually present in the second decade of life. HGGs may arise from transformation of LGGs and there exist reports of long-term survivors, suggesting a more favorable prognosis relative to patients with sporadic HGGs [12]. MB is the most common CNS tumor in the setting of Gorlin syndrome and develops earlier compared to sporadic tumors. Most patients are younger than 3 years of age, with tumor histology showing medulloblastoma with extensive nodularity (MBEN), which is almost pathognomonic for the syndrome in young children. Several reports have documented the development of intracranial meningiomas in patients with Gorlin syndrome with or without prior craniospinal radiation therapy [13]. MBs are the most common brain tumors in FAP patients (60%), followed by astrocytomas (14%) and ependymoma (10%). The lifetime risk of developing a primary CNS tumor is roughly 1% in the context of FAP, but the risk of developing MBs is 92 times higher than in the general population [14]. Brain tumors are found in about 14% of the patients with *TP53* germline mutations, with an average of onset of 16 years. The frequency of brain tumors is high (21%) in patients with mutations in the L2 and L3 loops of *TP53* that mediate the binding to the minor groove of DNA. Among associated CNS tumors, choroid plexus carcinoma affects LFS carriers in the first decade of life and MBs usually in the second, while malignant gliomas can occur throughout childhood but more commonly in young adults. HGGs are the most common CNS tumor in the context of LFS [15].

As for family risk, a higher risk of developing CNS tumors was observed among siblings diagnosed with medulloblastoma and other CNS embryonal tumors; in general, there is limited evidence for an association between family history of cancer and non-syndromic PBTs. The genetic architecture of familial PBTs has not been extensively studied due to their extreme rarity. About 10% of sporadic PBT cases harbor a germline predisposition mutation; yet to date, studies have mainly focused on high-penetrant germline mutations in known cancer predisposition genes.

1.6 Non-genetic Risk Factors

1.6.1 Pollution

The increased CNS cancer burden due to environmental factors is linked to a country's degree of industrialization. *Pagano C* et al. discussed the impact of environmental carcinogens on modulating the risk of brain tumorigenesis. Continuous exposure to pesticides, heavy metals, and industrial-generated microparticles (such as PM2.5) can have an impact on pediatric brain cancer, and there is a scientific association between environmental pollutants and brain tumors [16]. Early development (e.g., prenatal and early childhood) seems to be a vulnerable window of exposure [17]. There is an increased risk of astrocytoma in children living in the border areas between urban and industrial areas [18, 19].

Some studies have focused on the association between maternal exposure to environmental pollutants and brain tumors, concluding that there is an increased risk for astrocytoma for maternal employment in diesel engine exhaust industries. Moreover, there is an increased risk of having a child affected by astrocytoma in the first 5 years of life for mothers living within 1.6 km of sites that release carcinogens into the environment. Increased risk has been observed for mothers living within 1 mile of a facility releasing carcinogens compared to ones living >1 mile from a facility [20, 21].

1.7 Ionizing and Non-ionizing Radiations

It is well known that children are more radiosensitive than adults and that children who received radiation therapy for acute lymphoblastic leukemia have an increased risk of brain tumor development later in life. [22]. Fetal exposure to moderate doses of ionizing radiation between weeks 8 and 25 of gestation may increase CNS developmental defects and later brain tumor risk [23]. The effects of non-ionizing radiation on the risk of PBTs are not supported by sufficient data, so that IARC concluded that there are not sufficient data to classify ELFs as a risk factor for brain tumors [22, 24].

1.8 Child Characteristics

There is no consistent evidence for an association between allergic and atopic conditions and decreased risk of PBTs. High birth weight and neurological anomalies seem to be correlated with an increased risk of pediatric CNS tumors, particularly astrocytoma and embryonal tumors [24].

References

1. Sung H, Ferlay J, Siegel RL. Global Cancer Statistics 2020: GLOBOCAN estimates of incidence and mortality worldwide for 36 cancers in 185 countries; First published: 04 February 2021. https://doi.org/10.3322/caac.21660
2. Fahmideh MA, Scheurer ME. Pediatric brain tumors: descriptive epidemiology, risk factors, and future directions. Cancer Epidemiol Biomarkers Prev. 2021;30(5):813–21. https://doi.org/10.1158/1055-9965.EPI-20-1443. Epub 2021 Mar 2
3. Louis DN, Perry A, Wesseling P, et al. The 2021 WHO classification of tumors of the central nervous system: a summary. Neuro-Oncology. 2021;23:1231–51.
4. Sturm D, Pfister SM, Jones DTW. Pediatric gliomas: current concepts on diagnosis, biology, and clinical management. J Clin Oncol. 2017;35:2370–7.
5. McKean-Cowdin R, Razavi P, Barrington-Trimis J, et al. Trends in childhood brain tumor incidence, 1973–2009. J Neuro-Oncol. 2013;115:153–60.
6. Cohen AR. Brain tumors in children. N Engl J Med. 2022;386(20):1922–31. Published May 18, 2022. https://doi.org/10.1056/NEJMra2116344.
7. Price M, Ballard CAP, Benedetti JR, Kruchko C, Barnholtz-Sloan JS, Ostrom QT. CBTRUS statistical report: primary brain and other central nervous system tumors diagnosed in the United States in 2018–2022. Neurooncol. 2025;27(Suppl_4):iv1–iv66. https://doi.org/10.1093/neuonc/noaf194.
8. Subramanian S, Ahmad T. Childhood brain tumors; Last Update: August 8, 2023.
9. Sait SF, Walsh MF, Karajannis MA. Genetic syndromes predisposing to pediatric brain tumors. Neurooncol Pract. 2021;8(4):375–90. https://doi.org/10.1093/nop/npab012. Advance Access date 13 February 2021
10. Ruggieri M, Iannetti P, Polizzi A, et al. Earliest clinical manifestations and natural history of neurofibromatosis type 2 (NF2) in childhood: a study of 24 patients. Neuropediatrics. 2005;36(1):21–34.
11. Roach ES, Gomez MR, Northrup H. Tuberous sclerosis complex consensus conference: revised clinical diagnostic criteria. J Child Neurol. 1998;13(12):624–8.
12. Wimmer K, Etzler J. Constitutional mismatch repair-deficiency syndrome: have we so far seen only the tip of an iceberg? Hum Genet. 2008;124(2):105–22.
13. Askaner G, Lei U, Bertelsen B, et al. Novel SUFU frameshift variant leading to meningioma in three generations in a family with Gorlin syndrome. Case Rep Genet. 2019;2019:9650184.
14. Attard TM, Giglio P, Koppula S, et al. Brain tumors in individuals with familial adenomatous polyposis: a cancer registry experience and pooled case report analysis. Cancer. 2007;109(4):761–6.
15. Olivier M, Goldgar DE, Sodha N, et al. Li-Fraumeni and related syndromes: correlation between tumor type, family structure, and TP53 genotype. Cancer Res. 2003;63(20):6643–50.
16. Pagano C e a, Navarra G, Coppola C, et al. Impacts of environmental pollution on brain tumorigenesis. Int J Mol Sci. 2023;24(5):5045. https://doi.org/10.3390/ijms24055045.
17. Parenteau AM, Hang S, Swartz JR, Wexler AS, Hostinar CE. Clearing the air: a systematic review of studies on air pollution and childhood brain outcomes to mobilize policy change. Dev Cogn Neurosci. 2024;69:101436. https://doi.org/10.1016/j.dcn.2024.101436.
18. Ramis R, Tamayo-Uria I, Gómez-Barroso D, et al. Risk factors for central nervous system tumors in children: new findings from a case-control study. PLoS One. 2017;12(2):e0171881.
19. Danysh HE, Mitchell LE, Zhang K, Scheurer ME, Lupo PJ. Traffic-related air pollution and the incidence of childhood central nervous system tumors: Texas, 2001-2009. Pediatr Blood Cancer. 2015;62(9):1572–8. https://doi.org/10.1002/pbc.25549. Epub 2015 May 11
20. Volk J, Heck JE, Schmiegelow K, Hansen J. Parental occupational exposure to diesel engine exhaust in relation to childhood leukaemia and central nervous system cancers: a register-based nested case-control study in Denmark 1968-2016. Occup Environ Med. 2019;76(11):809–17.
21. Choi HS, Shim YK, Wendy E, et al. Potential residential exposure to toxics release inventory chemicals during pregnancy and childhood brain cancer. Environ Health Perspect. 2006;114, 7
22. Ostrom QT, AdelFahmideh M, Cote DJ, Muskens IS, Schraw JM, Scheurer ME, et al. Risk factors for childhood and adult primary brain tumors. Neuro-Oncology. 2019;21:1357–75.
23. Adel Fahmideh M, Lavebratt C, Schuz J, Roosli M, Tynes T, Grotzer MA, et al. Common genetic variations in cell cycle and DNA repair pathways associated with pediatric brain tumor susceptibility. Oncotarget. 2016;7:63640–50.
24. Cooney T, Fisher PG, Tao L, Clarke CA, Partap S. Pediatric neuro-oncology survival disparities in California. J Neuro-Oncol. 2018;138:83–97.

Clinical Presentation and Diagnosis

2

Valentina Di Martino and Daniele Bertin

2.1 Introduction

Clinical manifestations of brain tumors vary and depend on their site, histological type, patient's age, and the presence of increased intracranial pressure.

Frequently, brain tumors manifest with a constellation of non-specific symptoms with the risk of delay in diagnosis. Some studies show that specific and localising signs occur in the late phases of the disease process, while early non-specific symptoms could not trigger suspicion of a brain tumor. A prolonged interval between symptom onset and diagnosis correlates with a greater likelihood of life-threatening complications; moreover, those experiencing a delayed diagnosis often exhibit irreversible neurological deficits at the time of diagnosis, including visual impairment and endocrinopathies, or cognitive impairments later in life. It is important to note that not only the tumor itself but also associated hydrocephalus could significantly impair neurodevelopment and have severe long-term sequelae [1, 2].

The second problem that delays the diagnosis is that many initial symptoms and signs of central nervous system (CNS) tumors overlap with those of more prevalent and less severe childhood ills, such as gastroenteritis, migraine, and behavioural disorders.

Finally, the age of the patient is important for the risk of a delayed diagnosis for the ability to express a symptom: an older patient could describe a new onset headache or a visual loss, while younger children are not able to localise the pain or have not the skills to understand a particular condition [2].

The CNS tumors typically present with symptoms indicative of raised intracranial pressure related to tumor mass effect or concomitant hydrocephalus; these include the classical triad (early morning headache, vomiting, and papilledema), sometimes coupled with focal neurological deficits. In these cases, an emergency brain CT scan or, if possible, MRI should be conducted [1].

However, additional symptoms may also be present, including motor, verbal, and behavioural deficits, which can be progressive. These symptoms are often related to the exact location of the tumor: for example, in the most frequent tumors, such as those located in the posterior fossa, there is often ataxia, fine motor dysfunction, and balance disorders. Sometimes there are also cranial nerve deficits. Lastly, the brainstem could be involved with respiratory and circulatory disorders [1–3].

In this chapter, we will outline the primary clinical patterns observed in childhood brain

V. Di Martino · D. Bertin (✉)
Paediatric Haematology Oncology Department – Ospedale Infantile Regina Margherita, Turin, Italy
e-mail: dbertin@cittadellasalute.to.it

A. Mastronuzzi, A. Carai (eds.), *Navigating Pediatric Brain Tumors*,
https://doi.org/10.1007/978-3-032-18992-9_2

tumors, categorizing them based on the specificity of their signs and symptoms and then based on their location.

2.2 Non-Specific Signs & Symptoms

The most common non-specific signs and symptoms are related to increased intracranial pressure (ICP). This depends on the obstruction of cerebrospinal fluid drainage and manifests as the classical triad including headache, vomiting, and lethargy. Other non-specific symptoms include anisocoria, impaired vision, delayed or regressive development, decreased academic performance, and behaviour changes [1, 2] (Fig. 2.1).

Symptoms related to increased intracranial pressure are present in up to the 80% of cases of posterior fossa tumors, 60% of midline tumors, 60% of hemispheric tumors, 30% of brainstem tumors, and 7% of spinal cord tumors [3].

The headache is typically morning-related, may cause night-time awakenings during sleep, is non-well localized, and lasts less than 4–6 months. It could be associated with vomit, with or less commonly without nausea, and with visual alteration.

In cases of known headache patients, it is described as a headache different from usual. Sometimes it presents as a sudden, new-onset, and severe new-onset headache [2, 4, 5].

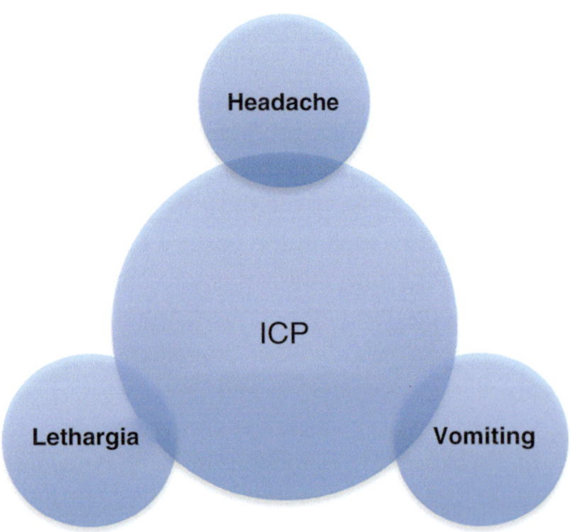

Fig. 2.1 Non-specific symptoms

When a suspected headache occurs, fundoscopy is mandatory: if intracranial pressure increases, the papilledema typically occurs. However, it could be absent in the early days. In case of slow-growing lesions, optic pallor may be present [6].

In case of severe and acute intracranial hypertension, the Cushing reflex occurs: it is characterised by the triad of widened pulse pressure (increasing systolic, decreasing diastolic), bradycardia, and irregular respiration pattern. This is an emergency case and requires a prompt diagnosis and therapy [7].

Among visual symptoms, it should be considered that papilledema in the initial phase is often asymptomatic. Sometimes there may be a mild central visual acuity loss, transient visual blurring, visual field defects, and diplopia if isolated sixth cranial nerve palsy occurs due to compression of the sixth cranial nerve by transverse branches of the basilar artery at the skull base [8].

As described in the dedicated paragraph, neonates and infants (less than 3 years old) with increasing intracranial pressure may have a different pattern of symptoms related to ICP: there is an increase in head circumference, bulging fontanelle, the setting sun phenomenon, and other non-specific symptoms such as irritability with moaning, crying, and lethargy [9].

In some cases of hypertension with dilation of the third ventricle or direct compression of the tectal region due to a midline tumor, the setting sun phenomenon could appear. It is due to upward-gaze paresis. This condition causes the eyes to be driven downward, with the sclera visible between the upper eyelid and the iris, and the lower pupil partially covered by the lower eyelid [1].

2.3 Specific Signs & Symptoms

Depending on the location of the tumor, there are specific symptoms, and the combination of these can support the experienced clinician in finding the diagnosis without delay. For example, in the case of the most frequent tumors, that is, those at the level of the posterior fossa, cerebellar symptoms, such as ataxia, coordination and balance disorders, and those related to long pathway involvement prevail. In contrast, in the case of tumors at the hemispheric level, seizures and focal deficits are more frequent. On the other hand, when the hypothalamochiasmatic region is involved, there are early field defects and endocrinological alterations. If the pineal gland and tectal region are involved, oculomotor deficits predominate, while extrapyramidal defects indicate involvement of the basal ganglia [1, 2, 5].

2.3.1 Posterior Fossa Tumors

The most common symptoms are nausea and vomiting, present in 75% of cases, headache in 67%, abnormal gait and coordination difficulties in 60%, papilledema in 34%, abnormalities in eye movements in 20%, lethargy in 13% of cases, and, less frequently, nausea without vomiting, weight loss, focal motor weakness, macrocephaly, impaired consciousness, dizziness or auditory symptoms, squint, stiff neck, head tilt, and accidental head injury [3].

At least 75% of cerebellar tumors obstruct the flow of cerebrospinal fluid through the aqueduct and into the fourth ventricle, so they also present with symptoms and signs of raised intracranial pressure, but typical symptoms of this type of tumor include cerebellar signs, cranial nerve palsies, and long tract deficits [1].

The cerebellar signs are:

- Lateralized ataxia in gait or ataxia with Romberg test positive: the patient does not have the capacity to stand with his feet placed together and eyes open.
- Dysmetria demonstrable with the finger-nose test.
- Dysdiadochokinesia with impaired ability to perform rapid, alternating movement.

Particularly, in case of a lesion of the central/vermian cerebellum without invasion of the brainstem, central ataxia may occur, while in case of lesions in the cerebellar hemispheres, such as astrocytoma, lateralized cerebellar deficits, a combination of dysmetria, kinetic tremor, hypotonia, and dysdiadochokinesia, are more frequent [1, 10].

2.3.2 Brainstem Tumors

Brainstem tumors predominantly present with abnormal gait and coordination difficulties in 78% of cases, cranial nerve palsies (unspecified) in 52% of cases, pyramidal signs (unspecified) in 33% of cases, headache (23%), squint (19%), and less frequently facial palsy, papilledema, nonspecific symptoms of increased intracranial pressure, abnormalities in eye movements, and behavioural alterations or learning difficulties [3].

Cranial nerve dysfunction is thus a common sign of brainstem disease: the brainstem contains the nuclei of the third to the twelfth cranial nerves, and multiple or single nerves may be involved in a disease process; signs are typically asymmetrical [11].

The classic cranial nerve involvement is the sixth nerve palsy: this occurs in cases of increased intracranial pressure, but sometimes the sixth nerve palsy could be associated with the involvement of the third and fourth nerve, with deficits in conjugate eye movements, oculomotor weakness, strabismus, and resting pupillary changes [1].

In the case of cerebellopontine angle lesions, such as ependymoma, deficits of the sixth, seventh, and eighth cranial nerves may occur with unilateral cerebellar deficits. In the case of isolated seventh cranial nerve deficit, complete or peripheral paralysis is more typical of ependymoma, while incomplete or central paralysis is typical of brainstem infiltrating lesions [2] (Fig. 2.2).

2.3.3 Hemispheric Tumors

Supratentorial tumors present in 47% of cases with nonspecific symptoms of increased intracra-

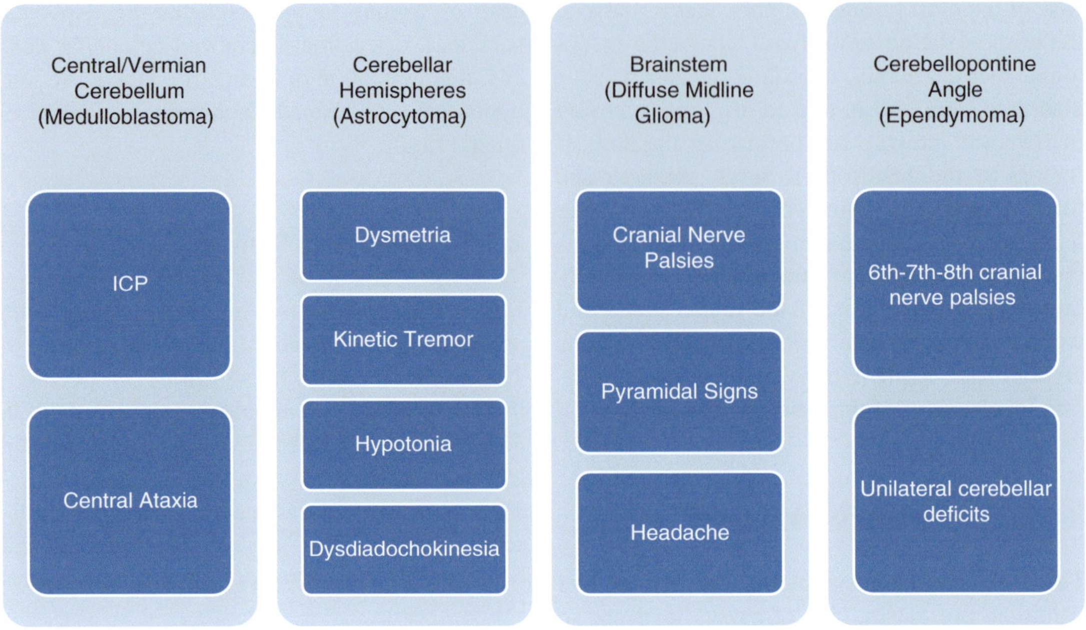

Fig. 2.2 Most common symptoms related to specific infratentorial locations and their typical histology

nial pressure, 38% with epileptic seizures, 21% with papilledema, 17% with focal neurological symptoms, 11% with headache, 10% with hemiplegia, and less frequently with nausea and vomiting, macrocephaly, and behavioural alterations [3].

Particularly, primary brain tumors frequently present with seizures and cause epilepsy with a prevalence of 10–19% with the risk of reduced quality of life and long-term cognitive impairment. The seizures occur in 50% of low-grade gliomas (LGG) and 20% of high-grade gliomas (HGG), with the predominance of histologies as low-grade astrocytomas, oligodendrogliomas, and dysembryoplastic neuroepithelial tumors (DNET).

They are complex-partial seizures, mainly affecting the temporal lobe. This location contributes to a good prognosis, because the seizure freedom after surgery is better for temporal and right-side lesions, especially in the case of total resection.

Patients with pre-existing epilepsy, such as those with type I neurofibromatosis and tuberous sclerosis, have seizures that are difficult to control [1, 2, 12].

Focal neurological deficits are typical of high-grade tumors such as anaplastic astrocytomas and primitive neuro-ectodermal tumors (PNETs). Pyramidal motor disorders, characterised by hemiparesis and hyperreflexia, are predominantly observed, while sensory disturbances are less frequent [2].

Behavioural alterations mainly occur in silent area lesions or cases of subacute intracranial hypertension. They can also manifest as mood disorders, concentration difficulties leading to reduced study capacity, neuromotor developmental delay or regression of already acquired milestones [3].

2.3.4 Midline/Central Tumors

The most frequent onset symptom is headache (49% of cases). They present with abnormal eye movement and squint in 21% of cases, nausea and vomiting in 19%, papilledema in 8%, reduced visual acuity in 6%, non-specific symptoms of increased intracranial pressure in 13%, diabetes insipidus in 12%, abnormal gait and coordination difficulties in 10%, and less frequently, behavioural alterations, altered level of consciousness, reduced visual fields, epileptic seizures, hemiplegia, focal motor deficits, developmental delay, short stature, weight loss, vertigo, and auditory and visual symptoms [3].

Typically, in the case of hypothalamic-chiasmatic gliomas, there is a complex visual field loss and/or proptosis [13].

In cases of tumors involving the hypothalamus and pituitary gland, such as gliomas, germ cell tumors, craniopharyngioma, and prolactinoma, endocrinological changes are also present: the most common are diabetes insipidus, GH deficiency, hypothyroidism, and precocious puberty [1, 13].

In some cases of hypothalamus involvement, a diencephalic syndrome could appear: it is characterised by a general condition deterioration with weight loss despite adequate nutrition and normal linear growth, nystagmus, developmental delay, and irritability. Sometimes it could also present other symptoms, such as hyperactivity and euphoria, hydrocephalus, and vomiting [14].

If the tumor is in the pineal region or causes dilation of the third ventricle, it may manifest as Parinaud's syndrome: it is characterised by gaze elevation, altered accommodation, and abnormalities of the pupillary reflex [13] (Fig. 2.3).

2.3.5 Spinal Tumor

Spinal cord tumors and masses can present with a variety of clinical signs and symptoms. Typically, they manifest with back pain in 67% of cases, abnormal gait or coordination difficulties in 42%, spinal deformities in 39%, focal motor weakness in 21%, sphincter disturbance in 20%, decreased upper limb movement in 17% of cases, and less frequently developmental delay, head tilt, and headache [3].

2.4 Neonatal/Prenatal and Infant Tumor

The clinical presentation of neonatal CNS tumors is extremely variable. It is a commonly agreed upon to define congenital tumors when symptoms appear in the prenatal period or at birth, probably congenital if symptoms appear within the first week of life, and possibly congenital if symptoms appear within 6 months of birth.

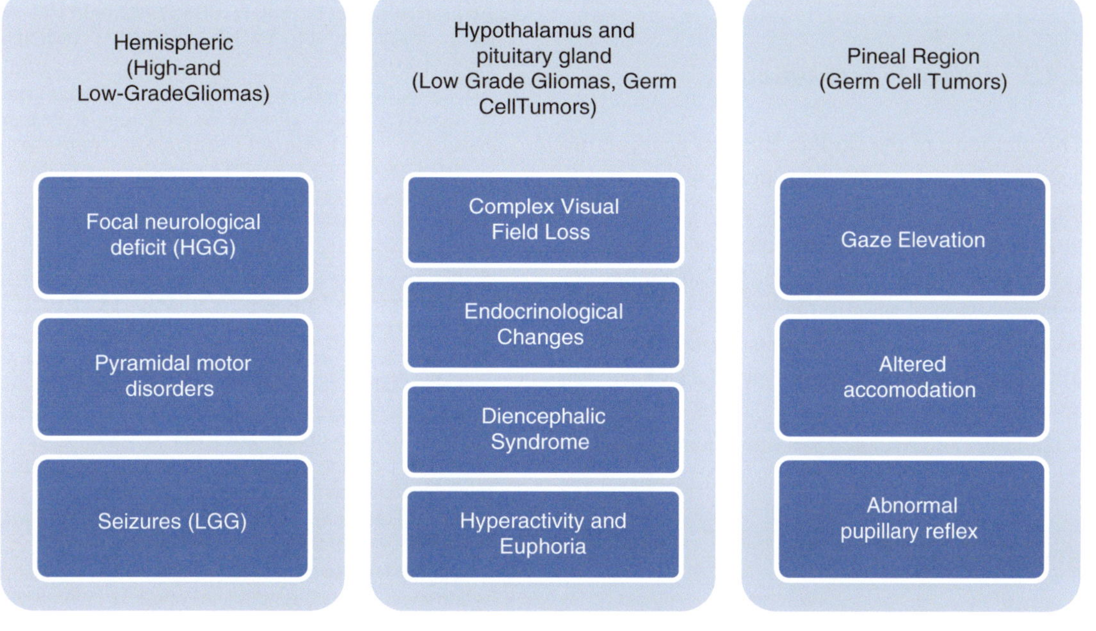

Fig. 2.3 Most common symptoms related to specific supratentorial locations and their typical histology

2.4.1 Foetal Presentation

During pregnancy foetal ultrasounds are routinely performed and can lead to early detection of abnormalities or suspicious features that may unveil the presence of an intracranial mass and provide an indication for further diagnostic tests. The most common signs are polyhydramnios, macrocephaly, or intracranial haemorrhage. All these findings frequently lead to serious impairment of the normal brain development, and if the congenital brain tumor reaches a size that causes hydrops or miscarriage, the diagnosis is made post-mortem [9].

2.4.2 Neonatal Presentation

Complications during labour due to cephalopelvic disproportion may lead to a suspected neonatal brain tumor. A caesarean section is required in 60% of cases, since the main sign of a neonatal brain tumor is macrocephaly, often asymptomatic. Nevertheless, elevated intracranial pressure can manifest as bulging fontanelles, irritability, lethargy, even apnoeic episodes, and seizures. Rarely, large and highly vascular masses may present with high-output heart failure [9].

2.4.3 Infant Presentation

The plasticity of the skull in the first years of life could lead to a more insidious onset, with an ongoing presence of macrocephaly or exponential growth of the head circumference without acute symptoms, except for bulging fontanelles or delayed fusion of sutures. Other symptoms may be non-specific, such as drowsiness, irritability, vomiting, apnoea, developmental delay, lack of growth, or abnormal eye movements. Tumor bleeding or seizures are often related to a more acute onset [9].

Bibliography

1. Walker D, Perilongo G, Punt J, Taylor R. Brain and spinal tumors of childhood. London: Oxford University Press; 2004.
2. Packer R, MacDonald T, Rood B, et al. Neoplastic disease. In: David RB, editor. Child and adolescent neurology. Malden: Blackwell Publishing; 2005.
3. Wilne S, Collier J, Kennedy C, et al. Presentation of childhood CNS tumors: a systematic review and meta-analysis. Lancet Oncol. 2007;8:685–95.
4. Wilne S, Koller K, Collier J, et al. The diagnosis of brain tumours in children: a guideline to assist healthcare professionals in the assessment of children who may have a brain tumour. Arch Dis Child. 2010;95:534–9.
5. Dinallo S, Waseem M. Cushing reflex. In: StatPearls [Internet]. Treasure Island: StatPearls Publishing; 2023. PMID: 31747208.
6. Kawar RA, Gross I, Biro Y, et al. The yield of ophthalmoscopy as a screening tool for intracranial pathology in pediatric headache. Eur J Pediatr. 2023;182(2):609–14. https://doi.org/10.1007/s00431-022-04708-0. Epub 2022 Nov 19. PMID: 36401633.
7. Goldman RD, Cheng S, Cochrane DD. Improving diagnosis of pediatric central nervous system tumours: aiming for early detection. CMAJ. 2017;189(12):E459–63. https://doi.org/10.1503/cmaj.160074. Epub 2016 Nov 28. PMID: 27895146; PMCID: PMC5367991.
8. Rigi M, Almarzouqi SJ, Morgan ML, et al. Papilledema: epidemiology, etiology, and clinical management. Eye Brain. 2015;7:47–57. https://doi.org/10.2147/EB.S69174. PMID: 28539794; PMCID: PMC5398730.
9. Toniutti M, Sasso AL, Carai A, et al. Central nervous system tumours in neonates: what should the neonatologist know? Eur J Pediatr. 2024;183(4):1485–97. https://doi.org/10.1007/s00431-023-05404-3. Epub 2024 Jan 11. PMID: 38206395; PMCID: PMC11001680.
10. Sridhar K, Sridhar R, Venkatprasanna G. Management of posterior fossa gliomas in children. J Pediatr Neurosci. 2011;6(Suppl 1):S72–7. https://doi.org/10.4103/1817-1745.85714. PMID: 22069433; PMCID: PMC3208911.
11. March PA. Diseases of the brain and cranial nerves. In: Saunders manual of small animal practice; 2006. p. 1249–76. https://doi.org/10.1016/B0-72-160422-6/50128-5. Epub 2009 May 15. PMCID: PMC7149320.
12. Katlowitz KA, Athukuri P, Sharma H, et al. Seizure outcomes after resection of primary brain tumors in pediatric patients: a systematic review and meta-analysis. J Neuro-Oncol. 2023;164:525–33.
13. Gan HW, Cerbone M, Bulwer C, et al. Pituitary and hypothalamic tumor syndromes in childhood. In: Endotext [Internet]. South Dartmouth: MDText.com, Inc; 2022. PMID: 2590537.
14. La Spina M, Caruso M, Gulizia C, et al. Diencephalic syndrome: misleading clinical onset of low-grade glioma. Curr Oncol. 2023;30(9):8401–10. https://doi.org/10.3390/curroncol30090610. PMID: 37754525; PMCID: PMC10529672.

3 Neuroimaging

Shivaram Avula

3.1 Introduction

Neuroimaging plays a vital role in the management of pediatric brain tumors at every stage of the patient journey, including diagnosis, preoperative assessment, intraoperative assessment, therapy planning and follow-up. This is usually the earliest method of confirming an intracranial neoplasm. Improvement in access to neuroimaging and public education has enabled earlier diagnosis. Advances in neuroimaging, particularly in the field of magnetic resonance imaging, have enabled the differentiation of neoplastic from non-neoplastic lesions to be more efficient. Imaging biomarkers have been identified that correlate with not only the histological diagnosis but also tumor subgroups and molecular diagnosis, which were incorporated in the 2021 WHO classification of central nervous system tumors [1, 2]. There has been a steady improvement in the quality of imaging with high-quality volumetric imaging available on most MRI scanners, including 1.5 tesla MRI scanners, enabling effective surgical planning, neuro navigation and radiotherapy treatment planning. There has been a greater emphasis on harmonising image acquisition and adopting paediatric-specific response assessment in the last decade, facilitating multicentre trials. This chapter will provide an overview of the imaging techniques available for neuroimaging in the setting of paediatric brain tumor, their indications and the recent advances.

S. Avula (✉)
Alder Hey Children's NHS Foundation Trust, Liverpool, UK
e-mail: shivaram.avula@alderhey.nhs.uk

3.2 Imaging Techniques

3.2.1 Ultrasound

Ultrasound (US) is a safe, convenient and relatively inexpensive imaging modality that is widely available and employs sound waves to generate images of the body. As US cannot penetrate bone, its use in clinical neuroimaging is restricted to the neonatal period or early infancy when the open fontanelles aid in visualisation of the intracranial contents. On rare occasions, foetal US can demonstrate intracranial lesions, which often need follow-up foetal MRI or postnatal imaging [3]. US plays a very practical role in the initial investigation of infants or neonates who present with signs of raised intracranial pressure or hydrocephalus. Neonatal brain tumors most commonly present with macrocephaly (50–60%), and trans fontanelle ultrasound is the first diagnostic test [4]. The rapid access to US scans, including bedside assessment, can expedite management when there is direct or indirect evidence of an intracranial tumor. Ultrasound can provide information including the size of the location, tumor, vascular-

A. Mastronuzzi, A. Carai (eds.), *Navigating Pediatric Brain Tumors*,
https://doi.org/10.1007/978-3-032-18992-9_3

ity using doppler imaging, presence of calcification, solid/cystic components and involvement of adjacent structures. The disadvantages of US are that it is operator-dependent, the resolution is limited, especially for structures away from the fontanelle, and the sensitivity is poor for detecting smaller lesions. Ultrasound has gained popularity as a very practical tool in the intraoperative setting and will be discussed in detail in the intraoperative section of the chapter.

3.2.2 CT Scans

CT scan is often the first modality of imaging where a brain tumor is identified. It is more easily accessible than an MRI scan, less expensive and quick to perform, making it an ideal imaging modality when screening for a space-occupying lesion. This is particularly true in resource-poor settings. The spatial and contrast resolution of the CT scan images are inferior compared to that of MRI, but it does provide clinically useful information. It can reveal an intracranial space-occupying lesion or its side effects that need urgent neurosurgical intervention, such as hydrocephalus drainage. CT scan is often performed as a volumetric scan of the brain, thereby aiding in neuro navigation for these emergency procedures. The CT imaging characteristics can indicate the type of tumor or provide a differential diagnosis. Brighter lesions that demonstrate increased density are suggestive of a relatively cellular tumor, such as a medulloblastoma (Fig. 3.1a) or other embryonal tumors [5]. A contrast-enhanced CT scan can provide information on the enhancement characteristics of the tumor, but this is often not performed as a non-contrast scan demonstrating a tumor is usually followed by an MRI scan with contrast. A study to determine the accuracy of CT in diagnosing paediatric brain tumors in 120 children showed an agreement of 87% between the CT diagnosis and histopathology, with 83% of medulloblastomas and 92% of astrocytomas being diagnosed accurately on CT scan. CT is very sensitive in identifying intra-tumoral calcification compared to MRI

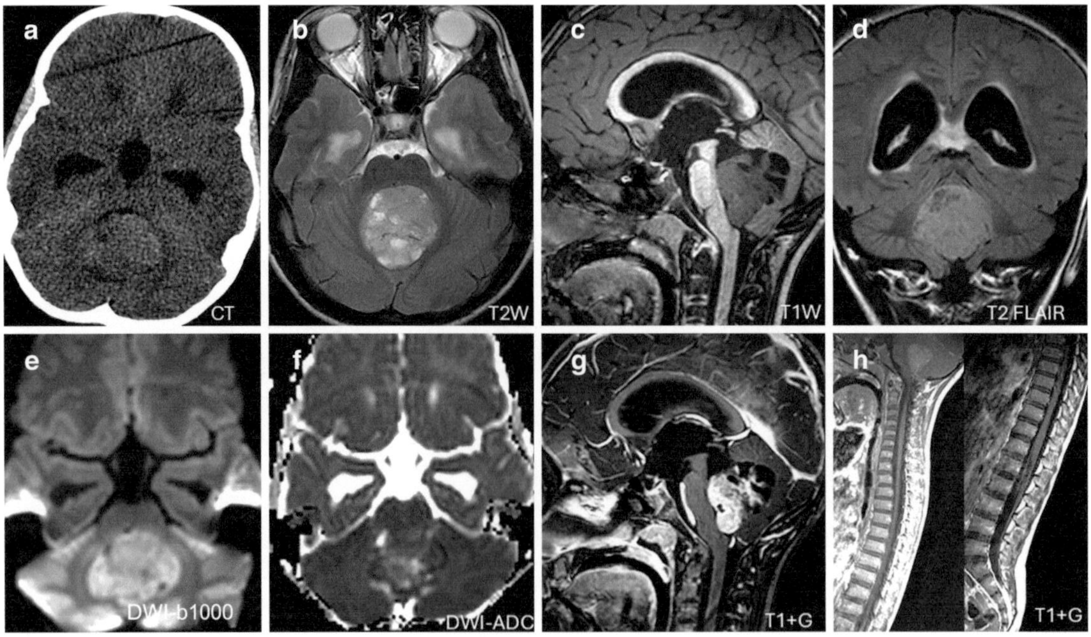

Fig. 3.1 Neuroimaging of a 12-year-old boy with a medulloblastoma identified initially on the CT scan that demonstrates increased density of the fourth ventricular mass (**a**). B-H demonstrates the tumor using standard MRI imaging performed in accordance with the SIOPE brain tumor imaging protocol. The tumor demonstrates typical characteristics of medulloblastoma appearing isointense to grey matter on T2 (**b**) and diffusion restriction (E &F) in keeping with the increased cellularity of the tumor. The T1 post-contrast scan of the spine (H) is performed as two segments to include the posterior fossa

and can help distinguish a suprasellar pilocytic astrocytoma from a craniopharyngioma. Using the Hounsfield units, one can differentiate between intratumoral calcification and haemorrhage. CT is extremely helpful in detecting bony changes and is better than MRI in assessing bone involvement in tumors that extend to the skull vault. Slow-growing tumors tend to scallop the skull vault as opposed to more aggressive tumors showing destructive changes to the bone. Evaluating the skull using the bone window settings also helps assess bony landmarks, including foramina, that transmit important neurovascular structures.

The main disadvantage of CT scans is the cranial radiation involved, but the newer CT scans deliver a lower dose compared to those employed a decade ago. A multicentre study involving children and young adults observed a significant dose-response relationship between CT-related radiation exposure and brain tumors [6]. Every effort should be made to keep the CT dose as low as reasonably possible without compromising the quality of the scan. One also should be aware that CT has a reduced sensitivity in identifying small lesions with a density similar to brain parenchyma. This is particularly true in the posterior fossa, where the surrounding bones can result in beam hardening artefacts causing multiple dark streaking bands (streaking artefacts) or reduced image density in the middle of the image (cupping artefact).

3.2.3 Magnetic Resonance Imaging

The superior signal, contrast and spatial resolution that MRI provides make it the ideal imaging modality to assess brain tumors. It provides not only structural imaging information, including the size, location, architecture, signal characteristics of the tumor, and involvement of local and distant structures, but also functional information, including vascularity, diffusion characteristics, metabolite profiles, and identification of eloquent regions using techniques such as functional MRI.

MRI scans can vary in strength, with a 1.5 tesla scan being the most commonly used. A high field strength 3-Tesla MRI scanner can produce better quality images due to an increased signal-to-noise ratio and is relatively quicker than a 1.5-tesla scanner for similar quality images. The duration of the scan can vary based on the field strength of the scanner and the number of sequences performed. MRI scans consisting of a set of sequences can range between 30 min for the basic structural sequences to 60 min when advanced imaging such as MR spectroscopy, perfusion imaging and diffusion tensor imaging is used. Spine imaging may be required in some scenarios and adds to the time. The longer the scan time, the greater the chances of motion artefact, particularly affecting sequences lasting 5 min or more. Regular encouragement during the scan, audiovisual distraction, and the use of play therapists can help patients cooperate during the scan. Children less than 5–6 years of age will often require general anaesthesia or sedation for the scan.

A standard MRI protocol is encouraged to enable the comparison of scans for an individual across various time points and to compare across multiple centres. Standardisation of image acquisition is vital for multi-institutional research. For European brain tumor studies, a standard imaging protocol (Fig. 3.1) has been published by the Brain Tumor Imaging Working Group of the European Society of Paediatric Oncology (SIOPE) [7, 8]. This contains information on the essential and optional sequences of the brain and spine for 1.5 and 3 Tesla MRI scanners. The Response Assessment in Pediatric Neuro-Oncology (RAPNO) working groups have published imaging protocols for medulloblastoma, low-grade glioma, high-grade glioma, diffuse midline glioma (formerly DIPG), Ependymoma and craniopharyngioma [9–14]. All the published protocols follow the principle that the essential sequences can be adopted widely and do not require advanced imaging capabilities.

The essential sequences consist of T1-weighted sequences before and after gadolinium contrast agent, T2-weighted, T2-weighted fluid-attenuated inversion recovery (T2 FLAIR) and diffusion-weighted imaging. The T1-weighted sequences are performed as 2D or 3D volumetric sequences. The T1 3D volumetric sequences produce high-resolution images that can be reconstructed in multiple planes and help identify and characterise small lesions. They can be helpful in volumetric analysis of the tumor and serve as a neuronavigational data set to aid surgery. There has been concern regarding the long-term effects of gadolinium deposition in the brain, and the European medicines agency has recommended using macrocyclic gadolinium-based contrast agents to minimise long-term effects [15]. Good quality T2 weighted images are important in characterising and measuring tumors. Response assessment in paediatric tumors relies on the T2 characteristics that can be obtained from T2 weighted images or T2 FLAIR images. If measurements are required in 3 orthogonal planes, combining 2D T2 and 2D T2 FLAIR sequences in at least two different planes will be helpful. Volumetric T2 weighted sequences are advantageous in aiding neuro navigation and volumetric tumor measurements, but their role in response assessment has not been validated. A balance steady-state free precession (bSSFP) scan produces a heavily T2-weighted image and has superior contrast resolution that can delineate structures within and close to CSF. Depending on the MRI vendor, the sequences are known by acronyms: CISS, FIESTA, BFFE, T2 DRIVE. The sequences have been included in the RAPNO and SIOPE guidelines as optional sequences, which are particularly helpful in identifying small metastatic lesions in the extra-axial space, ventricles (Fig. 3.2), and spinal canal. T2 FLAIR sequences

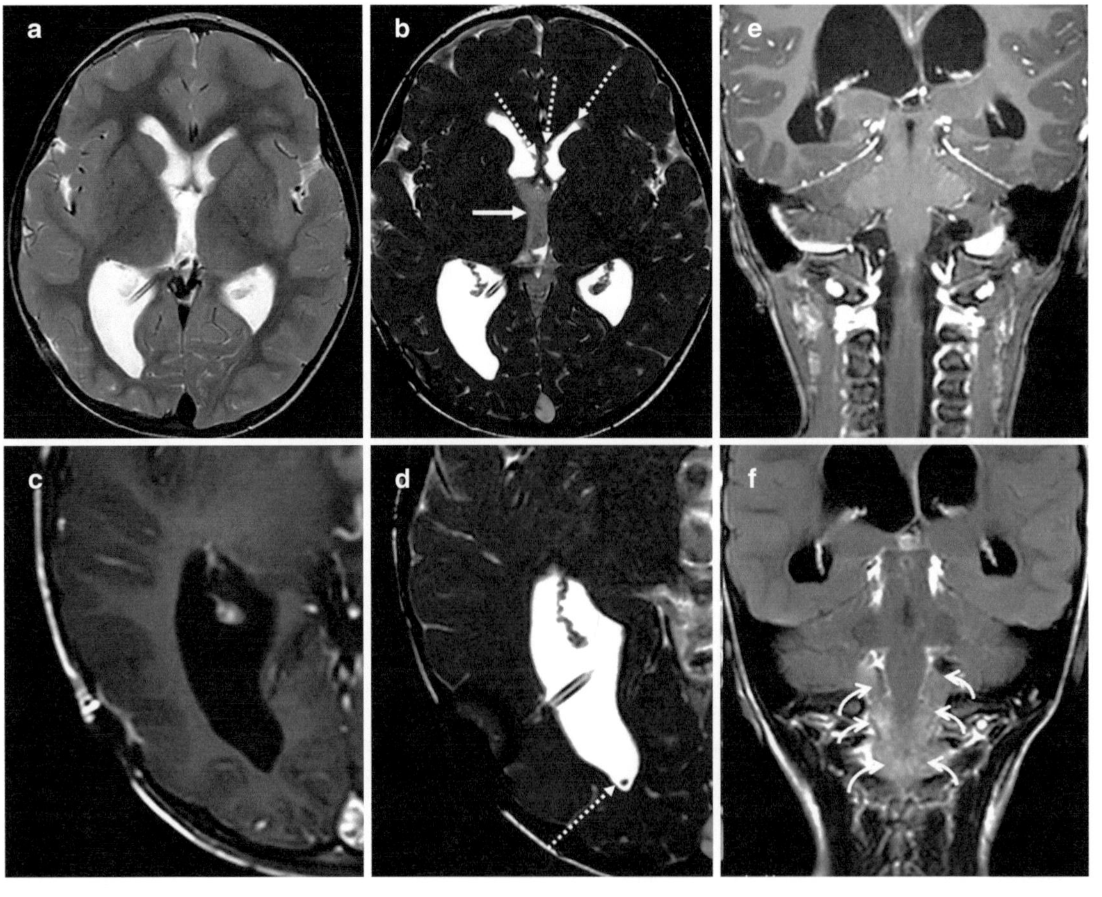

Fig. 3.2 MRI scan of a 4-year-old girl demonstrating the primary lesion within the third ventricle (white arrow), which is seen on the heavily T2 weighted- bSSFP sequence (**b**) but not on the standard T2 weighted image (**a**). The bSSFP sequence also shows multiple nodules along the ventricular margin and septum pellucidum (dotted arrows on **b**), which are not visible on the T2 weighted image (**a**). The bSSFP sequence also showed intraventricular metastatic nodules (**d**) that were not visible on T1 post-contrast scans (**c**). The T2 FLAIR post-contrast image (**f**) demonstrates diffuse enhancement of the leptomeninges and extra-axial spaces around the brain stem and the cervical cord (curved arrows), which was not visible on the T1 post-contrast scan (**e**). On pathological assessment, post-biopsy, the tumor was shown to represent an FGFR-altered Pilocytic astrocytoma

obtained following contrast administration (Fig. 3.2f)have been shown to be highly sensitive in identifying leptomeningeal metastasis [16, 17]. This has been incorporated as an essential or optional method in acquiring T2 FLAIR on multiple RAPNO guidelines. Postcontrast T2 FLAIR sequences may also show areas of nonspecific enhancement that may cause challenges in image interpretation, and it is good practice to have a pre-contrast T2 FLAIR sequence for comparison. Diffusion-weighted imaging (DWI) has become integral in assessing brain tumors. DWI is based on the mobility of water molecules, which in turn depends on the surrounding cellular architecture. It is extremely helpful in the assessment of tumor cellularity, differential diagnosis, treatment response, and identification of metastatic lesions [18, 19]. DWI is usually performed with at least 2 *b*-values ($b = 0$ s/mm^2 $b = 1000$ s/mm^2), and the ADC map should be available for interpretation. Susceptibility-weighted imaging (SWI) or T2 gradient imaging are useful adjuncts to evaluate intratumoral haemorrhage and vascularity. They are also helpful in postoperative imaging in differentiating haemorrhage from residual tumor tissue.

Imaging of the spine is recommended at the time of diagnosis with sagittal T1 post-contrast and an optional sagittal T2 sequence when the tumor is intracranial. T2 weighted sequences and pre-contrast T1 are mandatory for primary tumors of the spine. Dedicated axial sequences through the tumor are essential. It is best practice to image the spine in two segments (upper and lower), including the posterior fossa and the sacral-cul-de-sac as delayed enhancement of posterior fossa tumors is sometimes better appreciated on spine imaging. Heavily T2-weighted bSSFP imaging is useful in identifying drop metastasis <3 mm [20]. It is best practice to obtain spine imaging prior to surgery as early post-operative spine imaging findings can be challenging to interpret due to intraspinal subdural collections.

Advanced MRI sequences can complement standard imaging, providing microstructural, haemodynamic and metabolic information related to the tumor and surrounding brain.

Diffusion tensor imaging (DTI) not only measures the mobility of water molecules like DWI but also the direction of water diffusion. DTI works on the principle that water diffusion in the white matter is anisotropic, following the direction of the axon, as opposed to isotropic, where diffusion is equal in all directions. In DTI, magnetic field gradient pulses are applied in multiple directions (at least 6), usually between 16 and 32 in clinical practice, to obtain fractional anisotropy (FA) in a voxel. FA is a diffusion metric where 0 represents fully isotropic diffusion, and 1 represents fully anisotropic diffusion. The higher the number of directions, the greater the resolution of the DTI data, but the longer the duration of the scan is an important consideration when imaging the paediatric population. 3-dimensional diffusion tensor tractography (3D-tractography) is a mathematical method of creating 3-D trajectories of white matter fibres based on the FA values within a brain region. There is a standardised colour coding for the direction of the tracts where red corresponds to transverse fibres, green to anteroposterior fibres and blue to craniocaudal fibres. Tractography can help understand the structural relationship between brain tumors and adjacent tracts. White matter tracts displaced by the tumor maintain their anisotropy. Anisotropy can be reduced in areas of tumor infiltration or oedema. Anisotropy can be completely lost when the white matter tracts are destroyed [21]. 3-D tractography is valuable in surgical planning, particularly in deep-seated tumors, to determine the neurosurgical path, understand the eloquent regions around the tumor and complement intraoperative neurophysiological monitoring [22] (Figs. 3.3 and 3.5).

Magnetic resonance spectroscopy (MRS) is a non-invasive method of assessing the metabolic profile of the brain tissue. Proton MRS (H^1-MRS) detects signals from the hydrogen attached to various molecules in the chemical environment of the tissue in question, and the output is displayed in a graph with the X-axis depicting the chemical shift or the frequency shift of the proton from a reference compound (at 0 parts per million) and the y- axis depicting the signal intensity of the metabolites. The metabolites are identified

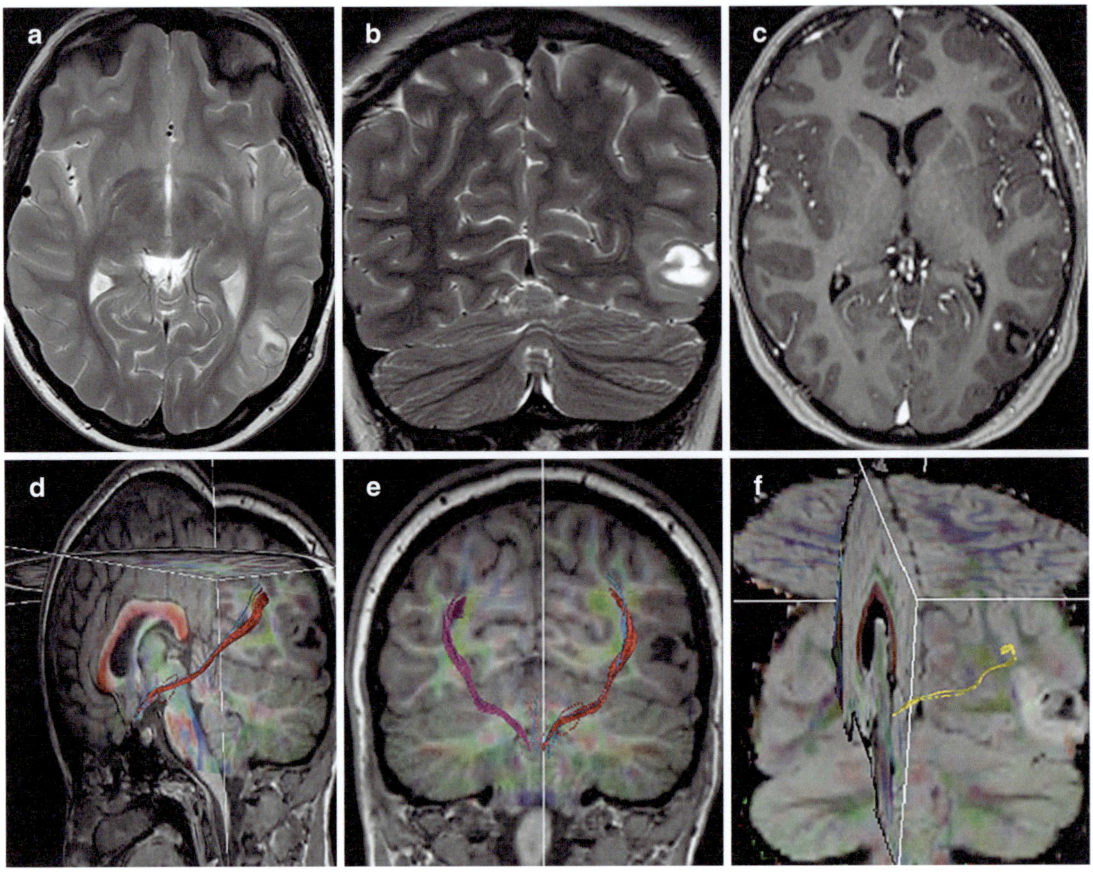

Fig. 3.3 16-year-old girl presenting with seizures demonstrated a left parietal solid/cystic tumor shown on the axial (**a**) and coronal (**b**) T2 weighted images with focal enhancement on the T1 post-contrast sequence (**c**). Tractography of the optic radiation was performed using DTI data (32-diffusion directions), demonstrating the relationship between the left optic radiation to the Tumor on the T1 weighted sequence (**d** and **e**) and T2 FLAIR sequence (**f**). The tumor histology following resection demonstrated a dysembryoplastic neuroepithelial tumor

based on their position on the x-axis as they have a certain chemical shift, and the volume under the curve denotes their concentration. N-acetyl-aspartate (NAA) is a marker for neuronal function, and its concentration decreases with various brain pathologies where the neuronal density or function is impaired. Choline (Cho) is involved in the phospholipid metabolism of cell membranes and is raised with increased cell membrane turnover associated with tumor growth (Fig. 3.4e). Although elevated in neoplastic lesions, it can be normal in slow-growing tumors. Creatine (Cr) is involved in cellular energy metabolism and is regarded as an internal standard. Myo inositol (mI) is thought to be a product of myelin degradation located mainly in glial cells and is elevated in certain tumors such as ependymomas and inflammatory/demyelinating disorders. The concentration of mI can distinguish choroid plexus papilloma from carcinoma [23]. Lactate (Lac) is a product of anaerobic glycolysis and is elevated in high-grade tumors. Lipids (Lip) are also elevated in a variety of tumors. Certain metabolites are also regarded to be elevated in specific tumors, such as Taurine in medulloblastomas. Recent studies have shown that Taurine varied between subgroups of medulloblastoma, appearing low in the Sonic Hedgehog subgroup [24]. The metabolite levels are often expressed in ratios such as Naa: Cr, Cho: Cr, and Naa: Cho, as absolute quantification can be challenging. Single voxel spectroscopy (SVS) is a

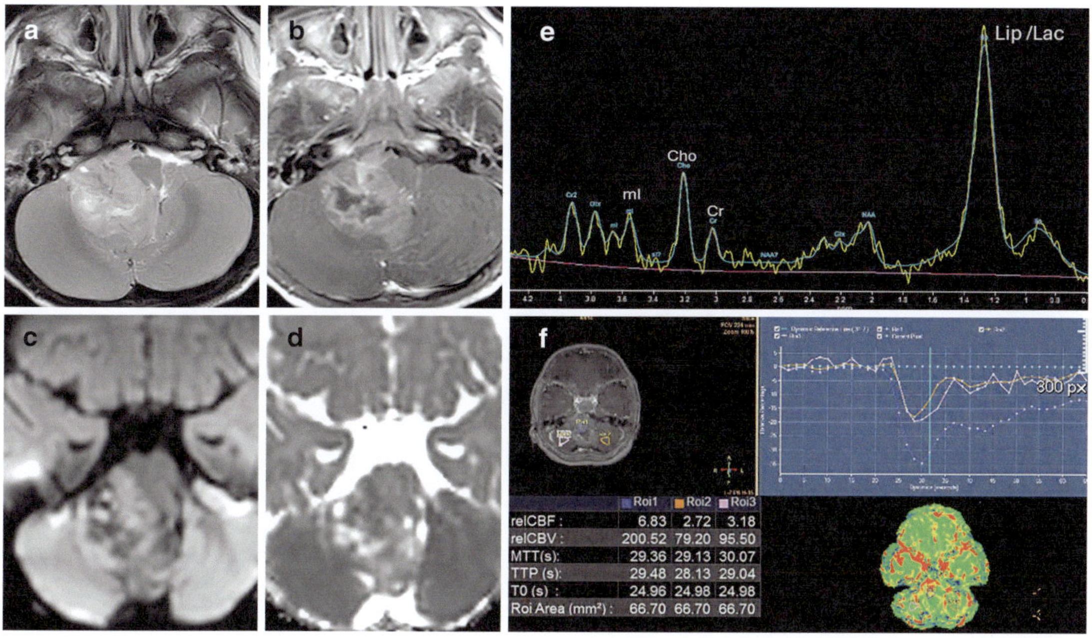

Fig. 3.4 MRI imaging on an 18-month-old boy with a history of vomiting and irritability demonstrated a mass centred over the right foramen of Luschka and extending into the right cerebellopontine angle and fourth ventricle. It demonstrated heterogeneous T2 signal characteristics (**a**) and heterogeneous enhancement (**b**). The diffusion-weighted sequences show heterogeneous diffusion characteristics on the b-1000 image (**c**) and ADC map (**d**) with areas of restricted and unrestricted diffusion. Single voxel spectroscopy (short echo time—35 ms) over the lesion (**e**) demonstrated an elevated choline (Cho) and lipid/lactate (Lip/Lac) peak in relation to creatine (Cr). The myoinositol (mI) level is also elevated in relation to creatine. DSC perfusion imaging performed during contrast administration shows an increase in relative cerebral blood volume (rCBV) and flow (rCBF) within the tumor (Roi1) compared to the normal cerebellar tissue (Roi 2 & Roi 3). The MRI and spectroscopy characteristics are typical of an Ependymoma confirmed on histopathological assessment

technique where a region of interest or voxel is placed over the tumor to sample the metabolite profile in that volume of tumors. This can be performed using a short echo time (TE) of 35 milliseconds or an Intermediate TE of 135–145 milliseconds. The short TE MRS demonstrates additional metabolites such as mI, glutamate/glutamine, taurine and alanine, which may help characterise the tumor. The intermediate TE MRS demonstrates the main metabolites, i.e. NAA, Cho, Cr and Lip/Lac. Multivoxel spectroscopy (MVS), or chemical shift imaging (CSI), can be used to sample a larger area, obtaining the metabolite profiles in multiple voxels.This is often helpful in assessing diffuse infiltrating tumors with heterogeneous signal characteristics. MRS can be a valuable tool in surgical planning or choosing a biopsy site. MRS is a valuable problem-solving tool in neurooncology, helping differentiate tumors from non-tumor pathologies such as infection, inflammation or post-treatment changes.

The vascularity of the brain tumor and its haemodynamic status can be determined using Perfusion imaging. Whilst contrast enhancement within the brain tumor only relates to the leakiness of the blood vessels, it does not provide quantitative information on the blood flow or volume in the tumor. This information can be useful in differentiating tumors from non-tumor lesions, separating low-grade from high-grade lesions, and monitoring treatment response. Perfusion imaging can be performed using contrast-enhanced techniques, such as dynamic susceptibility perfusion (DSC) or dynamic contrast-enhanced (DCE) perfusion, and a non-contrast technique, as in arterial spin labelling (ASL). DSC perfusion imaging or T2* perfusion

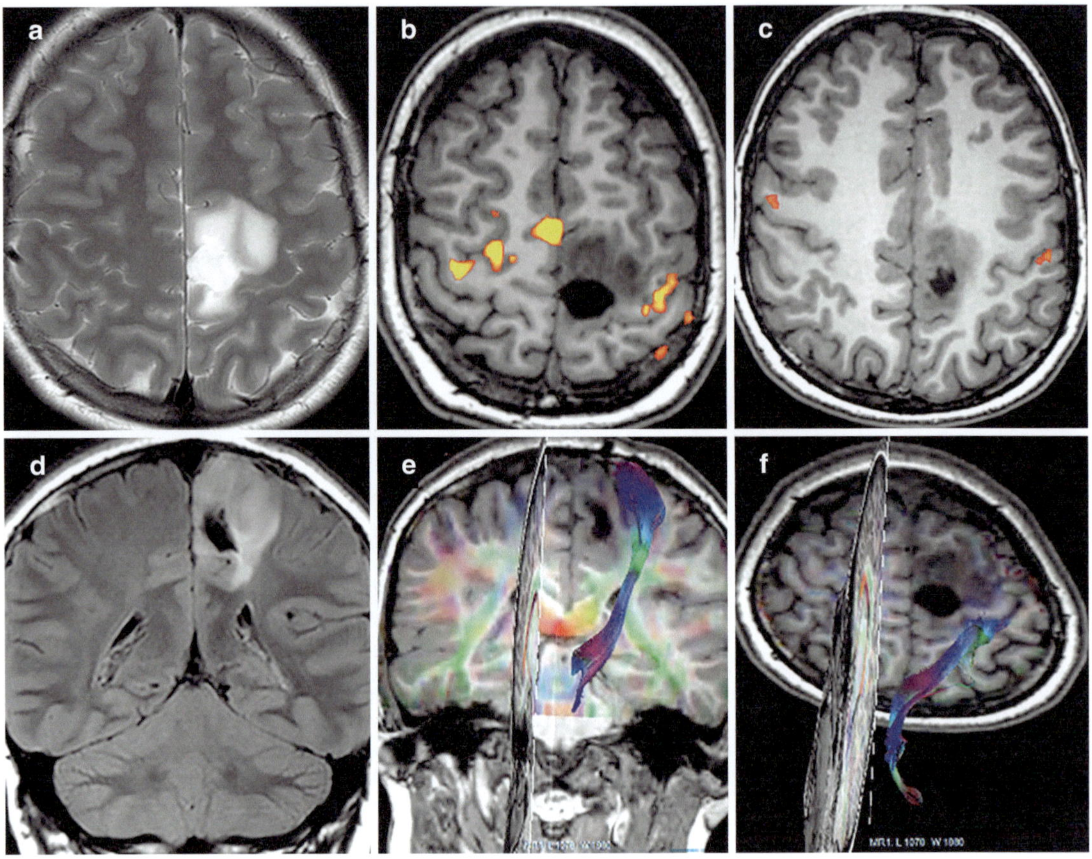

Fig. 3.5 MRI scan of a 15-year-old boy with a progressive gemistocytic astrocytoma around the previous surgical cavity in the left cerebral hemisphere demonstrated the axial T2 (**a**) and coronal T2 FLAIR (**d**) sequences. Preoperative assessment included fMRI and DTI (32-direction)-Tractography. Right finger-tapping paradigm (**b**) and tongue movement paradigm (**c**) demonstrate bilateral activation around the central sulcus which is situated posterior to the lesion. Tractography performed using ROIs from the fMRI demonstrates the relationship of the left corticospinal tract located posterolateral to the lesion (**e** and **f**)

is the commonly used contrast-enhanced technique where the first pass of Gadolinium-based contrast agent within the tumor is captured, and haemodynamic parameters such as relative cerebral blood volume (rCBV), relative cerebral blood flow (rCBF), time to peak (TTP) and mean transit time (MTT) can be calculated (Fig. 3.4f). DCE perfusion is a T1-weighted permeability imaging technique where the endothelial permeability or the transfer coefficient K_{trans} can be obtained. ASL is a non-invasive technique where magnetically labelled water protons in arterial blood are used as an endogenous tracer to determine the absolute CBF within the tumor. ASL is gaining popularity, particularly in the paediatric age group, as it is a non-invasive technique, and it is suitable in patients with decreased renal function. Each technique has its limitations. DSC offers better signal-to-noise (SNR) and contrast-to-noise (CNR) ratios than ASL and is relatively quicker to acquire. Its disadvantages are that it requires an intravenous contrast agent and a large bore cannula with pump injection. In the DSC perfusion technique, the results can be affected by leakage of contrast into the parenchyma, necessitating leakage correction methods. In a study of 63 paediatric brain tumors, a maximum rCBV (the maximum CBV in the tumor divided by the CBV in the contralateral white matter) of 1.38 had a high negative predictive value (88%) to exclude high-grade neoplasms with a sensitivity of 925 and specificity of 40% [25]. The low specificity was due to the considerable overlap between low-grade tumors, such as pilocytic astrocytomas, and high-grade tumors, such as medulloblastomas, due to the high vascularity of the low-grade tumors. ASL is an attractive technique in children as the high water content of the paediatric brain improves the ASL signal, and the sequences are also repeatable within the same session. The disadvantages of ASL are the longer acquisition time, poor SNR, and age-related and sedation-related CBF changes that can pose interpretation challenges [26]. Among the various ASL techniques, pseudocontinuous ASL (pCASL) is recommended for clinical use [27]. In a cohort of 54 children, the maximal rCBF of high-grade tumors was significantly higher than that of low-grade tumors ($P < 0.001$), but it did not distinguish between individual tumor histology [28]. In a cohort of 129 children with brain tumors, the mean CBF was significantly greater in high-grade tumors, and a cut-off of >50 mL/min/100 g demonstrated sensitivity and specificity of 90% and 93% for cerebral hemispheric tumors, 100% and 80% for thalamic tumors and 65% and 94% for posterior fossa tumors [29]. The popularity of ASL in paediatric use has increased despite some of its limitations, and a systematic review found ASL to be comparable and not inferior to the DSC perfusion technique in assessing paediatric brain tumors [30]. A study of 15 paediatric brain tumor patients revealed a strong relationship between DSC and ASL when leakage correction was applied to the DSC data in enhancing tumors [31].Perfusion imaging is still not routinely used in clinical practice due to the additional time involved and the post-processing that requires specific expertise still, it is a valuable problem-solving tool in paediatric brain tumor management.

Functional MRI (fMRI) is an imaging method of mapping eloquent brain areas using paradigms when the subject performs a task in the scanner. It works on the principle that the task stimulates neuronal activity in the eloquent region of the brain, causing an increase in blood flow. fMRI exploits the differences in the magnetic properties of oxyhaemoglobin, which is diamagnetic (weaker magnetic susceptibility) and deoxyhemoglobin, which is paramagnetic (greater magnetic susceptibility). The increased blood flow causes oxyhaemoglobin to displace deoxyhaemoglobin, increasing the MR signal due to a phenomenon known as the blood-oxygen dependent (BOLD) effect. fMRI is often performed during preoperative planning to identify the eloquent areas in relation to the tumor. Tasks such as finger tapping, toe movement or tongue movement may be used to map the sensorimotor cortex. Language paradigms may be used to identify the dominant hemisphere for language function (Fig. 3.5b and c). A systematic review of the use of fMRI in preoperative mapping for children with CNS tumors showed that task-based fMRI located eloquent cortex with more than 80% success rate [32]. As there are numerous fMRI paradigms that can be performed, the American Society of Functional Neuroradiology has published useful recommendations on fMRI paradigms for presurgical language lateralisation for children and adults [33]. As fMRI needs considerable cooperation from the patient, it can be challenging for younger children who may not be able to understand the task, cooperate during the scan or lie still. The help of neuropsychologists and play therapists can be beneficial in preparing the child for the scan. One must exhibit caution when estimating the distance between the tumor and the region of activation, as these regions can increase or decrease in size to an extent based on statistical threshold values used in the analysis. Another potential pitfall of interpreting fMRI in individuals with brain tumors is the phenomenon of neurovascular uncoupling (NVU). Neurovascular coupling comprises the biochemical process that regulates blood flow due to neuronal activation, and tumors can alter the vascularity and extracellular matrix of the adjacent brain parenchyma, causing NVU. This could result in false negative BOLD activation during fMRI, which one has to be aware of in its interpretation. Some centres perform cerebrovascular reactivity mapping (CVR) that can demonstrate reduced CVR due to NVU. This can, in turn, guide the interpretation of fMRI when NVU can pose challenges [34]. Combined multiparametric mapping with combinations of fibre tracking, fMRI, and multivolex spectroscopy may help in the surgical planning of complex tumors close to eloquent areas.

3.2.4 Nuclear Imaging

Positron Emission Tomography (PET) is a nuclear medicine imaging technique which employs the use of radiopharmaceuticals that interact with tissues to emit positrons, which, when combined with electrons, annihilate and emit two photons in opposite directions as gamma rays that are captured by detectors. PET images are combined with CT (PET-CT) or MRI (PET-MRI) to obtain hybrid images that facilitate accurate lesion localisation. The most commonly used radiotracer for PET is ^{18}F-Fluorodeoxyglucose (^{18}F-FDG). Still, its use in neuro-oncology is limited as there is increased physiological uptake of FDG in the cerebral cortex that can mask tumor uptake. In addition, its uptake is increased in inflammatory lesions and reduced in low-grade neoplasms. Some studies have demonstrated the value of 18F-FDG PET in the grading of tumors with a greater uptake in higher-grade neoplasms and reduced survival in brain stem gliomas [35, 36]. Recently, amino acid PET tracers have gained popularity as they demonstrate increased uptake in brain tumors, including low-grade neoplasms. These include L-methyl-^{11}C-methionine (^{11}C–MET), 3,4-dihydroxy-6-[^{18}F] fluoro-l-phenylalanine (^{18}F-DOPA) and ^{18}F -Fluoroethyl-l-tyrosine (^{18}FFET). The joint European Association of Nuclear Medicine (EANM), the European Society of Pediatric Neuro-Oncology (SIOPE), The Society of Nuclear Medicine and Molecular Medicine (SNMMI) and The Response Assessment in Pediatric Neuro-oncology (RAPNO) have published the standards for imaging paediatric gliomas using PET [37]. PET imaging can be used in various clinical scenarios. At the time of diagnosis, it can complement MRI in distinguishing neoplastic from non-neoplastic lesions. In a study of 30 children with epilepsy with brain lesions, ^{11}C–MET PET demonstrated significant differences in lesion-to-grey mater ratio between tumors and focal cortical dysplasia (FCD) [38]. It can help in the preoperative grading of tumors and prognostication [35, 39]. In a study of 26 children with diffuse astrocytic tumors, ^{18}F-DOPA PET uptake correlated better with progression-free survival than ADC and rCBF obtained using ASL. Combining the MRI and PET data provided the best prediction for tumor progression [40]. ^{11}C-Methionine PET helped identify non-enhancing tumor regions at high risk for recurrence in pediatric high-grade glioma [41]. PET can complement MRI information in identifying a suitable biopsy site [39, 42]. PET can be beneficial during patient follow-up, helping distinguish residual tumor or tumor recurrence from post-surgical or treatment-related changes. In a cohort of 22 children, ^{18}F-FET PET combined with MRI discriminated residual tumors from post-surgical changes with a higher specificity than MRI alone [43]. In a study of 26 children with new or worsening MRI abnormalities that were concerning for tumor recurrence, ^{11}C-methionine PET showed slightly greater sensitivity and accuracy in predicting tumor recurrence than MRI with a better interobserver agreement [44]. The use of PET in paediatric neurooncology is rapidly growing, but there is a relative paucity of data supporting its clinical role compared to MRI. One has to be aware of pitfalls due to increased tracer uptake related to developmental venous anomalies, low-grade tumors during increased epileptogenic activity and increased striatal uptake of [^{18}F]DOPA [37]. Co-registration with MRI is essential in properly analysing PET imaging, and a good level of interaction between the neuroradiologist and nuclear medicine physician is vital for effective interpretation of the imaging.

3.3 Indications for Imaging

3.3.1 Diagnosis and Treatment Planning

Imaging is the primary mode of identifying and diagnosing a brain tumor. Due to resource constraints, the need for sedation/anaesthesia or urgency, some children undergo a CT scan in the first instance when there is a suspicion of an intracranial space-occupying lesion. As discussed earlier, CT can provide helpful information on the cellularity, presence of haemorrhage/calcification, extent of disease and tumor-related pathology such as hydrocephalus. MRI scan remains the mainstay for characterising the lesion, estimating its size and extent, differentiating from non-tumor pathology, evaluating for metastasis and, in some cases, predicting the subgroup of the tumor as in medulloblastomas [45]. It is crucial to adopt one of the recommended MRI protocols [7, 9–13, 14] and this is often based on local practice or participation in clinical trials. As discussed earlier, imaging of the spine should ideally be performed before surgery as post-operative subdural collections or haemorrhage can pose diagnostic problems. It is good practice to provide a differential diagnosis for the lesion and comment on features suggestive of an aggressive or benign aetiology. This often involves a combination of location, structural, and functional characteristics such as diffusion, perfusion and MR spectroscopy. A provisional tumor diagnosis based on imaging before surgery can help plan treatment, including surgical timing, approach and extent of resection. Some tumors, such as optic pathway gliomas in patients with type 1 neurofibromatosis, bifocal germinomas, marker positive cell tumors, and classical diffuse midline gliomas affecting the pons (formerly diffuse intrinsic pontine glioma-DIPG) may not need biopsies for confirmation. Often, there are instances where the tumor characteristics are atypical, necessitating the need for biopsies, particularly where surgical resections may be challenging. Diffuse midline gliomas are a good example where atypical MRI findings are often present, necessitating a biopsy. Where possible, a central neuroimaging review can improve the accuracy of diagnosis, as noted in the analysis of the DIPG registry, where there was a 9.5% discordance of the diagnosis between local and central reviews [46]. The tumors wrongly diagnosed as DIPG often represented non-diffuse low-grade gliomas or embryonal tumors [47]. A provisional tumor diagnosis may also help in prognostication and predicting the risk of postoperative complications such as paediatric cerebellar mutism syndrome (pCMS). The diagnosis of medulloblastoma increases the risk of CMS based on clinical studies and risk prediction tools [48, 49]. Advanced MR sequences such as DTI, perfusion, fMRI and spectroscopic imaging are optional sequences on the recommended SIOPE brain tumor protocol. Still, they are often very helpful in surgical planning, particularly involving tumors adjacent to eloquent areas. DTI and functional MRI can identify the relationship between the tumor and vital structures, including the optic radiation, corticospinal tract and arcuate fasciculus. The surgical approach to deep-seated thalamic tumors often benefits from multiparametric imaging. Functional characteristics of the tumor, such as diffusion, perfusion and spectroscopy, can also help guide biopsy planning.

3.3.2 Imaging for Neuronavigation

Neuronavigation is an important tool in improving the accuracy of surgical resection and has gained popularity in the last two decades. An important pre-requisite for neuronavigation is a high-resolution volumetric dataset, ideally with slice thickness ≤1 mm thick with no gaps between the slices such that it can be reconstructed in any plane without compromising the quality of the image. Post-contrast Volumetric T1 weighted images are often used to delineate the enhancing and non-enhancing components of the tumor and its relationship to the surrounding brain parenchyma. On some occasions, volumetric T2 or T2 FLAIR sequences may also be used depending on the tumor's characteristics. Overlapping advanced imaging data, including DTI, FMRI, and MR spectroscopy, could add more functional information to the neuronavigation system. The field of view, the anatomy coverage and the MRI data's compatibility with the neuronavigational software will be crucial in setting up the neuronavigation system. Volumetric data from CT scans have also been used when access to volumetric data is limited.

3.3.3 Early Postoperative Imaging

The optimum period for early postoperative imaging is the first 48 h, as nonspecific intracranial enhancement is often seen 72 h following surgery [50, 51]. This may be compounded by the presence of haemostatic material and electrocoagulation. Using identical sequences on the preoperative and postoperative imaging is ideal for accurate comparison. Techniques such as SWI to identify blood products, heavily T2-weighted sequences to identify residual tumor nodules within the CSF spaces, and diffusion-weighted imaging to identify areas of residual restricting tumor or ischaemic injury can be useful in postoperative image interpretation. Often, postoperative appearances can be challenging, and consensus with the neurosurgical team will help interpret such cases. In situations where the early postoperative scan is inconclusive for residual tumor, an early follow-up scan in 2–3 weeks after surgery will be helpful to evaluate for residual disease. The SIOPE and RAPNO guidelines support this recommendation. A similar approach can be adopted if the spine imaging performed in the early postoperative period is inconclusive. There is no unified definition for the categories of postoperative residual intracranial disease across the various tumors. Gross total resection (GTR) can be generally regarded as no radiological evidence of disease, but the definitions for near-total resection (NTR), subtotal or partial resection vary between tumor types, and the practice varies regionally or adapted to clinical trials where applicable. If the postoperative scan is to be used as a baseline before adjuvant therapy or the start of a clinical trial, some of the RAPNO guidelines recommend that it be within 4–6 weeks before the start of the intervention [9, 11, 14].

3.3.4 Intraoperative Imaging

There has been an exponential increase in intraoperative MRI (ioMRI) use in aiding paediatric brain tumor resection over the last decade. This has been aided by the improvements in technology with dedicated coils and the availability of high-field strength (3 Tesla) MRI scans in an intraoperative setting. The main advantage of ioMRI is the ability to compensate for brain shift following craniotomy and surgery by updating neuronavigation and identifying residual tumor tissue that can be safely resected. This is particularly advantageous in the paediatric brain tumor population where complete resection of the tumor has prognostic significance, as in ependymoma or pilocytic astrocytomas. Setting up an ioMRI facility can be expensive, and the option of dual room intraoperative facilities where the scanner is located adjacent to the neurosurgical theatre introduces flexibility in using the scanner as a cost-effective and valuable radiological resource. A successful ioMRI facility needs close collaboration between the neurosurgical, radiological and anaesthetic teams and relies on strict adherence to the MRI safety guidelines. The MRI protocol for intraoperative imaging can be adapted based on the neurosurgical indication, but adherence to the brain tumor imaging guidelines is recommended as best practice. The preoperative and intraoperative sequences need to be comparable to aid evaluation. One must be aware of the pitfalls of interpreting ioMRI, such as surgically induced contrast enhancement and haemorrhage in the surgical field [52]. Intracranial air is a source of susceptibility artefact degrading echo planar sequences such as DWI. Adequate irrigation of the surgical cavity with saline can help mitigate this problem, or the use of non-echoplanar sequences can also help [53, 54]. The use of advanced MRI sequences in ioMRI can help in specific circumstances. Intraoperative MR spectroscopy can help characterise areas that are equivocal for tumor remnants [55]. The final ioMRI scan can be used as a postoperative baseline (only validated on 3 T) as long as the standard brain tumor protocol is followed, is supervised by a radiologist experienced in children's brain tumors and is reported in consensus with the operating neurosurgeon [56]. The indications and use of ioMRI vary between different neurosurgical centres based on the need for ioMRI and surgical experience. There is also variability in the rates of extension of resection or after ioMRI, ranging between 9% and 43% [53, 57, 58]. This can depend on the varying threshold for the neurosurgeon on when to perform the scan, as ioMRI can be used to confirm the completeness of resection, determine its extent or update neuronavigation. The rate of GTR is shown to be greater with ioMRI compared to conventional surgery without ioMRI based on a review [59]. IoMRI has been shown to be effective in avoiding unnecessary early repeat surgery where complete resection of the tumor was decided [57, 60]. A similar beneficial impact has been noted with low-grade glioma surgery, where ioMRI resulted in significantly better complete resection rates compared to the pre-ioMRI population [61]. There is limited evidence on the influence of ioMRI on overall survival in the paediatric brain tumor population. One study showed better progression-free survival (PFS) rates in children with low-grade gliomas but not a significant difference compared to conventional surgery without ioMRI. However, there was a significant difference in PFS in subjects with complete resection versus those with incomplete resection [61].

Intraoperative ultrasound (ioUS) is a more widely used intraoperative imaging technique than ioMRI, mainly due to its low cost and easier implementation. It also has the advantage of being performed during surgery in real-time with minimal risk and quicker with minimal additional operative time. The limitation when compared to ioMRI is that the imaging is operator-dependent, and the spatial resolution, the contrast resolution and the field of view are poorer in ioUS. There is also a need for fluid or CSF as an interface between the ultrasound (US) probe and the tissue of interest, and pockets of intracranial air can cause artefacts as US does not travel through air. Ultrasound transducers with small footprints are most suited for ioUS. A linear array transducer with higher frequencies of 7–15 MHz provides high-resolution images at a depth of 2–7 cm, and sector array probes with a curved footprint have frequencies ranging from 4 to 8 MHz can be used in small craniotomies and are capable of higher penetration with lesser resolution of images [62]. US transducers can be referenced to a neuronavigation system that combines preoperative MRI with real-time ioUS. A 2D ultrasound scan produce an image in a single plane, but a 3D ultrasound can produce a 3D volume that has advantages over navigated 2D ultrasonography [63]. IoUS is initially used before the dural incision to confirm the tumor's location, characterise it, and identify its relation to adjacent structures, including blood vessels. In a study of 365 adult patients operated for neoplastic and non-neoplastic brain lesions, ioUS showed a significantly better definition of tumor edges, contours, necrosis, calcification and cystic components than T1-weighted MRI [64]. A study of 24 paediatric patients undergoing brain tumor resection showed that the tumor volume obtained from ioUS before resection correlates with the preoperative MRI [65]. It can guide the shortest and safest surgical route when coregistered to neuronavigation [66]. Contrast-enhanced ultrasound (CEUS) involves intravenous injection of microbubble contrast agents prior to scanning and is reported to be helpful in the localisation and resection of hypervascular lesions [67]. There is limited published literature on the paediatric population. One of the important uses of ioUS is to assess the extent of resection (EOR). In a study of 24 paediatric patients, the accuracy of residual tumor detection was similar to that of ioMRI [65].

There are ethical challenges in undertaking randomised controlled studies on the utility of ioUS versus ioMRI in aiding brain tumor surgery. A review of the literature comparing publications on ioUS and ioMRI concluded that for the majority of brain tumors, ioUS is comparable to ioMRI in estimating EOR based on the rate of GTR (70% in ioMRI and 77% in ioUS) [68]. The article does not take into consideration the studies where low-field strength MRI (<1.5 T MRI) has been used and factor the number of cases where the intention was GTR. The utility of both techniques can vary based on the indication, experience and technical factors. In a review of experiences across four international paediatric neurosurgical centres, 111 operations used ioUS, and 182 used ioMRI in the resection of low-grade gliomas. Both modalities facilitated the intended complete resection in almost all cases. It was felt that in more deep-seated tumors, ioMRI had advantages over ioUS in visualising residual tumors. Factors limiting complete resection due to eloquent or neighbouring brain tissue affected both modalities similarly, In long-term follow-up, both ioUS and ioMRI showed complete resection, significantly lowering disease recurrence. The authors recommend using ioUS in any surgery independent of the intended extent of resection and the availability of ioMRI.

3.3.5 Response Assessment

During the patient journey, most of the imaging occurs during follow-up to evaluate for evidence of disease recurrence or response to treatment. The frequency and duration of imaging surveillance is variable, depending on several factors, including the type and grade of tumor, the patient's age, the kind of treatment, local practice and participation in research trials. A review of literature evaluating the imaging schedule of children and adolescents with low-grade glioma could not identify the optimal frequency and duration of surveillance with further influencing factors such as the tumor location, the histological type and molecular characteristics [69]. In general, surveillance imaging is done more frequently in the first 2 years following surgery and adjuvant therapy with annual or biannual scans thereafter. The frequency of scans can be higher in tumors of a higher grade. It is good practice to include spine imaging in children with tumors with a risk of intraspinal metastasis. With growing concerns about long-term gadolinium deposition in the brain, there are increasing debates over the routine use of contrast MRI in surveillance imaging. There has been no consensus on this matter, but there are efforts to identify tumor types or clinical scenarios where routine intravenous contrast administration can be avoided or reduced. It is recommended that the SIOPE or the RAPNO guidelines for tumor imaging be followed, as discussed earlier in this chapter.

The measurement of the residual or relapsed tumors varies between institutions and geographic regions. For SIOPE trials, measurements are obtained in the three standard Planes, i.e. Anteroposterior, transverse and craniocaudal and the tumor volume is calculated based on the spherical volume formula $a \times b \times c \times ½$. The RAPNO guidelines commonly recommend a 2D measurement approach with the products of the largest diameter and the maximum perpendicular diameter for the measurement of the tumor area. The RAPNO LGG guidelines include the 3D approach of calculating tumor size in addition to the 2D approach [11]. The gold standard will be to obtain volumetric measurements with accurate segmentation of tumors. However, manual segmentation is time-consuming and automated segmentation of paediatric brain tumors is still a technical challenge to accomplish. When measuring tumors for clinical trials, lesions are defined as measurable if they are $\geq$10 in both perpendicular diameters in the axial plane or $\geq$2 times the MRI slice thickness + interslice gap as defined in the Response assessment in Neurooncology (RANO) criteria [70]. In clinical practice, non-measurable lesions that are too small or ill-defined are qualitatively assessed for response to treatment. Unlike the RANO criteria, where the T1 post-contrast sequences are mainly used to determine measurable disease, the RAPNO recommendations rely more on the T2 weighted sequence to assess response. This is particularly relevant in targeted therapy where the tumor enhancement can resolve without significant change in size and is best appreciated on T2 / T2 FLAIR sequences. A detailed description of the RAPNO criteria is beyond the scope of this chapter, and the salient points are discussed here. The definitions of response vary slightly between the different RAPNO recommendations [71]. The main categories are Complete response (CR), where there is complete resolution of enhancing and non-enhancing disease; Partial response (PR), where there is $\geq$50% decrease; and progressive disease (PD), where there is $\geq$25% increase in disease, clear progression of the non-measurable disease or clinical deterioration not attributable to other causes. Additional response criteria of minor response (The HGG and LGG) for 25–49% decrease in disease and major response (LGG) for ≥75% decrease in disease have also been recommended. The response is categorised as stable disease (SD) when none of the other criteria are met. The LGG and Craniopharyngioma RAPNO recommendations have advised on the measurements of cysts associated with the tumors [11, 12]. In Craniopharyngiomas, both the solid and cystic components are included in the measurement. In contrast, in LGGs, the cysts are included if it is a true tumor cyst or a part of a mixed solid-cystic tumor. Response to immunotherapy has gained increasing interest, and immunotherapy RANO (iRANO) recommendations were published by the RANO working group in 2015 [72]. The response criteria are like RANO except that where there is evidence of radiological progression within 6 months of therapy and no clinical progression, repeat imaging after 3 months with continuation of treatment is recommended to confirm PD, provided there is no clinical decline during this period. No specific guidelines for the paediatric population have been published.

The phenomenon of pseudoprogression is well recognised, particularly in within the first 3 months after chemoradiotherapy when the imaging demonstrates a transient increase in the size of the tumor either due to increased blood-brain barrier permeability or increased oedema. In such cases, provided the patient can tolerate treatment, progression is confirmed on the subsequent MRI scan and the date of progression is back-dated if there is true and sustained progressive disease [70]. Pseudoresponse is a phenomenon where there is a reduction in the size of the tumor or the enhancement characteristics following antiangiogenic agents often seen in the adult high-grade glioma population. It is less common in the paediatric population, and the T2 weighted imaging will help assess the true response. Radionecrosis or radiation-induced changes can often mimic disease recurrence or progression. Advanced imaging such as DWI, MRS and perfusion imaging can help in some cases differentiate post-radiation change from tumor, but follow-up imaging is often the only way to differentiate the two.

3.4 Novel Techniques of Imaging and Analysis

Magnetic resonance elastography (MRE) is an advanced MRI-based technique that generates quantitative images based on the material properties of tissue [73]. It is a non-invasive form of palpation and could be a surrogate marker for tissue stiffness and viscosity. The images are acquired using a special MRI-phase contrast technique that can detect tissue motion in response to an applied excitation, and the viscoelastic property is reconstructed from the measured displacement [74]. MRE can help characterise the tumor consistency and adherence to normal brain tissue, which can help improve surgical planning, including the surgical approach and instrument selection. A study on meningiomas in adults using MRE showed that tumor consistency was an important factor in surgical outcomes, with a higher grade of tumor consistency resulting in significantly lesser GTR rates, longer duration of surgery and higher perioperative complications [75]. In another study, the shear stiffness of meningiomas, pituitary adenomas, vestibular schwannomas and gliomas correlated well with the surgeon's qualitative assessment of the tumor consistency [76]. There is limited evidence on the use of MRE in paediatric brain tumors. In a study on 23 children with primary LGG or with Type 1 neurofibromatosis (NF1), the gliomas were significantly softer and of lower viscosity than reference tissue and focal abnormal signal intensities (FASI) associated with NF1 were stiffer though not significantly [77]. Further research will be required to evaluate this technique's utility in managing brain tumors in children.

Chemical exchange saturation transfer (CEST) imaging is a form of MRI technique providing molecule-specific contrast by detecting mobile proteins and peptides. In CEST imaging, a chemical of interest that is capable of exchanging its hydrogen protons with those of water is magnetically saturated using a radiofrequency pulse. This magnetic saturation is transferred to water over time, decreasing the water signal. This signal is captured by MRI, providing an indirect measure of the chemical [78]. Amide proton transfer (APT) is a form of CEST imaging where exchangeable amide protons from proteins and peptides, through their interaction with the surrounding water, are detected through the CEST mechanism. As HGGs are associated with increased expression of cellular proteins and peptides compared to LGGs, APT MRI can be used as a technique to differentiate them. A systematic review and meta-analysis showed significantly higher APT in HGG compared to LGG [79]. APT MRI was also a significant predictor of overall survival in HGGs, and IDH-wildtype HGGS were significantly associated with high APT signals [80]. In the paediatric populations, one study showed APT values that were significantly higher in LGG and HGG compared to normal white matter [81], and another study showed significantly higher values in patients with HGG versus those with LGG [82]. Future studies will help evaluate the use of APT MRI in clinical decision-making during managing children with brain tumors.

3.5 Advances in Image Analysis

Radiology data can be mined to obtain a vast amount of quantitative information that is not easily perceived by the human eye. Radiomics is an emerging field that involves extracting an extensive array of features from medical imaging, including size, shape and texture and using machine learning models to aid management by improving the accuracy of diagnosis, assessing risk, prognostication and response assessment in the context of neurooncology. Radiomic analysis requires expert radiology and computer vision knowledge to extract quantitative features based on computational techniques. Multiple studies have shown accurate and reproducible image extraction methods to capture brain tumor characteristics such as shape and texture [83–85]. Associating these radiomic imaging biomarkers with the genomic characteristics of the disease has led to growth in the field of radiogenomics. A radiomic and radiogenomic pipeline typically involves image acquisition and registration, segmentation of the region of interest, preprocessing, feature extraction and selection, machine learning and developing radiogenomic associations [86]. Radiomics has been used in a wide variety of research studies in paediatric neurooncology. It has been used to distinguish tumors of varying histology and overlapping imaging features. In a cohort of 231 children with supratentorial tumors, radiomic features from T2 and T1 post-contrast scans could distinguish embryonal tumors, high-grade gliomas and ependymomas [87]. Similarly, radiomic features have been shown to distinguish atypical teratoid/rhabdoid tumors from medulloblastomas [88]. Radiogenomics has shown promise in distinguishing tumor subgroups. MRI-based machine learning models have been developed to identify the WNT, SSH, group 3 and group 4 medulloblastomas [89, 90]. In a cohort of 107 midline paediatric HGGs, including 79 with H3K27 mutation, a combination of radiomic features and ring enhancement had the ability to predict H3K27 mutation in midline pHGGs [91]. Similarly, the feasibility of identifying BRAF status of pediatric LGGs using radiomics has been demonstrated by different groups [92, 93]. Machine learning models can also help in predicting prognosis in multiple tumor types. Three immunologically different clusters were identified on radiogenomic analysis of pLGGs, integrating MRI and RNA sequencing data. This could predict the immune profile, PFS and treatment response [94].In addition to identifying medulloblastoma subgroups, radiogenomics-based machine learning models could predict prognosis and improve risk stratification [90, 95]. Radiomics based machine learning model has also been shown to prognosticate Diffuse Intrinsic pontine gliomas (Diffuse midline gliomas) [96].

3.6 Conclusions

Imaging has proven vital in the management of pediatric CNS tumors, from diagnosis to surveillance following treatment. Over the past two decades, imaging quality and imaging technology improvement has exponentially increased, contributing to high-quality structural and functional information. This has also increased the complexity of image assessment and interpretation. A close interaction between the various clinic clinical teams managing the patient becomes highly relevant in incorporating the imaging findings within the patient journey. While the demand for imaging and the number of techniques have increased, the quality of imaging studies should not be compromised. It is vital that the basic imaging protocol is in line with the agreed international guidelines. With increasing importance being laid on imaging in therapeutic decision-making, a central review of imaging has shown to be beneficial, particularly in challenging cases. Advanced imaging techniques and image analysis methods, including machine learning techniques, are proving to be valuable tools in decision-making. These methods are still in their early phase of development within the paediatric neuro Oncology population. Validation with multicentre and large population studies will be important going forward.

References

1. Louis DN, Perry A, Wesseling P, Brat DJ, Cree IA, Figarella-Branger D, et al. The 2021 WHO classification of tumors of the central nervous system: a summary. Neuro-Oncology. 2021;23(8):1231–51.
2. McNamara C, Mankad K, Thust S, Dixon L, Limback-Stanic C, D'Arco F, et al. 2021 WHO classification of tumours of the central nervous system: a review for the neuroradiologist. Neuroradiology. 2022;64(10):1919–50.
3. Cornejo P, Feygin T, Vaughn J, Pfeifer CM, Korostyshevskaya A, Patel M, et al. Correction to: imaging of fetal brain tumors. Pediatr Radiol. 2021;51(3):492.
4. Toniutti M, Sasso AL, Carai A, Colafati GS, Piccirilli E, Del Baldo G, et al. Central nervous system tumours in neonates: what should the neonatologist know? Eur J Pediatr. 2024;183(4):1485–97.
5. Tortori-Donati P, Fondelli MP, Rossi A, Cama A, Caputo L, Andreussi L, et al. Medulloblastoma in children: CT and MRI findings. Neuroradiology. 1996;38(4):352–9.
6. Hauptmann M, Byrnes G, Cardis E, Bernier MO, Blettner M, Dabin J, et al. Brain cancer after radiation exposure from CT examinations of children and young adults: results from the EPI-CT cohort study. Lancet Oncol. 2023;24(1):45–53.
7. Avula S, Peet A, Morana G, Morgan P, Warmuth-Metz M, Jaspan T, et al. European Society for Paediatric Oncology (SIOPE) MRI guidelines for imaging patients with central nervous system tumours. Child Nerv Syst. 2021;37(8):2497–508.
8. Avula S, Peet A, Morana G, Morgan P, Warmuth-Metz M, Jaspan T, et al. Correction to: European Society for Paediatric Oncology (SIOPE) MRI guidelines for imaging patients with central nervous system tumours. Childs Nerv Syst. 2021;37(8):2509–10.
9. Cooney TM, Cohen KJ, Guimaraes CV, Dhall G, Leach J, Massimino M, et al. Response assessment in diffuse intrinsic pontine glioma: recommendations from the Response Assessment in Pediatric Neuro-Oncology (RAPNO) working group. Lancet Oncol. 2020;21(6):e330–e6.
10. Erker C, Tamrazi B, Poussaint TY, Mueller S, Mata-Mbemba D, Franceschi E, et al. Response assessment in paediatric high-grade glioma: recommendations from the Response Assessment in Pediatric Neuro-Oncology (RAPNO) working group. Lancet Oncol. 2020;21(6):e317–e29.
11. Fangusaro J, Witt O, Hernaiz Driever P, Bag AK, de Blank P, Kadom N, et al. Response assessment in paediatric low-grade glioma: recommendations from the Response Assessment in Pediatric Neuro-Oncology (RAPNO) working group. Lancet Oncol. 2020;21(6):e305–e16.
12. Hoffman LM, Jaimes C, Mankad K, Mirsky DM, Tamrazi B, Tinkle CL, et al. Response assessment in pediatric craniopharyngioma: recommendations from the Response Assessment in Pediatric Neuro-Oncology (RAPNO) Working Group. Neuro-Oncology. 2023;25(2):224–33.
13. Warren KE, Vezina G, Poussaint TY, Warmuth-Metz M, Chamberlain MC, Packer RJ, et al. Response assessment in medulloblastoma and leptomeningeal seeding tumors: recommendations from the Response Assessment in Pediatric Neuro-Oncology committee. Neuro-Oncology. 2018;20(1):13–23.
14. Lindsay HB, Massimino M, Avula S, Stivaros S, Grundy R, Metrock K, et al. Response assessment in paediatric intracranial ependymoma: recommendations from the Response Assessment in Pediatric Neuro-Oncology (RAPNO) working group. Lancet Oncol. 2022;23(8):e393–401.
15. Agency EM. PRAC concludes assessment of gadolinium agents used in body scans and recommends regulatory actions, including suspension for some marketing authorisations; 2017. Available from: https://www.ema.europa.eu/en/news/prac-

concludes-assessment-gadolinium-agents-used-body-scans-recommends-regulatory-actions-including-suspension-some-marketing-authorisations.
16. Utz MJ, Tamber MS, Mason GE, Pollack IF, Panigrahy A, Zuccoli G. Contrast-enhanced 3-dimensional fluid-attenuated inversion recovery sequences have greater sensitivity for detection of leptomeningeal metastases in pediatric brain tumors compared with conventional spoiled gradient echo sequences. J Pediatr Hematol Oncol. 2018;40(4):316–9.
17. Fukuoka H, Hirai T, Okuda T, Shigematsu Y, Sasao A, Kimura E, et al. Comparison of the added value of contrast-enhanced 3D fluid-attenuated inversion recovery and magnetization-prepared rapid acquisition of gradient echo sequences in relation to conventional postcontrast T1-weighted images for the evaluation of leptomeningeal diseases at 3T. AJNR Am J Neuroradiol. 2010;31(5):868–73.
18. Ramaglia A, Tortora D, Mankad K, Lequin M, Severino M, D'Arco F, et al. Role of diffusion weighted imaging for differentiating cerebral pilocytic astrocytoma and ganglioglioma BRAF V600E-mutant from wild type. Neuroradiology. 2020;62(1):71–80.
19. Kan P, Liu JK, Hedlund G, Brockmeyer DL, Walker ML, Kestle JR. The role of diffusion-weighted magnetic resonance imaging in pediatric brain tumors. Childs Nerv Syst. 2006;22(11):1435–9.
20. Buch K, Caruso P, Ebb D, Rincon S. Balanced steady-state free precession sequence (CISS/FIESTA/3D driven equilibrium radiofrequency reset pulse) increases the diagnostic yield for spinal drop metastases in children with brain tumors. AJNR Am J Neuroradiol. 2018;39(7):1355–61.
21. Jellison BJ, Field AS, Medow J, Lazar M, Salamat MS, Alexander AL. Diffusion tensor imaging of cerebral white matter: a pictorial review of physics, fiber tract anatomy, and tumor imaging patterns. AJNR Am J Neuroradiol. 2004;25(3):356–69.
22. Kim JH, Phi JH, Lee JY, Kim KH, Park SH, Choi YH, et al. Surgical outcomes of thalamic tumors in children: the importance of diffusion tensor imaging, neuro-navigation and intraoperative neurophysiological monitoring. Brain Tumor Res Treat. 2018;6(2):60–7.
23. Krieger MD, Panigrahy A, JG MC, Nelson MD, Liu X, Gonzalez-Gomez I, et al. Differentiation of choroid plexus tumors by advanced magnetic resonance spectroscopy. Neurosurg Focus. 2005;18(6A):E4.
24. Kohe S, Bennett C, Burte F, Adiamah M, Rose H, Worthington L, et al. Metabolite profiles of medulloblastoma for rapid and non-invasive detection of molecular disease groups. EBioMedicine. 2024;100:104958.
25. Ho CY, Cardinal JS, Kamer AP, Lin C, Kralik SF. Contrast leakage patterns from dynamic susceptibility contrast perfusion MRI in the grading of primary pediatric brain tumors. AJNR Am J Neuroradiol. 2016;37(3):544–51.
26. Proisy M, Bruneau B, Rozel C, Treguier C, Chouklati K, Riffaud L, et al. Arterial spin labeling in clinical pediatric imaging. Diagn Interv Imaging. 2016;97(2):151–8.
27. Alsop DC, Detre JA, Golay X, Gunther M, Hendrikse J, Hernandez-Garcia L, et al. Recommended implementation of arterial spin-labeled perfusion MRI for clinical applications: a consensus of the ISMRM perfusion study group and the European consortium for ASL in dementia. Magn Reson Med. 2015;73(1):102–16.
28. Yeom KW, Mitchell LA, Lober RM, Barnes PD, Vogel H, Fisher PG, et al. Arterial spin-labeled perfusion of pediatric brain tumors. AJNR Am J Neuroradiol. 2014;35(2):395–401.
29. Dangouloff-Ros V, Deroulers C, Foissac F, Badoual M, Shotar E, Grevent D, et al. Arterial spin labeling to predict brain tumor grading in children: correlations between histopathologic vascular density and perfusion MR imaging. Radiology. 2016;281(2):553–66.
30. Vella S, Lauri J, Grech R. Comparison of arterial spin-labeling and DSC perfusion MR imaging in pediatric brain tumors: a systematic review and meta-analysis. AJNR Am J Neuroradiol. 2025;46(1):178–85.
31. Novak J, Withey SB, Lateef S, MacPherson L, Pinkey B, Peet AC. A comparison of pseudo-continuous arterial spin labelling and dynamic susceptibility contrast MRI with and without contrast agent leakage correction in paediatric brain tumours. Br J Radiol. 2019;92(1094):20170872.
32. Manan HA, Aidilla Sahrizan NS, Palaniandy K, Hamid HA, Yahya N. The utilisation of fMRI for pre-operative mapping in the paediatric population with central nervous system tumours: a systematic review. Neuroradiology. 2024;
33. Black DF, Vachha B, Mian A, Faro SH, Maheshwari M, Sair HI, et al. American society of functional neuroradiology-recommended fMRI paradigm algorithms for presurgical language assessment. AJNR Am J Neuroradiol. 2017;38(10):E65–73.
34. Agarwal S, Welker KM, Black DF, Little JT, DeLone DR, Messina SA, et al. Detection and mitigation of neurovascular uncoupling in brain gliomas. Cancers (Basel). 2023;15(18)
35. Borgwardt L, Hojgaard L, Carstensen H, Laursen H, Nowak M, Thomsen C, et al. Increased fluorine-18 2-fluoro-2-deoxy-D-glucose (FDG) uptake in childhood CNS tumors is correlated with malignancy grade: a study with FDG positron emission tomography/magnetic resonance imaging coregistration and image fusion. J Clin Oncol. 2005;23(13):3030–7.
36. Zukotynski KA, Fahey FH, Kocak M, Alavi A, Wong TZ, Treves ST, et al. Evaluation of 18F-FDG PET and MRI associations in pediatric diffuse intrinsic brain stem glioma: a report from the Pediatric Brain Tumor Consortium. J Nucl Med. 2011;52(2):188–95.
37. Piccardo A, Albert NL, Borgwardt L, Fahey FH, Hargrave D, Galldiks N, et al. Joint EANM/SIOPE/RAPNO practice guidelines/SNMMI procedure standards for imaging of paediatric gliomas using PET with radiolabelled amino acids and [(18)F]

FDG: version 1.0. Eur J Nucl Med Mol Imaging. 2022;49(11):3852–69.
38. Phi JH, Paeng JC, Lee HS, Wang KC, Cho BK, Lee JY, et al. Evaluation of focal cortical dysplasia and mixed neuronal and glial tumors in pediatric epilepsy patients using 18F-FDG and 11C-methionine pet. J Nucl Med. 2010;51(5):728–34.
39. Rosenfeld A, Etzl M, Bandy D, Carpenteri D, Gieseking A, Dvorchik I, et al. Use of positron emission tomography in the evaluation of diffuse intrinsic brainstem gliomas in children. J Pediatr Hematol Oncol. 2011;33(5):369–73.
40. Morana G, Piccardo A, Tortora D, Puntoni M, Severino M, Nozza P, et al. Grading and outcome prediction of pediatric diffuse astrocytic tumors with diffusion and arterial spin labeling perfusion MRI in comparison with 18F-DOPA PET. Eur J Nucl Med Mol Imaging. 2017;44(12):2084–93.
41. Lucas JT Jr, Serrano N, Kim H, Li X, Snyder SE, Hwang S, et al. (11)C-Methionine positron emission tomography delineates non-contrast enhancing tumor regions at high risk for recurrence in pediatric high-grade glioma. J Neuro-Oncol. 2017;132(1):163–70.
42. Pirotte BJ, Lubansu A, Massager N, Wikler D, Goldman S, Levivier M. Results of positron emission tomography guidance and reassessment of the utility of and indications for stereotactic biopsy in children with infiltrative brainstem tumors. J Neurosurg. 2007;107(5 Suppl):392–9.
43. Marner L, Nysom K, Sehested A, Borgwardt L, Mathiasen R, Henriksen OM, et al. Early postoperative (18)F-FET PET/MRI for pediatric brain and spinal cord tumors. J Nucl Med. 2019;60(8):1053–8.
44. Bag AK, Wing MN, Sabin ND, Hwang SN, Armstrong GT, Han Y, et al. (11)C-methionine PET for identification of pediatric high-grade glioma recurrence. J Nucl Med. 2022;63(5):664–71.
45. Perreault S, Ramaswamy V, Achrol AS, Chao K, Liu TT, Shih D, et al. MRI surrogates for molecular subgroups of medulloblastoma. AJNR Am J Neuroradiol. 2014;35(7):1263–9.
46. Leach JL, Roebker J, Schafer A, Baugh J, Chaney B, Fuller C, et al. MR imaging features of diffuse intrinsic pontine glioma and relationship to overall survival: report from the International DIPG Registry. Neuro-Oncology. 2020;22(11):1647–57.
47. Lazow MA, Fuller C, DeWire M, Lane A, Bandopadhayay P, Bartels U, et al. Accuracy of central neuro-imaging review of DIPG compared with histopathology in the International DIPG Registry. Neuro-Oncology. 2022;24(5):821–33.
48. Bae D, Mlc VV, Catsman-Berrevoets CE. Preoperative prediction of postoperative cerebellar mutism syndrome. Validation of existing MRI models and proposal of the new Rotterdam pCMS prediction model. Childs Nerv Syst. 2020;36(7):1471–80.
49. Sidpra J, Marcus AP, Lobel U, Toescu SM, Yecies D, Grant G, et al. Improved prediction of postoperative pediatric cerebellar mutism syndrome using an artificial neural network. Neurooncol Adv. 2022;4(1):vdac003.
50. Bette S, Gempt J, Huber T, Boeckh-Behrens T, Ringel F, Meyer B, et al. Patterns and time dependence of unspecific enhancement in postoperative magnetic resonance imaging after glioblastoma resection. World Neurosurg. 2016;90:440–7.
51. Lescher S, Schniewindt S, Jurcoane A, Senft C, Hattingen E. Time window for postoperative reactive enhancement after resection of brain tumors: less than 72 hours. Neurosurg Focus. 2014;37(6):E3.
52. Knauth M, Aras N, Wirtz CR, Dorfler A, Engelhorn T, Sartor K. Surgically induced intracranial contrast enhancement: potential source of diagnostic error in intraoperative MR imaging. AJNR Am J Neuroradiol. 1999;20(8):1547–53.
53. Tejada S, Avula S, Pettorini B, Henningan D, Abernethy L, Mallucci C. The impact of intraoperative magnetic resonance in routine pediatric neurosurgical practice-a 6-year appraisal. Childs Nerv Syst. 2018;34(4):617–26.
54. Thorpe JC, Thust SC, CHM G, Rowe S, Swain CE, DC MA, et al. Comparison of echo planar and turbo spin echo diffusion-weighted imaging in intraoperative MRI. J Magn Reson Imaging. 2024;
55. Roder C, Skardelly M, Ramina KF, Beschorner R, Honneger J, Nagele T, et al. Spectroscopy imaging in intraoperative MR suite: tissue characterization and optimization of tumor resection. Int J Comput Assist Radiol Surg. 2014;9(4):551–9.
56. Avula S, Jaspan T, Pizer B, Pettorini B, Garlick D, Hennigan D, et al. Comparison of intraoperative and post-operative 3-T MRI performed at 24-72 h following brain tumour resection in children. Neuroradiology. 2021;63(8):1367–76.
57. Shah MN, Leonard JR, Inder G, Gao F, Geske M, Haydon DH, et al. Intraoperative magnetic resonance imaging to reduce the rate of early reoperation for lesion resection in pediatric neurosurgery. J Neurosurg Pediatr. 2012;9(3):259–64.
58. Roessler K, Winter F, Kiesel B, Shawarba J, Wais J, Tomschik M, et al. Current aspects of intraoperative high-field (3T) magnetic resonance imaging in pediatric neurosurgery: experiences from a recently launched unit at a tertiary referral center. World Neurosurg. 2024;182:e253–e61.
59. Wu O, Clift GW, Hilliard S, Ip M. Evaluating the use of intraoperative magnetic resonance imaging in paediatric brain tumour resection surgeries: a literature review. J Med Radiat Sci. 2023;70(4):479–90.
60. Avula S, Pettorini B, Abernethy L, Pizer B, Williams D, Mallucci C. High field strength magnetic resonance imaging in paediatric brain tumour surgery--its role in prevention of early repeat resections. Childs Nerv Syst. 2013;29(10):1843–50.
61. Roder C, Breitkopf M, Ms, Bisdas S, Freitas RS, Dimostheni A, et al. Beneficial impact of high-field intraoperative magnetic resonance imaging on the efficacy of pediatric low-grade glioma surgery. Neurosurg Focus. 2016;40(3):E13.

62. El Beltagy MA, Elbaroody M. The value of intraoperative ultrasound in brain surgery. Adv Tech Stand Neurosurg. 2024;50:185–99.
63. Yeole U, Singh V, Mishra A, Shaikh S, Shetty P, Moiyadi A. Navigated intraoperative ultrasonography for brain tumors: a pictorial essay on the technique, its utility, and its benefits in neuro-oncology. Ultrasonography. 2020;39(4):394–406.
64. Elmesallamy WAEA. Gross pathology of brain mass lesions by intraoperative ultrasonography: a comparative study. Egypt J Neurosurg. 2024;39(24)
65. Klein Gunnewiek K, van Baarsen KM, Graus EHM, Brink WM, Lequin MH, Hoving EW. Navigated intraoperative ultrasound in pediatric brain tumors. Childs Nerv Syst. 2024;40(9):2697–705.
66. Frassanito P, Stifano V, Bianchi F, Tamburrini G, Massimi L. Enhancing the reliability of intraoperative ultrasound in pediatric space-occupying brain lesions. Diagnostics (Basel). 2023;13(5)
67. Tao AY, Chen X, Zhang LY, Chen Y, Cao D, Guo ZQ, et al. Application of intraoperative contrast-enhanced ultrasound in the resection of brain tumors. Curr Med Sci. 2022;42(1):169–76.
68. Giussani C, Trezza A, Ricciuti V, Di Cristofori A, Held A, Isella V, et al. Intraoperative MRI versus intraoperative ultrasound in pediatric brain tumor surgery: is expensive better than cheap? A review of the literature. Childs Nerv Syst. 2022;38(8):1445–54.
69. Roka K, Kersbergen KJ, Schouten-van Meeteren AYN, Avula S, Sehested A, Otth M, et al. Towards a risk-based follow-up surveillance imaging schedule for children and adolescents with low-grade glioma. Curr Oncol. 2024;31(11):7330–51.
70. Ellingson BM, Wen PY, Cloughesy TF. Modified criteria for radiographic response assessment in glioblastoma clinical trials. Neurotherapeutics. 2017;14(2):307–20.
71. Geraldo AF, Maldonado F, Severino M, Mankad K, Dahmoush H, Soares B, et al. Response assessment in pediatric neurooncology (RAPNO) criteria revisited: a practical navigation guide for neuroradiologists. Neuroradiology. 2024;66(12):2117–42.
72. Okada H, Weller M, Huang R, Finocchiaro G, Gilbert MR, Wick W, et al. Immunotherapy response assessment in neuro-oncology: a report of the RANO working group. Lancet Oncol. 2015;16(15):e534–e42.
73. Manduca A, Bayly PJ, Ehman RL, Kolipaka A, Royston TJ, Sack I, et al. MR elastography: principles, guidelines, and terminology. Magn Reson Med. 2021;85(5):2377–90.
74. Yin Z, Romano AJ, Manduca A, Ehman RL, Huston J 3rd. Stiffness and beyond: what MR elastography can tell us about brain structure and function under physiologic and pathologic conditions. Top Magn Reson Imaging. 2018;27(5):305–18.
75. Itamura K, Chang KE, Lucas J, Donoho DA, Giannotta S, Zada G. Prospective clinical validation of a meningioma consistency grading scheme: association with surgical outcomes and extent of tumor resection. J Neurosurg. 2019;131(5):1356–60.
76. Sakai N, Takehara Y, Yamashita S, Ohishi N, Kawaji H, Sameshima T, et al. Shear stiffness of 4 common intracranial tumors measured using MR elastography: comparison with intraoperative consistency grading. AJNR Am J Neuroradiol. 2016;37(10):1851–9.
77. McIlvain G, Hayes LL, Walter AW, Averill LW, Kandula V, Johnson CL, et al. Mechanical properties of pediatric low-grade gliomas in children with and without neurofibromatosis type 1. Neuroradiology. 2024;66(12):2301–11.
78. Wu B, Warnock G, Zaiss M, Lin C, Chen M, Zhou Z, et al. An overview of CEST MRI for non-MR physicists. EJNMMI Phys. 2016;3(1):19.
79. Suh CH, Park JE, Jung SC, Choi CG, Kim SJ, Kim HS. Amide proton transfer-weighted MRI in distinguishing high- and low-grade gliomas: a systematic review and meta-analysis. Neuroradiology. 2019;61(5):525–34.
80. Joo B, Han K, Ahn SS, Choi YS, Chang JH, Kang SG, et al. Amide proton transfer imaging might predict survival and IDH mutation status in high-grade glioma. Eur Radiol. 2019;29(12):6643–52.
81. Obdeijn IV, Wiegers EC, Alic L, Plasschaert SLA, Kranendonk MEG, Hoogduin HM, et al. Amide proton transfer weighted imaging in pediatric neuro-oncology: initial experience. NMR Biomed. 2024;37(6):e5122.
82. Zhang H, Yong X, Ma X, Zhao J, Shen Z, Chen X, et al. Differentiation of low- and high-grade pediatric gliomas with amide proton transfer imaging: added value beyond quantitative relaxation times. Eur Radiol. 2021;31(12):9110–9.
83. Chaddad A, Desrosiers C, Hassan L, Tanougast C. A quantitative study of shape descriptors from glioblastoma multiforme phenotypes for predicting survival outcome. Br J Radiol. 2016;89(1068):20160575.
84. Czarnek N, Clark K, Peters KB, Mazurowski MA. Algorithmic three-dimensional analysis of tumor shape in MRI improves prognosis of survival in glioblastoma: a multi-institutional study. J Neuro-Oncol. 2017;132(1):55–62.
85. Kickingereder P, Burth S, Wick A, Gotz M, Eidel O, Schlemmer HP, et al. Radiomic profiling of glioblastoma: identifying an imaging predictor of patient survival with improved performance over established clinical and radiologic risk models. Radiology. 2016;280(3):880–9.
86. Beig N, Bera K, Tiwari P. Introduction to radiomics and radiogenomics in neuro-oncology: implications and challenges. Neurooncol Adv. 2020;2(Suppl 4):iv3–iv14.
87. Zhang M, Tam L, Wright J, Mohammadzadeh M, Han M, Chen E, et al. Radiomics can distinguish pediatric supratentorial embryonal tumors, high-grade gliomas, and ependymomas. AJNR Am J Neuroradiol. 2022;43(4):603–10.
88. Zhang M, Wong SW, Lummus S, Han M, Radmanesh A, Ahmadian SS, et al. Radiomic phenotypes distinguish atypical teratoid/rhabdoid tumors from medulloblastoma. AJNR Am J Neuroradiol. 2021;42(9):1702–8.

89. Zhang M, Wong SW, Wright JN, Wagner MW, Toescu S, Han M, et al. MRI radiogenomics of pediatric medulloblastoma: a multicenter study. Radiology. 2022;304(2):406–16.
90. Liu Z, Ren S, Zhang H, Liao Z, Liu Z, An X, et al. Multiparametric MRI-based machine learning system of molecular subgroups and prognosis in medulloblastoma. Eur Radiol. 2025;35:5053.
91. Wu C, Zheng H, Li J, Zhang Y, Duan S, Li Y, et al. MRI-based radiomics signature and clinical factor for predicting H3K27M mutation in pediatric high-grade gliomas located in the midline of the brain. Eur Radiol. 2022;32(3):1813–22.
92. Wagner MW, Hainc N, Khalvati F, Namdar K, Figueiredo L, Sheng M, et al. Radiomics of pediatric low-grade gliomas: toward a pretherapeutic differentiation of BRAF-mutated and BRAF-fused tumors. AJNR Am J Neuroradiol. 2021;42(4):759–65.
93. Haldar D, Kazerooni AF, Arif S, Familiar A, Madhogarhia R, Khalili N, et al. Unsupervised machine learning using K-means identifies radiomic subgroups of pediatric low-grade gliomas that correlate with key molecular markers. Neoplasia. 2023;36:100869.
94. Kazerooni AF, Kraya A, Rathi KS, Kim MC, Kesherwani V, Corbett R, et al. Imaging clusters of pediatric low-grade glioma are associated with distinct molecular characteristics. AJNR Am J Neuroradiol. 2025;
95. Zheng H, Li J, Liu H, Ting G, Yin Q, Li R, et al. MRI radiomics signature of pediatric medulloblastoma improves risk stratification beyond clinical and conventional MR imaging features. J Magn Reson Imaging. 2023;58(1):236–46.
96. Tam LT, Yeom KW, Wright JN, Jaju A, Radmanesh A, Han M, et al. MRI-based radiomics for prognosis of pediatric diffuse intrinsic pontine glioma: an international study. Neurooncol Adv. 2021;3(1):vdab042.

4 Pathology and Molecular Biology

Sabrina Rossi, Evelina Miele, and Manila Antonelli

4.1 Introduction

Within a few years, genome-wide methylation profiling has had a revolutionary impact on CNS tumor classification. Historically, brain tumors were classified based on morphology. Nowadays the integration of molecular information has improved the diagnostic process, overcoming the extreme heterogeneity in terms of histology and molecular features. Molecular alterations provide significant prognostic and therapeutic implications beyond the morphologic examination alone, and different tumors may harbor similar molecular alterations with diagnostic and therapeutic implications.

This chapter aims to summarize the advances in pediatric CNS tumors with a distinction between glial/glioneuronal and embryonal tumors, focusing on the integration of molecular data with histologic, clinical, and radiographic features to reach the most accurate diagnosis.

4.1.1 Pediatric-Type Diffuse Low-Grade Gliomas

The World Health Organization (WHO) Classification of Tumors of the Central Nervous System incorporate significant molecular diagnostics, with the aim to recognize new tumor types, and new grading schemes for existing tumor types. Low-grade gliomas and glioneuronal tumors (pLGGs/GNTs) are the most common tumors of the central nervous system (CNS), accounting for 30% of pediatric CNS neoplasms [60]. The etiology was largely understood in the last 10 years in terms of new insights into their genetic drivers, thanks to the advance of technology and novel applications. However, about 5% of these tumors were attributed to genetic syndromes. In many cases, the different histologic entities are easy to distinguish; however, cases of overlapping morphology are sometimes difficult to identify.

pLGG/GNTs include several entities, which over the last decades were detailed by histological and immunohistochemical examination with overlapping morphology that was tricky for pathologists. Molecular characterization has overcome these difficulties by defining tumor entities with specific molecular alterations.

Ryall et al. in 2020 [74] published the largest cohort of pLGGs/GNTs with respect to clinical

S. Rossi
Pathology Unit, Department of Laboratories, Bambino Gesù Children's Hospital, IRCCS, Rome, Italy

E. Miele
Area of Hematology-Oncology, Cell Therapy, Gene Therapies, and Hematopoietic Transplantation, Bambino Gesù Children's Hospital, IRCCS, Rome, Italy

M. Antonelli (✉)
Department of Radiological, Oncological and Anatomic Pathology, Sapienza University, Rome, Italy
e-mail: manila.antonelli@uniroma1.it

A. Mastronuzzi, A. Carai (eds.), *Navigating Pediatric Brain Tumors*,
https://doi.org/10.1007/978-3-032-18992-9_4

molecular data and found specific driver alterations in neoplasms arising in various locations throughout the CNS and identified them. Most of these tumors are characterized by aberrant MAPK and/or mTOR activation, including KIAA1549::BRAF, BRAF p.V600E mutation, and FGFR gene family alterations. a fraction harbor instead non-canonical driver alterations such as (MYB family rearrangements) and rare non MAPK related alteration such as PDGFRA codon 385 mutations in myxoid glioneuronal tumors (MGT).

Epigenetic and genetic studies identified three new tumor types: diffuse glioneuronal tumor with oligodendroglioma-like features and nuclear clusters, the myxoid glioneuronal tumor and the multinodular and vacuolating neuronal tumor. pLGGs/GNTs could be diffuse or circumscribed and different type of tumor has a specific molecular alteration resulting in clinical implications in trials for specific inhibitors such as BRAF p. V600E- and MEK-inhibitors [74].

Diffuse astrocytoma MYB- or MYBL1-altered Diffuse astrocytoma MYB- or MYBL1-altered is a diffusely infiltrative glial neoplasm, composed of monomorphous cells with diffuse growth pattern and genetic alterations in MYB or MYBL1 gene (grade 1 sec. CNS WHO 2021). Most commonly, the tumor is located in the cerebral hemispheres, preferentially in the temporal lobe [92]. Rarely, it may also occur in the brainstem [74].

Diffuse astrocytoma, MYB- or MYBL1-altered are low-grade gliomas, usually epilepsy-associated tumors and have good prognosis [92]. At the MRI, the tumor appears mostly in a well-defined way but may also have, at least focally, a diffuse growth pattern (Fig. 4.1a) [32]. Tumors harboring these molecular alterations are classified as angiocentric glioma (AG) or diffuse astrocytoma (DA) according to their histology.

Histologically, the tumor is moderately cellular, and neoplastic cells are GFAP-positive, MAP2, OLIG2-, IDH1R132H-, CD34-negative, were detected and nuclear ATRX-expression was retained. The proliferation index was low. In

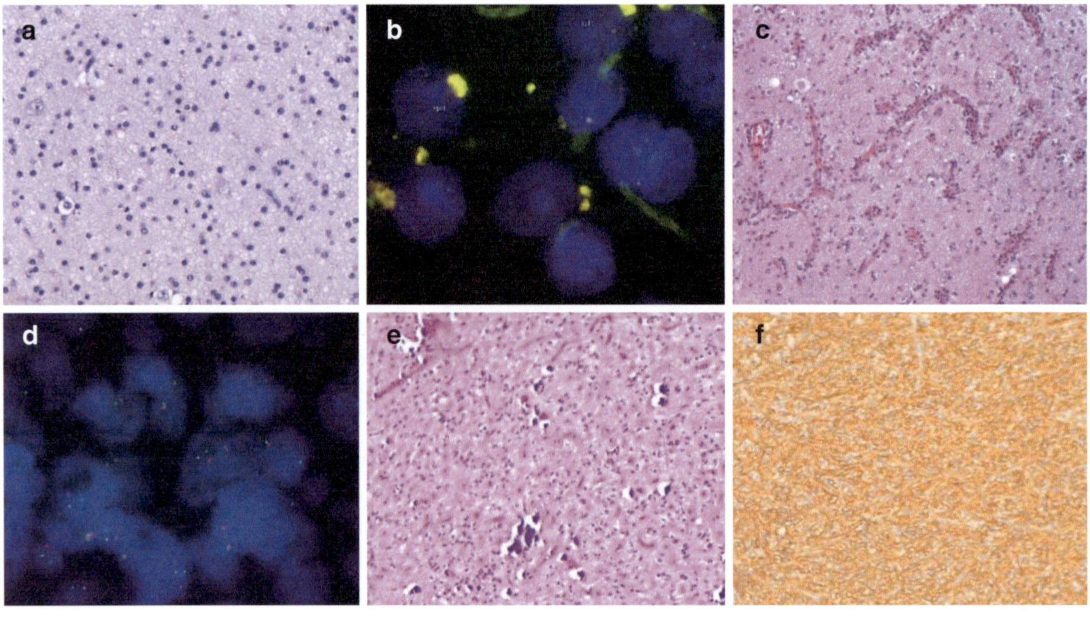

Fig. 4.1 Tumors show minimally pleomorphic cells, often with speckled chromatin. The cell density is slightly (**a**). FISH analysis confirms fusion between the MYB gene and a partner gene (**b**). Monomorphous cells with characteristic perivascular growth pattern and diffuse infiltrative fashion with and neurons in the cerebral cortex (**c**). Fish analysis confirms rearrangement of MYB (**d**). The neoplasm is characterized by cells with oligodendroglia-like features and nuclear pleomorphism, spindled glial elements and calcification (**e**). By immunohistochemistry the tumor cells were diffusely positive for diffuse CD34 (**f**)

older adolescents and young adults, this tumor must be distinguish from IDH-mutant and IDH-wildtype diffuse gliomas with similar histomorphological features but more aggressive behavior.

Molecular diagnostic testing that demonstrates fusion between the MYB or MYBL1 genes and a partner gene confirms the diagnosis (Fig. 4.1a). DNA methylation profile matching to diffuse astrocytoma, MYB- or MYBL1-altered further supports the diagnose.

MYB and its related family member MYBL1 are transcriptional transactivators for cell proliferation and differentiation; these gene undergo rearrangements resulting in truncation of the C-terminal negative-regulatory domain of protein [92].

On t-SNE of methylation analysis, MYB and MYBL1 tumors cluster together, reflecting a single tumor entity

Angiocentric glioma Angiocentric glioma (AG) is a rare tumor that occurs in children and young adults and commonly presents with seizures. They occur in the cerebral cortex or brainstem and on imaging are characteristically a well-delineated, non-enhancing, T2-FLAIR hyperintense [32] tumor. Tumors consist of monomorphous cells and a characteristic perivascular growth pattern; cells are bland and the patterns is diffusely infiltrative with and neurons in the cerebral cortex (Fig. 4.1b). Tumor cells are GFAP-positive but negative for OLIG2 and neuronal markers. EMA immunohistochemistry usually reveals a dot-like or ring-like (i.e., microlumina) positivity, which is similar to ependymomas [91]. AG has recurrent rearrangement of MYB, with MYB–QKI fusions as a specific driver event (Fig. 4.1b). QKI encodes the signaling and activation protein related to RNA binding Quaking, which is widely expressed in the nervous system and plays an important role in oligodendroglial differentiation [91]. Diffuse astrocytoma with MYB- or MYBL1-fusion and angiocentric glioma with MYB-QKI fusion share many morphologic, genetic, and epigenetic similarities, but are considered separate tumor types in the current WHO classification. Rarely *MYB* shows other fusion partners such as *PCDHGA1*. Angiocentric glioma is a low-grade diffuse glioma with indolent growth and is designated CNS WHO grade 1 [4].

Polymorphous low-grade neuroepithelial tumors of the young (PLNTY) Polymorphous low-grade neuroepithelial tumor of the young (PLNTY) is an epileptogenic tumor that originates from the cortex layer and subcortical white matter. PLNTY is a diffusely infiltrating glioma occurring mostly in children and young adults and in older patients, and it has been first described in 2017 by Huse et al. and included as a new entity in the 2021 classification with a CNS WHO grade 1 [36]. On MRI, their appearance is solid and cystic with T2 hyperintensity and frequent calcification; focal contrast enhancement can be present [36].

They are a low-grade glial neoplasm characterized morphologically by cells with oligodendroglia like features, neuronal nuclear pleomorphism, spindle-shaped astroglial elements, and calcification. By immunohistochemistry (IHC), the tumor cells were diffusely positive for GFAP and diffuse CD34 immunopositivity. Calcifications are typically observable and are usually confluent. Low proliferative activity was observed (Ki67 < 2%) [36]. *BRAF* p.V600E represents the most common genetic mutation, but fusions regarding *FGFR2* and *FGFR3* genes are also encountered [7]. FGFR fusions are mutually exclusive with BRAF V600E mutations. *FGFR3::TACC3* fusion, usually associated with a rare subtype of adult-type diffuse glioma, IDH-wildtype, has also been reported in a single case of PLNTY [7], even if the DNA methylation profile was not assessed. For these reasons, pathologists and oncologists must always remember that *BRAF* and *FGFR3* alterations are not specific of PLNTYs but may also be encountered in high-grade gliomas, showing PLNTY-like morphological features [7].

Diffuse low-grade glioma, MAPK pathway altered Diffuse low-grade glioma, MAPK pathway-altered is a group of gliomas with infiltrative growth pattern composed by bland cells with astrocytic, oligo-like, or mixed morphology. Moreover, tumor cells are typically located in the subpial region in a radial fashion. This tumor occurs mostly in children and are related to activation of the MAPK pathway such as *BRAF* p.V600E mutations or *FGFR1* alterations, in the form of *FGFR1* internal tandem duplication (ITD), tyrosine kinase domain (TKD) mutation, or fusion gene [74].

Tumor cells are immunopositive for GFAP and OLIG2 and negative for neuronal markers, extravascular CD34 immunostaining is usually limited to vessels. IDH1 is negative and exclude adult-type diffuse glioma. A CNS WHO grade has not yet been assigned, and DNA methylation profiling does not assign these tumors into a single group but instead into several distinct tumor types.

4.1.2 Pediatric-Type Diffuse High-Grade Gliomas

Pediatric-type diffuse high-grade gliomas are less common than their low-grade counterpart, and different types are defined depending on typical location, age and molecular alterations. They comprise four main entities: (1) Diffuse midline glioma H3 K27-altered; (2) Diffuse hemispheric glioma H3 G34-mutant; (3) Diffuse pediatric-type high-grade glioma H3-wildtype and IDH-wildtype; and (4) Infant-type hemispheric glioma. This tumor family is defined as "pediatric-type diffuse high-grade gliomas" and this designation reflects their general characteristics. However, although they are qualified as "diffuse", a circumscribed pattern of growth is typically found in the infant type [9, 10, 33] 3,4 and may be also encountered in the H3-wildtype and IDH-wildtype type. Secondly, with respect to the definition of "high-grade", the H3K27-altered type sometimes appears remarkably hypocellular without evidence of mitotic activity 5 or the infant type may show low-grade glioneural features with a ganglionic differentiation. Regardless of the morphological features, the pediatric-type diffuse high-grade gliomas are biologically aggressive tumors with a dismal prognosis and are designated as grade 4, except for the infant-type to which a formal grade has not been assigned due to limited experience. Finally, although classified as "gliomas", they sometimes show morphological and phenotypic features typical of the embryonal tumors, especially if belonging to the H3 G34-mutant type or to the H3-wildtype and IDH-wildtype type.

For the clinico-radiological features and the pathogenesis of each type of this tumor family, also refer to the dedicated chapter of this book.

Diffuse midline glioma H3 K27-altered Diffuse midline glioma (DMG) is an aggressive astrocytic tumor occurring in the brainstem or the midline structures of the brain, recognized as a CNS WHO grade 4 malignancy regardless of its histological features. In children it is located mostly in the pons (diffuse intrinsic pontine glioma—DIPG) or it may be bithalamic, whereas in adolescents and adults, it is usually monothalamic or spinal. It is characterized by the loss of H3K27me3 and is molecularly defined into three subtypes: (1) DMG, with H3K27M/I mutation, encompassing H3.3-mutant and H3.1 or H3.2-mutant cases; (2) DMG, H3-wildtype with overexpression of EZHIP; and (3) DMG, with EGFR alteration, including either mutation, e.g. EGFRvIII, or amplification. Recently, an additional subgroup showing the co-occurrence of H3.3K27M with BRAF or FGFR1 alterations has recently emerged. Notably, it forms a distinct methylation cluster, harbors atypical radiological and histological features and tends to have a better prognosis [6]. The majority of DMGs look like grade 3 or 4 astrocytomas with a morphologic spectrum varying from cells with hyperchromatic oval to elongated nuclei with scant cytoplasm, to cells with epithelioid features, or, rarely, giant cells 24. Mitotic figures are frequently observed and microvascular proliferation and/or necrosis may be present. Cases of grade 2 histology also have been described [9, 10]. The immunophenotype is consistent with the glial nature of this tumor. Thus, neoplastic cells are reactive for OLIG2 and S100 and variably for

GFAP. Of note, antibodies for H3K27M (mutated protein), H3K27me3 (trimethylated protein) and EZHIP represent a valuable molecular surrogate to identify DMG subtypes (Fig. 4.2a). A subset of tumors, in addition to H3K27me3 loss, can also show p53 expression and/or nuclear loss of ATRX immunostaining resulting from TP53 or ATRX mutations [12]. The differential diagnosis includes circumscribed glial/glioneural tumors, i.e. pilocytic astrocytoma and ganglioglioma, and the distinction from DMG is particularly challenging for those cases carrying H3K27M mutation, relying only on a morphological ground 26. Diffuse gliomas are also in the differential. The possibility of an infratentorial IDH-mutant astrocytoma, although rare in children, has to be considered. Notably, in this context, the immunohistochemistry for IDH1 Arg132His mutant and ATRX is of limited use, as the infratentorial IDH-mutant astrocytomas frequently carry alternative nonArg132His IDH1 mutations, and usually lack ATRX mutations [8]. Hence, sequencing of IDH1 and IDH2 hot spot region is warranted [8]. Moreover, in pediatric IDH-mutant astrocytoma a possible association with a mismatch repair deficiency syndrome has to be evaluated [82]. Cases of high-grade glioma, H3-wildtype and IDH-wildtype with MYCN amplification arising in the brainstem have also been described and should be considered in the differential diagnosis [83]. Beside glioneural and glial tumors, even embryonal tumors such as atypical teratoid/rhabdoid tumor and embryonal tumor with multilayered rosettes enter in the differential diagnosis, which may be addressed by immunohistochemistry.

Diffuse hemispheric glioma, H3 G34-mutant Diffuse hemispheric glioma, H3 G34–mutant, is a CNS WHO grade 4 astrocytoma, diffusely infiltrative, arising in the cerebral hemispheres. It affects children and young adults with a median age of 15 years. The driver alteration is a point mutation at codon 35 of the histone H3.3 gene H3-3A, corresponding to glycine 34 of the mature H3.3 protein [77, 95], 33. Concurrent TP53 and ATRX mutations are present in ~90% of cases. Between 50% and 70% of diffuse hemispheric glioma H3 G34-mutant harbor PDGFRA mutations, which may offer new therapeutic opportunities for these patients [14, 15]. Histologically it may display a classic glioblastoma appearance or an embryonal (PNET-like) appearance (Fig. 4.2b). The glioblastoma-like pattern shows a strong expression of GFAP; the PNET-like variant is diffusely positive for synaptophysin and exhibits a focal expression of GFAP. Both variants are negative for OLIG2. The absence of OLIG2 and ATRX expression together with the presence of a diffuse p53 expression is the typical phenotypic constellation of this entity and strongly suggests the diagnosis in the appropriate clinic-pathological context. However, it is not highly specific as it may be encountered in rare cases of diffuse pediatric-type high-grade glioma, H3-wildtype and IDH-wildtype. Hence, molecular confirmation of the H3-3A driver mutation is needed to address the differential.

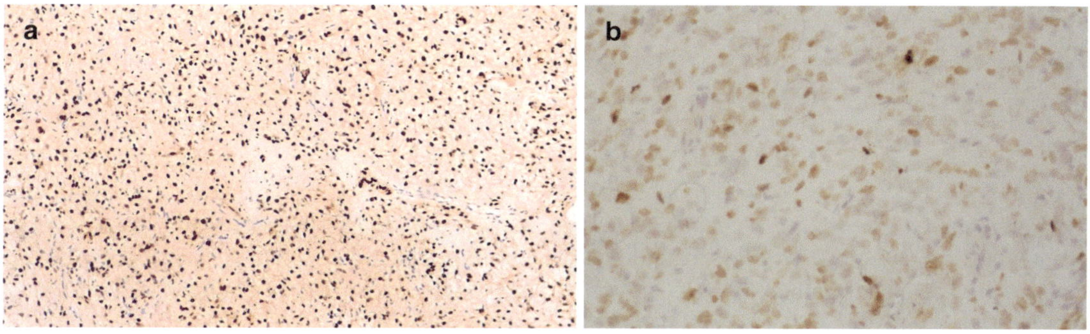

Fig. 4.2 EZHIP immunopositivity in a DMG tumor (**a**). H3 G34 antibody stains tumor cells in a diffuse hemispheric glioma H3 G34-mutant (**b**)

Diffuse pediatric-type high-grade glioma, H3-wildtype and IDH-wildtype Diffuse pediatric-type high-grade glioma H3-wildtype and IDH-wildtype (pHGG H3/IDH WT) is a heterogeneous entity currently defined by the combination of a high-grade morphology, either glial or primitive/undifferentiated, and the following molecular features: (i) the absence of IDH1/2 mutations, (ii) the absence of oncohistone alterations, e.g., H3.3/H3.1/H3.2 pK27M, (iii) the alignment of the tumor with one of three pediatric high-grade glioma (pHGG) methylation groups, i.e., pHGG RTK1, pHGG RTK2, pHGG MYCN 40, or, alternatively, the identification of genetic alterations that are considered characteristic of these groups, affecting PDGFRA, EGFR or MYCN, respectively (Table 4.1). The documentation of the absence of IDH and H3 abnormalities even when occurring in an appropriate clinicopathological context is not per se sufficient to make a diagnosis and the alignment of the tumor methylation profile with the pHGG RTK1, pHGG RTK2, pHGG MYCN or the occurrence of PDGFRA, EGFR or MYCN alterations are essential WHO diagnostic criteria. It has to be highlighted that PDGFRA, EGFR or MYCN/MYC alterations are neither sensitive nor specific of the pHGG RTK1, pHGG RTK2, pHGG MYCN methylation groups, cautioning against embracing the diagnosis of pHGG H3/IDH WT upon the identification of PDGFRA, EGFR or MYCN/MYC alterations [35, 84] and indicating that the methylation analysis is the diagnostic gold standard for this entity. Another issue regarding this entity as currently defined is related to the substantial amount of cases encountered in our daily diagnostic practice that are wildtype for IDH and H3, negative for receptor tyrosine kinase (RTK) fusions and do not classify as pHGG RTK1, pHGG RTK2, pHGG MYCN. These tumors are designated as 'NEC' according to the WHO classification after thorough molecular characterization 2. There are a few studies investigating the clinicopathological features correlated with pHGG H3/IDH WT. Notably, the pHGG RTK1 subgroup includes most of the radiation-induced gliomas developing in patients previously treated for medulloblastomas or acute lymphoblastic leukemia as well as most of the gliomas arising in syndromic contexts (e.g., Li Fraumeni, constitutional mismatch repair deficiency and Lynch syndrome) [19, 20, 48]. As for the location, the vast majority of pHGG H3/IDH WT occur in the supratentorial anatomic compartment. A minority of pHGG MYCN (about 15%) arise in the brainstem [9, 10, 41]. pHGG RTK1 may also occur in infratentorial/brainstem structures, for instance in patients treated for medulloblastoma who received the highest radiotherapy dose in the posterior fossa [4, 19, 20, 48]. As for the outcome, the overall prognosis of pHGG H3/IDH WT is poor (WHO grade 4). pHGG and MYCN are associated with the lowest survival rates. Within the pHGG RTK1 subgroup, survivals of the radiation-induced pHGG RTK1 are remarkably shorter than the sporadic counterpart. pHGG RTK2 has been shown to be the least aggressive. Furthermore, the occurrence of TP53, ATRX and mismatch repair genes mutations in the context of pHGG H3/IDH WT have been associated with adverse outcomes [35]. Microscopically, pHGG H3/IDH WT may feature classical diffuse astrocytic morphology, with brisk mitotic activity, foci of necrosis and microvascular proliferation, showing a conventional phenotype with the expression of glial markers, i.e., GFAP and OLIG2. Some cases, especially those belonging to pHGG MYCN or, more rarely, to pHGG RTK1, may display a primitive/embryonal morphology and pushing borders with only minimal infiltration of the surrounding parenchyma. In such cases, the expression of the glial markers may be focal or even absent, whereas neuronal markers may be diffusely expressed, e.g., synaptophysin. A biphasic pattern may also be present, and embryonal nodules may be found in a background of an infiltrating high-grade astrocytoma [83]. A remarkable nuclear pleomorphism may be seen in pHGG H3/IDH WT arising in syndromic contexts, i.e., Li Fraumeni syndrome [89]. As for the immunophenotype, p53 is commonly found overexpressed in pHGG H3/IDH WT. ATRX is lost in a minority of cases, which, in combination with p53 overexpression, may suggest the possibility of an astrocytoma IDH-mutant.

Infant-type hemispheric glioma The essential diagnostic criteria for infant-type hemispheric glioma are a combination of clinicopathological and molecular characteristics. Cellular astrocytic morphology, presentation in early childhood (usually before age 5), and hemispheric location are fundamental to the diagnosis. Infant-type hemispheric glioma is typically driven by a fusion involving a receptor tyrosine kinase (RTK) gene, i.e., NTRK 1/2/3, ALK, ROS1, and MET, as 3′ partner. Either the presence of the fusion or the methylation profile of infant-type hemispheric glioma is also required for the diagnosis (Table 4.1). It is worth highlighting that although the RTK fusion identification has relevant therapeutic implications, its identification within the context of a glioma does not equate to a diagnosis of infant-type hemispheric glioma, as RTK fusions may be found in other well-established or emerging entities. First, RTK fusions are occasionally detected in other types of HGG (e.g., adult-type glioblastoma IDH-WT, diffuse pediatric-type HGG H3/IDH WT, diffuse midline H3-altered) [24, 55, 94] where they likely represent additional molecular events, resulting from clonal evolution. Furthermore, RTK fusions may characterize a subset of low-grade gliomas (e.g., PA, diffuse LGG with MAPKinase-altered). Moreover, RTK fusions also drive emerging molecular tumor groups. Among those, a novel methylation group of glioneuronal tumors driven by a kinase fusion, typically affecting children and presenting with an oligodendroglioma-like morphology with no/low mitoses, has been recently described. An additional epigenetic group of glioneuronal tumors with anaplastic features showing the co-occurrence of a kinase fusion and ATRX inactivation and typically affecting adolescents and young adults has also been identified [57]. The clinicopathological features (infancy or childhood), the genomic landscape of the tumor (e.g., absence of other gene variants, quiet copy number variation profile), and the methylation profile, beside the presence of the RTK fusion, should be considered to address the differential diagnosis.

Infant-type hemispheric glioma typically shows sharp demarcation from the adjacent parenchyma and a uniform astrocytic cytomorphology, consisting of monotonous sheets of gemistocytes/minigemistocytes or fascicles of spindle cells [16, 33]. The majority of cases show a high-grade morphology sometimes associated with a low-grade component with ganglionic differentiation [16, 33]. As for the immunophenotype, infant-type hemispheric gliomas express glial markers, i.e., OLIG2 and GFAP, and sometimes EMA with a dot-like pattern. The differential diagnosis includes other entities occurring during infancy, such as desmoplastic infantile ganglioglioma/astrocytoma (DIG/DIA), supratentorial ependymoma, astroblastoma MN1-altered, CNS tumor with BCOR internal tandem duplication (ITD), and, for cases with a low-grade morphology, ganglioglioma [16, 33]. As to the prognosis, a formal grade has not been assigned to infant-type hemispheric glioma, as follow-up data are still limited. However, the outcome of infant-type hemispheric glioma, even in cases with high-grade features, seems favorable compared with other gliomas with similar morphology but different underlying biology. However, the morbidity is high, calling into question the current approach of maximal surgical resection and chemotherapy for children affected by this tumor type. On the basis of data reported in a single study, ALK-rearranged tumors show the best prognosis (53.8% 5-year OS) as compared with the intermediate prognosis of NTRK-fused tumors (42.9% 5-year OS) and the poorer prognosis of tumors harboring ROS1 alterations (25% 5-year OS) [33], but more data are needed to draw definitive conclusions. What is unquestioned is the importance of identifying the 3′ gene partner of the fusion to predict tumor response to targeted therapy and choose the most appropriate molecular agent, e.g., Larotrectinib for NTRK rearrangement or, for instance, Alectinib for ALK rearrangement [13].

4.1.3 Circumscribed Astrocytic Gliomas

Pilocytic astrocytoma Pilocytic astrocytomas (PA) are low-grade, slow-growing, well-circumscribed brain tumors with cystic component, though they can infiltrate the surrounding

Table 4.1 List of embryonal tumors according to CNS5 with main features

			Age	Location	Histology	Immunohistochemistry	Subgroups	Genetics	Chromosomal abnormalities	Outcome of subgroups (5 years survival)
Medulloblastomas	Medulloblastoma, WNT-activated		Childhood	Central, frequently contiguous to brainstem	Mostly classic, rarely large cell anaplastic	Nuclear beta-catenin, Filamin A positive, YAP1 positive, GAB1 negative	α, βl	CTNNB1, DDX3X, SMARCA4, and TP53 mutations	Monosomy of chromosome 6	97% (α), 100% (β)
	Medulloblastoma, SHH-activated, and TP53-wildtype		Infancy/ Adulthood		Desmoplastic/ Large cell/ anaplastic	P53 negative		PTCH1, SMO, SUFU, TP53 mutations	9q deletion, 10q loss	69.8% (α), 67.3% (β), 88% (γ), 88.5% (δ)
	Medulloblastoma, SHH-activated, and TP53-mutant		Childhood	Hemispheric (rarely midline)	Nodular	Cytoplasmic beta catenin, Filamin A positive, YAP1 positive, GAB1 positive, p53 positive	α, β, γ, δ	TERT promoter mutations	MYCN amplification, GLI2 amplification, 17p loss	
	Medulloblastoma, non-WNT/ non-SHH	Group 3	Childhood	Midline (filling 4th ventricle)	Classic, Large cell anaplastic	Cytoplasmic beta catenin, Filamin A negative, YAP1 negative, GAB1 negative	II, III, IV (Group 3)	MYC, OTX2, SMARCA4, NOTCH, TGF-β mutations	MYC amplification, isodicentric 17q, 1q gain, and 5q and 10q loss	50% (II) 43% (III) 80% (IV) 77% (I) 59% (V) 85% (VII)
							I, V, VII (Group 3/4)			
		Group 4	All age groups	Midline (filling 4th ventricle)	Classic, Large cell anaplastic		VI, VIII (Group 4)	MYCN, KDM6A, CDKNA mutation, SNCAIP duplications	MYC amplification; isodicentric 17q; 8, 10, and 11 loss; 4, 7, 17, and 18 gain	81% (VI) 81% (VIII)

Other CNS embryonal tumors	Atypical teratoid/rhabdoid tumor	Infancy/ childhood	More frequently supratentorial	Poorly differentiated cells, focal or diffuse rhabdoid features, polyphenotypic differentiation	INI1 negative (BRG1-negative in rare cases)	AT/RT-SHH, AT/RT-TYR, AT/RT-MYC	SMARCB1 point mutations/focal deletions	In TYR subtype complete or partial loss chr22	
	Cribriform neuroepithelial tumor	Infancy	Periventricular areas	Strands and ribbons conferring a cribriform pattern of nonrhabdoid cells	Strong positivity for EMA and loss of SMARCB1 expression				
	Embryonal tumor with multilayered rosettes	Infancy/ childhood	Cerebral hemispheres or infratentorial compartment	Multilayered mitotically active rosettes of embryonal cells	Strong and diffuse cytoplasmic LIN28A		Biallelic DICER1 mutations	C19MC amplification	24%
	CNS neuroblastoma, FOXR2-activated	Childhood	Supratentorial	Embryonal cells with hyperchromatic nuclei and inconspicuous cytoplasm arranged in a sheet-like pattern	Strong immunopositivity for OLIG2 and GFAP, and vimentin negativity			FOXR2 rearrangements	85%
	CNS tumor with BCOR internal tandem duplication (ITD)	Infancy/ Adulthood	Cerebral or cerebellar hemispheres	Uniform oval or spindleshaped cells, with round or oval nuclei showing a delicate chromatin pattern	Vimentin and CD56 positive, OLIG2, GFAP, or S100 negative or scarce			Heterozygous ITD in exon 15 of the BCOR gene	<50%
	CNS embryonal tumor NOS			Embryonal			No alteration that would classify it as one of the other CNS embryonal tumors	No alteration that would classify it as one of the other CNS embryonal tumors	

Adapted from Gianno et al. [29]

brain parenchyma [91]. It occurs in the cerebellum, along the optic pathways, hypothalamus, brainstem and in the cerebral hemispheres. PAs are characterized by MAPK pathway alterations (typically, *KIAA1549*::*BRAF* gene fusion). Other mutations include *BRAFV600E* point mutations more prevalent in supratentorial tumors and FGFR1 mutations. Up to 20% of patients with NF1 develop a pilocytic astrocytoma, most commonly along the optic pathway. PAs typically have low-to-moderate cellularity, and cells have long and bipolar processes. Rosenthal fibers, which are elongated eosinophilic bundles, and eosinophilic granular bodies are characteristic. Multinucleated giant cells with peripheral nuclei can be present. Calcifications and areas of necrosis and microvascular proliferation may also be observed. Histological diagnosis may be particularly challenging in tumors with an infiltrative component, even in classically well-circumscribed pilocytic astrocytoma. PAs stain positive for glial fibrillary acidic protein (GFAP), S100, and OLIG2 and SYN while being negative for CD34. There are two subtypes: pilomyxoid astrocytoma and pilocytic astrocytoma with histological features of anaplasia. Pilomyxoid astrocytoma develops in the hypothalamic/chiasmatic area and has a worse prognosis with tendency to spread throughout the CSF fluid. A diffusely myxoid background is the hallmark of the tumor. Rosenthal fibers and eosinophilic granular bodies are often absent. Pilocytic astrocytoma with histological features of anaplasia has the same morphological features of pilocytic astrocytoma but with sparkling mitotic activity and sometimes necrosis and/or anaplasia. Necrosis, alternative telomere lengthening, and ATRX deletion are associated with poorer survival.

High-grade astrocytoma with piloid features High-grade astrocytoma with piloid features (HGAP) is a brain tumor defined by a specific DNA methylation profile and recently added to the last WHO classification of central nervous system tumors. HGAP rarely happens in the pediatric population, and median age is 40 years (range: 4–88 years) [26]. This tumor is sporadic and reported cases in patients with *NF1* gene alterations are on record. CNS WHO grade currently is not assigned, and clinical behavior is similar to CNS WHO grade 3. This tumor is a circumscribed astrocytic glioma with high-grade piloid or glioblastoma-like histological features that can occur throughout the entire CNS, mostly in the posterior fossa, particularly cerebellum, and more rarely in supratentorial or spinal location. Histologically this tumor has moderately cellular density, pleomorphic cells with multiple eosinophilic granular bodies, mitotic figures, and a Rosenthal fiber (Fig. 4.3). Genes of the MAPK pathway are the most commonly reported, involving most frequently NF1 alteration, followed by *KIAA1549*::*BRAF* fusions and *FGFR1* mutations. *BRAF* p. V600E mutation can occur with a very low percentage. Furthermore, nearly all tumors harbor *CDKN2A/B* homozygous deletion, rarely *CDK4* amplification, are *IDH1* wild-type and have alterations in ATRX gene [71]. HGAP forms a separate DNA methylation cluster, and outcome analysis confirmed an unfavorable clinical course in comparison to PA, but better than IDH wildtype glioblastoma [71].

Pleomorphic xanthoastrocytoma Pleomorphic xanthoastrocytomas (PXA) are epileptogenic tumors accounting for about 1% of primary brain tumors, mostly located in temporal, parietal and frontal lobes. It can be WHO grade 2 or 3 and arises in young patients, with a peak incidence in the second to third decades of life. They are typically located superficially with a cystic component and contrast enhancement, most commonly in the temporal lobe and firmly associated

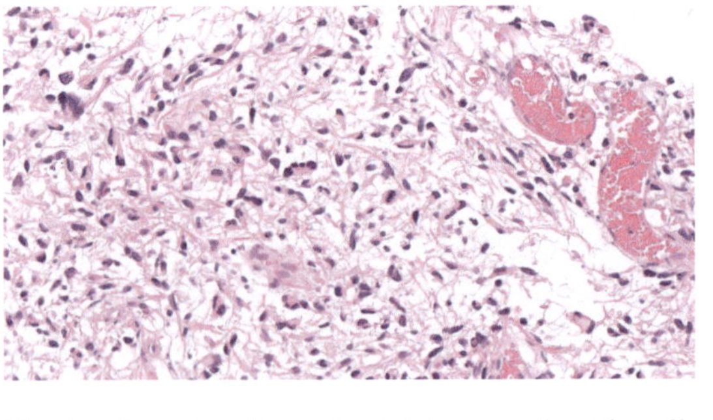

Fig. 4.3 Hematoxylin–eosin staining a moderately cell-rich, moderately pleomorphic glial with mitotic activity, without vascular proliferation or necrosis

with the leptomeninges. They grow slowly and are circumscribed tumors, such that no surrounding edema is present. The tumor is highly cellular with pleomorphic cells and with occasional bizarre-looking nuclei; it also presents a component of spindle neoplastic and neoplastic cells with bizarre nuclei or multinucleation and neoplastic cells with multivacuolated cytoplasm. The cytoplasm of the tumor cells is eosinophilic and contains varying amounts of hyaline protein and lipid droplets. Pericellular reticulin deposition is also present. Lymphoplasmacytic infiltration and eosinophilic granular bodies are present. Scattered mitotic figures could be observed (<5 mitoses/10 high-powered fields) in CNS WHO grade 2. Anaplastic PXA (CNS WHO grade 3) is defined by the presence of increased cellularity, necrosis and high mitotic activity >5 mitoses/10 high-powered fields. Grade 3 PXA could be composed mostly of monomorphic tumor cells with increased cellularity. Tumor cells are positive for GFAP, vimentin and S100. The most frequently found mutated gene in PXAs is *BRAF*. BRAF mutations can be found in 70% of typical PXA and are less common in aPXAs (17–65%). Moreover, CDKN2A/B deletion could be present in similar proportion of PXA grade 2 and grade 3, suggesting its involvement in biology of PXA and not in tumor grade or BRAF mutation [47].

Subependymal giant cell astrocytoma Subependymal giant cell astrocytomas (SEGA) are benign tumors (CNS WHO grade 1), with a typical glioneuronal origin, distinct from astrocytomas. They occur almost exclusively seen in TSC patients, and the diagnosis should prompt confirmatory genetic testing; a small percentage of SEGAs have been reported in the absence of TSC, suggesting that these solitary SEGAs may be secondary to somatic mosaicism [26]. SEGAs arise from the ependymal lining of the ventricles and are typically located adjacent to the caudate nuclei. These tumors are composed of large polygonal cells with plentiful cytoplasm admixed with smaller cells with oval nuclei and elongated cytoplasmic processes. Giant cells with a ganglionic appearance are present, with eccentric, vesicular nuclei with distinct nucleoli and glassy eosinophilic cytoplasm. Scattered calcifications could be present. The cells are immunoreactive for GFAP and NFP. TSC is caused by mutations in the TSC1 or TSC2 tumor suppressor genes, encoding for the proteins hamartin and tuberin, respectively. The dysfunctional hamartin and tuberin seen in TSC allow for constitutive activation of the mTOR pathway.

Chordoid glioma Chordoid glioma is a slow-growing and well-circumscribed tumor (CNS WHO grade 2) characterized by a specific histology and typically arising from the anterior wall or roof of the third ventricle and frequently adherent to the hypothalamus and extending to the suprasellar region and lateral ventricles [2]. They are non-invasive, slow-growing tumors and occur in adults, predominantly in females [69]. On MRI, it appears as an isointense multilobulated mass on T1-weighted images, with homogeneous enhancement [69]. Tanycytes of the third ventricle have been proposed as the cell of origin owing to its location. Microscopically, these tumors are composed of cords of epithelioid cells, which are embedded in mucoid/myxoid matrix. Lymphoplasmacytic infiltrates with Russell bodies are frequently observed. Tumor cells are positive for GFAP and vimentin, and focally positive for EMA, pan-cytokeratin, S-100 protein, and TTF-1. They are characterized by recurrent *PRKCA p.D463H* missense mutation.

Astroblastoma MN1-altered Astroblastoma is an uncommon glial brain tumor arising more frequently in children (median age 15 years), with a female predominance and occurring predominantly in the cerebral hemispheres, although the cases of the brainstem and spinal cord have been recorded. The histologic characteristic of *MN1*-altered astroblastoma is the "astroblastic" pseudorosette, a perivascular structuring of neoplastic cells that are radially arrayed, often with a papillary or pseudopapillary growth. Vascular and stromal sclerosis is another typical feature of this tumor (Fig. 4.4). Neoplastic cells have elongated nuclei and abundant eosinophilic cytoplasm with a prominent process extending to central hyalin-

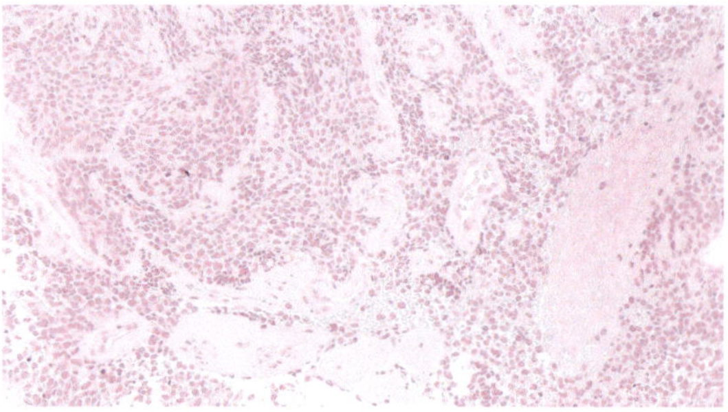

Fig. 4.4 Neoplastic cells have elongated nuclei and abundant eosinophilic cytoplasm with a prominent process extending to central hyalinized vessels. Vascular and stromal sclerosis is another typical feature of this tumor

ized vessels. Neoplastic cells are usually immunoreactive for GFAP, with focal nuclear OLIG2 expression. Cytoplasmic positivity for EMA is regularly seen with variable distribution. MN1-altered astroblastoma has no CNS WHO grade assigned. Astroblastoma displays a distinct DNA methylation pattern, and the characteristic molecular aberration is the MN1 rearrangement at chromosome band 22q12.1 with fusion partner genes, such as *BEND2*. In the spinal cord, tumors with astroblastoma-like morphology have been described, harboring different gene fusions involving chromosome X and 22q12 breakpoint regions as EWSR1::BEND2 fusion [56]. Patients with MN1-altered astroblastomas have a high rate of local recurrence but good overall survival.

4.1.4 Glioneuronal and Neuronal Tumors

Glioneuronal tumors (WHO grade 1/2) are a group of rare neoplasms strongly associated with seizures and affect infants, children and young adults, but are also described in adults and the elderly. Glioneuronal tumors are rare tumors composed of both neural and glial components in different proportions. Both glial and neuronal cells are highlighted by GFAP, Olig2, and synaptophysin. They include central, extraventricular, and lipo-neurocytoma; desmoplastic infantile astrocytoma and ganglioglioma (DIA/DIG), diffuse leptomeningeal glioneuronal tumor (DLGNT), dysembryoplastic neuroepithelial tumor (DNET), papillary glioneuronal tumor (PGNT), rosette-forming glioneuronal tumor of the fourth ventricle (RGNT), rosetted glioneuronal tumor with neuropil-like islands (GNTNI), gangliocytoma (GC), and ganglioglioma (GG). Most glioneuronal tumors fall within two major groups: group 1 containing a higher proportion of tumors with a ganglioglioma-like appearance displaying more BRAF-V600E mutations, while group 2 tumors are more DNET-like in appearance and display more FGFR1 mutations [79]. Other mutations include PIK3CA (RGNTs and mixed RGNT/DNET) [30] with implications for targeting the PI3K/AKT/mTOR pathway, FGFR1 mutations, SLC44A1-PRKCA, and NOTCH1-PRKCA fusion [59].

The WHO CNS5 comprises three new entities: multinodular and vacuolating neuronal tumor (MNVNT), diffuse glioneuronal tumor with oligodendroglioma-like features and nuclear clusters (DGONC), which is a provisional type, and myxoid glioneuronal tumor (MGT).

Multinodular and vacuolating neuronal tumor (MVNT) is a CSN WHO grade 1 neoplasm, arising in the temporal/frontal lobe of adult patients, with few pediatric examples. Histologically, MVNTs are characterized by hypomyelinated nodules with a fibrillary matrix, prominent vacuolar alteration, and monomorphic neuronal cells. Neoplastic cells are positive for OLIG2, synaptophysin, and MAP2.

Diffuse glioneuronal tumor with oligodendroglioma-like features and nuclear clusters (DGONC) [18] occurs in pediatric age and is localized in the cerebral hemispheres. Histopathological features are diffuse growth of oligo-like and multinucleated cells, with nuclear clusters disposed as "pennies on a plate" (Fig. 4.5). Tumor cells display diffuse positivity for OLIG-2, synaptophysin, and MAP2, and variable positivity for GFAP. The mitotic index is variable, and the Ki-67 labeling index can be up to 30%. The molecular hallmark of DGONC is monosomy of chromosome 14. Due to the low number of cases with an available follow-up, DGONC was not assigned to a CNS WHO grade.

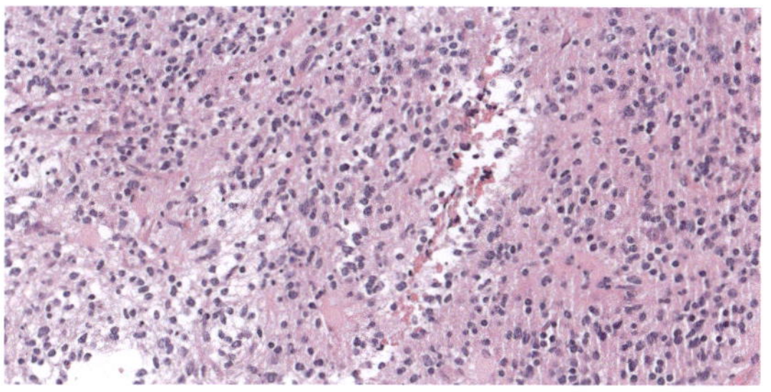

Fig. 4.5 Neoplasm shows diffuse growth of oligo-like and multinucleated cells, with nuclear clusters disposed as "pennies on a plate"

Myxoid glioneuronal tumor (MGT) (CNS WHO grade 1) is typically located in septum pellucidum and deep periventricular white matter [51]. These are uncommon primary brain tumors with a peak incidence in the second and third decades of life. Histologically, MGT is a circumscribed tumor composed of oligo-like cells immersed in a myxoid stroma. Some cases may show floating neurons and perivascular neuropil, which are similar to DNTs. The oligo-like cells are immunoreactive for OLIG2, GFAP, and MAP2 and negative for synaptophysin. Floating neurons, perivascular neuropil, and neurocytic rosettes are synaptophysin-positive. MGT shows a recurrent *PDGFRA* p.K385L/I dinucleotide somatic mutation [51].

4.1.5 Ependymal Tumors

Ependymomas are circumscribed glial tumors with histological features of ependymal cells and are classified according to morphological features and molecular characteristics across three anatomic compartments: supratentorial, posterior fossa, and spinal. Ependymomas represent the third most common brain tumor in children, the large majority (about 90%) being intracranial tumors, with the two-thirds arising in the posterior fossa. Within the pediatric population, infratentorial ependymomas tend to occur more frequently in younger children, supratentorial lesions in older children, and spinal ones in preteens [53]. Surgical resection is a relevant prognostic factor, and second-look surgery of residual tumor is highly recommended [54]. Post-surgical focal radiotherapy is the mainstay of care for most cases, whereas the role of chemotherapy is still controversial [17, 54]. The family of ependymal tumors generally includes lesions ranging from CNS WHO grade 1 (i.e., subependymomas) to grade 3 (formerly designated as anaplastic ependymomas), and brisk mitoses and/or microvascular proliferation are currently used as histological grading criteria. However, the correlation between histological grading and patients' outcome is controversial, and a variable degree of inter-observer variability in distinguishing grade 2 from grade 3 ependymomas has been reported [44]. While the existence of unambiguously grade 2 and grade 3 ependymomas associated with progression-free survival is acknowledged [17, 54, 72], there is a grey zone of "indeterminate malignancy" whose prognostic significance is unclear.

Both gene expression and methylation data support the idea that supratentorial, posterior fossa and spinal cord ependymomas are different entities with distinct molecular alterations and clinicopathologic characteristics [63, 87]. This chapter will focus on those ependymomas typical of the pediatric age.

Supratentorial ependymomas Supratentorial ependymomas represent about 30% of all intracranial ependymomas, occurring more frequently in children than in adults. They show clear-cut ependymal differentiation: sharp circumscription, perivascular pseudorosettes, true rosettes/canals, combined with GFAP positivity, no or focal OLIG2 expression and EMA dot-like staining. The current WHO classification of the CNS tumors recognizes two types of supratentorial ependymomas: supratentorial ependymoma ZFTA fusion-positive, and supratentorial ependymoma YAP1 fusion-positive. According to the WHO, the diagnosis of supratentorial ependymoma not elsewhere classified (NEC) and not otherwise specified (NOS) is used when the fusions of *ZFTA* or *YAP1* are not detected or the molecular analysis is not feasible, respectively.

Supratentorial ependymoma *ZFTA* fusion-positive (ST-EPN-ZFTA) is driven by a gene fusion between *ZFTA* as 3′ partner and frequently *RELA* as 5′ partner, encoding the p65 subunit of the NF-κB transcription factor complex, leading to pathological activation of NF-κB signaling. *ZFTA* and *RELA* both map on chromosome 11q13, and chromothripsis of chromosome 11 has been indicated as the causative event of the rearrangement, at least in a proportion of cases. Other 5′ partners (e.g., *MAML2/3, NCOA1/2, CTNNA2, MN1*) are also rarely encountered. ST-EPN-ZFTA accounts for 20–58% of supratentorial ependymomas in adults and for 66–84% in children (WHO 2021 subchapter ZFTA). They are typically hemispheric, mostly affecting the frontal and the parietal lobes with less frequent involvement of the occipital and temporal lobes [25, 61]. However, ST-EPN-ZFTA may rarely occur in the midline region and/or infratentorial compartment [11, 39]. The outcome of the ST-EPN-ZFTA is still debated: ST-EPN-ZFTA was originally described as a highly malignant tumor with a 10-year progressive-free survival of 19% [63], whereas later studies demonstrated good survival rates, unless *CDKN2A* homozygous deletion was present [38, 40, 46, 62, 88]. Frequent pathological key features include a clear cell morphology with a rich network of branching delicate capillaries, associated with nuclear expression of p65 (mostly restricted to the cases harboring the canonical *ZFTA::RELA* fusion) and cytoplasmic expression of L1CAM [25, 27, 85]. Notably, compared to PF and spinal ependymomas that are invariably OLIG2 negative, ST-EPN-ZFTA may show focal expression of OLIG2. Although p65 and L1CAM represent reliable markers of this entity (Fig. 4.6), the demonstration of *ZFTA* fusion is required for the diagnosis according to the current WHO classification of CNS tumors. Notably, cases bearing non-canonical *ZFTA* fusions form separate satellite clusters proximal to the main group of *ZFTA::RELA* supratentorial ependymomas on methylation analysis and may either show a typical ependymoma morphology or different histologies, including pleomorphic xanthoastrocytoma-like tumors, astroblastoma-like tumors, and even primitive-looking tumors with mesenchymal or embryonal differentiation [44, 85]. The latter subset of ZFTA-rearranged tumors with a non-ependymal phenotype currently lacks a proper nosological WHO definition [44].

Supratentorial ependymoma *YAP1* fusion-positive (ST-EPN-YAP1) are very rare lesions, which typically occur during infancy and present as large, well-demarcated, cystic hemispheric lesions often spatially related to the lateral ventricles [3, 64]. The differential diagnosis includes other infantile tumors, i.e., infant-type hemispheric glioma and desmoplastic infantile glioma/astrocytoma. Compared to ST-EPN-ZFTA, they seem to show a more indolent course [88]. Histologically, they are well-circumscribed, consist of monomorphic cells embedded in a fibrillary matrix, and often show PAS-positive eosinophilic granular bodies. Compared to ST-EPN-ZFTA, they do not express p65/RELA and L1CAM, and essential to the diagnosis is the demonstration of *YAP1* fusion most frequently

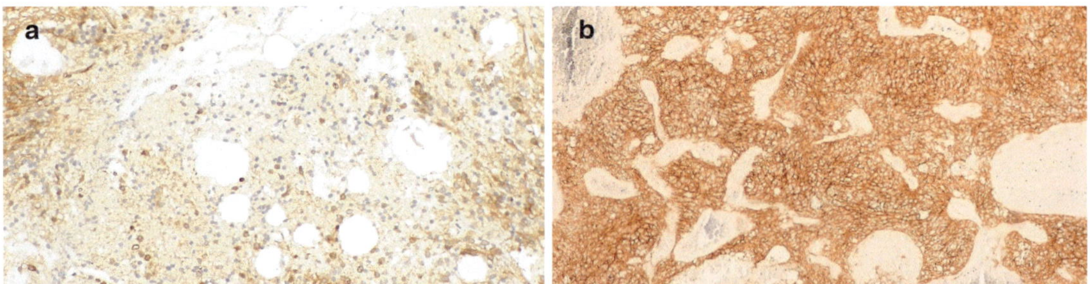

Fig. 4.6 Supratentorial ependymoma with p65 (**a**) and L1CAM (**b**) immunopositivity in a case of ST-EPD ZFTA subtype

rearranged with *MAMLD1* [3, 64]. The differential diagnosis of supratentorial ependymoma is wide and includes astroblastoma MN1-altered and recent or emerging entities. Among those, CNS tumors with BCOR internal tandem duplication (ITD) have to be considered. CNS tumors with BCOR ITD affect young children (median age 4 years), and, although clinical data are limited, most tumors relapse. BCOR ITD mainly features a circumscribed growth pattern, ependymoma-like perivascular pseudorosettes, delicate branching capillaries, microcystic pattern, focal-to-absent immunostaining for GFAP, and variable expression of OLIG2 and neural markers [5]. Tumors carrying BCOR(L1) fusions with EP300/CREBBP show a morphology similar to BCOR ITD tumors but seem to differ from a clinical standpoint, as they affect older patients (median age 30 years) and have a better prognosis than CNS tumors with BCOR ITD. Although non-specific, BCOR nuclear expression may help in the diagnosis of the BCOR ITD tumors but not in the BCOR(L1)-rearranged tumors. Furthermore, an ependymal phenotype is often shown by groups of tumors with a distinctive methylation signature that have recently emerged, i.e., PATZ1-rearranged tumors and PLAGL1-rearranged tumors [1, 80]. Notably, due to their marked clinicopathological heterogeneity, they have not been included as distinct entities in the 2021 WHO Classification of CNS tumors. They typically occur in the pediatric age (median age 11 and 6, respectively) [1, 80], and, although information on their biological behavior is limited, they seem to follow an intermediate course. PATZ1-rearranged tumors often present as a juxtaventricular lesion consisting of extensive low proliferative monotonous oligo-like areas and a rich network of variably hyalinized capillaries somewhat reminiscent of ST-EPN-ZFTA. Notably, they show a polyphenotypic profile with focal/patchy GFAP, OLIG2, and synaptophysin variably associated to CD34 expression and sparse desmin-positive cells [1, 73]. PLAGL1-rearranged tumors may show a moderate/high cellularity in a mostly fine neurofibrillary matrix with prominent microcystic changes and a diffuse expression of GFAP combined with a limited expression of OLIG2 [80].

Posterior fossa ependymomas Posterior fossa (PF) ependymomas arise within the fourth ventricle or in the cerebellopontine angle and include two main molecular groups according to WHO: PFA and PFB. PFA mainly develops in infants and young children, compared to PFB arising in teenagers and adults. Overall, PFAs tend to show a lateral localization, and gross total resection is hard to achieve with a consequent high recurrence rate and low survival, compared to PFB, which shows a more favorable prognosis. The implementation of H3K27me3 and EZHIP immunostains allows the identification of the PFA ependymomas: loss of H3K27me3 is the hallmark of this entity, which is usually underlined by EZHIP expression except for a few cases showing pathogenic mutations in the gene (Fig. 4.7) [52, 66]. PFB ependymomas maintain H3K27me3 and lack EZHIP expression, but this combination is not specific, and the diagnosis of PFB ependymomas requires the alignment with the corresponding methylation class. When dealing with a PFA ependymoma, it is also of paramount importance to assess the 1q and 6q status, as 1q gain and 6q loss are well-established negative prognostic markers [21]. Within the PFA group, 2 subgroups and 9 epigenetic subtypes have been further identified. Remarkably, one of them, i.e., PFA2c, shows a good outcome, pointing at DNA methylation profiling as an invaluable tool for accurate prognostic stratification of the patients affected by PFA ependymomas (Pajtler KW). As for PFB ependymomas, 13q loss has been indicated as predictor of PFS (but not OS) [65]

From a histological point of view, both PFA and PFB ependymomas are usually circumscribed tumors characterized by perivascular pseudorosettes which may be associated with true rosettes, expression of GFAP and dot-like EMA in absence of OLIG2 positivity. Notably, the PFA group typically shows areas of high cellular density and proliferation, which appear well-demarcated from the less cellular and low-

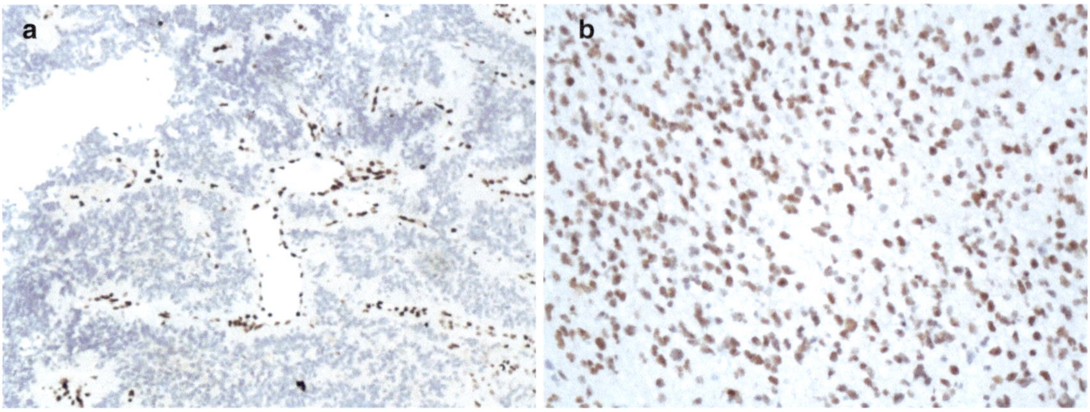

Fig. 4.7 PFA ependymoma (**a**, **b**). Ependymoma cells with loss of H3K27me3 (**a**) and EZHIP expression (**b**)

proliferative background lesion. It has been demonstrated that these areas are enriched of 1q gain and 6q loss, likely reflecting the clonal evolution of the tumor, and their presence in high proportion (>70%) correlates with poor survival [31].

While the clinico-pathological features and the immunophenotype of the PFA ependymomas are straightforward, PFB ependymomas should be distinguished from rare forms of ependymomas ZFTA fusion-positive arising in the PF and brainstem [11, 39] and from ependymomas aligning with the methylation class of subependymomas. Notably, the latter group of tumors, typically presenting during adulthood, seems to follow a more aggressive course of the PFB ependymomas, especially when showing a pure ependymoma morphology (versus mixed ependymoma/subependymoma or pure subependymoma morphology) and harboring chromosome 6 loss and *TERT* promoter mutation [87].

4.2 Embryonal Tumors

The evolution of the classification of embryonal tumors in the central nervous system (CNS) highlights the significant impact of advanced molecular profiling techniques on understanding these neoplasms. Historically, embryonal tumors were broadly categorized into medulloblastomas and supratentorial primitive neuroectodermal tumors (PNETs). This classification, however, became less precise as new molecular insights emerged [49, 81].

With the advent of DNA methylation and gene expression profiling, researchers discovered that some tumors previously classified as PNETs harbored genetic features associated with glial tumors rather than the primitive neuroectodermal lineage [81]. This led to the 2016 WHO classification of CNS tumors eliminating the term "PNET" due to its misleading nature in describing the molecular heterogeneity of these tumors. These profiling techniques have revealed distinct genetic and epigenetic signatures, which have contributed to more accurate tumor classification and a deeper understanding of tumor biology [50].

The integration of molecular characteristics into the classification of CNS embryonal tumors has indeed transformed our understanding and management of these complex neoplasms, offering a more refined framework that better captures the diversity of these tumors based on their molecular characteristics. The fifth edition of the WHO classification of CNS tumors (WHO CNS5) reflects these advancements by incorporating molecular profiles into the classification system. This updated classification includes both medulloblastomas and other CNS embryonal tumors.

The WHO CNS5 classification has significantly refined the categorization of medulloblastomas as well as atypical teratoid/rhabdoid tumor (AT/RT), integrating both molecular and histopathological features (Table 4.1). Among other embryonal tumors, two newly recognized entities were introduced: central nervous system neuroblastoma, activated by FOXR2, and central nervous system tumor with BCOR internal tandem duplication (ITD). Finally, embryonic multilayer rosette tumor (ETMR) presents a subdivision into the previously known C19MC and the newly discovered DICER1 altered.

This refined classification not only enhances our ability to predict patient outcomes and tailor treatments but also guides ongoing research into more effective and less harmful therapies. For example, by distinguishing between different molecular subgroups and their specific clinical implications, the CNS5 classification facilitates a more personalized approach to treating medulloblastoma, ultimately aiming to improve patient outcomes and advance the field of neuro-oncology. Clinical trials are increasingly focusing on targeting specific genetic alterations and molecular pathways identified through profiling, aiming to provide more effective and less toxic treatment options for patients, especially those with high-risk profiles [58].

Moreover, the complexity of these tumors, involving both histopathological and molecular features, underscores the necessity of a comprehensive diagnostic report. The recommended tiered reporting method provides a structured framework for integrating different types of data, with diagnosis integrated at the top and layers below that include histological, molecular and other essential details [49].

New emerging entities are being characterized and will be included in the next WHO classification.

4.2.1 Medulloblastoma

The WHO CNS5 classification has provided a more granular understanding of medulloblastomas by incorporating molecular profiling into the diagnostic framework [68, 76]. Medulloblastoma is now recognized into four main molecular and morphologic subtypes, recognizing shared features that are clinically relevant [23, 30, 43, 68, 70, 76, 78, 93, 96].

The principal molecular groups are:

WNT-Activated (Wingless): Characterized by alterations in the WNT signaling pathway, this group has a generally favorable prognosis and is typically associated with specific histopathological features (classic histology, nuclear beta-catenin, Filamin A and YAP1 expression; GAB1 negative) and molecular markers (mutations in CTNNB1, DDX3X, SMARCA4, and TP53; and monosomy of chromosome 6 shown in Fig. 4.8a). They mostly occur in childhood and in central locations, often near the brainstem.

SHH-Activated (Sonic Hedgehog): Tumors in this group are driven by the SHH signaling pathway. This category is further subdivided based on *TP53* status in *TP53*-mutant and *TP53*-wildtype. TP53-mutant SHH medulloblastomas are associated with worse clinical outcomes than their wild-type counterparts, and they also display characteristic immunohistochemical markers and chromosomal alterations, including MYCN amplification, GLI2 amplification, and 17p loss (Fig. 4.8b).

Non-WNT/Non-SHH: This includes Group 3 and Group 4 medulloblastomas, which do not fall into the WNT or SHH categories. These tumors have been further classified into eight subgroups based on DNA methylation profiling. Both groups have common locations (midline, filling the fourth ventricle), histology, and are characterized by peculiar rearrangements, including MYC amplification (Fig. 4.8c) and isocentric chromosome 17q (Fig. 4.8d). The two groups, however, present different immunohistochemical markers.

These groups are further stratified into subgroups: SHH-activated medulloblastomas are subdivided into four subgroups differing in their clinical behavior, prognostic outcomes, and response to treatment.

Non-WNT/non-SHH medulloblastomas are divided into eight subgroups, which include Group 3 and Group 4 medulloblastomas. These subgroups reveal additional molecular heterogeneity and have different implications for prognosis and treatment strategies. The CNS5 classification does not include these 12 molecular subgroups, focusing instead on integrating histological features.

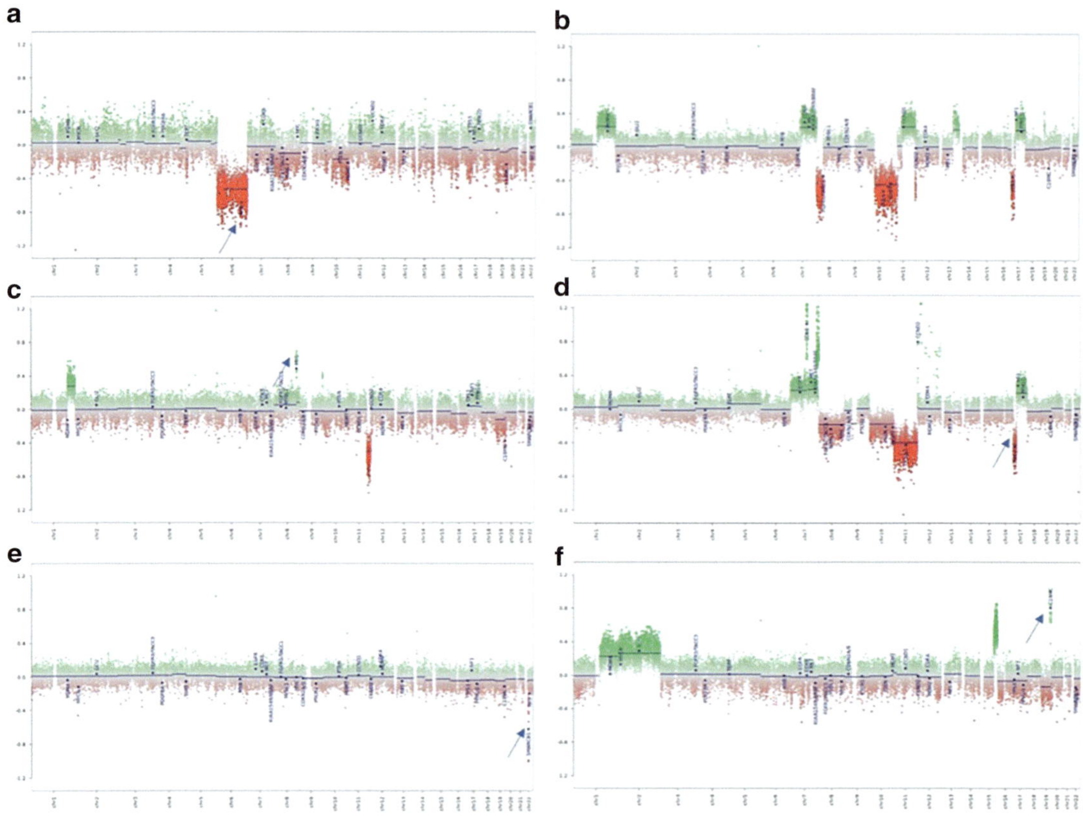

Fig. 4.8 Examples of copy number profiles of medulloblastoma WNT with chromosome 6 loss (**a**), medulloblastoma SHH with TP53 mutation (**b**), medulloblastoma G3 with MYC amplification (**c**), medulloblastoma G4 with isodicentric 17q (**d**), AT/RT with SMARCB1 deletion (**e**) and ETMR with C19MC amplification (**f**). Relevant copy number alterations are signaled by blue arrows

DNA methylation profiling is the gold standard for accurately identifying the specific group or subgroup of medulloblastoma [67, 68]. However, immunohistochemistry remains a valuable tool for distinguishing between different types of medulloblastomas, such as those driven by WNT, SHH, and the non-WNT/non-SHH categories [20]. For WNT-activated medulloblastomas, the presence of beta-catenin in the nucleus is a key marker, though its expression can sometimes be weak or inconsistent. SHH-activated medulloblastomas, on the other hand, are characterized by the presence of GAB1 and YAP1 proteins in the cytoplasm. Both WNT and SHH medulloblastomas also show cytoplasmic staining for Filamin A. In contrast, non-WNT/non-SHH tumors typically exhibit beta-catenin in the cytoplasm but lack GAB1 and YAP1.

Histologically, four types of medulloblastoma are now consolidated: classic, desmoplastic/nodular, medulloblastoma with extensive nodularity, and large cell/anaplastic with a recognized correlation between histological patterns and molecular subgroups. For instance, desmoplastic/nodular medulloblastomas and those with extensive nodularity are typically associated with the SHH molecular group, often falling into SHH-1 or SHH-2 subgroups. WNT tumors generally present with classic morphology, while large cell/anaplastic tumors are usually part of the SHH-3 subgroup or the non-WNT/non-SHH (Group 3/4) subgroups [23, 86].

4.2.2 Atypical Teratoid/Rhabdoid Tumor (AT/RT)

AT/RT, or atypical teratoid/rhabdoid tumor, is defined by the WHO CNS5 as a highly aggressive malignancy characterized by poorly differentiated cells that often exhibit rhabdoid features, either focal or widespread. These tumors are marked by polyphenotypic differentiation and are genetically defined by the biallelic inactivation of the SMARCB1 gene, also known as hSNF5, INI1, or BAF47 [22] (Fig. 4.8e). In rare cases—less than 5%—the tumor may involve the inactivation of the SMARCA4 gene, also referred to as BRG1 [34, 75].

CNS5 recognizes three distinct molecular subgroups of AT/RT: SHH (driven by SHH and Notch signaling), TYR (characterized by tyrosinase upregulation), and MYC (with MYC oncogene expression) [37]. This classification provides a deeper understanding of the tumor's biological behavior and potential responses to treatment, thus impacting prognostic assessments and therapeutic decisions [30].

4.2.3 Cribriform Neuroepithelial Tumor

Cribriform neuroepithelial tumor is a provisional entity in WHO CNS5, which is described as "a nonrhabdoid neuroectodermal tumor characterized by cribriform strands and ribbons and showing loss of nuclear SMARCB1 expression". This exceptionally rare cancer occurs mostly in infants in periventricular areas. Histologically, they show strong positivity for EMA and loss of SMARCB1 expression. Their DNA methylation profile is undistinguishable from the AT/RT molecular subtype AT/RT-TYR.

4.2.4 Embryonal Tumor with Multilayered Rosettes (ETMR)

ETMR was present in previous classifications but named after its hallmark alteration of the microRNA cluster on chromosome 19 (C19MC) [42]. In CNS5, this tumor has received an updated nomenclature due to the identification of new genetic alterations. In fact, the discovery that ~10% of ETMR lack the previously recognized C19MC alterations but present biallelic DICER1 alteration [45] refines the classification of this tumor and improves diagnostic accuracy. This tumor is mostly found in the cerebral hemispheres but can also develop in the infratentorial compartment and grows in a peculiar pattern of mitotically active multilayered rosettes, composed of a pseudostratified epithelium of embryonal cells organized around a lumen [28]. Another useful diagnostic marker is the strong and diffuse cytoplasmic immunoreactivity for LIN28A.

4.2.5 CNS Neuroblastoma (FOXR2-Activated)

CNS neuroblastoma with FOXR2 activation has been identified as a distinct entity thanks to DNA methylation profiling. This subtype is characterized by chromosomal rearrangements leading to an increased expression of the forkhead box R2 (FOXR2) gene, which is critical for diagnosis and may influence therapeutic strategies. CNS NB-FOXR2 tumors tend to present in slightly older children, in supratentorial locations, and respond well to treatment with a reported 5-year OS of 85% [90]. Histologically, these neoplasms are composed of densely packed embryonal cells with hyperchromatic nuclei and inconspicuous cytoplasm, arranged in a sheet-like pattern, with frequent mitotic figures, apoptotic bodies, and areas of necrosis. Most cases are strongly immunopositive for OLIG2 but negative for GFAP and vimentin [81].

4.2.6 CNS Tumor with BCOR Internal Tandem Duplication (ITD)

Despite their rarity and limited clinical characterization, CNS tumors with BCOR ITD are associated with a unique set of clinical and molecular features, warranting separate classification for accurate diagnosis and management. While they display a peculiar histological/immunohistochemical pattern, the only specific diagnostic marker is the heterozygous ITD in exon 15 of the BCOR gene, which is also associated with a specific DNA methylation profile [81].

4.3 Conclusions

Classification of CNS tumors during the last 10 years has improved thanks to molecular pathology that has enhanced our understanding of CNS tumors, providing new elements to integrate diagnosis. This approach allows us to define new tumoral entities and define alterations that correlate with clinical behavior and response to therapy.

This approach, together with having a pediatric neuro-oncology multidisciplinary tumor board, improves the management of patients, particularly of the pediatric age, which is based on a personalized approach and the interaction of many specialists.

References

1. Alhalabi OT, et al. A novel patient stratification strategy to enhance the therapeutic efficacy of dasatinib in glioblastoma. Neuro-Oncology. 2022;24(1):39–51.
2. Ampie L, Choy W, Lamano JB, Kesavabhotla K, Mao Q, Parsa AT, et al. Prognostic factors for recurrence and complications in the surgical management of primary chordoid gliomas: a systematic review of literature. Clin Neurol Neurosurg. 2015;138:129–36. https://doi.org/10.1016/j.clineuro.2015.08.011.
3. Andreiuolo F, Lisner T, Zlocha J, et al. H3F3A-G34R mutant high grade neuroepithelial neoplasms with glial and dysplastic ganglion cell components. Acta Neuropathol Commun. 2019;7(1):78. https://doi.org/10.1186/S40478-019-0731-5.
4. Andrey K, Jakobiec FA, Eberhart CG, et al. Comparative integrated molecular analysis of intraocular medulloepitheliomas and central nervous system embryonal tumors with multilayered rosettes confirms that they are distinct nosologic entities. Neuropathology. 2015;35(6):538–44. https://doi.org/10.1111/NEUP.12227.
5. Appay R, Macagno N, Padovani L, Korshunov A, Kool M, André N, Scavarda D, Pietsch T, Figarella-Branger D. HGNET-BCOR Tumors of the cerebellum: clinicopathologic and molecular characterization of 3 cases. Am J Surg Pathol. 2017;41(9):1254–60. https://doi.org/10.1097/PAS.0000000000000866.
6. Auffret L, Ajlil Y, Tauziède-Espariat A, Kergrohen T, Puiseux C, Riffaud L, Blouin P, Bertozzi AI, Leblond P, Blomgren K, Froelich S, Picca A, Touat M, Sanson M, Beccaria K, Blauwblomme T, Dangouloff-Ros V, Boddaert N, Varlet P, Debily MA, Grill J, Castel D. A new subtype of diffuse midline glioma, H3 K27 and BRAF/FGFR1 co-altered: a clinico-radiological and histomolecular characterisation. Acta Neuropathol. 2023;147(1):2. https://doi.org/10.1007/s00401-023-02651-4. PMID: 38066305; PMCID: PMC10709479.
7. Bale TA. FGFR- gene family alterations in low-grade neuroepithelial tumors. Acta Neuropathol Commun. 2020;8:21. https://doi.org/10.1186/s40478-020-00898-6.
8. Banan R, Stichel D, Bleck A, et al. Infratentorial IDH-mutant astrocytoma is a distinct subtype. Acta Neuropathol. 2020;140(4):569–81. https://doi.org/10.1007/S00401-020-02194-Y.
9. Buczkowicz P, Bartels U, Bouffet E, Becher O, Hawkins C. Histopathological spectrum of pediatric diffuse intrinsic pontine glioma: diagnostic and therapeutic implications. Acta Neuropathol. 2014a;128(4):573. https://doi.org/10.1007/S00401-014-1319-6.
10. Buczkowicz P, Hoeman C, Rakopoulos P, et al. Genomic analysis of diffuse intrinsic pontine gliomas identifies three molecular subgroups and recurrent activating ACVR1 mutations. Nat Genet. 2014b;46(5):451–6. https://doi.org/10.1038/NG.2936.
11. Cardoni A, Barresi S, Piccirilli E, Alesi V, Miele E, Giovannoni I, Genovese S, Del Baldo G, Diomedi-Camassei F, Antonelli M, Giangaspero F, Puggioni C, Carai A, Colafati GS, Mastronuzzi A, Gessi M, Alaggio R, Rossi S. A non-hemispheric transtentorial ZFTA fusion-positive ependymoma in a 6-month-old boy. Neuropathol Appl Neurobiol. 2023;49(1):e12886. https://doi.org/10.1111/nan.12886. PMID: 36709981
12. Castel D, Kergrohen T, Tauziède-Espariat A, et al. Histone H3 wild-type DIPG/DMG overexpressing EZHIP extend the spectrum diffuse midline gliomas with PRC2 inhibition beyond H3-K27M mutation. Acta Neuropathol. 2020;139(6):1109–13. https://doi.org/10.1007/S00401-020-02142-W.
13. Ceglie G, Vinci M, Carai A, et al. Infantile/congenital high-grade gliomas: molecular features and therapeutic perspectives. Diagnostics (Basel, Switzerland). 2020;10(9) https://doi.org/10.3390/DIAGNOSTICS10090648.
14. Chen CCL, Deshmukh S, Jessa S, et al. Histone H3.3G34-mutant interneuron progenitors co-opt PDGFRA for Gliomagenesis. Cell. 2020;183(6):1617–1633.e22. https://doi.org/10.1016/J.CELL.2020.11.012.
15. Cheng Z, Cheung P, Kuo AJ, et al. A molecular threading mechanism underlies Jumonji lysine demethylase KDM2A regulation of methylated H3K36. Genes

Dev. 2014;28(16):1758–71. https://doi.org/10.1101/GAD.246561.114.
16. Clarke M, Mackay A, Ismer B, et al. Infant high-grade gliomas comprise multiple subgroups characterized by novel targetable gene fusions and favorable outcomes. Cancer Discov. 2020;10(7):942–63. https://doi.org/10.1158/2159-8290.CD-19-1030.
17. Crotty E, Gust J. Pediatric ependymoma: new perspectives on older trials. Neuro-Oncology. 2022;24(6):949–50. https://doi.org/10.1093/neuonc/noac060. PMID: 35325202; PMCID: PMC9159413
18. Deng MY, Sill M, Sturm D, Stichel D, Witt H, Ecker J, Wittmann A, Schittenhelm J, Ebinger M, Schuhmann MU, Figarella-Branger D, Aronica E, Staszewski O, Preusser M, Haberler C, Lauten M, Schüller U, Hartmann C, Snuderl M, Dunham C, Jabado N, Wesseling P, Deckert M, Keyvani K, Gottardo N, Giangaspero F, von Hoff K, Ellison DW, Pietsch T, Herold-Mende C, Milde T, Witt O, Kool M, Korshunov A, Wick W, von Deimling A, Pfister SM, Jones DTW, Sahm F. Diffuse glioneuronal tumor with oligodendroglioma-like features and nuclear clusters (DGONC) - a molecularly defined glioneuronal CNS tumor class displaying recurrent monosomy 14. Neuropathol Appl Neurobiol. 2020;46(5):422–30. https://doi.org/10.1111/nan.12590. Epub 2020 Feb 5.
19. Deng MY, Sturm D, Pfaff E, et al. Radiation-induced gliomas represent H3-/IDH-wild type pediatric gliomas with recurrent PDGFRA amplification and loss of CDKN2A/B. Nat Commun. 2021;12(1) https://doi.org/10.1038/S41467-021-25708-Y.
20. DeSisto J, Lucas JT, Xu K, et al. Comprehensive molecular characterization of pediatric radiation-induced high-grade glioma. Nat Commun. 2021;12(1) https://doi.org/10.1038/S41467-021-25709-X.
21. Donson AM, Bertrand KC, Riemondy KA, Gao D, Zhuang Y, Sanford B, Norris GA, Chapman RJ, Fu R, Willard N, Griesinger AM, Ribeiro de Sousa G, Amani V, Grimaldo E, Hankinson TC, Booker F, Sill M, Grundy RG, Pajtler KW, Ellison DW, Foreman NK, Ritzmann TA. Significant increase of high-risk chromosome 1q gain and 6q loss at recurrence in posterior fossa group A ependymoma: a multicenter study. Neuro-Oncology. 2023;25(10):1854–67. https://doi.org/10.1093/neuonc/noad096. PMID: 37246777; PMCID: PMC10547517
22. Eaton KW, Tooke LS, Wainwright LM, Judkins AR, Biegel JA. Spectrum of SMARCB1/INI1 mutations in familial and sporadic rhabdoid tumors. Pediatr Blood Cancer. 2011;56(1):7–15. https://doi.org/10.1002/pbc.22831.
23. Ellison DW, et al. Medulloblastoma: clinicopathological correlates of SHH, WNT, and non-SHH/WNT molecular subgroups. Acta Neuropathol. 2011;121(3):381–96. https://doi.org/10.1007/s00401-011-0800-8.
24. Ferguson SD, Zhou S, Huse JT, et al. Targetable gene fusions associate with the IDH wild-type astrocytic lineage in adult gliomas. J Neuropathol Exp Neurol. 2018;77(6):437–42. https://doi.org/10.1093/JNEN/NLY022.
25. Figarella-Branger D, Lechapt-Zalcman E, Tabouret E, Jünger S, de Paula AM, Bouvier C, Colin C, Jouvet A, Forest F, Andreiuolo F, Quintin-Roue I, Machet MC, Heitzmann A, Milin S, Sevestre H, Godfraind C, Labrousse F, Metellus P, Scavarda D, Pietsch T. Supratentorial clear cell ependymomas with branching capillaries demonstrate characteristic clinicopathological features and pathological activation of nuclear factor-kappaB signaling. Neuro-Oncology. 2016;18(7):919–27. https://doi.org/10.1093/neuonc/now025. Epub 2016 Mar 15. PMID: 26984744; PMCID: PMC4896549
26. Franz DN, Belousova E, Sparagana S, Bebin EM, Frost MD, Kuperman R, et al. Long-term use of Everolimus in patients with tuberous sclerosis complex: final results from the EXIST-1 study. PLoS One. 2016;11:e0158476. https://doi.org/10.1371/journal.pone.0158476.
27. Gessi M, Giagnacovo M, Modena P, Elefante G, Gianno F, Buttarelli FR, Arcella A, Donofrio V, Diomedi Camassei F, Nozza P, Morra I, Massimino M, Pollo B, Giangaspero F, Antonelli M. Role of immunohistochemistry in the identification of supratentorial C11ORF95-RELA fused ependymoma in routine neuropathology. Am J Surg Pathol. 2019;43(1):56–63. https://doi.org/10.1097/PAS.0000000000000979.
28. Gessi M, et al. Embryonal tumors with abundant neuropil and true rosettes: a distinctive CNS primitive neuroectodermal tumor. Am J Surg Pathol. 2009;33(2):211–7. https://doi.org/10.1097/PAS.0b013e318186235b.
29. Gianno F, Miele E, Antonelli M, Giangaspero F. Embryonal tumors in the WHO CNS5 classification: a review. Indian J Pathol Microbiol. 2022;65(Supplement):S73–82. https://doi.org/10.4103/ijpm.ijpm_1049_21.
30. Gibson P, et al. Subtypes of medulloblastoma have distinct developmental origins. Nature. 2010;468(7327):1095–9. https://doi.org/10.1038/nature09587.
31. Gödicke S, Kresbach C, Ehlert M, Obrecht D, Altendorf L, Hack K, von Hoff K, Carén H, Melcher V, Kerl K, Englinger B, Filbin M, Pajtler KW, Gojo J, Pietsch T, Rutkowski S, Schüller U. Clinically relevant molecular hallmarks of PFA ependymomas display intratumoral heterogeneity and correlate with tumor morphology. Acta Neuropathol. 2024;147(1):23. https://doi.org/10.1007/s00401-023-02682-x. PMID: 38265527; PMCID: PMC10808473
32. Guerin JB, Kaufmann TJ, Eckel LJ, Morris JM, Vaubel RA, Giannini C, Johnson DR. A radiologist's guide to the 2021 WHO central nervous system tumor classification: part 2-newly described and revised tumor types. Radiology. 2023;307(5):e221885. https://doi.org/10.1148/radiol.221885. Epub 2023 May 16. PMID: 37191486.
33. Guerreiro Stucklin AS, Ryall S, Fukuoka K, et al. Alterations in ALK/ROS1/NTRK/MET drive

a group of infantile hemispheric gliomas. Nat Commun. 2019;10(1) https://doi.org/10.1038/S41467-019-12187-5.
34. Hasselblatt M, et al. SMARCA4-mutated atypical teratoid/rhabdoid tumors are associated with inherited germline alterations and poor prognosis. Acta Neuropathol. 2014;128(3):453–6. https://doi.org/10.1007/s00401-014-1323-x.
35. Hong L, Shi ZF, Li KKW, et al. Molecular landscape of pediatric type IDH wildtype, H3 wildtype hemispheric glioblastomas. Lab Investig. 2022;102(7) https://doi.org/10.1038/S41374-022-00769-9.
36. Huse JT, Snuderl M, Jones DTW, Brathwaite CD, Altman N, Lavi E, et al. Polymorphous low-grade neuroepithelial tumor of the young (PLNTY): an epileptogenic neoplasm with oligodendroglioma-like components, aberrant CD34 expression, and genetic alterations involving the MAP kinase pathway. Acta Neuropathol. 2017;133:417–29. https://doi.org/10.1007/s00401-016-1639-9.
37. Johann PD, et al. Atypical teratoid/rhabdoid tumors are comprised of three epigenetic subgroups with distinct enhancer landscapes. Cancer Cell. 2016;29(3):379–93. https://doi.org/10.1016/j.ccell.2016.02.001.
38. Jünger ST, Andreiuolo F, Mynarek M, et al. Ependymomas in infancy: underlying genetic alterations, histological features, and clinical outcome. Childs Nerv Syst. 2020;36(11):2693–700. https://doi.org/10.1007/S00381-020-04655-X.
39. Keenan C, Graham RT, Harreld JH, Lucas JT Jr, Finkelstein D, Wheeler D, Li X, Dalton J, Upadhyaya SA, Raimondi SC, Boop FA, DeCuypere M, Zhang J, Vinitsky A, Wang L, Chiang J. Infratentorial C11orf95-fused gliomas share histologic, immunophenotypic, and molecular characteristics of supratentorial RELA-fused ependymoma. Acta Neuropathol. 2020;140(6):963–5. https://doi.org/10.1007/s00401--020-02238-3. Epub 2020 Oct 24. PMID: 33099686; PMCID: PMC8611811
40. Khatua S, Ramaswamy V, Bouffet E. Current therapy and the evolving molecular landscape of paediatric ependymoma. Eur J Cancer. 2017;70:34–41. https://doi.org/10.1016/j.ejca.2016.10.013. Epub 2016 Nov 18
41. Korshunov A, Ryzhova M, Hovestadt V, et al. Integrated analysis of pediatric glioblastoma reveals a subset of biologically favorable tumors with associated molecular prognostic markers. Acta Neuropathol. 2015;129(5):669–78. https://doi.org/10.1007/S00401-015-1405.
42. Korshunov A, et al. Focal genomic amplification at 19q13.42 comprises a powerful diagnostic marker for embryonal tumors with ependymoblastic rosettes. Acta Neuropathol. 2010;120(2):253–60. https://doi.org/10.1007/s00401-010-0688-8.
43. Korshunov A, et al. Molecular progression of SHH-activated medulloblastomas. Acta Neuropathol. 2019;138(2):327–30. https://doi.org/10.1007/s00401-019-02022-y.
44. Kresbach C, Neyazi S, Schüller U. Updates in the classification of ependymal neoplasms: the 2021 WHO classification and beyond. Brain Pathol. 2022;32(4):e13068. https://doi.org/10.1111/bpa.13068. Epub 2022 Mar 21. PMID: 35307892; PMCID: PMC9245931
45. Lambo S, et al. The molecular landscape of ETMR at diagnosis and relapse. Nature. 2019;576(7786):274–80. https://doi.org/10.1038/s41586-019-1815-x.
46. Lillard JC, Venable GT, Khan NR, Tatevossian RG, Dalton J, Vaughn BN, Klimo P. Pediatric supratentorial ependymoma: surgical, clinical, and molecular analysis. Neurosurgery. 2019;85(1):41–9. https://doi.org/10.1093/neuros/nyy239.
47. Lin Y, Luo YK, Li J, Ren XY, Wang HW. [Diagnostic Value of American Thyroid Association Guidelines, American College of Radiology Thyroid Imaging Reporting and Data System, and Chinese thyroid imaging reporting and data system alone and combined with BRAFV600E mutation in atypia of undetermined significance/follicular lesion of undetermined significance]. Zhongguo Yi Xue Ke Xue Yuan Xue Bao. 2023;45(6):921–8. Chinese. https://doi.org/10.3881/j.issn.1000-503X.15754.
48. López GY, Van Ziffle J, Onodera C, et al. The genetic landscape of gliomas arising after therapeutic radiation. Acta Neuropathol. 2019;137(1):139–50. https://doi.org/10.1007/S00401-018-1906-Z.
49. Louis DN, et al. International Society of Neuropathology-Haarlem Consensus Guidelines for nervous system tumor classification and grading. Brain Pathol. 2014;24(5):429–35. https://doi.org/10.1111/bpa.12171.
50. Louis DN, et al. The 2016 World Health Organization classification of tumors of the central nervous system: a summary. Acta Neuropathol. 2016;131(6):803–20. https://doi.org/10.1007/s00401-016-1545-1.
51. Lucas CG, Villanueva-Meyer JE, Whipple N, Oberheim Bush NA, Cooney T, Chang S, McDermott M, Berger M, Cham E, Sun PP, Putnam A, Zhou H, Bollo R, Cheshier S, Poppe MM, Fung KM, Sung S, Glenn C, Fan X, Bannykh S, Hu J, Danielpour M, Li R, Alva E, Johnston J, Van Ziffle J, Onodera C, Devine P, Grenert JP, Lee JC, Pekmezci M, Tihan T, Bollen AW, Perry A, Solomon DA. Myxoid glioneuronal tumor, PDGFRA p.K385-mutant: clinical, radiologic, and histopathologic features. Brain Pathol. 2020;30(3):479–94. https://doi.org/10.1111/bpa.12797. Epub 2019 Nov 6. PMID: 31609499; PMCID: PMC7780370.
52. Mariet C, Castel D, Grill J, Saffroy R, Dangouloff-Ros V, Boddaert N, Llamas-Guttierrez F, Chappé C, Puget S, Hasty L, Chrétien F, Métais A, Varlet P, Tauzière-Espariat A. Posterior fossa ependymoma H3 K27-mutant: an integrated radiological and histomolecular tumor analysis. Acta Neuropathol Commun. 2022;10(1):137. https://doi.org/10.1186/s40478-022-01442-4. PMID: 36104744; PMCID: PMC9476256

53. McGuire CS, Sainani KL, Fisher PG. Both location and age predict survival in ependymoma: a SEER study. Pediatr Blood Cancer. 2009;52(1):65–9. https://doi.org/10.1002/pbc.21806.
54. Merchant TE, Bendel AE, Sabin ND, Burger PC, Shaw DW, Chang E, Wu S, Zhou T, Eisenstat DD, Foreman NK, Fuller CE, Anderson ET, Hukin J, Lau CC, Pollack IF, Laningham FH, Lustig RH, Armstrong FD, Handler MH, Williams-Hughes C, Kessel S, Kocak M, Ellison DW, Ramaswamy V. Conformal radiation therapy for pediatric ependymoma, chemotherapy for incompletely resected ependymoma, and observation for completely resected, supratentorial ependymoma. J Clin Oncol. 2019;37(12):974–83. https://doi.org/10.1200/JCO.18.01765. Epub 2019 Feb 27. PMID: 30811284; PMCID: PMC7186586
55. Meredith DM, Cooley LD, Dubuc A, Morrissette J, Sussman RT, Nasrallah MP, Rathbun P, Yap KL, Wadhwani N, Bao L, Wolff DJ, Ida C, Sukhanova M, Horbinski C, Jennings LJ, Farooqi M, Gener M, Ginn K, Kam KL, Sasaki K, Kanagal-Shamanna R, Alexandrescu S, Brat D, Lu X. ROS1 alterations as a potential driver of gliomas in infant, pediatric, and adult patients. Mod Pathol. 2023;36(11):100294. https://doi.org/10.1016/j.modpat.2023.100294. Epub 2023 Jul 31
56. Mhatre R, Sugur HS, Nandeesh BN, Chickabasaviah Y, Saini J, Santosh V. MN1 rearrangement in astroblastoma: study of eight cases and review of literature. Brain Tumor Pathol. 2019;36:112–20. https://doi.org/10.1007/s10014-019-00346-x.
57. Miele E, Barresi S, Colafati GS, Pedace L, Cardoni A, Nardini C, Tancredi C, Patrizi S, Del Baldo G, Megaro G, Muccio CF, Sievers P, Alaggio R, Mastronuzzi A, Rossi S, Locatelli F. A case of glioneuronal tumor with ATRX alteration, kinase fusion and anaplastic features showing rapid ependymal and leptomeningeal dissemination. Neuropathol Appl Neurobiol. 2024;50(4):e13001. https://doi.org/10.1111/nan.13001.
58. Mynarek M, et al. Nonmetastatic medulloblastoma of early childhood: results from the prospective clinical trial HIT-2000 and an extended validation cohort. J Clin Oncol. 2020;38(18):2028–40. https://doi.org/10.1200/JCO.19.03057.
59. Nagaishi M, Nobusawa S, Matsumura N, Kono F, Ishiuchi S, Abe T, Ebato M, Wang Y, Hyodo A, Yokoo H, Nakazato Y. SLC44A1-PRKCA fusion in papillary and rosette-forming glioneuronal tumors. J Clin Neurosci. 2016;23:73–5. https://doi.org/10.1016/j.jocn.2015.04.021. Epub 2015 Aug 7. PMID: 26260115.
60. Ostrom QT, Patil N, Cioffi G, Waite K, Kruchko C, Barnholtz-Sloan JS. CBTRUS statistical report: primary brain and other central nervous system tumors diagnosed in the United States in 2013–2017. Neuro Oncol. 2020;22(12 Suppl 2):iv1–iv96. https://doi.org/10.1093/neuonc/noaa200. Erratum in: Neuro Oncol. 2022 Jul 1;24(7):1214. https://doi.org/10.1093/neuonc/noaa269. PMID: 33123732; PMCID: PMC7596247
61. Pagès M, Pajtler KW, Puget S, Castel D, Boddaert N, Tauzière-Espariat A, Picot S, Debily MA, Kool M, Capper D, Sainte-Rose C, Chrétien F, Pfister SM, Pietsch T, Grill J, Varlet P, Andreiuolo F. Diagnostics of pediatric supratentorial RELA ependymomas: integration of information from histopathology, genetics, DNA methylation and imaging. Brain Pathol. 2019;29(3):325–35. https://doi.org/10.1111/bpa.12664. Epub 2018 Nov 28. PMID: 30325077; PMCID: PMC7379587
62. Pajtler KW, Mack SC, Ramaswamy V, Smith CA, Witt H, Smith A, Hansford JR, von Hoff K, Wright KD, Hwang E, Frappaz D, Kanemura Y, Massimino M, Faure-Conter C, Modena P, Tabori U, Warren KE, Holland EC, Ichimura K, Giangaspero F, Castel D, von Deimling A, Kool M, Dirks PB, Grundy RG, Foreman NK, Gajjar A, Korshunov A, Finlay J, Gilbertson RJ, Ellison DW, Aldape KD, Merchant TE, Bouffet E, Pfister SM, Taylor MD. The current consensus on the clinical management of intracranial ependymoma and its distinct molecular variants. Acta Neuropathol. 2017;133(1):5–12. https://doi.org/10.1007/s00401--016-1643-0. Epub 2016 Nov 17. PMID: 27858204; PMCID: PMC5209402
63. Pajtler KW, Pfister SM, Kool M. Molecular dissection of ependymomas. Oncoscience. 2015;2(10):827–8. https://doi.org/10.18632/oncoscience.202. PMID: 26682265; PMCID: PMC4671940
64. Pajtler KW, Wei Y, Okonechnikov K, Silva PBG, Vouri M, Zhang L, Brabetz S, Sieber L, Gulley M, Mauermann M, Wedig T, Mack N, Imamura Kawasawa Y, Sharma T, Zuckermann M, Andreiuolo F, Holland E, Maass K, Körkel-Qu H, Liu HK, Sahm F, Capper D, Bunt J, Richards LJ, Jones DTW, Korshunov A, Chavez L, Lichter P, Hoshino M, Pfister SM, Kool M, Li W, Kawauchi D. YAP1 subgroup supratentorial ependymoma requires TEAD and nuclear factor I-mediated transcriptional programmes for tumorigenesis. Nat Commun. 2019;10(1):3914. https://doi.org/10.1038/s41467-019-11884-5. PMID: 31477715; PMCID: PMC6718408
65. Pajtler KW, Wen J, Sill M, Lin T, Orisme W, Tang B, Hübner JM, Ramaswamy V, Jia S, Dalton JD, Haupfear K, Rogers HA, Punchihewa C, Lee R, Easton J, Wu G, Ritzmann TA, Chapman R, Chavez L, Boop FA, Klimo P, Sabin ND, Ogg R, Mack SC, Freibaum BD, Kim HJ, Witt H, Jones DTW, Vo B, Gajjar A, Pounds S, Onar-Thomas A, Roussel MF, Zhang J, Taylor JP, Merchant TE, Grundy R, Tatevossian RG, Taylor MD, Pfister SM, Korshunov A, Kool M, Ellison DW. Molecular heterogeneity and CXorf67 alterations in posterior fossa group A (PFA) ependymomas. Acta Neuropathol. 2018;136(2):211–26. https://doi.org/10.1007/s00401-018-1877-0. Epub 2018 Jun 16. PMID: 29909548; PMCID: PMC6105278
66. Panwalkar P, Clark J, Ramaswamy V, Hawes D, Yang F, Dunham C, Yip S, Hukin J, Sun Y, Schipper MJ, Chavez L, Margol A, Pekmezci M, Chung C,

Banda A, Bayliss JM, Curry SJ, Santi M, Rodriguez FJ, Snuderl M, Karajannis MA, Saratsis AM, Horbinski CM, Carret AS, Wilson B, Johnston D, Lafay-Cousin L, Zelcer S, Eisenstat D, Silva M, Scheinemann K, Jabado N, PD MN, Kool M, Pfister SM, Taylor MD, Hawkins C, Korshunov A, Judkins AR, Venneti S. Immunohistochemical analysis of H3K27me3 demonstrates global reduction in group-A childhood posterior fossa ependymoma and is a powerful predictor of outcome. Acta Neuropathol. 2017;134(5):705–14.https://doi.org/10.1007/s00401--017-1752-4. Epub 2017 Jul 21. PMID: 28733933; PMCID: PMC5647236
67. Phillips CL, Miles L, Jones BV, Sutton M, Crone K, Fouladi M. Medulloblastoma with melanotic differentiation: case report and review of the literature. J Neuro-Oncol. 2011;103(3):759–64. https://doi.org/10.1007/s11060-010-0436-x.
68. Pietsch T, Haberler C. Update on the integrated histopathological and genetic classification of medulloblastoma - a practical diagnostic guideline. Clin Neuropathol. 2016;35(6):344–52. https://doi.org/10.5414/NP300999.
69. Pomper MG, Passe TJ, Burger PC, Scheithauer BW, Brat DJ. Chordoid glioma: a neoplasm unique to the hypothalamus and anterior third ventricle. AJNR Am J Neuroradiol. 2001;22(3):464–9. PMID: 11237967; PMCID: PMC7976835.
70. Ramaswamy V, et al. Recurrence patterns across medulloblastoma subgroups: an integrated clinical and molecular analysis. Lancet Oncol. 2013;14(12):1200–7. https://doi.org/10.1016/S1470-2045(13)70449-2.
71. Reinhardt A, Stichel D, Schrimpf D, Sahm F, Korshunov A, Reuss DE, et al. Anaplastic astrocytoma with piloid features, a novel molecular class of IDH wildtype glioma with recurrent MAPK pathway, CDKN2A/B and ATRX alterations. Acta Neuropathol. 2018;136:273–91. https://doi.org/10.1007/s00401-018-1837-8.
72. Ritzmann TA, Chapman RJ, Kilday JP, Thorp N, Modena P, Dineen RA, Macarthur D, Mallucci C, Jaspan T, Pajtler KW, Giagnacovo M, Jacques TS, Paine SML, Ellison DW, Bouffet E, Grundy RG. SIOP ependymoma I: final results, long-term follow-up, and molecular analysis of the trial cohort-A BIOMECA consortium study. Neuro-Oncology. 2022;24(6):936–48. https://doi.org/10.1093/neuonc/noac012. PMID: 35018471; PMCID: PMC9159435
73. Rossi S, Barresi S, Colafati GS, et al. Pediatric astroblastoma-like neuroepithelial tumor of the spinal cord with a MAMLD1-BEND2 rearrangement. Neuropathol Appl Neurobiol. 2022; https://doi.org/10.1111/NAN.12814.
74. Ryall S, Zapotocky M, Fukuoka K, Nobre L, Guerreiro Stucklin A, Bennett J, Siddaway R, Li C, Pajovic S, Arnoldo A, Kowalski PE, Johnson M, Sheth J, Lassaletta A, Tatevossian RG, Orisme W, Qaddoumi I, Surrey LF, Li MM, Waanders AJ, Gilheeney S, Rosenblum M, Bale T, Tsang DS, Laperriere N, Kulkarni A, Ibrahim GM, Drake J, Dirks P, Taylor MD, Rutka JT, Laughlin S, Shroff M, Shago M, Hazrati LN, D'Arcy C, Ramaswamy V, Bartels U, Huang A, Bouffet E, Karajannis MA, Santi M, Ellison DW, Tabori U, Hawkins C. Integrated molecular and clinical analysis of 1,000 pediatric low-grade gliomas. Cancer Cell. 2020;37(4):569–583.e5. https://doi.org/10.1016/j.ccell.2020.03.011. PMID: 32289278; PMCID: PMC7169997.
75. Schneppenheim R, et al. Germline nonsense mutation and somatic inactivation of SMARCA4/BRG1 in a family with rhabdoid tumor predisposition syndrome. Am J Hum Genet. 2010;86(2):279–84. https://doi.org/10.1016/j.ajhg.2010.01.013.
76. Schwalbe EC, et al. Novel molecular subgroups for clinical classification and outcome prediction in childhood medulloblastoma: a cohort study. Lancet Oncol. 2017;18(7):958–71. https://doi.org/10.1016/S1470-2045(17)30243-7.
77. Schwartzentruber J, Korshunov A, Liu XY, et al. Driver mutations in histone H3.3 and chromatin remodelling genes in pediatric glioblastoma. Nature. 2012;482(7384):226–31. https://doi.org/10.1038/NATURE10833.
78. Shih DJH, et al. Cytogenetic prognostication within medulloblastoma subgroups. J Clin Oncol. 2014;32(9):886–96. https://doi.org/10.1200/JCO.2013.50.9539.
79. Sievers P, Appay R, Schrimpf D, Stichel D, Reuss DE, Wefers AK, Reinhardt A, Coras R, Ruf VC, Schmid S, de Stricker K, Boldt HB, Kristensen BW, Petersen JK, Ulhøi BP, Gardberg M, Aronica E, Hasselblatt M, Brück W, Bielle F, Mokhtari K, Lhermitte B, Wick W, Herold-Mende C, Hänggi D, Brandner S, Giangaspero F, Capper D, Rushing E, Wesseling P, Pfister SM, Figarella-Branger D, von Deimling A, Sahm F, Jones DTW. Rosette-forming glioneuronal tumors share a distinct DNA methylation profile and mutations in FGFR1, with recurrent co-mutation of PIK3CA and NF1. Acta Neuropathol. 2019;138(3):497–504. https://doi.org/10.1007/s00401-019-02038-4. Epub 2019 Jun 27. PMID: 31250151.
80. Sievers P, Sill M, Schrimpf D, et al. A subset of pediatric-type thalamic gliomas share a distinct DNA methylation profile, H3K27me3 loss and frequent alteration of EGFR. Neuro-Oncology. 2021;23(1):34–43. https://doi.org/10.1093/NEUONC/NOAA251.
81. Sturm D, Orr BA, Toprak UH, et al. New brain tumor entities emerge from molecular classification of CNS-PNETs. Cell. 2016;164(5):1060–72. https://doi.org/10.1016/J.CELL.2016.01.015.
82. Suwala AK, Stichel D, Schrimpf D, et al. Primary mismatch repair deficient IDH-mutant astrocytoma (PMMRDIA) is a distinct type with a poor prognosis. Acta Neuropathol. 2021;141(1):85–100. https://doi.org/10.1007/S00401-020-02243-6.
83. Tauziède-Espariat A, Debily MA, Castel D, et al. An integrative radiological, histopathological and molecular analysis of pediatric pontine histone-wildtype

glioma with MYCN amplification (HGG-MYCN). Acta Neuropathol Commun. 2019;7(1):87. https://doi.org/10.1186/S40478-019-0738-Y.
84. Tauziède-Espariat A, Debily MA, Castel D, et al. The pediatric supratentorial MYCN-amplified high-grade gliomas methylation class presents the same radiological, histopathological and molecular features as their pontine counterparts. Acta Neuropathol Commun. 2020;8(1) https://doi.org/10.1186/S40478-020-00974-X.
85. Tauziède-Espariat A, Siegfried A, Nicaise Y, Kergrohen T, Sievers P, Vasiljevic A, Roux A, Dezamis E, Benevello C, Machet MC, Michalak S, Puiseux C, Llamas-Gutierrez F, Leblond P, Bourdeaut F, Grill J, Dufour C, Guerrini-Rousseau L, Abbou S, Dangouloff-Ros V, Boddaert N, Saffroy R, Hasty L, Wahler E, Pagès M, Andreiuolo F, Lechapt E, Chrétien F, Blauwblomme T, Beccaria K, Pallud J, Puget S, Uro-Coste E, Varlet P, RENOCLIP-LOC, the BIOMECA (Biomarkers for Ependymomas in Children, Adolescents) consortium. Supratentorial non-RELA, ZFTA-fused ependymomas: a comprehensive phenotype genotype correlation highlighting the number of zinc fingers in ZFTA-NCOA1/2 fusions. Acta Neuropathol Commun. 2021;9(1):135. https://doi.org/10.1186/s40478-021-01238-y. PMID: 34389065; PMCID: PMC8362233
86. Teo W-Y, et al. Implications of tumor location on subtypes of medulloblastoma. Pediatr Blood Cancer. 2013;60(9):1408–10. https://doi.org/10.1002/pbc.24511.
87. Thomas AG, Chattopadhyay A, Dineen RA. Ependymal tumors. Neuroimaging Clin N Am. 2026;36(1):69–83. https://doi.org/10.1016/j.nic.2025.08.008. Epub 2025 Oct 23
88. Upadhyaya SA, Robinson GW, Onar-Thomas A, Orr BA, Billups CA, Bowers DC, Bendel AE, Hassall T, Crawford JR, Partap S, Fisher PG, Tatevossian RG, Seah T, Qaddoumi IA, Vinitsky A, Armstrong GT, Sabin ND, Tinkle CL, Klimo P, Indelicato DJ, Boop FA, Merchant TE, Ellison DW, Gajjar A. Molecular grouping and outcomes of young children with newly diagnosed ependymoma treated on the multi-institutional SJYC07 trial. Neuro-Oncology. 2019;21(10):1319–30. https://doi.org/10.1093/neuonc/noz069. PMID: 30976811; PMCID: PMC6784269
89. Viaene AN, Santi M, Hawkins C. Pediatric glial tumors. Pediatr Dev Pathol. 2022;25(1):46–58. https://doi.org/10.1177/10935266211009101.
90. von Hoff K, et al. Therapeutic implications of improved molecular diagnostics for rare CNS embryonal tumor entities: results of an international, retrospective study. Neuro-Oncology. 2021;23(9):1597–611. https://doi.org/10.1093/neuonc/noab136.
91. Wang M, Tihan T, Rojiani AM, Bodhireddy SR, Prayson RA, Iacuone JJ, et al. Monomorphous angiocentric glioma: a distinctive epileptogenic neoplasm with features of infiltrating astrocytoma and ependymoma. J Neuropathol Exp Neurol. 2005;64:875–81. https://doi.org/10.1097/01.jnen.0000182981.02355.10.
92. Wefers AK, Stichel D, Schrimpf D, Coras R, Pages M, Tauziède-Espariat A, Varlet P, Schwarz D, Söylemezoglu F, Pohl U, Pimentel J, Meyer J, Hewer E, Japp A, Joshi A, Reuss DE, Reinhardt A, Sievers P, Casalini MB, Ebrahimi A, Huang K, Koelsche C, Low HL, Rebelo O, Marnoto D, Becker AJ, Staszewski O, Mittelbronn M, Hasselblatt M, Schittenhelm J, Cheesman E, de Oliveira RS, Queiroz RGP, Valera ET, Hans VH, Korshunov A, Olar A, Ligon KL, Pfister SM, Jaunmuktane Z, Brandner S, Tatevossian RG, Ellison DW, Jacques TS, Honavar M, Aronica E, Thom M, Sahm F, von Deimling A, Jones DTW, Blumcke I, Capper D. Isomorphic diffuse glioma is a morphologically and molecularly distinct tumor entity with recurrent gene fusions of MYBL1 or MYB and a benign disease course. Acta Neuropathol. 2020;139(1):193–209. https://doi.org/10.1007/s00401-019-02078-w. Epub 2019 Sep 28. PMID: 31563982; PMCID: PMC7477753.
93. Wefers AK, et al. Subgroup-specific localization of human medulloblastoma based on pre-operative MRI. Acta Neuropathol. 2014;127(6):931–3. https://doi.org/10.1007/s00401-014-1271-5.
94. Woo HY, Na K, Yoo J, et al. Glioblastomas harboring gene fusions detected by next-generation sequencing. Brain Tumor Pathol. 2020;37(4):136–44. https://doi.org/10.1007/S10014-020-00377-9.
95. Wu G, Broniscer A, McEachron TA, et al. Somatic histone H3 alterations in pediatric diffuse intrinsic pontine gliomas and non-brainstem glioblastomas. Nat Genet. 2012;44(3):251–3. https://doi.org/10.1038/NG.1102.
96. Zhao F, et al. Distinctive localization and MRI features correlate of molecular subgroups in adult medulloblastoma. J Neuro-Oncol. 2017;135(2):353–60. https://doi.org/10.1007/s11060-017-2581-y.

Cancer Predisposition Syndromes 5

Selene Cipri, Tiziano Zinicola, Luigi Boccuto, Giovanna Stefania Colafati, Federica D'Antonio, Claudia D'Orazio, Emanuele Agolini, and Angela Mastronuzzi

5.1 Introduction

Cancer predisposition syndromes (CPSs) are recognized as a central aspect of oncogenesis, particularly for central nervous system (CNS) tumors in both pediatric and adult patients [1, 2]. CPSs account for a significant proportion of pediatric tumors, with currently an estimated 10% of childhood cancers linked to germline pathogenic variants in cancer-predisposition genes [1, 3]. These syndromes are characterized by hereditary genetic variants that increase the risk of developing tumors, including those affecting the CNS [1, 2]. CPSs encompass a variety of genetic conditions in which alterations in tumor suppressor genes or DNA repair mechanisms predispose individuals to early-onset tumors [1, 2].

The advent of next-generation sequencing (NGS) has revolutionized the diagnosis of CPSs by enabling the identification of pathogenic variants in genes associated with CNS tumors, such as *SMARCB1*, *SMARCA4*, and *TP53* [1, 4, 5]. These variants are often implicated in the development of aggressive brain tumors, such as atypical teratoid/rhabdoid tumors (AT/RT) and gliomas, which tend to manifest at an early age, especially in pediatric patients, with a generally poor prognosis [6]. Timely diagnosis of these genetic alterations is crucial for initiating targeted treatments and personalized surveillance strategies [7].

S. Cipri · T. Zinicola · F. D'Antonio
Area of Hematology-Oncology, Cell Therapy, Gene Therapies, and Hematopoietic Transplantation, Bambino Gesù Children's Hospital, IRCCS, Rome, Italy

L. Boccuto
School of Nursing, College of Behavioral, Social and Health Sciences, Clemson University, Clemson, SC, USA

G. S. Colafati · C. D'Orazio
Oncological Neuroradiology and Advanced Diagnostics Unit, Bambino Gesù Children's Hospital, IRCCS, Rome, Italy

E. Agolini
Laboratory of Medical Genetics, Bambino Gesù Children's Hospital, IRCCS, Rome, Italy

A. Mastronuzzi (✉)
Area of Hematology-Oncology, Cell Therapy, Gene Therapies, and Hematopoietic Transplantation, Bambino Gesù Children's Hospital, IRCCS, Rome, Italy

Department of Life Sciences and Public Health, Università Cattolica del Sacro Cuore, Rome, Italy
e-mail: angela.mastronuzzi@opbg.net

A. Mastronuzzi, A. Carai (eds.), *Navigating Pediatric Brain Tumors*,
https://doi.org/10.1007/978-3-032-18992-9_5

CPSs, such as Li-Fraumeni syndrome (LFS) and phacomatoses, a group of neurocutaneous syndromes including neurofibromatosis type 1 (NF1), tuberous sclerosis complex (TSC), and von Hippel-Lindau disease (VHL), play a key role in the management of childhood CNS tumors [1, 2]. These syndromes are associated with the development of both benign and malignant tumors, including gliomas and astrocytomas [2, 8, 9]. Children with phacomatoses are at a higher risk of developing CNS tumors due to underlying deleterious variants affecting cell growth pathways [10]. Early genetic testing and careful monitoring are essential to prevent complications related to tumor progression [11, 12].

In adults, syndromes such as Lynch syndrome, caused by germline variants in mismatch repair (MMR) genes, and hereditary breast and ovarian cancer (HBOC), often associated with mutated *BRCA1*, *BRCA2*, and other BRCA-related DNA repair genes, also increase the risk of secondary CNS tumors [13]. Recognizing these genetic predispositions allows clinicians to implement more effective surveillance strategies, including cascade testing to identify asymptomatic carriers among family members. This proactive surveillance can significantly improve outcomes by identifying high-risk individuals before tumors develop. Guidelines for managing CPSs recommend the use of next-generation sequencing to identify molecular defects in genes such as *TP53*, *SMARCB1*, *NF1*, and *VHL*, which are crucial for early recognition of the syndromes and for initiating preventive strategies. Cascade testing is strongly encouraged for family members of patients with pathogenic variants, helping to identify asymptomatic at-risk individuals and initiate appropriate preventive measures [14].

For surveillance, the guidelines establish syndrome-specific protocols. In patients with LFS or NF1, regular monitoring through magnetic resonance imaging (MRI) of the brain and spine is recommended, as it is preferred over computed tomography (CT) to avoid exposure to ionizing radiation [12, 15]. Phacomatoses like NF1 require continuous surveillance to detect the early development of optic gliomas or other CNS tumors, with scan frequency varying based on age and individual risk [11, 12].

The guidelines also recommend the use of whole-body or focused MRI to monitor not only the CNS but also other organs, such as the kidneys and liver, in syndromes like VHL [16]. These approaches are continuously updated based on new research and technological advances, such as the emerging use of pulmonary MRI to monitor lung blastomas in DICER1 syndrome [17].

Finally, genetic counseling is essential in managing CPSs (Fig. 5.1). Before and after genetic testing, patients and families should receive detailed information about genetic risks and the implications of the test, as well as support in making informed decisions [18]. Genetic counseling facilitates cascade testing, which helps identify asymptomatic carriers within the family and allows for the initiation of personalized prevention and management plans [18].

In summary, cancer predisposition syndromes, including pediatric phacomatoses, play a crucial role in the development of CNS tumors throughout life. Advances in genetic sequencing and targeted therapies, along with advanced surveillance protocols, provide patients with new opportunities for early diagnosis, personalized treatments, and significant improvements in clinical outcomes. In this chapter, we will discuss the known CPSs associated with the development of CNS tumors.

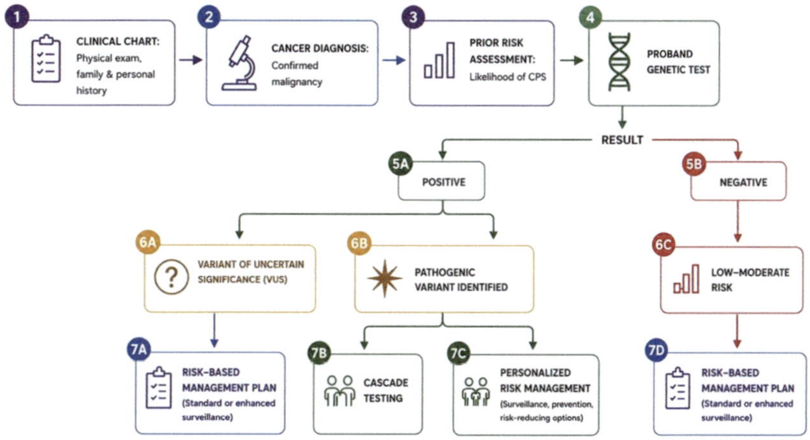

Fig. 5.1 Cascade testing is strongly encouraged for all first-degree relatives of patients with identified pathogenic variants, enabling early intervention in asymptomatic carriers

5.2 Common Genetic Tumor Predisposition Syndromes and CNS Tumors

5.2.1 Facomatosis

5.2.1.1 Neurofibromatosis Type 1

Neurofibromatosis type 1 (NF1) is an autosomal dominant disorder affecting approximately 1 in 2500–3000 individuals [19, 20]. It is caused by pathogenic alterations in *NF1* on chromosome 17 encoding neurofibromin, a negative regulator of RAS signaling [19, 21]. NF1 shows complete penetrance and variable expressivity, and approximately 50% of cases arise de novo [19, 22].

In addition, it is important to point out that clinical diagnosis is very efficient. Consequently, many patients do not perform genetic testing, so the percentage of cases with pathogenic variants of NF1 is likely to be underestimated.

Clinical manifestations include café-au-lait macules, axillary or inguinal freckling, cutaneous and plexiform neurofibromas, and Lisch nodules [19, 21, 23–26].

Malignant peripheral nerve sheath tumors (MPNSTs) are the most common NF1-associated malignancies and often arise from plexiform neurofibromas [19, 27, 28]. Rapid growth and persistent pain should raise suspicion for malignant transformation [19, 27, 28].

NF1-associated optic pathway gliomas are frequently indolent or asymptomatic and may remain stable or regress spontaneously [19, 29]. Symptomatic tumors usually occur before 6 years of age [19, 29].

Non-optic gliomas are usually incidental low-grade lesions with slow growth, although symptomatic or high-grade tumors may rarely occur [19, 30, 31].

The pediatric population with *NF1* gene defects also includes patients at risk for developing hematopoietic malignancies such as acute or chronic leukemias or different types of lymphomas [32]. Furthermore, patients might also develop neoplasms affecting the endocrine system, such as pheochromocytomas or multiple gastrointestinal stromal tumors (GISTs). Melanomas can also occur, as can breast cancer in adult women [33].

5.2.1.1.1 Diagnosis

The diagnosis of NF1 is established in an individual with two or more of the clinical features: six or more café au lait macules: >5 mm in greatest diameter in prepubertal individuals and >15 mm in greatest diameter in postpubertal individuals; freckling in the axillary or inguinal regions; two or more neurofibromas of any type or one plexiform neurofibroma; presence of glioma in the optic pathway; two or more Lisch nodules identified by slit-lamp examination or two or more choroidal abnormalities detected by Optical Coherence Tomography/near-infrared (OCT/NIR) reflectance imaging; a distinctive osseous lesion such as sphenoid dysplasia, anterolateral bowing of the tibia, or pseudarthrosis of a long bone; a parent who meets the diagnostic criteria for NF1; detection of a germline *NF1* pathogenic variant [19, 34]. Table 5.1 summarizes the diagnostic criteria to establish a diagnosis of NF1.

Table 5.1 Establishing the diagnosis of Neurofibromarosis type 1

Diagnostic criterion	Description
Two or more suggestive findings	Diagnosis of NF1 is established in a proband with two or more characteristic clinical features.
Legius syndrome consideration	Individuals with Legius syndrome may meet the pigmentary criteria for NF1 but do not have neurofibromas, optic pathway gliomas, Lisch nodules, or typical osseous lesions of NF1.
Bilateral features	CALMs, intertriginous freckling, cutaneous neurofibromas, and Lisch nodules are usually bilateral in NF1. If present only on one side, consider mosaic *NF1*.
Sphenoid wing dysplasia	Not a separate criterion if ipsilateral orbital plexiform neurofibromas are present.
Germline *NF1* pathogenic variant	A germline *NF1* pathogenic variant must be identified for genetic testing to serve as a diagnostic criterion. Variants only in tumor tissue or of uncertain significance do not count.
Possible negative genetic testing	Negative *NF1* genetic testing does not rule out a diagnosis of NF1. Some individuals diagnosed clinically do not have detectable pathogenic variants with current technology.

Table modified and adapted from Genereviews [19]

Genetic testing includes NF1 sequencing and deletion/duplication analysis. CMA or multigene panels may be considered in selected cases, particularly in patients with atypical phenotypes or suspected mosaicism [19, 34–36].

If CMA fails to detect a chromosomal alteration and no pathogenic variants are detected in either the gDNA or cDNA of *NF1* and no targeted deletion of the gene, a karyotype may be performed with a clinical diagnosis of NF1 due to the possibility of balanced translocations encompassing the *NF1* locus. When the diagnosis needs to be differentiated due to phenotype overlap with other diseases characterized, for example, by neoplasia or hyperpigmentation, a multigene panel, such as a panel on tauopathies, should be performed [19, 34–36].

Prenatal and preimplantation genetic testing may be offered when the familial pathogenic variant is known [19].

5.2.1.1.2 Surveillance

Annual check-ups by a physician knowledgeable about the condition are essential [12, 19]. Recommended surveillance is reported in Table 5.2.

5.2.1.2 NF2-Related Schwannomatosis

NF2-related schwannomatosis (NF2), formerly known as Neurofibromatosis type 2, is an autoso-

Table 5.2 Recommended surveillance for cildren and adults with neurofibromatosis 1

Surveillance area	Annual frequency	As needed frequency
Eyes	Ophthalmologic exam until adolescence or as recommended by ophthalmologist	Older children
Tumors	Physical exam for neurofibromas, new or changing plexiform neurofibromas, & other signs/symptoms of malignancy by a clinical provider familiar w/the patient	/
Neurologic system	Neurologic evaluation for adults and children with NF1 whole-gene deletions	Brain MRI only is recommended based on signs or symptoms.
Neurodevelopment	/	Developmental assessment by screening questionnaire for children
Neuropsychiatric	Assessment for cognitive issues & depression for adults	Assessment as needed
Skeletal	Clinical assessment for asymmetry & scoliosis throughout childhood until growth is complete	/
	Assess for increased fractures for children	/
	/	Serum vitamin D levels for adults
Cardiovascular	Blood pressure, monitoring and clinical assessment, for both children and adults	Blood pressure, monitoring and clinical assessment, for both children and adults before surgical procedures
Growth deficiency	Assessment height and head circumference on NF1-specific growth charts throughout childhood	
Endocrine manifestations	Assessment pubertal development. Throughout early childhood	
Breast cancer (in women w/NF1)	Mammography beginning at age 30 years.	
	Contrast-enhanced breast MRI between ages 30 and 50 years.	

Table modified and adapted from Genereviews [19]

mal dominant disorder caused by pathogenic variants in the NF2 gene on chromosome 22, encoding merlin, a regulator of cell growth and cytoskeletal organization [37–40]. Alterations of these genes are most frequently truncating and lead to severe forms of NF2, yet single- and multiple-exon deletions/duplications are also common [37]. Tumorigenesis in individuals with NF2 follows a two-hit model [10, 37]. These result in a loss of merlin, leading to unfettered cell growth [10, 37]. Truncating variants are generally associated with more severe disease and poorer prognosis [37, 41]. The hallmark of NF2 is the development of unilateral or bilateral vestibular schwannomas, typically occurring by early adulthood [38, 42, 43].

The hallmark of NF2 is the development of monoliteral or bilateral vestibular schwannomas (acoustic neuromas), seen in 90 to 95 percent of patients, usually by age 30 [37, 42, 44]. NF2 patients also frequently develop other brain tumors, notably meningiomas [37, 43, 45]. Approximately half of NF2 patients have meningiomas [37]. NF2-related meningiomas often appear at a younger age and are more likely to be atypical or anaplastic compared to sporadic cases. In addition, about 25% of patients develop an ependymoma [37, 46].

5.2.1.2.1 Diagnosis

NF2 can be diagnosed if the proband has bilateral vestibular schwannomas or an identical *NF2* pathogenic variant in two or more different NF2-related tumors, such as schwannomas, meningiomas, or ependymomas [11, 37, 47, 48].

The diagnosis can be confirmed with either two major criteria or one major and two minor criteria (Table 5.3).

Table 5.3 Major criteria and minor criteria for diagnosis of Neurofibromarosis type 2

Category	Criterion	Description
Major criteria		
	Unilateral vestibular Schwannoma	Presence of a vestibular schwannoma on one side
	First-degree relative with NF2	Having a first-degree relative (excluding a sibling) with NF2
	Two or more meningiomas	Presence of two or more meningiomas
	NF2 pathogenic variant in unaffected tissue	Identification of the *NF2* pathogenic variant in unaffected tissues (e.g., blood)—It is important to note that if the variant allele fraction (VAF) is clearly <50%, the diagnosis is mosaic NF2
Minor criteria		
	Ependymoma, Schwannoma (non-vestibular)	Presence of ependymoma or non-vestibular schwannoma. Two ependymomas or two non-vestibular schwannomas count as two minor criteria
	Single meningioma	Presence of a single meningioma. Two meningiomas count as a major criterion
	Juvenile subcapsular or cortical cataract, retinal hamartoma, Epiretinal membrane in a person age <40 years	Each bilateral ocular manifestation counts as one minor criterion

Table modified and adapted from Genereviews [37]

Genetic testing usually includes NF2 sequencing and deletion/duplication analysis using NGS and MLPA approaches. Mosaicism is relatively common, particularly in de novo and asymmetric presentations, and should be considered in patients with negative blood testing despite a suggestive phenotype [11, 37, 47, 48]. Postzygotic mosaicism is detected, particularly in cases with later onset and asymmetric presentation [49]. Prenatal and preimplantation genetic testing may be offered when the familial pathogenic variant is known [11, 37, 47, 48].

Table 5.4 Recommended surveillance for Neurofibromarosis type 2

	Management strategies
Surveillance	Neurologic examination: annual check-ups by a provider experienced in NF2.
	Brain MRI: annual scans starting at age 10–12 years and continuing until at least the fourth decade of life.
	Hearing evaluation: annual assessments, including brainstem auditory evoked response (BAER) testing.
	Ophthalmology examination: annual complete eye exams.

Table modified and adapted from Genereviews [37]

5.2.1.2.2 Surveillance

The surveillance guidelines recommended neurological, earing and ophthalmology examination and an annual brain MRI starting at age 10–12 years old, as reported in Table 5.4 [11, 37].

5.2.1.3 *LZTR1*- and *SMARCB1*-Related Schwannomatoses

LZTR1- and SMARCB1-related schwannomatoses are autosomal dominant disorders with reduced penetrance caused by pathogenic alterations in the *LZTR1* or *SMARCB1* genes [47, 50]. They are characterized by the development of multiple schwannomas, most commonly affecting peripheral and spinal nerves, and typically present between the third and fifth decades of life with pain, neurological symptoms, or asymptomatic masses [47, 50]. However, a recent study in which cases without a molecular diagnosis of bilateral schwannomas were excluded reported a 72% frequency of de novo *NF2* variants, and nearly 50% of these were mosaics [47, 50]. Furthermore, the study emphasizes the difficult clinical differentiation of *LZTR1*- and *SMARCB1*-related schwannomatoses versus NF2; in case of negative germline testing for the studied genes, it is appropriate to screen for somatic variants. In a study of 51 individuals with *LZTR1*- or *SMARCB1*-related schwannomatosis who underwent whole-body MRI, 36 (71%) had internal nerve sheath tumors, 81% of which were discrete; three individuals (8%) had plexiform neurofibromas; and the rest had both tumor types [50, 51]. Meningiomas have only been documented in those with *SMARCB1*-related schwannomatosis [50, 52]. Malignancy risk exists in *SMARCB1*-related schwannomatosis, with malignant transformation of schwannomas being a concern [50, 53]. Rapid growth of a schwannoma and severe, unrelenting pain should prompt suspicion of malignancy. Pain is a prevalent comorbid condition in individuals with *LZTR1*- or *SMARCB1*-related schwannomatosis and may not always correspond to the location of the schwannoma.

5.2.1.4 Diagnosis

The diagnosis of *LZTR1*- or *SMARCB1*-related schwannomatosis is made in the presence of characteristic clinical signs and when an *LZTR1* or *SMARCB1* germline pathogenic alteration is found (Table 5.5). Genetic testing usually includes sequencing of *LZTR1, SMARCB1*, and *NF2* through multigene panels. Mosaic *NF2* should be considered in patients with negative germline testing, particularly when bilateral schwannomas or multiple anatomically distinct tumors are present [47, 50]. When feasible, analysis of both blood and tumor tissue may improve diagnostic accuracy. Future challenges include identifying other genetic factors involved in familial SWN, as no germline pathogenic alterations in *SMARCB1* or *LZTR1* genes are found in 20–30% of this case series. In addition, even in some cases diagnosed with sporadic SWN, no germline pathogenic alterations are found in *SMARCB1* or *LZTR1* genes, but identical *NF2* pathogenic variants were found on two anatomically unrelated tumors in 37%–57% of these patients; in this case, mosaic *NF2* variants are confirmed [47, 50]. Consequently, whenever possible, it is best to analyze blood and at least two tumors for genetic diagnosis [47, 50].

Table 5.5 Suggestive findings and diagnostic criteria

Category and criteria	Description
Suggestive findings	
Multiple schwannomas	The presence of two or more non-intradermal tumors indicative of schwannomas
Absence of bilateral vestibular schwannomas	Lack of bilateral vestibular schwannomas
Family history	Family history of schwannomatosis consistent with autosomal dominant inheritance (e.g., affected males and females across several generations). The absence of family history does not exclude the diagnosis
Establishing the diagnosis	
Genetic testing	Diagnosis of *LZTR1*- or *SMARCB1*-related schwannomatosis is confirmed in a proband with suggestive findings by identifying a heterozygous germline pathogenic (or likely pathogenic) variant in *LZTR1* or *SMARCB1* through molecular genetic testing (see Table 5.1) or by identifying identical pathogenic (or likely pathogenic) variants in *SMARCB1* or *LZTR1* in two or more anatomically distinct schwannomatosis-related tumors

Table modified and adapted from Genereviews [50]

5.2.1.5 Surveillance

The surveillance guidelines for *LZTR1*- and *SMARCB1*-related schwannomatosis are listed in Table 5.6 and recommended neurologic and neuropsychiatric evaluation [47, 50].

5.2.1.6 Tuberous Sclerosis Complex

Tuberous Sclerosis Complex (TSC) is an autosomal dominant neurocutaneous disorder caused by pathogenic alterations in *TSC1* or *TSC2*, encoding hamartin and tuberin, key regulators of the mTOR pathway [54–56]. Approximately two-thirds of cases arise de novo [54–56]. TSC is characterized by multisystem involvement affecting the skin, brain, kidneys, heart, and lungs [57, 58]. CNS manifestations,

Table 5.6 Surveillance guidelines

System/concern	Annual frequency	Other frequency
Neurologic	Neurologic and pain assessment	/
	/	Brain and spine MRI or whole-body MRI every 2–3 years beginning at age 12 years
	/	Whole-body MRI exam at age 18–20 years, then as needed
Neuropsychiatric	Assessment for anxiety/ depression	Assessment for anxiety/depression as needed

Table modified and adapted from Genereviews [50]

including TSC-associated neuropsychiatric disorders (TAND), epilepsy, cortical dysplasia, and subependymal giant cell astrocytomas (SEGAs), represent the major cause of morbidity [57–59]. Epilepsy is common and frequently drug resistant, often presenting with infantile spasms in early childhood [54, 60, 61]. Typical extracranial manifestations include hypomelanotic macules, angiofibromas, renal angiomyolipomas, and lymphangioleiomyomatosis [54, 60]. mTOR inhibitors have significantly improved the management of TSC-associated tumors and neurologic manifestations [54, 57, 62]. In Fig. 5.2 illustrates an MRI on subependymal giant cell astrocytoma in an 8-year-old boy with Tuberous Sclerosis.

5.2.1.6.1 Diagnosis

The clinical diagnosis of TSC can be confirmed in an individual based on clinical diagnostic criteria or through a molecular diagnosis by identifying a heterozygous pathogenic (or likely pathogenic) variant in the *TSC1* or *TSC2* genes [54, 63]. A definitive clinical diagnosis of TSC can be established if the individual presents with two major features or one major feature along with two or more minor features (see Suggestive Findings in Table 5.7) [54, 63]. Table 5.7 summarizes the major and minor features used to establish the clinical diagnosis of TSC. A definitive diagnosis can be made with either two major features, or one major feature accompanied by two or more minor features [54, 63].

De novo pathogenic variants have been found in 2/3 of affected patients with TSC. Affected individuals with TSC should be offered genetic testing for *TSC1* and *TSC2* and genetic counselling [54, 63]. If a pathogenic variant is found in the proband, genetic testing should be offered to at least first-degree relatives [54, 63]. Genetic testing may include sequence and targeted deletion/duplication analysis of the *TSC1* and *TSC2* genes [54, 63]. If a pathogenic variant is not detected, somatic mosaicism for a pathogenic variant should be hypothesized [54, 63]. Instead, a multigenic panel including *TSC1*, *TSC2*, and other genes of interest may be considered when the diagnosis of TSC is uncertain [54, 63].

5.2.1.6.2 Surveillance

Surveillance (Table 5.8) is crucial for monitoring existing manifestations, evaluating the individual's response to supportive care, and detecting new manifestations [54, 63]. This table outlines the recommended surveillance protocols for individuals with Tuberous Sclerosis Complex (TSC) [54, 63].

5.2.1.7 Von Hippel-Lindau Syndrome

The *von Hippel-Lindau* (*VHL*) gene, mapped to chromosome 3p25 and cloned in the early 1990s, has been the subject of extensive research over the past 20 years [58, 64] . Its product, the VHL protein, functions as a tumor suppressor [58, 64]. This model involves a germline loss-of-function variant that inactivates one copy of the VHL gene in all cells [16, 58, 64]. For VHL-associated tumors to develop, the second normal allele must also be lost, either through somatic changes, deletion of the second allele, or promoter hypermethylation [58, 64]. In sporadic renal cell cancers, inactivation of both VHL alleles through somatic changes is very common [16, 65].

Significant advances have been made in the past two decades in understanding the biology of

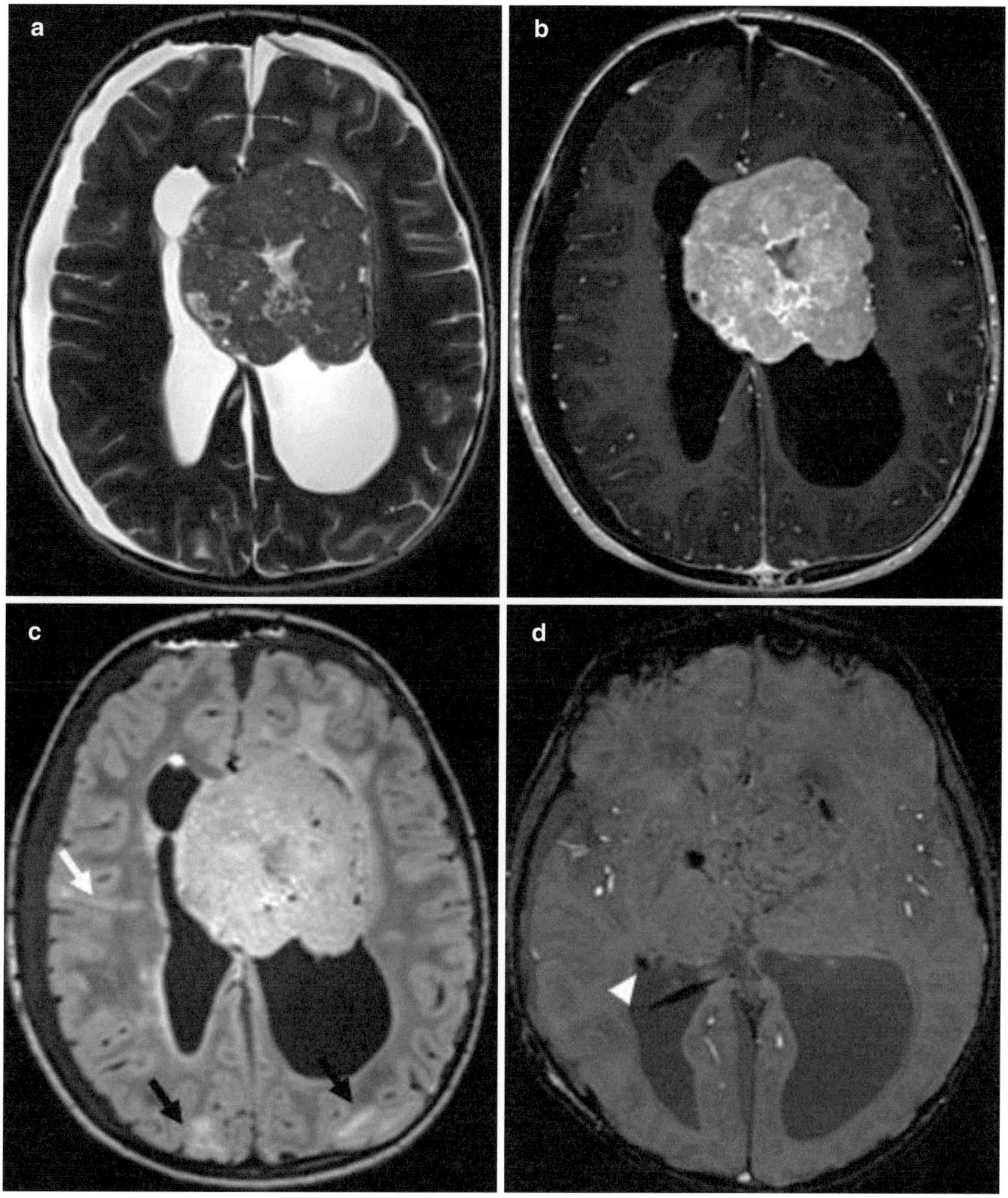

Fig. 5.2 Subependymal giant cell astrocytoma in an 8-year-old boy with Tuberous Sclerosis. MRI shows a voluminous intraventricular mass with inhomogeneous T2 signal (**a**) and intense contrast enhancement (**b**). Small subependymal nodular lesion with calcifications (**d**, arrowhead), cortico-subcortical hamartomas (**c**, black arrows) and radial bands (**c**, white arrow). Presence of thin subdural collection and minimal amount of pneumocephalus following recent ventricular catheter placement

Table 5.7 Major and minor features used to establish the clinical diagnosis of Tuberous Sclerosis Complex

Major features	Minor features
Hypomelanotic macules (≥3 macules at least 5 mm in diameter) Angiofibromas (≥3) or fibrous cephalic plaque Shagreen patch Ungual fibromas (≥2) Subependymal nodules (SENs) (≥2) Multiple cortical tubers and/or radial migration lines Subependymal giant cell astrocytoma (SEGA) Renal angiomyolipomas (≥2) Cardiac rhabdomyoma Lymphangioleiomyomatosis (LAM) Multiple retinal nodular hamartomas	"Confetti" skin lesions (numerous 1- to 3-mm hypopigmented macules scattered over regions such as the arms and legs) Sclerotic bone lesions Dental enamel pits (>3) Intraoral fibromas (≥2) Multiple renal cysts (≥2) Extrarenal hamartomas Retinal achromic patch

Table modified and adapted from Genereviews [54]

VHL-associated tumors [16, 66]. The VHL protein forms a stable complex with several other proteins, including elongin B, elongin C, and cullin 2 [16, 66]. These complexes target specific proteins for proteasomal degradation, thereby regulating their cellular levels [16, 66]. The VHL component functions as an E3 ubiquitin ligase for these target molecules, tagging them with ubiquitin, which facilitates their degradation by the proteasome [16, 66].

Besides its role as an E3 ubiquitin ligase, VHL is involved in several other critical cellular functions, such as maintaining the primary cilium, regulating cytokinesis, controlling microtubule function, ensuring extracellular matrix integrity, and regulating the cell cycle [16, 66]. Pathogenic variants in the VHL gene have also been linked to congenital forms of polycythemia vera [16, 67]. Genotype-phenotype correlations are reported in the literature [16, 68]. VHL1 seems to be caused by pathogenic missense variants that disrupt HIF regulation, while patho-

Table 5.8 Surveillance guidelines for Tuberous Sclerosis Complex-related conditions

Surveillance area	Frequency/details
Dermatologic examination	Annual detailed examination
SEGA	Brain MRI every 1–3 years in asymptomatic individuals with TSC under 25 years to monitor for new SEGAs
	Periodically in adulthood for those with asymptomatic SEGA in childhood
	More frequent for large/growing SEGAs or those causing ventricular enlargement
Seizures	Seizure assessment: At each visit by a neurologist
	EEG in infants: Every 6 weeks up to 12 months; every 3 months up to 24 months; as clinically indicated
	Video EEG: Prolonged video EEG for suspected seizures with normal routine EEG
TAND screening	At least annually with comprehensive formal evaluation at key developmental stages
Kidney function assessment	Annual assessment of glomerular filtration rate and blood pressure
	Abdominal MRI every 1–3 years to monitor for new or progressing
	Angiomyolipoma and cystic kidney disease
Echocardiogram	Every 1–3 years in asymptomatic infants and children with cardiac rhabdomyomas until regression
	For cardiology recommendations for symptomatic cardiac rhabdomyomas
Pulmonary evaluation	LAM symptoms screening: At each visit in females over 18 and individuals with respiratory symptoms
	High-resolution CT for LAM: Every 5–7 years in asymptomatic females without lung cysts starting after age 18 through menopause; follow-up intervals determined individually for those with LAM-related cystic lung disease

Table modified and adapted from Genereviews [54]

genic missense variants that do not disrupt HIF regulation have a higher probability of being associated with VHL2 [16, 66].

5.2.1.7.1 Diagnosis

The clinical diagnosis of VHL can be established according to the criteria specified in the Dutch or Danish guidelines (Table 5.9) [16, 69, 70]. Conversely, when clinical features are inconclusive, the finding of a germline pathogenic variant of *VHL* establishes the diagnosis [16, 69, 70]. VHL-related manifestations included in all 3 published criteria are for both Dutch and Danish criteria: Retinal HB, CNS HB, RCC, Pheo, PNET, ELST; while VHL-related manifestations specific to publish criteria are Paraganglioma, Multiple kidney cysts, Multiple pancreatic cysts only for Dutch criteria [16, 69, 70].

Approximately 20% of patients diagnosed with VHL have a de novo germline pathogenic variant or as de novo postzygotic in an unaffected mosaic parent. VHL is an autosomal dominant syndrome [16, 69, 70]. At the time a pathogenic variant is identified in the proband, cascade genetic testing can be performed on asymptomatic family members at risk, and it is very important to test asymptomatic subjects during childhood as early diagnosis could apply medical management of the at-risk subject [16, 69, 70].

In addition, it is relevant to note that when a pathogenic variant is not identified at the level of the coding regions of the *VHL* gene in the proband, there is a need for intron 1 sequence analysis because certain pathogenic variants in this region can lead to the inclusion of a cryptic exon [16, 69, 70].

Table 5.9 von Hippel-Lindau diagnostic criteria

VHL published diagnostic criteria	VHL published diagnostic criteria	Clinical diagnostic criteria
Positive family	Dutch criteria	1 VHL-related tumor AND 1st- or second-degree relative with VHL diagnosis
	Danish criteria	1 VHL-related manifestation AND first-degree relative with VHL diagnosis
Unknown family history	Dutch criteria	≥2 VHL-related manifestations
	Danish criteria	≥2HB*OR*1HB&1*VHL-*

Table modified and adapted from Genereviews [16]

5.2.1.7.2 Surveillance

Table 5.10 outlines the recommended surveillance activities and their frequencies for individuals with von Hippel-Lindau (VHL) disease. Regular monitoring is crucial for early detection and management of disease manifestations, tailored to different age groups and clinical needs [16, 69, 70].

5.2.2 Li-Fraumeni Syndrome

The Li-Fraumeni syndrome (LFS), also known as sarcoma, breast, leukemia, and adrenal gland (SBLA) syndrome, is a rare autosomal dominant cancer predisposition syndrome caused by pathogenic variants in the TP53 tumor suppressor (*TP53*) gene on chromosome 17p13 [70–72]. The *TP53* encodes a nuclear transcription factor that

Table 5.10 Surveillance guidelines for von Hippel-Lindau syndrome

Age/stage	Surveillance activity	Frequency
Early childhood	Clinical assessments for neurological symptoms, vision problems, and hearing issues	Annually
Starting at age 1	Ophthalmology evaluations	Annually
Starting at age 5	Plasma or 24-hour urine tests for fractionated metanephrines	Annually
Starting at age 11	Brain and total spine MRIs	Every 2 years
Audiology evaluations	Every 2–3 years	
Starting at age 15	Abdominal MRIs	Every 2 years
MRI of the internal auditory canal (for asymptomatic individuals)	Between ages 15 and 20	

Table modified and adapted from Genereviews [16]

plays a central role in cell-cycle regulation, apoptosis, and DNA repair [70–72]. Most pathogenic variants are missense variants involving the DNA-binding domain of the protein, although nonsense and frameshift variants resulting in loss of function have also been described [71–74]. LFS is characterized by a markedly increased lifetime risk of multiple early-onset malignancies. Breast cancer is the most frequent tumor in affected women, whereas soft tissue sarcomas, osteosarcomas, adrenocortical carcinomas, leukemias, and CNS tumors are more commonly observed in children and adolescents [74] [75]. CNS manifestations include choroid plexus carcinoma, medulloblastoma, glioblastoma, and astrocytoma [8, 9]. *TP53* pathogenic variants are particularly associated with the SHH subgroup of medulloblastoma, whereas they are uncommon in Groups 3 and 4 [9, 76].

Germline *TP53* pathogenic variants account for a substantial proportion of specific pediatric malignancies, including diffuse anaplastic rhabdomyosarcoma, adrenocortical carcinoma, hypodiploid acute lymphoblastic leukemia, osteosarcoma, and pediatric brain tumors [77]. Mosaicism should be considered in patients presenting with highly suggestive sporadic tumors, particularly choroid plexus carcinoma or very early-onset breast cancer [78]. Cancer risk in LFS is extremely high, with many individuals developing malignancies during childhood or early adulthood [79, 80].

In 20% of patients, from 5 to 16 years old, with a germline PV in the *TP53* gene and diagnosed with MB sonic hedgehog (SHH) subgroup, a family history for LFS was relevant in 4% of them. In addition, a diagnosis of LFS is made in 56% of patients with a MB SHH/TP53 subgroup and a germinal PV in the *TP53* gene [76].

5.2.2.1 Diagnosis

The diagnosis of LFS is confirmed in a proband with all three of the classic LFS criteria and/or possesses a germline pathogenic (or likely pathogenic) variant in the *TP53* gene, as identified through molecular genetic testing [15, 74]. Table 5.11 details the classic criteria for diagnosing Li-Fraumeni Syndrome (LFS), emphasizing the importance of family history and the presence of specific cancers [15, 74]. Meeting these criteria, especially in conjunction with the identification of a germline *TP53* pathogenic variant, is critical for establishing an LFS diagnosis [15, 74]. In Fig. 5.3 MRI shows a high-grade glioma in a 9-year-old girl with LFS.

Table 5.11 Classic criteria for diagnosing Li-Fraumeni syndrome

Criteria	Description
Criterion 1	A proband with a sarcoma diagnosed before the age of 45 years
Criterion 2	A first-degree relative with any cancer diagnosed before the age of 45 years
Criterion 3	A first- or second-degree relative with any cancer diagnosed before age 45 years or a sarcoma diagnosed at any age

Table modified and adapted from Genereviews [74]

Peripheral blood analysis may fail to detect mosaic *TP53* alterations, particularly when the pathogenic alteration is confined to specific tissues; therefore, tumor testing may be useful in clinically suggestive cases [15, 74].

According to current recommendations, germline *TP53* testing should be considered in patients fulfilling the Chompret criteria, in children and adolescents with hypodiploid acute lymphoblastic leukemia, SHH-activated medulloblastoma, mandibular osteosarcoma, or second primary tumors within the *TP53* spectrum arising after radiotherapy [15, 74]. In pediatric patients from southern or southeastern Brazil, testing for the recurrent TP53 p.R337H variant should also be considered [15, 74].

Predictive testing may be offered to at-risk relatives of individuals carrying germline TP53 pathogenic variants, particularly in families with childhood-onset cancers [15, 74].

Finally, it is important to discuss with parents the appropriateness of testing for a germline causative variant of *TP53* in pediatric ages when there is a history of cancers in young adulthood (before age 31 years) within the family or when insufficient evidence is available to determine pediatric cancer risk in databases or registries [15, 74].

Outside of choroid plexus carcinoma, recommendations for *TP53* germline testing in patients

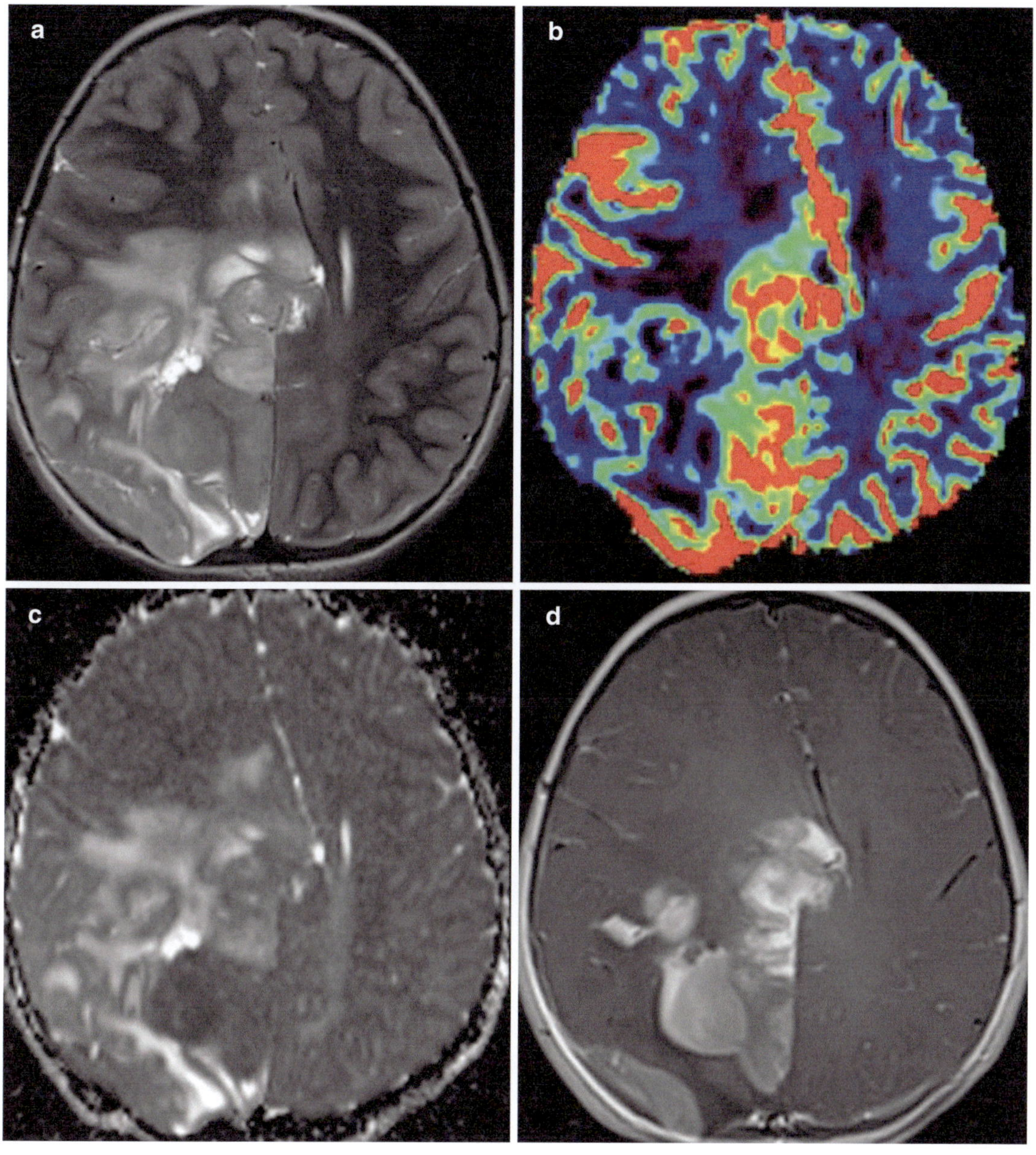

Fig. 5.3 High grade glioma in a 9-year-old girl with Li-Fraumeni Syndrome. MRI study shows a voluminous right fronto-parietal neoplasm with inhomogeneous T2 signal (**a**), hyperperfusion (**b**), restricted diffusivity (**c**) and contrast enhancement (**d**). Subfalcine herniation to the left

with brain tumors are not yet standardized. However, some experts suggest considering germline testing for specific brain tumor subtypes [15, 74]:

- Lower-grade choroid plexus tumors in children showing a mutant p53 pattern in tumor immunohistochemistry;
- TP53 SHH mutated MB in children, where germline *TP53* variants have been found in a significant proportion of cases;
- Astrocytomas with rare *isocitrate dehydrogenase type 1* (*IDH1*) p.R132C substitution, as this mutation has been associated with germline *TP53* variants.

Table 5.12 Recommended surveillance for Li-Fraumeni Syndrome

Age/stage	Surveillance activity	Frequency
Birth to age 18	Comprehensive physical examination and abdominal and pelvic ultrasound	Every 3–4 months
	Annual neurological assessments	Annually
	Whole-body MRI, including brain MRI	Annually
Age 18 and older	Comprehensive physical examination	Every 6 months
	Abdominal and pelvic ultrasound	Annually
	Dermatological evaluations	Annually
Age 20–25	Clinical breast examinations	Every 6–12 months
Age 20–30	Annual breast MRI	Annually
Age 30–75	Annual mammogram and breast MRI	Annually
Age 25 and older	Upper endoscopy	Every 2–5 years
	Colonoscopy	Every 2–5 years

Table modified and adapted from Genereviews [74]

5.2.2.2 Surveillance

Tumor surveillance presents difficulties due to the great variety of tumors associated with LFS, it plays a crucial role in early cancer detection [15, 74]. Table 5.12 outlines the recommended surveillance activities and their frequencies for individuals at various stages of life. Regular monitoring is essential for early detection and management of potential cancer risks and other health concerns [15, 74].

5.2.3 Lynch Syndrome and Constitutional Mismatch Repair Deficiency Syndrome

Lynch syndrome (LS) is caused by alterations of the mismatch repair (MMR) genes -specifically *MLH1, MSH2, MSH6* - and in addition *PMS2* gene, and characterized by the occurrence of hereditary non-polyposis colorectal cancer (HNPCC), along with other types of cancers like endometrial, urothelial, small intestine, and CNS tumors, most commonly gliomas [13]. Germline deletions of the last few *EPCAM* exons contribute to Lynch syndrome etiology [81].

LS is inherited as an autosomal dominant trait and is characterized by incomplete penetrance [77, 78, 82]. LS is considered primarily an adult-onset cancer predisposition syndrome, although pediatric cases have been reported [83].

Following the discovery of LS, a new unique autosomal recessive cancer predisposition syndrome, constitutional mismatch repair deficiency syndrome (CMMRD), was described as resulting from the inheritance of biallelic germline pathogenic variants in *MLH1, MSH2, MSH6, PMS2,* and in rare cases *EPCAM* [82, 84]. CMMRD is correlated to a high risk of developing tumors in early in life, including CNS tumors, as well as hematological and colonrectal cancers and other types of cancer typically seen in Lynch syndrome at older ages [82, 84, 85]. Moreover, patients with CMMRD frequently exhibit metachronous multiple brain lesions and brain vascular malformations, which are not adjacent to the primary tumor and are generally asymptomatic [82, 84, 85]. So, the tumor spectrum of the LS and CMMRD overlaps, and an earlier clinical onset (early childhood) is characteristic of the latter [82, 84].

5.2.3.1 Diagnosis

No standardized clinical diagnostic criteria for LS are currently available [82, 86, 87]. Table 5.13 outlines the key indicators that suggest a diagnosis of Lynch syndrome, including specific tumor types and tissue findings, as well as relevant cancer history. It highlights the presence of LS-associated tumors, diagnostic test results, and familial patterns that may warrant further investigation [82, 86, 87].

Specific brain MRI features of constitutional mismatch repair deficiency syndrome in children with high-grade gliomas have been described. Specifically, CMMRD-associated HGG generally shows hemispheric localization and ill-defined borders. They were also distinguished by a constant presence of developmental venous

Table 5.13 Suggestive Indicators for Lynch syndrome

	Indicator	Details
Tumor types	Presence of Lynch syndrome-associated tumors	Includes colorectal, endometrial, ovarian, stomach, small bowel, urinary tract (urothelial), biliary tract, prostate, brain (e.g., glioblastoma), skin (e.g., sebaceous adenomas, sebaceous carcinomas, keratoacanthomas), or pancreas
Tumor tissue findings	Microsatellite instability (MSI)	High MSI in the tumor
	Immunohistochemistry (IHC)	Loss of expression of mismatch repair (MMR) gene products (*MLH1, MSH2, MSH6, PMS2*)
	Next-generation sequencing	MSI revealed in the tumor tissue
	Pathogenic variant detection	Identification of a pathogenic variant in an MMR gene in the tumor tissue
Cancer history	Colorectal or endometrial cancer	
	Diagnosis before age 50	CRC or endometrial cancer diagnosed before age 50
	Synchronous/Metachronous Lynch syndrome-related cancers	Including colorectal, endometrial, ovarian, stomach, small bowel, urinary tract, biliary tract, prostate, brain, sebaceous adenomas, sebaceous carcinomas, keratoacanthomas, pancreatic cancers
	Colorectal tumor with MSI-high histology features	Such as poor differentiation, tumor-infiltrating lymphocytes, Crohn-like lymphocytic reaction, mucinous/signet-ring differentiation, medullary growth pattern
	Family history	At least one first-degree relative with Lynch syndrome-related cancer diagnosed before age 50. At least two first-degree relatives with any Lynch syndrome-related cancers, regardless of age. A family member with colorectal or endometrial cancer meeting one of the above criteria

Table modified and adapted from Genereviews [82]

anomalies and supra- and infratentorial areas of high FLAIR signal intensity NF1-like (Fig. 5.4) [88].

While the diagnostic criteria for CMMRD were established by Wimmer et al. in 2014 and are represented in Tables 5.14 and 5.15, which summarize the diagnostic criteria for CMMRD, along with clinical considerations for differentiating CMMRD from NF1 and indications for CMMRD testing, respectively [82, 86, 87]. In addition to a family history of cancer and/or consanguinity, specific radiological and histological findings can be critical for diagnosing CMMRD [82, 86, 87].

Finally, the diagnosis for LS and CMMRD can be established in a proband when a heterozygous or biallelic pathogenic (or likely pathogenic) germline variant, respectively, is found by genetic testing in one of the following genes: *MLH1*, *MSH2*, *MSH6*, *PMS2* [82, 86, 87]. Genetic testing for LS and CMMRD typically includes multigene panels targeting *MLH1, MSH2, MSH6, PMS2*, and *EPCAM*, together with deletion and methylation analyses when appropriate [82, 86, 87]. Broader genomic approaches, such as whole-exome or whole-genome sequencing, may also be considered in selected cases [82, 86, 87]. Immunohistochemical analysis of MMR proteins in tumor and normal tissues may help differentiate LS from CMMRD [82, 86, 87]. In LS-associated tumors, loss of MMR protein expression is generally restricted to tumor tissue, whereas in CMMRD, the loss is detectable in both tumor and normal cells [82, 86, 87]. Both disorders are characterized by high tumor mutation burden, although ultra-hypermutated tumors are more commonly associated with CMMRD [82, 86, 87].

CMMRD-associated gliomas may show distinctive histopathologic and molecular features, including loss of MMR protein expression, giant and pleomorphic glial cells, and secondary POLE/

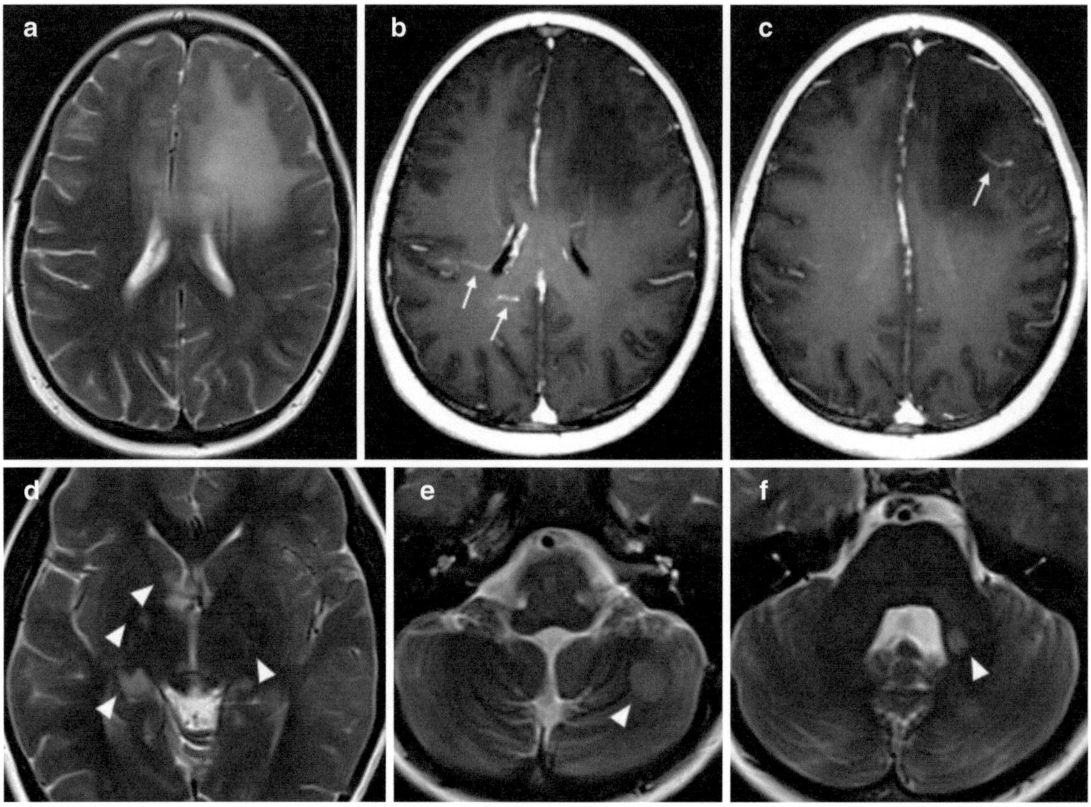

Fig. 5.4 High-grade glioma in a 10-year-old boy with mismatch repair deficiency syndrome. Axial T2 (**a**) and post-contrast T1 MRI images show an extensive bifrontal neoplasm with callosal involvement and ill-defined borders. Presence of some DVAs (**b** and **c**, arrows) and supra- and subtentorial NF1-like high T2 signal intensity (FASIs, **d–f**, arrowheads)

Table 5.14 Diagnostic criteria for constitutional mismatch repair deficiency syndrome - clinical considerations for differentiating CMMRD from Neurofibromatosis type 1

Clinical features similar to NF1:	Differentiation from NF1
Presence of CALM	CALM are common in both NF1 and CMMRD
Malignant tumors (e.g., brain tumors)	Malignant brain tumors are rare in NF1
Juvenile intestinal polyposis	If a child with CALM develops a malignant tumor, CMMRD should be considered before diagnosing NF1, especially with advanced therapeutic strategies available.

Table modified and adapted from Genereviews [82]

POLD1 mutations contributing to hypermutation [82, 86, 87]. Somatic POLE-mutated LS tumors may occasionally mimic the molecular profile of CMMRD-associated tumors [82, 86, 87].

The increasing use of large-scale sequencing platforms has improved the identification of pediatric LS and CMMRD cases, although the precise contribution of LS to childhood-onset tumors remains incompletely understood [83].

Although MMR deficiency and Lynch syndrome are uncommon in gliomas overall, they are more frequently observed in younger patients with IDH-wildtype glioblastomas [82, 86, 87]. These findings support the use of MMR testing in selected gliomas, particularly in patients younger than 50 years of age [82, 86, 87].

Table 5.15 Indication for constitutional mismatch repair deficiency syndrome testing. [a]Testing for CMMRD is indicated if the total score is ≥3 points

Criteria	Description	Points
Malignancies/premalignancies (one mandatory; add points if more than one present)		
Carcinoma from the Lynch syndrome (LS) spectrum[a]	At age <25 years	3 points
Multiple bowel adenomas or single high-grade dysplasia adenoma	At age <25 years, without APC/MUTYH variants	3 points
WHO grade III or IV glioma	At age <25 years	2 points
NHL (T-cell lineage) or sPNET	At age <18 years	2 points
Any malignancy	At age <18 years	1 point
Additional features (optional; add points if more than one present)		
NF1 clinical signs or ≥2 hyperpigmented/hypopigmented skin lesions	Lesions >1 cm	2 points
Diagnosis of LS in a first-degree or second-degree relative		2 points
Carcinoma from LS spectrum[a]	Before age 60 in a first, second, or third-degree relative	1 point
Sibling with carcinoma from LS spectrum[a], high-grade glioma, sPNET, or NHL		2 points
Sibling with any childhood malignancy		1 point
Multiple pilomatricomas	In the patient	2 points
One pilomatricoma	In the patient	1 point
Agenesis of corpus callosum or non-therapy-induced cavernoma	In the patient	1 point
Consanguineous parents		1 point
Deficiency/reduced levels of IgG2/4 and/or IgA		1 point

Table modified and adapted from Genereviews [87]
[a]*LS spectrum* lynch syndrome-associated cancers

Patients with MMR-deficient tumors should undergo genetic counseling and germline testing for LS-associated genes, as the diagnosis has important implications for surveillance, family screening, and reproductive counseling [82, 86, 87].In suspected cases of constitutional mismatch repair deficiency syndrome (CMMRD), counseling should also address the high risk of multiple malignancies and the 25% recurrence risk among siblings [82, 86, 87].

5.2.3.2 Surveillance

The surveillance recommendations for individuals with LS and CMMRD are reported in Tables 5.16 and 5.17, respectively [82, 86, 87]. In summary, LS association with MMR deficiency in gliomas, particularly IDH-wildtype glioblastomas in younger patients, highlights the necessity of genetic testing and counseling for appropriate management and surveillance [82, 86, 87].

5.2.4 Rhabdoid Tumor Predisposition Syndrome

Rhabdoid Tumor Predisposition Syndrome (RTPS) arises from germline loss-of-function variants in the *SMARCB1* gene and is phenotypically distinct from schwannomatosis despite both syndromes sharing a common genetic variant [89–91]. More recently, germline variants in the *SMARCA4* gene have also been linked to RTPS [92]. Both variants are inherited in an autosomal dominant manner [93, 94]. Patients with germline *SMARCB1* variants are classified as RTPS type 1, while those with germline *SMARCA4* variants are categorized as RTPS type 2 [93, 94] Patients with *SMARCB1* variants tend to develop more aggressive tumors, such as atypical teratoid rhabdoid tumors (AT/RT), intracranial meningiomas, schwannomas, and malignant peripheral nerve sheath tumors [93, 94]. Conversely, patients

Table 5.16 Surveillance recommendations for individuals with Lynch Syndrome

Area of surveillance	Procedure	Age	Frequency
Colorectal cancer	Colonoscopy	20–25 years or earlier if positive family history	Every 1–2 years
Gynecological cancer	Education for females	All ages	Annually
	Transvaginal ultrasound, CA125 test, and endometrial biopsy	From the age of 30–35 (ACG, USMSTF, ESMO) or 35–40 years (Mallorca group)	Every 1–2/3 years—several annual surveillance modalities have been proposed by many professional societies.
Gastric cancer	Upper endoscopy	30–35 years or earlier if positive family history	Every 3–5 years. Biopsies evaluated for H. Pylori infections
Small bowel cancer	Capsule endoscopy and small bowel Enterography	As needed	As needed
Urothelial cancer	Urine analysis with cytology	As needed	As needed
Pancreatic cancer	Pancreatic cancer screening	As needed	Alternating endoscopic ultrasound and/or MRI/magnetic resonance cholangiopancreatography as needed
Other cancers	No additional specific screening recommendations for other Lynch syndrome-associated cancers	Adhere to standard population screening recommendations. Obtain immediate medical evaluation for any health changes or ongoing symptoms. Modify screening schedules to start earlier if there is a family history of early onset of other cancer types.	If there is a family history of early onset of other cancer types, screening guidelines should be modified to initiate screening at a younger age.

Table modified and adapted from Genereviews [82]

Table 5.17 Surveillance recommendations for individuals with constitutional mismatch repair deficiency syndrome syndrome

Surveillance protocol for CMMRD	Details
Clinical examination	Every 6 months from the time of diagnosis
Brain MRI	Every 6–12 months starting at least by age 2
Ileocolonoscopy	Annually from age 6
Esophagogastroduodenoscopy/video capsule	Annually from age 10
Other annual procedures	To account for the increased risk of gynecological and urinary tract cancers
Family discussion	The benefits of surveillance protocols should be carefully analyzed and discussed with each family

Table modified and adapted from Genereviews [82]

with *SMARCA4* variants have a higher risk of developing ovarian and thoracic carcinoma, in addition to rhabdoid tumors [93, 94]. AT/RT can often be the first manifestation of RTPS, which is why current recommendations advise testing for germline variants in both genes in all newly diagnosed AT/RT cases [93, 94]. The presence of a germline *SMARCB1* variant generally indicates a poorer prognosis. An initial diagnosis of RTPS can be confirmed by identifying a germline heterozygous variant in either gene in a patient with a rhabdoid tumor anywhere in the body and/or a family history of rhabdoid tumors or other typical tumors as described above. Surveillance guidelines published by the American Association for Cancer Research (AACR) Childhood Cancer

Predisposition Workshop recommend an MRI of the brain and ultrasound of the abdomen every 3 months from diagnosis until the age of 5 years and a whole-body MRI at the age of five [95]. These recommendations apply specifically to truncating or loss-of-function variants in the *SMARCB1* gene [95]. There are no recommendations for brain imaging for *SMARCA4* variants or germline missense variants of *SMARCB1* [95]. The only recommendation for *SMARCA4* mutations is an abdominal ultrasound every 6 months and consideration of oophorectomy if deemed high-risk after childhood [95].

5.2.4.1 Diagnosis

The diagnosis of RTPS is established in individuals with rhabdoid tumors, a family history of rhabdoid tumors, or multiple SMARCB1- or SMARCA4-deficient tumors, together with the identification of a germline pathogenic variant in *SMARCB1* (RTPS1) or *SMARCA4* (RTPS2) (Table 5.18) [93, 94]. Most RTPS cases are associated with *SMARCB1* pathogenic variants, whereas SMARCA4-related RTPS is less frequent and appears to show incomplete penetrance [93, 94]. SMARCA4 pathogenic alterations may also be inherited from apparently unaffected parents [93, 94]. Both SMARCB1- and SMARCA4-related RTPS are associated with an aggressive clinical course and poorer prognosis compared with sporadic rhabdoid tumors, although long-term survival has been reported in selected cases [93, 94].

The penetrance of *SMARCB1*-related RTPS is >90% by age 5 years. Germline mosaicism is reported in 50% of families with this syndrome. Most of these individuals have a de novo germline variant [93, 94]. Germline and postzygotic mosaicism are increasingly recognized and may complicate diagnosis, especially in patients without a clear family history [93, 94, 96]. When the proband has a rhabdoid tumor and/or a family history of rhabdoid tumor and/or multiple SMARCB1- or SMARCA4-deficient tumors (synchronous or metachronous) and a germline pathogenic alteration in SMARCB1 or

Table 5.18 Suggesting finding: clinical features, genetic testing, and laboratory features of tumor tissue recommendations for rhabdoid tumors

Clinical features	*Details*
Congenital onset	Diagnosis before birth or symptoms occurring within the first 28 days of life.
Early age of onset	Rhabdoid tumors in individuals younger than 12 months.
Advanced disease stage	Diagnosis at a later stage, such as greater than M1 according to Chang classification or stage ≥II in extracranial malignant rhabdoid tumors.
Multiple tumors	Presence of more than one primary rhabdoid tumor simultaneously.
Family history	History of rhabdoid tumors, small-cell ovarian carcinoma (hypercalcemic type), or other malignant tumors, including cribriform neuroepithelial tumor, malignant peripheral nerve sheath tumor, myeloid sarcoma, epithelioid schwannoma, meningioma, benign myoepithelioma, chondrosarcoma, or ganglioglioma.
RTPS family history	Family history of rhabdoid tumor predisposition syndrome (RTPS).
Genetic testing	*Details*
Rhabdoid tumors	Testing is recommended for any rhabdoid tumor (at any age), familial rhabdoid tumors, multifocal tumors, or tumors with congenital onset.
SMARCB1 deficiency	Testing for tumors lacking SMARCB1 with a family history of rhabdoid tumors or early childhood cancer (before age 5).
SMARCA4 deficiency	Testing for tumors with absent SMARCA4 and a family history of rhabdoid tumors or early childhood cancer (before age 5).
Somatic testing	*Details*
Immunohistochemistry	The absence of SMARCB1 (INI-1) or SMARCA4 (BRG-1) staining indicates a lack of functional protein in the tumor tissue.
Molecular genetic testing	Identification of somatic *SMARCB1* or *SMARCA4* disease-causing variants in a rhabdoid tumor. Note: Fresh-frozen tumor is preferred; formalin-fixed, paraffin-embedded samples may also be acceptable.

Table modified and adapted from Genereviews [94]

SMARCA4, the diagnosis of RTPS is established in any proband [93, 94]. Sequence analysis and gene-targeted deletion/duplication analysis (MLPA) are recommended in individuals with the absence of SMARCB1 or SMARCA4 identified on tumor immunohistochemistry. A multi-gene panel can be performed [93, 94]. Advanced NGS approaches have improved the detection of low-level mosaic variants [93, 94, 96]. Genetic counseling and testing should be offered to parents and at-risk relatives, as siblings may also carry pathogenic variants and require surveillance [93, 94]. Prenatal and preimplantation genetic testing may be considered when the familial pathogenic variant is known [93, 94]. Specific brain MRI features on an atypical rhabdoid teratoid tumor (ATRT) in Rhabdoid Tumor Predisposition Syndrome in a 15-year-old boy is reported in Fig. 5.5.

5.2.4.2 Surveillance

RTPS1 is linked to the early onset of INI1-deficient rhabdoid tumors in childhood. A study involving 83 individuals identified 16 cases with RTPS1, some of whom underwent tumor monitoring. Three patients developed tumors between the ages of 9 and 17, partly detected through surveillance. A literature review highlighted an ongoing risk of tumor development beyond the age of five. Extending the surveillance period beyond this age could potentially improve outcomes for RTPS1 patients [97]. Table 5.19 outlines the recommended monitoring protocol for

Table 5.19 Surveillance for individuals with pathogenic germline variants in *SMARCB1* or *SMARCA4*

Age range	Examinations and imaging
Birth to 6 months	Monthly or every 2–3 months: Comprehensive clinical examination, including neurological assessment, abdominal and neck ultrasound, head ultrasound, brain and spine MRI, or whole-body MRI.
Seven to eighteen months	Every 2–3 months: Detailed clinical examination, including neurological evaluation and abdominal and neck ultrasound. Consider brain and spine MRI if whole-body MRI does not sufficiently visualize brain structures.
Nineteen months to five years	Every 3 months: Thorough clinical examination, including neurological assessment, abdominal and neck ultrasound, and brain and spine MRI.
After age 5 years	Every 6 months: Comprehensive clinical examination and neurological assessment.—annually: Whole-body MRI.—for those with SMARCA4-related SCCOHT: Abdominal and pelvic ultrasound every 6 months.

Table modified and adapted from Genereviews [94]

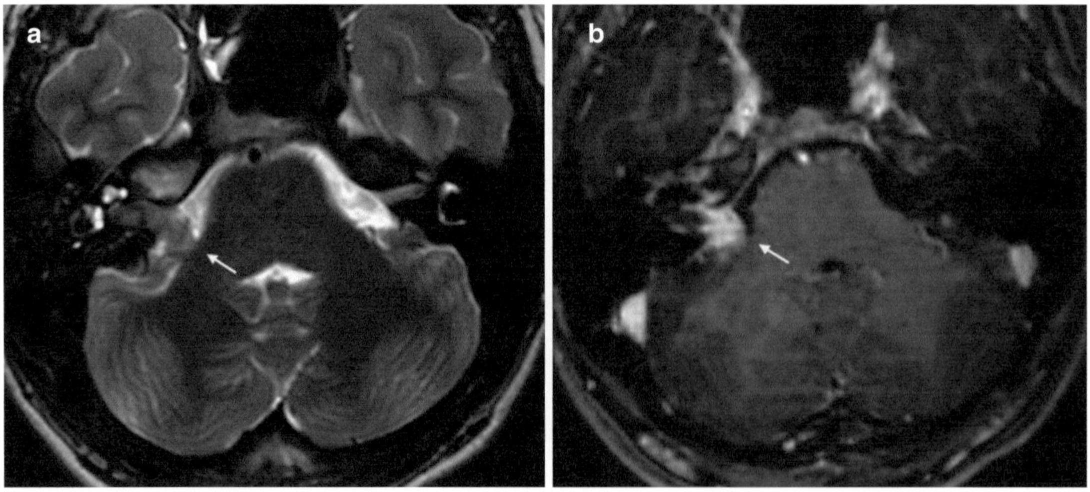

Fig. 5.5 Atypical rhabdoid teratoid tumor (ATRT) in Rhabdoid Tumor Predisposition Syndrome in a 15-year-old boy. Axial T2 and post-contrast T1 MRI images show a neoplasm in the right ponto-cerebellar angle (**a** and **b**, arrows) with low T2 signal and inhomogeneous contrast enhancement, extending into the external auditory canal, which appears enlarged

individuals with pathogenic germline variants in SMARCB1 or SMARCA4, including whole-body MRI and additional clinical evaluations at various age intervals [93, 94].

5.2.5 Familial Adenomatous Polyposis

Familial adenomatous polyposis (FAP) is an autosomal dominant disorder, part of a larger group of *APC*-associated polyposis conditions, characterized by pathogenic variants in the *APC* gene [98]. The penetrance appears to be complete in FAP; in contrast, little is known in attenuated FAP [99].

FAP presents the co-occurrence of brain tumors, primarily MBs [98]. It has been observed that affected FAP patients exhibiting the colonic polyposis phenotype present the tendency to develop the disease after the age of 17, while those without this phenotype may manifest the disease in the form of brain tumors by the age of 10 [100]. In FAP patients, a variant of the syndrome can manifest, characterized by the occurrence of brain tumors without concurrent polyposis, explained by the hypothesis that death occurs before adenomatous polyposis forms [101, 102]. Moreover, skin lesions, most commonly epidermal cysts, may also arise. In individuals with FAP, there is a 92% increased risk of developing MB, and its development has been reported in about 40% of patients affected by FAP. Specifically, certain recurring manifestations have been highlighted, including the development of the classic histological variant of MB, absence of metastasis at onset, and molecular subgroup WNT. Patients may also exhibit rarely pituitary, astrocytomas, or adenomas, and neurological manifestations can arise, varying on the base of the tumor's location [9, 103].

5.2.5.1 Diagnosis

Familial adenomatous polyposis and other APC-associated polyposis conditions should be suspected in individuals with multiple colorectal adenomatous polyps, particularly when associated with early-onset disease or a positive family history [102, 104]. The presence of a pathogenic APC variant, extracolonic manifestations, or characteristic tumors further supports the diagnosis [102, 104]. Extracolonic manifestations include congenital hypertrophy of the retinal pigment epithelium (CHRPE), desmoid tumors, osteomas, dental anomalies, duodenal adenomas, gastric polyposis, hepatoblastoma, thyroid carcinoma, and medulloblastoma [102, 104]. APC-associated polyposis may also present with early-onset colorectal cancer in patients with relatively few adenomas [102, 104]. Diagnosis is confirmed by identification of a pathogenic APC variant according to established clinical and molecular criteria (Table 5.20) [102, 104].

Genetic testing for FAP includes *APC* sequencing and deletion/duplication analysis, including evaluation of regulatory regions [102, 104]. In patients with negative germline testing but strong clinical suspicion, multigene panels or analysis of adenoma tissue may help identify somatic mosaicism [102, 104]. Approximately 25% of FAP cases arise de novo, and parental mosaicism should be considered in apparently sporadic cases [102, 105]. Genetic counseling and testing are recommended for parents, siblings, and at-risk relatives, as asymptomatic car-

Table 5.20 Familial adenomatous polyposis criteria

Condition	Diagnostic criteria
Classic FAP	Diagnosis is made with a heterozygous germline pathogenic variant in *APC* and one of the following:
	100 or more colorectal adenomatous polyps (younger individuals or those with colectomies may have fewer than 100 polyps)
	Multiple colorectal adenomatous polyps (fewer than 100) along with a family member with confirmed classic FAP
Attenuated FAP	Diagnosis is established with a heterozygous germline pathogenic variant in *APC* and one of the following:
	A relative with confirmed attenuated FAP
	Fewer than 100 colorectal adenomatous polyps
	More than 100 colorectal adenomatous polyps in individuals over 40 years old

Table modified and adapted from Genereviews [101]

Table 5.21 Surveillance guidelines for Familial adenomatous polyposis

Age group	Screening/examination	Frequency
Classic FAP	Colorectal screening (colonoscopy)	Every 1–2 years from age 10–15
Attenuated FAP	Colorectal screening (colonoscopy)	Late adolescence
Both classic and attenuated FAP	Esophagogastroduodenoscopy and small bowel examination	By age 20–25 or before colon surgery
Both classic and attenuated FAP	Annual thyroid palpation, thyroid ultrasound, neurological examination, and abdominal examination for desmoids	Annually
Under 5 years (for hepatoblastoma)	Liver palpation, liver ultrasound, serum alpha-fetoprotein measurement	Every 3–6 months

Table modified and adapted from Genereviews [101]

riers may occur due to reduced clinical expression or mosaicism [106, 107]. Offspring of affected individuals have a 50% risk of inheriting the pathogenic APC variant, and predictive testing is possible once the familial variant has been identified [102, 104].

5.2.5.2 Surveillance

Table 5.21 outlines the recommended surveillance protocols for individuals with Familial Adenomatous Polyposis (FAP) [102, 104]. It includes the frequency and type of screenings and examinations based on the individual's age and condition, with a particular focus on colorectal cancer, desmoid tumors, and hepatoblastoma [102, 104].

5.2.6 Cowden Syndrome

PTEN Hamartoma Tumor Syndrome (PHTS) is inherited as an autosomal dominant trait and typically linked to a germline alteration in the phosphatase and tensin homolog (*PTEN*) gene [108, 109]. PHTS encompasses several conditions, including Cowden Syndrome (CS), Bannayan-Riley-Ruvalcaba Syndrome (BRRS), and *PTEN*-related Proteus-like Syndrome. In 10–44% of PHTS index cases, pathogenic de novo variants were found in the *PTEN* gene [106–110]. The other non-*PTEN* genes are likely linked to distinct molecular genetic mechanisms. It has been suggested also to consider a germline KLLN epimutation and SDHB-D analysis, including PIK3CA, AKT1, SEC23B, and WWP1 [111–114].

CS, also known as multiple hamartoma syndrome, is an underdiagnosed genodermatosis and represents the most common phenotypical presentation of the PHTS spectrum [108, 115]. By their 40 s, nearly all affected individuals develop mucocutaneous manifestations, most commonly trichilemmomas and papillomatous papules, along with acral and plantar keratoses. Patients with CS also frequently exhibit macrocephaly and dolichocephaly [108, 115–117].

The majority of people with PHTS frequently develop hamartomatous and mixed gastrointestinal polyps, which elevate the risk for colorectal cancers. Individuals with CS face a heightened risk for breast, thyroid, renal, and endometrial cancers [108, 109, 118]. As with other hereditary cancer syndromes, there is an increased likelihood of multifocal and bilateral cancers, such as those affecting paired organs like the breasts [108, 109, 118]. Those with a germline *PTEN* pathogenic variant are seven times more likely to develop a second primary malignant tumor compared to the general population [108, 118].

Occasionally, individuals with CS may also develop brain tumors and vascular malformations affecting various organs [108, 119].

In Fig. 5.6, the MRI show a medulloblastoma in Cowden syndrome in a 3-year-old girl.

5.2.6.1 Diagnosis

For identifying CS or Cowden-like Syndrome (CLS), a scoring system developed from over 3000 cases helps evaluate the likelihood of a *PTEN* pathogenic variant based on clinical features (Table 5.22) and age at diagnosis [108, 115, 120].

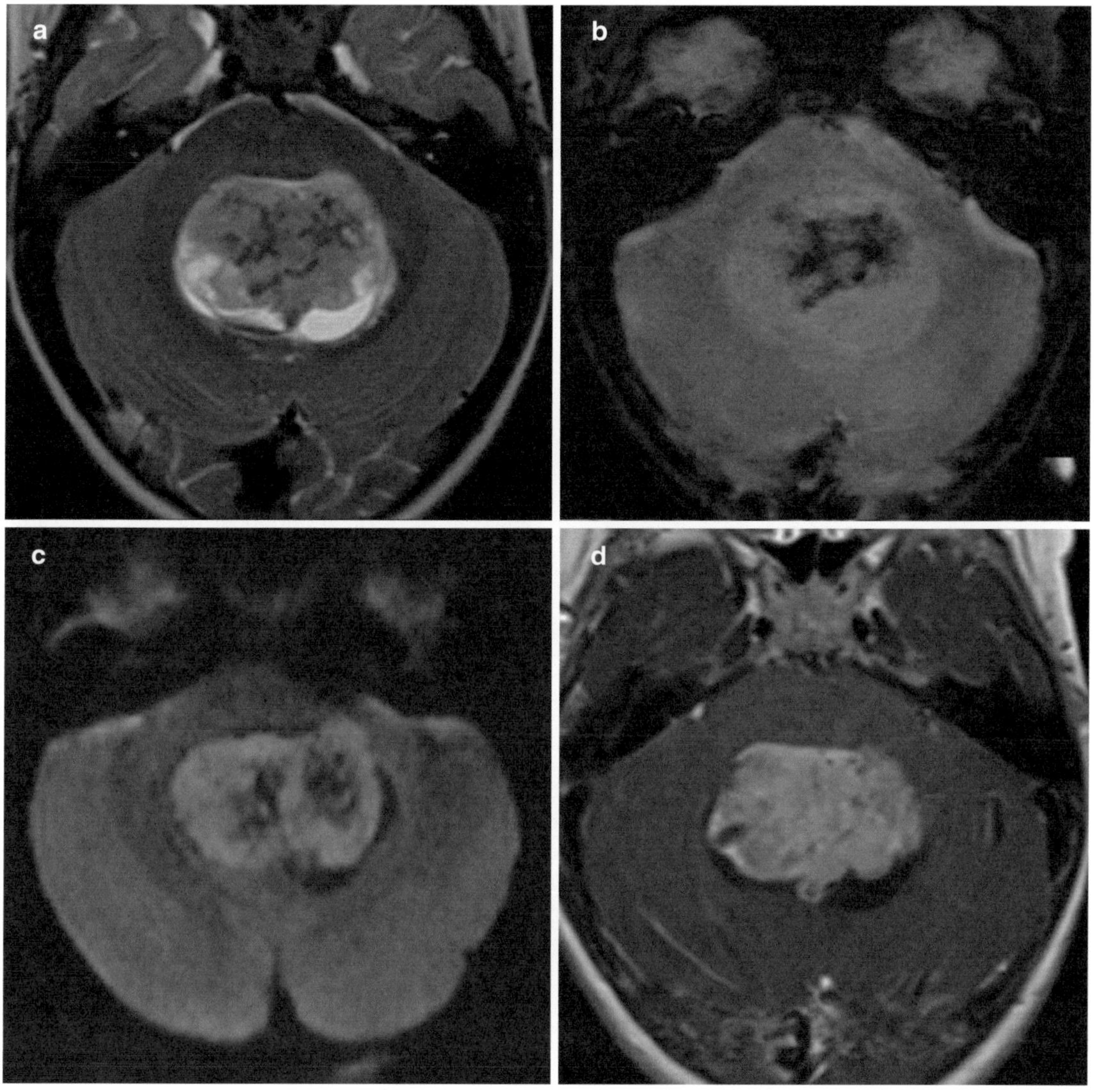

Fig. 5.6 Medulloblastoma in Cowden Syndrome in a 3-year-old girl. The MRI study shows a voluminous lesion of the posterior fossa occupying the fourth ventricle with inhomogeneous T2 signal (**a**), hemorrhage/mineralizations on SWI sequences (**b**), restricted diffusivity (**c**) and intense contrast enhancement (**d**)

Consensus clinical diagnostic criteria for CS, categorized into pathognomonic, major, and minor criteria, are updated annually by the National Comprehensive Cancer Network (see Table 5.23) [108, 115, 120].

A clinical diagnosis of CS is confirmed if an individual satisfies the conditions reported in Table 5.24 [108, 115, 120].

The first genetic test that is performed is *PTEN* gene analysis. In case the sequence analysis comes up negative, a deletion/duplication analysis of the gene should be performed. In the event that the deletion/duplication analysis is also negative, the *PTEN* promoter sequence is analyzed to identify possible variants that are responsible for the altered *PTEN* gene expression; in addition, a multigene panel analysis may also be performed [108, 115, 120].

Genetic testing is also recommended for the proband's parents, also to define whether or not the variant is inherited. Failure to find the variant in either parent may underscore that the variant is de novo or inherited from a lesser affected mosaic parent [108, 115, 120].

Table 5.22 Suggestive findings for Cowden Syndrome (CS)

	Criteria
Adults	Clinical threshold—A score of ten or above indicates the need to refer the individual to a genetic specialist for further PHTS evaluation.
Children	Consider PHTS if presenting with macrocephaly and one or more of the following:
	Autism or developmental delays
	Dermatologic features (lipomas, trichilemmomas, oral papillomas, penile freckling)
	Vascular issues (arteriovenous malformations, hemangiomas)
	Gastrointestinal polyps
	Pediatric-onset thyroid cancer or germ cell tumors

Table modified and adapted from Genereviews [108]

5.2.6.2 Surveillance

Table 5.25 outlines the recommended surveillance practices of PHTS generally to identify tumors at the earliest and most treatable stages based on age and specific circumstances [108, 115, 120, 121].

5.2.7 Nevoid Basal Cell Carcinoma (Gorlin) Syndrome

Gorlin Syndrome (GS), also known as Gorlin-Goltz syndrome or nevoid basal cell carcinoma syndrome (NBCCS), presents in 1/31,000–1/164,000 in Europe and has a prevalence at birth of 1/19,000 in the UK, the same frequency between males and females [122]. The Gorlin syndrome is genetically linked to hetero-

Table 5.23 Diagnostic criteria for Cowden syndrome

Criteria type	Criteria	Description
Major criteria	Breast cancer	Any form of breast cancer.
	Epithelial thyroid cancer	Includes non-medullary thyroid cancers, particularly follicular thyroid cancer.
	Macrocephaly	Occipital-frontal circumference ≥ 97th percentile.
	Endometrial carcinoma	Cancer of the endometrial lining of the uterus.
Minor criteria	Other thyroid lesions	Includes thyroid adenomas and multinodular goiter.
	Intellectual disability	IQ ≤75, indicating cognitive impairment.
	Hamartomatous intestinal polyps	Non-cancerous polyps in the intestines.
	Fibrocystic disease of the breast	A benign condition involving cysts and fibrosis in the breast tissue.
	Lipomas	Benign tumors of fatty tissue.
	Fibromas	Benign tumors of fibrous tissue.
	Genitourinary tumors	Includes tumors such as renal cell carcinoma.
	Genitourinary malformation	Abnormalities in the reproductive and urinary systems.
	Uterine fibroids	Benign tumors in the uterus
Pathognomonic criteria	Adult Lhermitte-Duclos disease	Presence of cerebellar dysplastic gangliocytoma [Zhou et al. 2003a]
	Mucocutaneous lesions	
	Trichilemmomas (facial)	Facial lesions typical of CS
	Acral Keratoses	Thickened patches on extremities
	Papillomatous lesions	Wart-like growths, seen on the skin
	Mucosal lesions	Lesions on mucous membranes, such as inside the mouth

Table modified and adapted from Genereviews [108]

Table 5.24 Diagnosis of Cowden Syndrome

Criteria type	Criteria
Pathognomonic mucocutaneous lesions	Six or more facial papules, with at least three being trichilemmomas
	Cutaneous facial papules combined with oral mucosal papillomatosis
	Oral mucosal papillomatosis along with acral keratoses
	Six or more palmoplantar keratoses
Two or more major criteria	
One major and three or more minor criteria	
Four or more minor criteria	

Table modified and adapted from Genereviews [108]

Table 5.25 Surveillance guidelines for early tumor detection of PTEN Hamartoma Tumor Syndrome

Age group/ circumstance	Surveillance recommendations
Children (under 18 years)	Conduct annual thyroid ultrasounds from diagnosis (earliest at age 7) and perform routine skin assessments
Adults	Annual thyroid ultrasounds and dermatological check-ups
Women (starting at age 30)	Monthly self-breast examinations and annual breast screenings, including at least mammograms (consider adding MRI). From age 35, consider transvaginal ultrasound or endometrial biopsy
Men and women	Start colonoscopy at age 35, with frequency based on polyposis level or family history of early-onset colon cancer (before age 40). Perform renal imaging (CT or MRI) every 2 years starting at age 40
Family history of early-onset cancer	Begin screening 5–10 years earlier than the age at which the youngest family member was diagnosed

Table modified and adapted from Genereviews [108]

zygous variants that result in the abnormal activation of SHH signaling and disruption of the normal functioning of the pathway crucial for brain development [123]. Pathogenic variants in *PTCH1* are the most frequently encountered, followed by *SUFU* variants, resulting in increased cellular growth and decreased cellular death [123, 124]. Recommendations for surveillance were proposed for individuals carrying these variants, including basal cell carcinoma screening every year by the age of 10, echocardiography in infancy, and MB screening with brain MRI, mainly in individuals carrying *SUFU* pathogenic variants [125]. The clinical phenotype includes patients with multiple keratocysts in the jaw, occurring during the second decade of life, and basal cell carcinomas (BCCs) usually begin to appear during the third decade of life [123–127]. Patients with *PTCH1* variants exhibit higher penetrance (90%) of BCCs and jaw keratocysts than those with *SUFU* variants [123–127]. A majority of affected individuals (60%) exhibit a characteristic phenotype, and several other manifestations have been recognized linked to this syndrome, most notably macrocephaly, congenital skeletal anomalies, facial abnormalities, and cutaneous changes [123–127]. Although the evidence of this syndrome may only become clear in adulthood, there are certain early clinical indicators important for the diagnosis, such as the presence of odontogenic keratocysts in children under 20 years old, basal cell carcinomas in individuals under 20 years old, pits on the palms or soles of the feet, calcification of the falx cerebri, and *DNMB* variant, associated with other criteria. MB is the most prevalent CNS tumor in the context of Gorlin syndrome (GS) and typically arises at an earlier age compared to sporadic tumors; it is estimated that GS is present in 5% of patients diagnosed with MB before the age of 5 and in 3.6% of patients at the age of 2 [123–127]. According to extensive population-based studies, the risk of developing an MB is less than 2% in *PTCH1*-mutated patients and 33% in individuals with *SUFU* variants [123–127].

5.2.7.1 Diagnosis

No widely accepted clinical diagnostic criteria for GS have been established. Proposed diagnostic criteria for GS have been put forward by various sources [123–125]. GS should be considered in individuals with the following findings, categorized into major and minor diagnostic criteria reported in Table 5.26 [123–125].

Table 5.26 Diagnostic criteria for Gorlin Syndrome

Criteria	Details
Major criteria	
Lamellar calcification	Sheet-like calcification of the falx or clear calcification evidence in individuals under 20 years old. Note: Falx calcification is usually present on anteroposterior skull radiographs after age 20
Jaw Keratocyst	Odontogenic keratocyst histologically; seen as translucency on orthopantomogram
Palmar/plantar pits	Two or more pits, more visible after soaking hands and feet in warm water for up to 10 minutes. Pits may appear as white "punched-out" or pink "pin-prick" lesions
Multiple basal cell carcinomas (BCCs)	More than five BCCs in a lifetime or a BCC before age 30. Risk factors include skin type and sun exposure
First-degree relative with GS	Diagnosis of GS in a first-degree relative
Minor criteria	
Childhood Medulloblastoma	Also known as primitive neuroectodermal tumor. Note: Suggestions exist to upgrade this to a major criterion with two minor criteria
Mesenteric lymphatic or pleural cysts	Presence of these cysts
Macrocephaly	Occipital-frontal circumference above the 97th percentile
Cleft lip/palate	Presence of cleft lip or palate
Rib/vertebral anomalies	Bifid, splayed, or extra ribs and bifid vertebrae observed on chest or spine radiographs
Preaxial or postaxial polydactyly	Presence of extra digits
Ovarian/cardiac fibromas	Fibromas in the ovaries or heart
Ocular anomalies	Includes cataracts, developmental defects, and pigmentary changes in the retinal epithelium

Table modified and adapted from Genereviews [124]

The Identification of a pathogenic variant in *PTCH1* or *SUFU* confirms the diagnosis of GS [123–125]. Mosaic PTCH1-related GS should be considered when the pathogenic variant is detected in tumor tissue but absent or present at low allele frequency in peripheral blood DNA [123–125]. Genetic testing typically includes sequencing and deletion/duplication analysis of *PTCH1* and *SUFU*, while multigene panels or broader genomic testing may be considered in atypical cases [123–125]. *PTCH1* testing is particularly indicated in individuals with odontogenic keratocysts, whereas *SUFU* analysis should be considered in patients with medulloblastoma without jaw cysts [123–125]. Most individuals with GS have an affected parent, although reduced penetrance and germline mosaicism may complicate family history assessment [123–125]. Genetic counseling and predictive testing are recommended for at-risk relatives, particularly during childhood, to allow early surveillance for complications such as medulloblastoma [123–125].

5.2.7.2 Surveillance

Table 5.27 outlines the recommended surveillance strategies for monitoring growth, development, and complications [123–125].

5.2.8 Others Cancer Predisposition Syndrome

5.2.8.1 *POT1* Tumor Predisposition

POT1 Tumor Predisposition (*POT1*-TPD) is inherited as an autosomal dominant trait and typically linked to a germline heterozygous alteration in the *POT1* gene [128]. The penetrance is unknown [128]. Most *POT1*-TPD cases are familial, while the proportion of diagnoses due to a de novo pathogenic variant is unknown [128]. Due to the insufficiency of studies performed on *POT1*-TPD case histories and functional studies, many of the variants found are classified as variants of uncertain significance [128].

Table 5.27 Recommended surveillance for Gorlin Syndrome

Surveillance area	Frequency and details
Head circumference	Track growth throughout childhood
Ophthalmology	Schedule evaluations with an ophthalmologist
Feeding, hearing, and speech	Assess as needed, particularly for individuals with a history of cleft lip/palate
Scoliosis	Conduct clinical exams for scoliosis as necessary
Skin examination	Perform annual skin checks
Jaw keratocysts	Obtain orthopantomograms every 12–18 months starting at age 8 to detect keratocysts
Developmental assessment	Conduct evaluations and physical examinations every 6 months until age five due to increased risk of medulloblastoma
Brain MRI	Perform MRIs every 3–4 months until age three, every 6 months until age five, annually until age eight for medulloblastoma, and every 3–5 years starting at age 30 for meningiomas
Ovarian ultrasound	Women should have an ultrasound at age 18

Table modified and adapted from Genereviews [124]

POT1-TPD involves a heightened lifetime risk for developing several conditions, including multiple cutaneous melanomas, chronic lymphocytic leukemia (CLL), angiosarcomas (notably cardiac angiosarcomas), and gliomas. While other cancers, such as colorectal cancer, thyroid cancer, and breast angiosarcomas, have been observed in individuals with *POT1*-TPD, the evidence is limited [128–130]. The initial occurrence of primary cutaneous melanoma can range from 15 to 80 years, with most *POT1*-related cancers being identified in adulthood [128–131].

5.2.8.2 *DICER1* Syndrome

DICER1 syndrome, formerly known as Pleuropulmonary Blastoma (PPB) syndrome, is caused by germline pathogenic variants in the *DICER1* gene, either through truncating variants or deletions [132, 133]. This pleiotropic tumor predisposition syndrome increases the risk of both malignant and benign neoplasms, typically manifesting in childhood [132–135]. Sporadic tumors, which exhibit two somatic *DICER1* variants, have been observed without any identified germline alteration; these tumors usually resemble those seen in individuals with *DICER1* syndrome [132–135]. Classic *DICER1*-associated tumors occurring outside the CNS include pleuropulmonary blastoma (PPB), cystic nephroma, Wilms tumor, Sertoli–Leydig cell tumor, uterine cervical embryonal rhabdomyosarcoma, multinodular goiter, nasal chondromesenchymal hamartoma, and other rare entities [132–135]. Metastatic PPB is considered the most commonly encountered *DICER1*-associated intracranial tumor, while primary *DICER1*-associated CNS tumors include pineoblastoma, pituitary blastoma, ciliary body medulloepithelioma (CBME), infantile cerebellar tumor with embryonal tumor with multilayered rosettes (ETMR)-like, and the newly described "primary *DICER1*-associated CNS sarcoma" (DCS) [132–135].

5.2.8.3 BRCA2-Associated Disorders

Patients with biallelic *BRCA2* variants exhibit the characteristic phenotype of Fanconi Anemia (FA), an autosomal recessive disorder characterized by a defect in DNA repair, leading to progressive failure of the bone marrow, congenital abnormalities, and an increased risk of cancer, including MB [136, 137]. While most solid tumors in FA patients typically manifest after the age of 20, brain tumors have been observed in children under 10 years old, sometimes appearing before the diagnosis [136–138]. FA is driven by pathogenic variants in at least 22 genes (FANCA-FANCW) that form the FA pathway. These genes are critical for repairing DNA crosslinks, and their impairment increases cellular sensitivity to damage from crosslinking agents like specific chemotherapies and radiation treatments [136–139]. The FA-D1 and FA-N complementation groups, caused by biallelic pathogenic variants in *FANCD1/BRCA2* and *FANCN/PALB2*, are rare and are linked to a very high risk of childhood cancers [136–139].

MBs and glioma tend to occur predominantly in individuals with both mutated copies of the *FANCD1/BRCA2* or *FANCN/PALB2* genes

[136–139]. Specifically, studies have demonstrated that BRCA2 biallelic variants exhibit worse PFS and OS compared to those with single heterozygous variants, which instead show a 100% survival rate without secondary tumors. It is particularly crucial to identify the specific variants present, as this information can guide appropriate cancer surveillance and medical management. Tumors harboring pathogenic variants in either BRCA1 or BRCA2 have shown increased sensitivity to PARP inhibitors [140, 141]. Moreover, molecular analysis has highlighted that many patients who develop MB belong to the SHH group, thus ensuring the utilization of target agent-based therapies, especially in the context of significant treatment-related toxicities in FA-affected patients [142, 143]. Furthermore, a connection has been observed between inherited alterations in the BRCA2 and PALB2 genes and a deficit in homologous recombination repair mechanisms (HRD), particularly in individuals with SHH group MB, indicating HRD as a possible biomarker, also useful for evaluating responsiveness to PARP inhibitor therapy [137].

5.3 Therapeutic Implications in CPSs Panorama

Over the past two decades, the recognition and treatment of hereditary cancer predispositions in pediatric and adult oncology have become pivotal aspects of modern clinical practices. Advances in genetic diagnostics and a deeper understanding of cancer-related genetic deleterious variants have enabled the early identification of at-risk children and young adults. This has led to the implementation of personalized monitoring strategies, timely interventions, and tailored therapies, which have improved treatment outcomes and provided families with appropriate support. The management of CPSs involves a combination of continuous surveillance, genetic counseling, and targeted treatments.

Managing CNS tumors associated with CPSs presents a significant challenge for oncologists due to the limited data on the natural progression of these diseases and the optimal therapeutic approaches. Further clinical trials are required to refine practical guidelines and assist oncologists and patients in making informed treatment decisions.

In the therapeutic realm, understanding a genetic predisposition allows for the selection of more precise treatments, reducing toxicity and enhancing prognosis. For instance, in patients with CNS tumors linked to alterations in genes like *TP53* or coding for MMR proteins, specific therapies, such as immune checkpoint inhibitors, may be recommended to exploit the genetic instability of the tumors [144, 145].

Targeted therapies, including PARP inhibitors for tumors with mutated BRCA and immune checkpoint inhibitors for tumors associated with LS, are offering new hope for patients with cancer predisposition syndromes by improving outcomes and minimizing side effects compared to traditional therapies [146, 147].

Additionally, a connection has been observed between inherited variants in *BRCA2* and *PALB2* and a deficiency in HRD, particularly in individuals with SHH-subgroup MB [136]. This suggests that HRD could serve as a valuable biomarker for assessing responsiveness to PARP inhibitors [148].

Genetic counseling plays a crucial role in helping patients and their families understand hereditary risks and therapeutic options, enabling them to make informed decisions about disease management and prevention [18].

This growing understanding of the genetic mechanisms underlying CNS tumors has paved the way for increasingly personalized medicine, where early diagnosis and treatments based on genetic profiling can significantly improve clinical outcomes [149].

5.4 Conclusions

CPSs represent a critical area of focus in oncology. Understanding the genetic basis, clinical manifestations, and appropriate management strategies is essential for improving patient outcomes. Advances in genetic testing and molecular diagnostics continue to enhance our ability to identify and manage these syndromes effectively, paving the way for personalized medicine approaches in oncology. Next-generation genetic technologies have expedited the identification of novel disease-causing genes and expanded our knowledge of the pathogenic mechanisms underlying several CPSs, suggesting new molecular-based categories. Advancement in our genetic understanding has also provided crucial information to develop biomarkers and outcome measures targeting key altered processes in individuals with CPSs, ultimately paving the way for more precise clinical management; early recognition, intensive surveillance, and targeted therapies are key components for the effective management of CPSs, improving the quality of life and survival prospects for patients.

References

1. Zhang J, Walsh MF, Wu G, Edmonson MN, Gruber TA, Easton J, et al. Germline mutations in predisposition genes in pediatric cancer. N Engl J Med. 2015;373(24):2336–46. https://doi.org/10.1056/NEJMoa1508054.
2. Patil P, Pencheva BB, Patil VM, Fangusaro J. Nervous system (NS) tumors in cancer predisposition syndromes. Neurotherapeutics. 2022;19(6):1752–71. https://doi.org/10.1007/s13311-022-01277-w.
3. ICGC PedBrain-Seq Project, ICGC MMML-Seq Project, Gröbner SN, Worst BC, Weischenfeldt J, Buchhalter I, et al. The landscape of genomic alterations across childhood cancers. Nature. 2018;555(7696):321–7. https://doi.org/10.1038/nature25480.
4. Eaton KW, Tooke LS, Wainwright LM, Judkins AR, Biegel JA. Spectrum of *SMARCB1/INI1* mutations in familial and sporadic rhabdoid tumors. Pediatr Blood Cancer. 2011;56(1):7–15. https://doi.org/10.1002/pbc.22831.
5. Price KS, Svenson A, King E, Ready K, Lazarin GA. Inherited cancer in the age of next-generation sequencing. Biol Res Nurs. 2018;20(2):192–204. https://doi.org/10.1177/1099800417750746.
6. Biswas A, Kashyap L, Kakkar A, Sarkar C, Julka P. Atypical teratoid/rhabdoid tumors: challenges and search for solutions. Cancer Manag Res. 2016;8:115–25. https://doi.org/10.2147/CMAR.S83472.
7. Johann PD, Altendorf L, Efremova EM, Holsten T, Steinbügl M, Nemes K, et al. Recurrent atypical teratoid/rhabdoid tumors (AT/RT) reveal discrete features of progression on histology, epigenetics, copy number profiling, and transcriptomics. Acta Neuropathol (Berl). 2023;146(3):527–41. https://doi.org/10.1007/s00401-023-02608-7.
8. Farouk Sait S, Walsh MF, Karajannis MA. Genetic syndromes predisposing to pediatric brain tumors. Neuro-Oncol Pract. 2021;8(4):375–90. https://doi.org/10.1093/nop/npab012.
9. Carta R, Del Baldo G, Miele E, Po A, Besharat ZM, Nazio F, et al. Cancer predisposition syndromes and medulloblastoma in the molecular era. Front Oncol. 2020;10:566822. https://doi.org/10.3389/fonc.2020.566822.
10. Tamura R. Current understanding of neurofibromatosis type 1, 2, and schwannomatosis. Int J Mol Sci. 2021;22(11):5850. https://doi.org/10.3390/ijms22115850.
11. Evans DG, Mostaccioli S, Pang D, Fadzil O Connor M, Pittara M, Champollion N, et al. ERN GENTURIS clinical practice guidelines for the diagnosis, treatment, management and surveillance of people with schwannomatosis. Eur J Hum Genet. 2022;30(7):812–7. https://doi.org/10.1038/s41431-022-01086-x.
12. Carton C, Evans DG, Blanco I, Friedrich RE, Ferner RE, Farschtschi S, et al. ERN GENTURIS tumour surveillance guidelines for individuals with neurofibromatosis type 1. eClinicalMedicine. 2023;56:101818. https://doi.org/10.1016/j.eclinm.2022.101818.
13. Lynch HT, Snyder CL, Shaw TG, Heinen CD, Hitchins MP. Milestones of Lynch syndrome: 1895-2015. Nat Rev Cancer. 2015;15(3):181–94. https://doi.org/10.1038/nrc3878. PubMed PMID: 25673086
14. Frey MK, Ahsan MD, Bergeron H, Lin J, Li X, Fowlkes RK, et al. Cascade testing for hereditary cancer syndromes: should we move toward direct relative contact? A systematic review and meta-analysis. J Clin Oncol. 2022;40(35):4129–43. https://doi.org/10.1200/JCO.22.00303.
15. The European Reference Network GENTURIS, Frebourg T, Bajalica Lagercrantz S, Oliveira C, Magenheim R, Evans DG. Guidelines for the Li–Fraumeni and heritable TP53-related cancer syndromes. Eur J Hum Genet. 2020;28(10):1379–86. https://doi.org/10.1038/s41431-020-0638-4.
16. van Leeuwaarde RS, Ahmad S, van Nesselrooij B, Zandee W, Giles RH. Von Hippel-Lindau syndrome. In: Adam MP, Feldman J, Mirzaa GM, Pagon RA, Wallace SE, Bean LJ, et al., editors. GeneReviews® [Internet]. Seattle (WA): University of Washington, Seattle; 1993 [cited 2024 Sep 28]. Available from: http://www.ncbi.nlm.nih.gov/books/NBK1463/. PubMed PMID: 20301636.
17. Bakhuizen JJ, Hanson H, Van Der Tuin K, Lalloo F, Tischkowitz M, Wadt K, et al. Surveillance recommendations for DICER1 pathogenic variant carriers: a report from the SIOPE Host Genome Working Group and CanGene-CanVar Clinical Guideline Working Group. Fam Cancer. 2021;20(4):337–48. https://doi.org/10.1007/s10689-021-00264-y.

18. Schienda J, Stopfer J. Cancer genetic counseling—current practice and future challenges. Cold Spring Harb Perspect Med. 2020;10(6):a036541. https://doi.org/10.1101/cshperspect.a036541.
19. Friedman JM. Neurofibromatosis 1. In: Adam MP, Feldman J, Mirzaa GM, Pagon RA, Wallace SE, Bean LJ, et al., editors. GeneReviews® [Internet]. Seattle (WA): University of Washington, Seattle; 1993 [cited 2024 Sep 28]. Available from: http://www.ncbi.nlm.nih.gov/books/NBK1109/. PubMed PMID: 20301288.
20. Ratner N, Miller SJ. A RASopathy gene commonly mutated in cancer: the neurofibromatosis type 1 tumour suppressor. Nat Rev Cancer. 2015;15(5):290–301. https://doi.org/10.1038/nrc3911.
21. Ferner RE. Neurofibromatosis 1 and neurofibromatosis 2: a twenty first century perspective. Lancet Neurol. 2007;6(4):340–51. https://doi.org/10.1016/S1474-4422(07)70075-3.
22. Rasmussen SA, Friedman JM. NF1 gene and Neurofibromatosis 1. Am J Epidemiol. 2000;151(1):33–40. https://doi.org/10.1093/oxfordjournals.aje.a010118.
23. Ferner RE, Gutmann DH. Neurofibromatosis type 1 (NF1). In: Handbook of clinical neurology [internet]. Elsevier; 2013 [cited 2024 Sep 28]. pp. 939–55. Available from: https://linkinghub.elsevier.com/retrieve/pii/B9780444529022000539 doi:https://doi.org/10.1016/B978-0-444-52902-2.00053-9.
24. DeBella K, Poskitt K, Szudek J, Friedman JM. Use of "unidentified bright objects" on MRI for diagnosis of neurofibromatosis 1 in children. Neurology. 2000;54(8):1646–51. https://doi.org/10.1212/WNL.54.8.1646.
25. Ozarslan B, Russo T, Argenziano G, Santoro C, Piccolo V. Cutaneous findings in neurofibromatosis type 1. Cancer. 2021;13(3):463. https://doi.org/10.3390/cancers13030463.
26. Albaghdadi M, Thibodeau ML, Lara-Corrales I. Updated approach to patients with multiple Café au Lait macules. Dermatol Clin. 2022;40(1):9–23. https://doi.org/10.1016/j.det.2021.08.002.
27. Sobczuk P, Teterycz P, Czarnecka AM, Świtaj T, Koseła-Paterczyk H, Kozak K, et al. Malignant peripheral nerve sheath tumors—outcomes and prognostic factors based on the reference center experience. Surg Oncol. 2020;35:276–84. https://doi.org/10.1016/j.suronc.2020.09.011.
28. Martin E, Coert JH, Flucke UE, Slooff WM, Van De Sande MAJ, Van Noesel MM, et al. Neurofibromatosis-associated malignant peripheral nerve sheath tumors in children have a worse prognosis: a nationwide cohort study. Pediatr Blood Cancer. 2020;67(4):e28138. https://doi.org/10.1002/pbc.28138.
29. Tang Y, Gutmann DH. Neurofibromatosis type 1-associated optic pathway gliomas: current challenges and future prospects. Cancer Manag Res. 2023;15:667–81. https://doi.org/10.2147/CMAR.S362678.
30. Sharif S, Ferner R, Birch JM, Gillespie JE, Gattamaneni HR, Baser ME, et al. Second primary tumors in neurofibromatosis 1 patients treated for optic glioma: substantial risks after radiotherapy. J Clin Oncol. 2006;24(16):2570–5. https://doi.org/10.1200/JCO.2005.03.8349.
31. Sellmer L, Farschtschi S, Marangoni M, Heran MKS, Birch P, Wenzel R, et al. Serial MRIs provide novel insight into natural history of optic pathway gliomas in patients with neurofibromatosis 1. Orphanet J Rare Dis. 2018;13(1):62. https://doi.org/10.1186/s13023-018-0811-9.
32. Tate JM, Gyorffy JB, Colburn JA. The importance of pheochromocytoma case detection in patients with neurofibromatosis type 1: a case report and review of literature. SAGE Open Med Case Rep. 2017;5:2050313X1774101. https://doi.org/10.1177/2050313x17741016.
33. Gorgel A, Cetinkaya DD, Salgur F, Demirpence M, Yilmaz H, Karaman EH, et al. Coexistence of gastrointestinal stromal tumors (GISTs) and pheochromocytoma in three cases of neurofibromatosis type 1 (NF1) with a review of the literature. Intern Med. 2014;53(16):1783–9. https://doi.org/10.2169/internalmedicine.53.2012. PubMed PMID: 25130111
34. Legius E, Messiaen L, Wolkenstein P, Pancza P, Avery RA, Berman Y, et al. Revised diagnostic criteria for neurofibromatosis type 1 and Legius syndrome: an international consensus recommendation. Genet Med. 2021;23(8):1506–13. https://doi.org/10.1038/s41436-021-01170-5.
35. Accetturo M, Bartolomeo N, Stella A. In-silico analysis of NF1 missense variants in ClinVar: translating variant predictions into variant interpretation and classification. Int J Mol Sci. 2020;21(3):721. https://doi.org/10.3390/ijms21030721.
36. De Luca A, Bottillo I, Dasdia MC, Morella A, Lanari V, Bernardini L, et al. Deletions of NF1 gene and exons detected by multiplex ligation-dependent probe amplification. J Med Genet. 2007;44(12):800–8. https://doi.org/10.1136/jmg.2007.053785.
37. Evans DG. NF2-related schwannomatosis. In: Adam MP, Feldman J, Mirzaa GM, Pagon RA, Wallace SE, Bean LJ, et al., editors. GeneReviews® [Internet]. Seattle (WA): University of Washington, Seattle; 1993 [cited 2024 Sep 28]. Available from: http://www.ncbi.nlm.nih.gov/books/NBK1201/. PubMed PMID: 20301380.
38. Curto M, McClatchey AI. Nf2/Merlin: a coordinator of receptor signalling and intercellular contact. Br J Cancer. 2008;98(2):256–62. https://doi.org/10.1038/sj.bjc.6604002.
39. Trofatter JA, MacCollin MM, Rutter JL, Murrell JR, Duyao MP, Parry DM, et al. A novel moesin-, ezrin-, radixin-like gene is a candidate for the neurofibromatosis 2 tumor suppressor. Cell. 1993;72(5):791–800. https://doi.org/10.1016/0092-8674(93)90406-g. PubMed PMID: 8453669

40. Rouleau GA, Merel P, Lutchman M, Sanson M, Zucman J, Marineau C, et al. Alteration in a new gene encoding a putative membrane-organizing protein causes neuro-fibromatosis type 2. Nature. 1993;363(6429):515–21. https://doi.org/10.1038/363515a0. PubMed PMID: 8379998
41. Kresak J, Walsh M. Neurofibromatosis: a review of NF1, NF2, and schwannomatosis. J Pediatr Genet. 2016;05(02):098–104. https://doi.org/10.1055/s-0036-1579766.
42. Evans D, Ramsden R, Gokhale C, Bowers N, Huson S, Wallace A. Should NF2 mutation screening be undertaken in patients with an apparently isolated vestibular schwannoma? Clin Genet. 2007;71(4):354–8. https://doi.org/10.1111/j.1399-0004.2007.00778.x.
43. Ruttledge MH, Sarrazin J, Rangaratnam S, Phelan CM, Twist E, Merel P, et al. Evidence for the complete inactivation of the NF2 gene in the majority of sporadic meningiomas. Nat Genet. 1994;6(2):180–4. https://doi.org/10.1038/ng0294-180. PubMed PMID: 8162072
44. Evans DR. Neurofibromatosis type 2 (NF2): a clinical and molecular review. Orphanet J Rare Dis. 2009;4(1):16. https://doi.org/10.1186/1750-1172-4-16.
45. Evans DGR. Multiple meningiomas: differential involvement of the NF2 gene in children and adults. J Med Genet. 2005;42(1):45–8. https://doi.org/10.1136/jmg.2004.023705.
46. Bachir S, Shah S, Shapiro S, Koehler A, Mahammedi A, Samy RN, et al. Neurofibromatosis type 2 (NF2) and the implications for vestibular schwannoma and meningioma pathogenesis. Int J Mol Sci. 2021;22(2):690. https://doi.org/10.3390/ijms22020690.
47. Plotkin SR, Messiaen L, Legius E, Pancza P, Avery RA, Blakeley JO, et al. Updated diagnostic criteria and nomenclature for neurofibromatosis type 2 and schwannomatosis: an international consensus recommendation. Genet Med. 2022;24(9):1967–77. https://doi.org/10.1016/j.gim.2022.05.007.
48. Halliday D, Emmanouil B, Evans DGR. Updated protocol for genetic testing, screening and clinical management of individuals at risk of *NF2* -related schwannomatosis. Clin Genet. 2023;103(5):540–52. https://doi.org/10.1111/cge.14310.
49. Kluwe L. Mosaicism in sporadic neurofibromatosis 2 patients. Hum Mol Genet. 1998;7(13):2051–5. https://doi.org/10.1093/hmg/7.13.2051.
50. Dhamija R, Plotkin S, Gomes A, Babovic-Vuksanovic D. LZTR1- and SMARCB1-related schwannomatosis. In: Adam MP, Feldman J, Mirzaa GM, Pagon RA, Wallace SE, Bean LJ, et al., editors. GeneReviews® [Internet]. Seattle (WA): University of Washington, Seattle; 1993 [cited 2024 Sep 28]. Available from: http://www.ncbi.nlm.nih.gov/books/NBK487394/. PubMed PMID: 29517885.
51. Plotkin SR, Bredella MA, Cai W, Kassarjian A, Harris GJ, Esparza S, et al. Quantitative assessment of whole-body tumor burden in adult patients with neurofibromatosis. Herholz K, editor. PLoS ONE. 2012;7(4):e35711. https://doi.org/10.1371/journal.pone.0035711.
52. Christiaans I, Kenter SB, Brink HC, Van Os TAM, Baas F, Van Den Munckhof P, et al. Germline SMARCB1 mutation and somatic NF2 mutations in familial multiple meningiomas. J Med Genet. 2011;48(2):93–7. https://doi.org/10.1136/jmg.2010.082420.
53. Eelloo JA, Smith MJ, Bowers NL, Ealing J, Hulse P, Wylie JP, et al. Multiple primary malignancies associated with a germline SMARCB1 pathogenic variant. Fam Cancer. 2019;18(4):445–9. https://doi.org/10.1007/s10689-019-00138-4.
54. Northrup H, Koenig MK, Pearson DA, Au KS. Tuberous Sclerosis Complex. In: Adam MP, Feldman J, Mirzaa GM, Pagon RA, Wallace SE, Bean LJ, et al., editors. GeneReviews® [Internet]. Seattle (WA): University of Washington, Seattle; 1993 [cited 2024 Sep 28]. Available from: http://www.ncbi.nlm.nih.gov/books/NBK1220/. PubMed PMID: 20301399.
55. Liang N, Zhang C, Dill P, Panasyuk G, Pion D, Koka V, et al. Regulation of YAP by mTOR and autophagy reveals a therapeutic target of tuberous sclerosis complex. J Exp Med. 2014;211(11):2249–63. https://doi.org/10.1084/jem.20140341. PubMed PMID: 25288394; PubMed Central PMCID: PMC4203941.
56. Crino PB, Nathanson KL, Henske EP. The tuberous sclerosis complex. N Engl J Med. 2006;355(13):1345–56. https://doi.org/10.1056/NEJMra055323. PubMed PMID: 17005952
57. Luo C, Ye WR, Shi W, Yin P, Chen C, He YB, et al. Perfect match: mTOR inhibitors and tuberous sclerosis complex. Orphanet J Rare Dis. 2022;17(1):106. https://doi.org/10.1186/s13023-022-02266-0.
58. Nordstrom-O'Brien M, van der Luijt RB, van Rooijen E, van den Ouweland AM, Majoor-Krakauer DF, Lolkema MP, et al. Genetic analysis of von Hippel-Lindau disease. Hum Mutat. 2010;31(5):521–37. https://doi.org/10.1002/humu.21219. PubMed PMID: 20151405.
59. Robinson CM, Ohh M. The multifaceted von Hippel–Lindau tumour suppressor protein. FEBS Lett. 2014;588(16):2704–11. https://doi.org/10.1016/j.febslet.2014.02.026.
60. Uysal SP, ŞahİN M. Tuberous sclerosis: a review of the past, present, and future. Turk J Med Sci. 2020;50(7):1665–76. https://doi.org/10.3906/sag-2002-133.
61. Kotulska K, Kwiatkowski DJ, Curatolo P, Weschke B, Riney K, Jansen F, et al. Prevention of epilepsy in infants with tuberous sclerosis complex in the EPISTOP trial. Ann Neurol. 2021;89(2):304–14. https://doi.org/10.1002/ana.25956.
62. Curatolo P, Moavero R. mTOR inhibitors in tuberous sclerosis complex. Curr Neuropharmacol. 2012;10(4):404–15. https://doi.org/10.2174/157015912804499537.

63. Northrup H, Aronow ME, Bebin EM, Bissler J, Darling TN, De Vries PJ, et al. Updated international tuberous sclerosis complex diagnostic criteria and surveillance and management recommendations. Pediatr Neurol. 2021;123:50–66. https://doi.org/10.1016/j.pediatrneurol.2021.07.011.
64. Hosoe S, Brauch H, Latif F, Glenn G, Daniel L, Bale S, et al. Localization of the von Hippel-Lindau disease gene to a small region of chromosome 3. Genomics. 1990;8(4):634–40. https://doi.org/10.1016/0888-7543(90)90249-t. PubMed PMID: 2276737
65. Moore LE, Nickerson ML, Brennan P, Toro JR, Jaeger E, Rinsky J, et al. Von Hippel-Lindau (VHL) inactivation in sporadic clear cell renal cancer: associations with germline VHL polymorphisms and etiologic risk factors. Maher ER, editor. PLoS Genet. 2011;7(10):e1002312. https://doi.org/10.1371/journal.pgen.1002312.
66. Kim WY, Kaelin WG. Role of *VHL* gene mutation in human cancer. J Clin Oncol. 2004;22(24):4991–5004. https://doi.org/10.1200/JCO.2004.05.061.
67. Hudler P, Urbancic M. The role of VHL in the development of von Hippel-Lindau disease and erythrocytosis. Genes. 2022;13(2):362. https://doi.org/10.3390/genes13020362.
68. Tamura K, Kanazashi Y, Kawada C, Sekine Y, Maejima K, Ashida S, et al. Variant spectrum of von Hippel–Lindau disease and its genomic heterogeneity in Japan. Hum Mol Genet. 2023;32(12):2046–54. https://doi.org/10.1093/hmg/ddad039.
69. Louise M, Binderup M, Smerdel M, Borgwadt L, Beck Nielsen SS, Madsen MG, Møller HU, et al. von Hippel-Lindau disease: updated guideline for diagnosis and surveillance. Eur J Med Genet. 2022;65(8):104538. https://doi.org/10.1016/j.ejmg.2022.104538.
70. Wolters WPG, Dreijerink KMA, Giles RH, Van Der Horst-Schrivers ANA, Van Nesselrooij B, Zandee WT, et al. Multidisciplinary integrated care pathway for von Hippel–Lindau disease. Cancer. 2022;128(15):2871–9. https://doi.org/10.1002/cncr.34265.
71. Malkin D, Li FP, Strong LC, Fraumeni JF, Nelson CE, Kim DH, et al. Germ line p53 mutations in a familial syndrome of breast cancer, sarcomas, and other neoplasms. Science. 1990;250(4985):1233–8. https://doi.org/10.1126/science.1978757. PubMed PMID: 1978757
72. Shete S, Amos CI, Hwang SJ, Strong LC. Individual-specific liability groups in genetic linkage, with applications to kindreds with Li-Fraumeni syndrome. Am J Hum Genet. 2002;70(3):813–7. https://doi.org/10.1086/339370. PubMed PMID: 11822026; PubMed Central PMCID: PMC384961
73. Hisada M, Garber JE, Fung CY, Fraumeni JF, Li FP. Multiple primary cancers in families with Li-Fraumeni syndrome. J Natl Cancer Inst. 1998;90(8):606–11. https://doi.org/10.1093/jnci/90.8.606. PubMed PMID: 9554443
74. Schneider K, Zelley K, Nichols KE, Schwartz Levine A, Garber J. Li-Fraumeni syndrome. In: Adam MP, Feldman J, Mirzaa GM, Pagon RA, Wallace SE, Bean LJ, et al., editors. GeneReviews® [Internet]. Seattle (WA): University of Washington, Seattle; 1993 [cited 2024 Sep 28]. Available from: http://www.ncbi.nlm.nih.gov/books/NBK1311/. PubMed PMID: 20301488.
75. Giacomazzi CR, Giacomazzi J, Netto CBO, Santos-Silva P, Selistre SG, Maia AL, et al. Pediatric cancer and Li-Fraumeni/Li-Fraumeni-like syndromes: a review for the pediatrician. Rev Assoc Med Bras. 2015;61(3):282–9. https://doi.org/10.1590/1806-9282.61.03.282. PubMed PMID: 26248253
76. Kolodziejczak AS, Guerrini-Rousseau L, Planchon JM, Ecker J, Selt F, Mynarek M, et al. Clinical outcome of pediatric medulloblastoma patients with Li–Fraumeni syndrome. Neuro-Oncol. 2023;25(12):2273–86. https://doi.org/10.1093/neuonc/noad114.
77. Wang C, Wang Y, Hughes KS, Parmigiani G, Braun D. Penetrance of colorectal cancer among mismatch repair gene mutation carriers: a meta-analysis. JNCI Cancer Spectr. 2020;4(5):pkaa027. https://doi.org/10.1093/jncics/pkaa027.
78. Donald N, Malik S, McGuire JL, Monahan KJ. The association of low penetrance genetic risk modifiers with colorectal cancer in lynch syndrome patients: a systematic review and meta-analysis. Fam Cancer. 2018;17(1):43–52. https://doi.org/10.1007/s10689-017-9995-8.
79. Bougeard G, Renaux-Petel M, Flaman JM, Charbonnier C, Fermey P, Belotti M, et al. Revisiting Li-Fraumeni syndrome from *TP53* mutation carriers. J Clin Oncol. 2015;33(21):2345–52. https://doi.org/10.1200/JCO.2014.59.5728.
80. Hanson H, Brady AF, Crawford G, Eeles RA, Gibson S, Jorgensen M, et al. UKCGG Consensus Group guidelines for the management of patients with constitutional *TP53* pathogenic variants. J Med Genet. 2021;58(2):135–9. https://doi.org/10.1136/jmedgenet-2020-106876.
81. Tutlewska K, Lubinski J, Kurzawski G. Germline deletions in the EPCAM gene as a cause of Lynch syndrome - literature review. Hered Cancer Clin Pract. 2013;11(1):9. https://doi.org/10.1186/1897--4287-11-9. PubMed PMID: 23938213; PubMed Central PMCID: PMC3765447
82. Idos G, Valle L Lynch Syndrome. In: Adam MP, Feldman J, Mirzaa GM, Pagon RA, Wallace SE, Bean LJ, et al., editors. GeneReviews® [Internet]. Seattle (WA): University of Washington, Seattle; 1993 [cited 2024 Sep 28]. Available from: http://www.ncbi.nlm.nih.gov/books/NBK1211/. PubMed PMID: 20301390.
83. Scollon S, Eldomery MK, Reuther J, Lin FY, Potter SL, Desrosiers L, et al. Clinical and molecular features of pediatric cancer patients with Lynch syndrome. Pediatr Blood Cancer. 2022;69(11):e29859.

https://doi.org/10.1002/pbc.29859. PubMed PMID: 35713195

84. Carrato C, Sanz C, Muñoz-Mármol AM, Blanco I, Pineda M, Del Valle J, et al. The challenge of diagnosing constitutional mismatch repair deficiency syndrome in brain malignancies from young individuals. Int J Mol Sci. 2021;22(9):4629. https://doi.org/10.3390/ijms22094629.
85. Guerrini-Rousseau L, Merlevede J, Denizeau P, Andreiuolo F, Varlet P, Puget S, et al. Glioma oncogenesis in the Constitutional mismatch repair deficiency (CMMRD) syndrome. Neuro-Oncol Adv. 2024;6(1):vdae120. https://doi.org/10.1093/noajnl/vdae120.
86. Seppälä TT, Latchford A, Negoi I, Sampaio Soares A, Jimenez-Rodriguez R, Sánchez-Guillén L, et al. European guidelines from the EHTG and ESCP for Lynch syndrome: an updated third edition of the Mallorca guidelines based on gene and gender. Br J Surg. 2021;108(5):484–98. https://doi.org/10.1002/bjs.11902.
87. Aronson M, Colas C, Shuen A, Hampel H, Foulkes WD, Baris Feldman H, et al. Diagnostic criteria for constitutional mismatch repair deficiency (CMMRD): recommendations from the international consensus working group. J Med Genet. 2022;59(4):318–27. https://doi.org/10.1136/jmedgenet-2020-107627.
88. Raveneau M, Guerrini Rousseau L, Levy R, Roux CJ, Bolle S, Doz F, et al. Specific brain MRI features of constitutional mismatch repair deficiency syndrome in children with high-grade gliomas. Eur Radiol. 2024; https://doi.org/10.1007/s00330-024-10885-3.
89. Sévenet N, Sheridan E, Amram D, Schneider P, Handgretinger R, Delattre O. Constitutional mutations of the hSNF5/INI1 gene predispose to a variety of cancers. Am J Hum Genet. 1999;65(5):1342–8. https://doi.org/10.1086/302639.
90. Versteege I, Sévenet N, Lange J, Rousseau-Merck MF, Ambros P, Handgretinger R, et al. Truncating mutations of hSNF5/INI1 in aggressive paediatric cancer. Nature. 1998;394(6689):203–6. https://doi.org/10.1038/28212.
91. Biegel JA, Zhou JY, Rorke LB, Stenstrom C, Wainwright LM, Fogelgren B. Germ-line and acquired mutations of INI1 in atypical teratoid and rhabdoid tumors. Cancer Res. 1999;59(1):74–9. PubMed PMID: 9892189
92. Schneppenheim R, Frühwald MC, Gesk S, Hasselblatt M, Jeibmann A, Kordes U, et al. Germline nonsense mutation and somatic inactivation of SMARCA4/BRG1 in a family with rhabdoid tumor predisposition syndrome. Am J Hum Genet. 2010;86(2):279–84. https://doi.org/10.1016/j.ajhg.2010.01.013.
93. Del Baldo G, Carta R, Alessi I, Merli P, Agolini E, Rinelli M, et al. Rhabdoid tumor predisposition syndrome: from clinical suspicion to general management. Front Oncol. 2021;11:586288. https://doi.org/10.3389/fonc.2021.586288.
94. Nemes K, Bens S, Bourdeaut F, Johann P, Kordes U, Siebert R, et al. Rhabdoid Tumor Predisposition Syndrome. In: Adam MP, Feldman J, Mirzaa GM, Pagon RA, Wallace SE, Bean LJ, et al., editors. GeneReviews® [Internet]. Seattle (WA): University of Washington, Seattle; 1993 [cited 2024 Sep 28]. Available from: http://www.ncbi.nlm.nih.gov/books/NBK469816/. PubMed PMID: 29215836.
95. Foulkes WD, Kamihara J, Evans DGR, Brugières L, Bourdeaut F, Molenaar JJ, et al. Cancer surveillance in Gorlin syndrome and rhabdoid tumor predisposition syndrome. Clin Cancer Res. 2017;23(12):e62–7. https://doi.org/10.1158/1078-0432.CCR-17-0595. PubMed PMID: 28620006
96. Thomson G, Filser M, Guerrini-Rousseau L, Tauziede-Espariat A, Bourneix C, Gauthier-Villars M, et al. Postzygotic mosaicism of *SMARCB1* variants in patients with rhabdoid tumors: a not-so-rare condition exposing to successive tumors. Neuro-Oncol. 2024:noae122. https://doi.org/10.1093/neuonc/noae122.
97. Nakano Y, Acker M, Druker H, Van Engelen K, Meyn MS, Wasserman JD, et al. Late-onset tumors in rhabdoid tumor predisposition syndrome type-1 (RTPS1) and implications for surveillance. Eur J Hum Genet. 2024; https://doi.org/10.1038/s41431-024-01674-z.
98. Balaguer F, Leoz M, Carballal S, Moreira L, Ocaña T. The genetic basis of familial adenomatous polyposis and its implications for clinical practice and risk management. Appl Clin Genet. 2015:95. https://doi.org/10.2147/TACG.S51484.
99. Bisgaard ML, Fenger K, Bülow S, Niebuhr E, Mohr J. Familial adenomatous polyposis (FAP): frequency, penetrance, and mutation rate. Hum Mutat. 1994;3(2):121–5. https://doi.org/10.1002/humu.1380030206.
100. Paraf F, Jothy S, Van Meir EG. Brain tumor-polyposis syndrome: two genetic diseases? J Clin Oncol. 1997;15(7):2744–58. https://doi.org/10.1200/JCO.1997.15.7.2744.
101. Menon G, Carr S, Kasi A. Familial adenomatous polyposis. In: StatPearls [Internet]. Treasure Island (FL): StatPearls Publishing; 2024 [cited 2024 Sep 28]. Available from: http://www.ncbi.nlm.nih.gov/books/NBK538233/. PubMed PMID: 30855821.
102. Yen T, Stanich PP, Axell L, Patel SG. APC-associated polyposis conditions. In: GeneReviews® [Internet] [Internet]. University of Washington, Seattle; 2022 [cited 2024 Sep 28]. Available from: https://www.ncbi.nlm.nih.gov/books/NBK1345/. PubMed PMID: 20301519.
103. Khattab A, Monga DK. Turcot syndrome. In: StatPearls [Internet]. Treasure Island (FL): StatPearls Publishing; 2024 [cited 2024 Sep 28]. Available from: http://www.ncbi.nlm.nih.gov/books/NBK534782/. PubMed PMID: 30521203.

104. Zaffaroni G, Mannucci A, Koskenvuo L, De Lacy B, Maffioli A, Bisseling T, et al. Updated European guidelines for clinical management of familial adenomatous polyposis (FAP), MUTYH-associated polyposis (MAP), gastric adenocarcinoma, proximal polyposis of the stomach (GAPPS) and other rare adenomatous polyposis syndromes: a joint EHTG-ESCP revision. Br J Surg. 2024;111(5):znae070. https://doi.org/10.1093/bjs/znae070.
105. Aretz S, Uhlhaas S, Caspari R, Mangold E, Pagenstecher C, Propping P, et al. Frequency and parental origin of de novo APC mutations in familial adenomatous polyposis. Eur J Hum Genet. 2004;12(1):52–8. https://doi.org/10.1038/sj.ejhg.5201088.
106. Lachlan KL, Lucassen AM, Bunyan D, Temple IK. Cowden syndrome and Bannayan Riley Ruvalcaba syndrome represent one condition with variable expression and age-related penetrance: results of a clinical study of PTEN mutation carriers. J Med Genet. 2007;44(9):579–85. https://doi.org/10.1136/jmg.2007.049981. PubMed PMID: 17526800; PubMed Central PMCID: PMC2597943
107. Marsh DJ, Kum JB, Lunetta KL, Bennett MJ, Gorlin RJ, Ahmed SF, et al. PTEN mutation spectrum and genotype-phenotype correlations in Bannayan-Riley-Ruvalcaba syndrome suggest a single entity with Cowden syndrome. Hum Mol Genet. 1999;8(8):1461–72. https://doi.org/10.1093/hmg/8.8.1461. PubMed PMID: 10400993
108. Yehia L, Eng C. PTEN hamartoma tumor syndrome. In: Adam MP, Feldman J, Mirzaa GM, Pagon RA, Wallace SE, Bean LJ, et al., editors. GeneReviews® [Internet]. Seattle (WA): University of Washington, Seattle; 1993 [cited 2024 Sep 28]. Available from: http://www.ncbi.nlm.nih.gov/books/NBK1488/. PubMed PMID: 20301661.
109. Blumenthal GM, Dennis PA. PTEN hamartoma tumor syndromes. Eur J Hum Genet EJHG. 2008;16(11):1289–300. https://doi.org/10.1038/ejhg.2008.162. PubMed PMID: 18781191; PubMed Central PMCID: PMC6939673
110. Martín-Valbuena J, Gestoso-Uzal N, Justel-Rodríguez M, Isidoro-García M, Marcos-Vadillo E, Lorenzo-Hernández SM, et al. PTEN hamartoma tumor syndrome: clinical and genetic characterization in pediatric patients. Childs Nerv Syst. 2024;40(6):1689–97. https://doi.org/10.1007/s00381-024-06301-2.
111. Bennett KL. Germline epigenetic regulation of KILLIN in Cowden and Cowden-like syndrome. JAMA. 2010;304(24):2724. https://doi.org/10.1001/jama.2010.1877.
112. Yehia L, Niazi F, Ni Y, Ngeow J, Sankunny M, Liu Z, et al. Germline heterozygous variants in SEC23B are associated with Cowden syndrome and enriched in apparently sporadic thyroid cancer. Am J Hum Genet. 2015;97(5):661–76. https://doi.org/10.1016/j.ajhg.2015.10.001.
113. Orloff MS, He X, Peterson C, Chen F, Chen JL, Mester JL, et al. Germline PIK3CA and AKT1 mutations in Cowden and Cowden-like syndromes. Am J Hum Genet. 2013;92(1):76–80. https://doi.org/10.1016/j.ajhg.2012.10.021.
114. Ni Y, He X, Chen J, Moline J, Mester J, Orloff MS, et al. Germline SDHx variants modify breast and thyroid cancer risks in Cowden and Cowden-like syndrome via FAD/NAD-dependant destabilization of p53. Hum Mol Genet. 2012;21(2):300–10. https://doi.org/10.1093/hmg/ddr459.
115. Garofola C, Jamal Z, Gross GP. Cowden disease. In: StatPearls [Internet]. Treasure Island (FL): StatPearls Publishing; 2024 [cited 2024 Sep 28]. Available from: http://www.ncbi.nlm.nih.gov/books/NBK525984/. PubMed PMID: 30252240.
116. Eng C. Will the real Cowden syndrome please stand up: revised diagnostic criteria. J Med Genet. 2000;37(11):828–30. https://doi.org/10.1136/jmg.37.11.828.
117. Nelen MR, Padberg GW, Peeters EAJ, Lin AY, Helm BVD, Frants RR, et al. Localization of the gene for Cowden disease to chromosome 10q22–23. Nat Genet. 1996;13(1):114–6. https://doi.org/10.1038/ng0596-114.
118. Ngeow J, Stanuch K, Mester JL, Barnholtz-Sloan JS, Eng C. Second malignant neoplasms in patients with Cowden syndrome with underlying germline *PTEN* mutations. J Clin Oncol. 2014;32(17):1818–24. https://doi.org/10.1200/JCO.2013.53.6656.
119. Hobert JA, Eng C. PTEN hamartoma tumor syndrome: an overview. Genet Med. 2009;11(10):687–94. https://doi.org/10.1097/GIM.0b013e3181ac9aea.
120. Takayama T, Muguruma N, Igarashi M, Ohsumi S, Oka S, Kakuta F, et al. Clinical guidelines for diagnosis and management of Cowden syndrome/PTEN hamartoma tumor syndrome in children and adults-secondary publication. J Anus Rectum Colon. 2023;7(4):284–300. https://doi.org/10.23922/jarc.2023-028.
121. Tischkowitz M, Colas C, Pouwels S, Hoogerbrugge N, PHTS Guideline Development Group, Bisseling T, et al. Cancer surveillance guideline for individuals with PTEN hamartoma tumour syndrome. Eur J Hum Genet. 2020;28(10):1387–93. https://doi.org/10.1038/s41431-020-0651-7.
122. Orphanet: Gorlin syndrome [Internet]. [cited 2024 Sep 28]. Available from: https://www.orpha.net/en/disease/detail/377
123. Onodera S, Nakamura Y, Azuma T. Gorlin syndrome: recent advances in genetic testing and molecular and cellular biological research. Int J Mol Sci. 2020;21(20):7559. https://doi.org/10.3390/ijms21207559.
124. Evans DG. Nevoid basal cell carcinoma syndrome. In: Adam MP, Feldman J, Mirzaa GM, Pagon RA, Wallace SE, Bean LJ, et al., editors. GeneReviews® [Internet]. Seattle (WA): University of Washington,

Seattle; 1993 [cited 2024 Sep 28]. Available from: http://www.ncbi.nlm.nih.gov/books/NBK1151/. PubMed PMID: 20301330.

125. Verkouteren BJA, Cosgun B, Reinders MGHC, Kessler PAWK, Vermeulen RJ, Klaassens M, et al. A guideline for the clinical management of basal cell naevus syndrome (Gorlin–Goltz syndrome). Br J Dermatol. 2022;186(2):215–26. https://doi.org/10.1111/bjd.20700.
126. Kimonis VE, Goldstein AM, Pastakia B, Yang ML, Kase R, DiGiovanna JJ, et al. Clinical manifestations in 105 persons with nevoid basal cell carcinoma syndrome. Am J Med Genet. 1997;69(3):299–308. PubMed PMID: 9096761
127. Kiran N, Tilak Raj T, Mukunda K, Reddy V. Nevoid basal cell carcinoma syndrome (Gorlin-Goltz syndrome). Contemp Clin Dent. 2012;3(4):514. https://doi.org/10.4103/0976-237X.107459.
128. Henry ML, Osborne J, Else T. POT1 tumor predisposition. In: Adam MP, Feldman J, Mirzaa GM, Pagon RA, Wallace SE, Bean LJ, et al., editors. GeneReviews® [Internet]. Seattle (WA): University of Washington, Seattle; 1993 [cited 2024 Sep 28]. Available from: http://www.ncbi.nlm.nih.gov/books/NBK563529/. PubMed PMID: 33119245.
129. Baptista Freitas M, Desmyter L, Badoer C, Smits G, Vandernoot I, t'Kint De Roodenbeke D. POT1 tumour predisposition: a broader spectrum of associated malignancies and proposal for additional screening program. Eur J Hum Genet. 2024;32(8):980–6. https://doi.org/10.1038/s41431-024-01611-0.
130. Wu Y, Poulos RC, Reddel RR. Role of POT1 in human cancer. Cancer. 2020;12(10):2739. https://doi.org/10.3390/cancers12102739.
131. Andreotti V, Vanni I, Pastorino L, Ghiorzo P, Bruno W. Germline POT1 variants: a critical perspective on POT1 tumor predisposition syndrome. Genes. 2024;15(1):104. https://doi.org/10.3390/genes15010104.
132. Kock L, Wu MK, Foulkes WD. Ten years of *DICER1* mutations: provenance, distribution, and associated phenotypes. Hum Mutat. 2019;40(11):1939–53. https://doi.org/10.1002/humu.23877.
133. Schultz KAP, Stewart DR, Kamihara J, Bauer AJ, Merideth MA, Stratton P, et al. DICER1 tumor predisposition. In: Adam MP, Feldman J, Mirzaa GM, Pagon RA, Wallace SE, Bean LJ, et al., editors. GeneReviews® [Internet]. Seattle (WA): University of Washington, Seattle; 1993 [cited 2024 Sep 28]. Available from: http://www.ncbi.nlm.nih.gov/books/NBK196157/. PubMed PMID: 24761742.
134. Brenneman M, Field A, Yang J, Williams G, Doros L, Rossi C, et al. Temporal order of RNase IIIb and loss-of-function mutations during development determines phenotype in pleuropulmonary blastoma / DICER1 syndrome: a unique variant of the two-hit tumor suppression model. F1000Res. 2015;4:214. https://doi.org/10.12688/f1000research.6746.2. PubMed PMID: 26925222; PubMed Central PMCID: PMC4712775
135. Caroleo AM, De Ioris MA, Boccuto L, Alessi I, Del Baldo G, Cacchione A, et al. DICER1 syndrome and cancer predisposition: from a rare pediatric tumor to lifetime risk. Front Oncol. 2021;10:614541. https://doi.org/10.3389/fonc.2020.614541.
136. Kastellan S, Kalb R, Sajjad B, McReynolds LJ, Giri N, Samuel D, et al. Germline biallelic BRCA2 pathogenic variants and medulloblastoma: an international cohort study. J Hematol OncolJ Hematol Oncol. 2024;17(1):26. https://doi.org/10.1186/s13045-024-01547-4.
137. McReynolds LJ, Biswas K, Giri N, Sharan SK, Alter BP. Genotype-cancer association in patients with Fanconi anemia due to pathogenic variants in *FANCD1* (*BRCA2*) or *FANCN* (*PALB2*). Cancer Genet. 2021;258(259):101–9. https://doi.org/10.1016/j.cancergen.2021.10.001.
138. Maxwell KN, Patel V, Nead KT, Merrill S, Clark D, Jiang Q, et al. Fanconi anemia caused by biallelic inactivation of BRCA2 can present with an atypical cancer phenotype in adulthood. Clin Genet. 2023;103(1):119–24. https://doi.org/10.1111/cge.14231.
139. Alter BP, Rosenberg PS, Brody LC. Clinical and molecular features associated with biallelic mutations in FANCD1/BRCA2. J Med Genet. 2006;44(1):1–9. https://doi.org/10.1136/jmg.2006.043257.
140. Kowalewski A, Szylberg Ł, Saganek M, Napiontek W, Antosik P, Grzanka D. Emerging strategies in BRCA-positive pancreatic cancer. J Cancer Res Clin Oncol. 2018;144(8):1503–7. https://doi.org/10.1007/s00432-018-2666-9.
141. Petrucelli N, Daly MB, Pal T. BRCA1- and BRCA2-associated hereditary breast and ovarian cancer. In: Adam MP, Feldman J, Mirzaa GM, Pagon RA, Wallace SE, Bean LJ, et al., editors. GeneReviews® [Internet]. Seattle (WA): University of Washington, Seattle; 1993 [cited 2024 Sep 28]. Available from: http://www.ncbi.nlm.nih.gov/books/NBK1247/. PubMed PMID: 20301425.
142. Kumar R, Liu APY, Northcott PA. Medulloblastoma genomics in the modern molecular era. Brain Pathol. 2020;30(3):679–90. https://doi.org/10.1111/bpa.12804.
143. Gold MP, Ong W, Masteller AM, Ghasemi DR, Galindo JA, Park NR, et al. Developmental basis of SHH medulloblastoma heterogeneity. Nat Commun. 2024;15(1):270. https://doi.org/10.1038/s41467-023-44300-0.
144. Bottosso M, Verret B, Caron O, Hamzaoui N, Pasmant E, Danlos FX, et al. Efficacy and safety of immune checkpoint blockade in patients with Li-Fraumeni syndrome. JCO Precis Oncol. 2024;8:e2400139. https://doi.org/10.1200/PO.24.00139.
145. Westdorp H, Kolders S, Hoogerbrugge N, De Vries IJM, Jongmans MCJ, Schreibelt G. Immunotherapy holds the key to cancer treatment and prevention in constitutional mismatch repair deficiency (CMMRD) syndrome. Cancer Lett. 2017;403:159–64. https://doi.org/10.1016/j.canlet.2017.06.018.

146. Hunia J, Gawalski K, Szredzka A, Suskiewicz MJ, Nowis D. The potential of PARP inhibitors in targeted cancer therapy and immunotherapy. Front Mol Biosci. 2022;9:1073797. https://doi.org/10.3389/fmolb.2022.1073797.
147. Alnahhas I, Rayi A, Ong S, Giglio P, Puduvalli V. Management of gliomas in patients with Lynch syndrome. Neuro-Oncol. 2021;23(1):167–8. https://doi.org/10.1093/neuonc/noaa227.
148. Wineland D, Le AN, Hausler R, Kelly G, Barrett E, Desai H, et al. Biallelic *BRCA* loss and homologous recombination deficiency in nonbreast/ovarian tumors in germline *BRCA1/2* carriers. JCO Precis Oncol. 2023;7:e2300036. https://doi.org/10.1200/PO.23.00036.
149. Bailey S, Davidson A, Parkes J, Tabori U, Figaji A, Epari S, et al. How can genomic innovations in pediatric brain tumors transform outcomes in low- and middle-income countries? JCO Glob Oncol. 2022;8:e2200156. https://doi.org/10.1200/GO.22.00156.

6 Principles of Neurosurgery

Pietro Spennato, Francesco Tengattini, Marianna Di Costanzo, Nicola Onorini, Giulia Meccariello, Giuseppe Mirone, and Giuseppe Cinalli

6.1 Introduction

Central nervous system tumors are the most common solid neoplasms in children. Surgical resection is the mainstay of therapy for most primary brain tumors in children: it reduces the size of the tumor mass and enables histologic and molecular diagnoses. The success of surgery is a balance between attempting to complete resection and preserving vital structures and eloquent brain regions ("maximal safe resection"). For some common tumors, such as pilocytic astrocytomas and ependymomas, surgical resection is the most important mode of therapy [1]; for most high-grade tumors, the extent of resection is correlated with prolonged survival. In recent years, image-guided techniques and intraoperative neurophysiological monitoring have allowed improved localization of the tumor to critical structures, making it possible to approach previously "untouchable" tumors, such as thalamic or brainstem neoplasms [2]. Unfortunately, in some cases, such as diffuse brainstem gliomas or infiltrating multilobar supratentorial tumors, resection is not feasible, and the role of surgery may be limited to biopsy (to obtain tissue for diagnosis) and to eventually treat associated conditions, such as hydrocephalus. Discussion within the multidisciplinary team allows for decisions to be made on whether observation, surgical resection, biopsy, radiation, chemotherapy, or a combination of these should be the best treatment for each case.

Pediatric neurosurgeons are usually involved in the early stages of the management of pediatric CNS tumors. Following proper evaluation of the tumor, neurosurgeons should have three main objectives in mind [3]:

- Maximal safe tumor resection when possible
- Histopathological diagnosis
- Treatment of associated conditions (e.g., hydrocephalus)

6.2 Tumor Resection

Craniotomy and resection of intracranial tumors, usually under microscopic magnification ("microsurgery"), are the most common surgical procedures in cases of brain tumors. Gross total

P. Spennato (✉) · N. Onorini · G. Meccariello
G. Mirone · G. Cinalli
Department of Pediatric Neurosciences, Pediatric Neurosurgery Unit, Santobono-Pausilipon Children's Hospital, AORN, Naples, Italy

F. Tengattini
Division of Neurosurgery, Department of Surgical Specialties, Radiological Sciences and Public Health, University of Brescia, Brescia, Italy

M. Di Costanzo
Department of Neurosciences and Reproductive and Dental Sciences, Division of Neurosurgery, Federico II University of Naples, Naples, Italy

A. Mastronuzzi, A. Carai (eds.), *Navigating Pediatric Brain Tumors*,
https://doi.org/10.1007/978-3-032-18992-9_6

resection (GTR) is usually the goal of surgery for those tumors amenable to surgical therapy, but microsurgery may also be used for "open" biopsy for histopathological diagnosis in cases of unresectable tumors, partial resection for tumors in which GTR is contraindicated (e.g., hypothalamic, chiasmatic tumors and some brainstem tumors), and to relieve symptoms with palliative purpose. GTR should be achieved without damaging important vascular and nervous structures and avoiding eloquent area injury. Modern tools, such as neuronavigation and neurophysiological monitoring, help neurosurgeons achieve GTR. Neuronavigation is a tool enabling three-dimensional reconstruction of preoperative digital neuroanatomical images (CT or MRI) of the brain. It synchronizes these images with the patient's actual skull and brain shape and dynamically visualizes the relationships between anatomical structures and the positions of various surgical instruments. Intraoperative imaging, such as ultrasound, CT, and MR imaging, further increases the safety of the surgical approach and verifies the extent of resection. Intraoperative neurophysiological monitoring (IONM) helps assess the integrity of neural structures during surgical procedures. It includes both continuous monitoring of neural tissue and the localization of vital neural structures [4]. Different modalities of intraoperative neurophysiological monitoring (IONM) are available, each monitoring a specific neural pathway; the most important are somatosensory evoked potential (SSEP), motor evoked potential (MEP), brainstem auditory evoked potential (BAEP), visual evoked potential (VEP), electroencephalography (EEG), and electromyography (EMG).

For different regions of the brain, a different surgical approach may be used. Accurate preoperative surgical planning is mandatory for the correct management of pediatric intracranial tumors, especially preoperative high-resolution MRI [5].

6.2.1 Posterior Fossa Tumors

The posterior fossa is the main location of pediatric central nervous system (CNS) tumors (60–70%) [6]. These neoplasms are also the ones that cause the most cancer-related deaths in children, and the extension of resection (EOR) is the main oncologic outcome predictor. Medulloblastoma, ependymoma, and pilocytic astrocytoma are the most prevalent, whereas atypical teratoid/rhabdoid tumor (AT/RT), hemangioblastoma, and ganglioglioma are less common [5].

6.2.1.1 Midline/Paramedian Suboccipital Craniotomy

The majority of posterior fossa tumors in children are approached via a midline or paramedian suboccipital craniotomy, usually in prone position. A linear incision along the midline and a wide craniotomy extended from the transverse sinuses to the foramen magnum, with or without the removal of the posterior arch of C1, guarantees the exposure of both the cerebellar hemispheres and tonsils. The subsequent steps vary depending on the lesion's location. The *transvermian approach* allows the surgeon to reach the dorsal aspect of the tumor in the middle portion and consists of an incision and lateral retraction of the inferior vermis. A neoplasm extending close to the foramen of Magendie (median 4th ventricle outflow) is reached via a telovelar approach, splitting the two tonsils and reaching the 4th ventricle. To access tumors that develop inferiorly across the ponto-medullary junction, *subtonsillar* (tonsils are dislocated above) or *transtonsillar* (tonsils are partially removed) *approaches* could be considered [5].

Hemispheric tumors can be removed via a *transcerebellar approach* with a trajectory studied preoperatively through the shortest way from the cerebellar surface to the tumor.

6.2.1.2 Retromastoid/Lateral Suboccipital Craniotomy

The *retromastoid (retrosigmoid) approach* is mainly used to approach tumors of the cerebellopontine angle (CPA). This area is full of vasculonervous structures such as cranial nerves from V to XII, arteries (e.g., posterior inferior cerebellar artery, vertebral artery, superior cerebellar artery), and veins (e.g., superior petrosal vein). A curvilinear incision behind the ear and delicate plane dissection expose the asterion, which is the center of the craniotomy (or craniectomy) and extends to the transverse sinus superiorly and the sigmoid sinus anteriorly. Before entering the CPA, a cisterna magna opening is mandatory to allow cerebrospinal fluid to drain and relax the cerebellum [5, 7].

6.2.2 Brainstem Tumors

Primary brainstem tumors are rare in children (7–16% of all CNS tumors) [8] and are deep and difficult to approach. Microsurgery has a role in focal, low-grade, and exophytic lesions. The approach chosen is based on the neoplasm location, considering the "anatomical safe entry zones" to access the lesion and avoid neurological deficits. A *unilateral suboccipital craniotomy* with occipital condyle resection (far lateral) could be considered for ventral tumors of the medulla; for lateral lesions, a retromastoid craniotomy is preferred, whereas a midline suboccipital craniotomy is most commonly used for dorsal tumors. The pons is accessed *via a transvermian or telovelar approach* for dorsal lesions, with a retromastoid craniotomy for lateral lesions, whereas a middle fossa *subtemporal craniotomy* with a tentorium incision provides access to ventrolateral pontine tumors (Fig. 6.1). The midbrain is approached ventrally via a *cranio-orbito-zygomatic approach* (the craniotomy is centered on the pterion, and the orbital rim, roof, and zygomatic process are removed to access the sylvian fissure), laterally via a *subtemporal approach,* and dorsally via an *infratentorial supracerebellar or occipital transtentorial approach* (as for "pineal region tumors") [5].

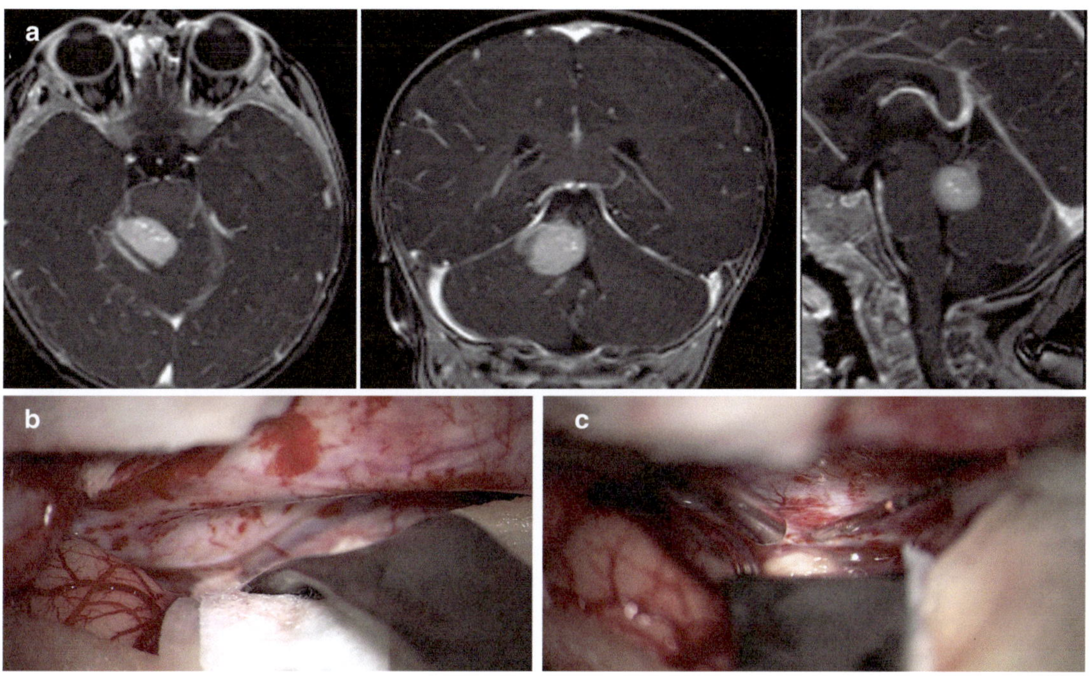

Fig. 6.1 A 2-year-old female patient. Torticollis and left arm hyposthenia. (**a**) Brain MR image showing a right superior cerebral peduncle tumor. It was decided to approach the tumor via a right subtemporal transtentorial microsurgical approach. (**b**) Elevation of the temporal lobe. (**c**) Identification of the tentorial incisura. (**d**) Arachnoid dissection. (**e**) Incision of the tentorium with LASER. F) Wide tentorial opening. (**g**) Tumor exposure. (**h** and **i**) Complete tumor resection. Histopathological examination revealed a nodular/desmoplastic medulloblastoma (WNT molecular subgroup)

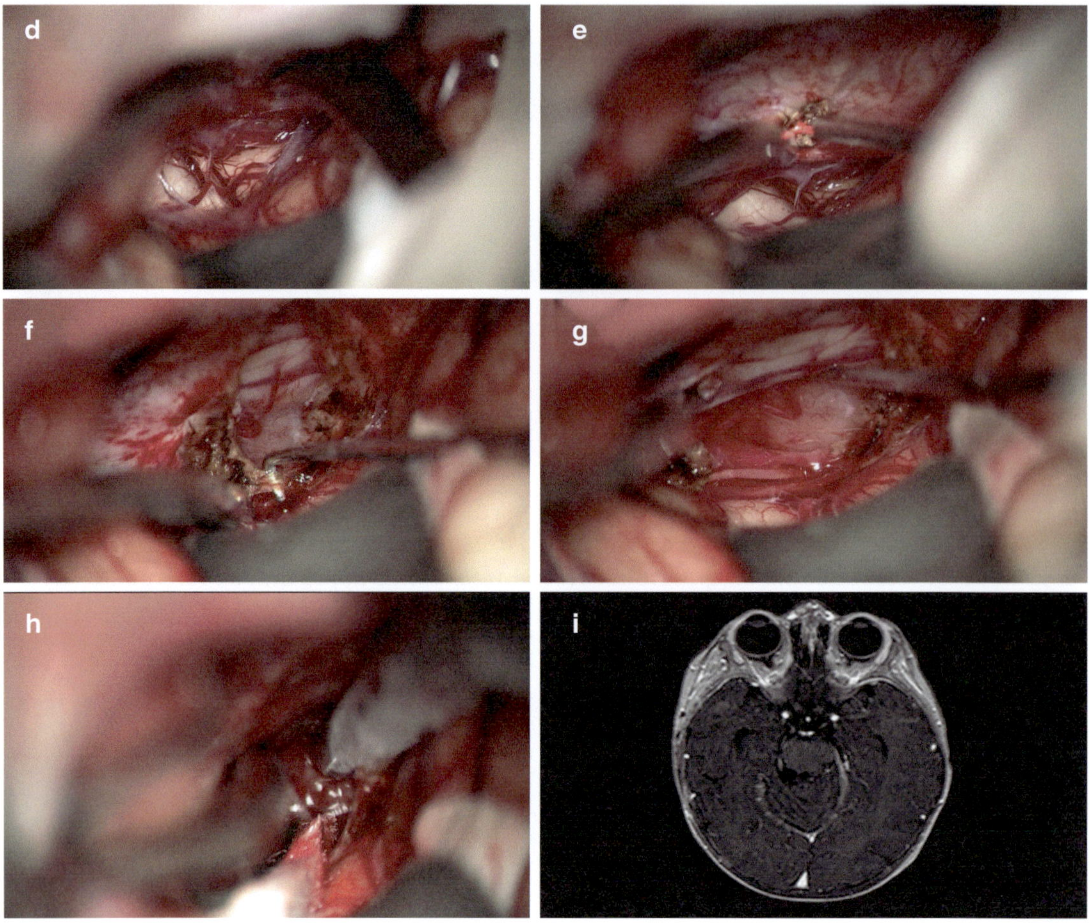

Fig. 6.1 (continued)

6.2.3 Pineal Region Tumors

Pineal region tumors represent between 0.4% and 2.7% of all primary CNS pediatric tumors [9]. For the majority of these lesions, biopsy is crucial for diagnosis to provide the best medical and/or surgical treatment. Because most tumors in this region are chemo- and radiosensitive, microsurgery is reserved for clearly resectable tumors if biopsy itself could be dangerous, for residual tumors following chemotherapy, and for rare nonchemosensitive tumors [5].

6.2.3.1 Infratentorial Supracerebellar Approach

The patient is placed in a seated or prone position, and a midline incision and a suboccipital craniotomy are performed. The cerebellum is retracted inferiorly, and the dorsal pineal region can be clearly identified. Although this approach provides the most direct route to the lesion, taking advantage of a natural supracerebellar corridor, the working space is long, the exposure is limited, and the risk of postoperative cerebellar edema, secondary to venous infarction, must be taken into consideration [5, 10].

6.2.3.2 Occipital Interhemispheric Transtentorial Approach

The *occipital transtentorial approach* with occipital parasagittal craniotomy allows to reach the pineal region and the quadrigeminal plate passing below and medially to the occipital lobe and above the tentorium; the tentorium is cut, and the pineal region is reached. The risk of visual deficits due to the need for greater retraction of the eloquent occipital lobe is the main disadvantage. These could be avoided by gently draining CSF and accurately positioning the patient's head, allowing the brain to fall by gravity [5, 11, 12].

6.2.4 Intraventricular Tumors

Intraventricular tumors are common in children, representing 16% of all pediatric intracranial tumors [6]. They can originate not only from neuroglial ventricular tissue but also from the surrounding cerebral parenchyma bulging into ventricular cameras. Gross total resection can be curative for most of these neoplasms [5].

6.2.4.1 Third Ventricle Approaches

6.2.4.1.1 Anterior Interhemispheric Approaches

Tumors located in the anterior-inferior part of the 3rd ventricle, not extending inside the sella turcica, can be approached via a *subfrontal approach* [13]. This approach can be performed bilaterally or unilaterally, depending on the tumor location and size, with bicoronal or hemicoronal skin incisions, respectively. A soft tissue flap is turned down to expose the supraorbital ridge, and craniotomy is performed. The interhemispheric fissure is accessed, and the frontal lobe is retracted, preserving the olfactory tract to avoid anosmia. The 3rd ventricle is reached through the lamina terminalis (for lesions located between the foramen of Monro and the sella turcica), the optico-carotid triangle, or via a subchiasmatic route.

An alternative to the subfrontal approach for midline anterior lesions is the *frontobasal interhemispheric approach* following a natural interhemispheric corridor. This approach permits less brain retraction and allows working in a larger surgical field. When the anterior communicating arteries are dislocated inferiorly by the tumor, superior dissection via a subcallosal corridor (subrostral approach) is preferred to avoid vascular injuries.

The *interhemispheric transcallosal* approach varies depending on the structures that must be crossed to reach the tumoral mass. The entry point for these approaches is precoronal; anterior callosotomy is performed and permits entry into the frontal horn of the lateral ventricle. Access to the third ventricle can be achieved through the fornix (*interforniceal approach*), foramen of Monro (*transforaminal approach*), or choroidal fissure (*transchoroidal and subchoroidal approaches*).

6.2.4.1.2 Antero-Lateral Approaches

These approaches are chosen for tumors placed near the lateral wall of the third ventricle or extended in the middle cranial fossa. The *pterional approach* (*fronto-temporal approach*) allows access to the third ventricle. The scalp incision is curvilinear, starting above the ear, proceeding back, and then turning in a frontal direction. Craniectomy and dural opening are performed to expose the Sylvian fissure, which is which is then dissected to separate the frontal and temporal lobes. Retractors are used to gently create a corridor and reach the ipsilateral olfactory and optic nerves, the anterior clinoid process, and the third ventricle.

The *orbitozygomatic approach* (the choice between these approaches is based on the surgeon's experience) is performed via the same head position and skin incision as the pterional approach. The craniotomy involves the frontotemporal pterional bone flap, the orbital rim, and a portion of the zygoma. The sylvian fissure and the optic and chiasmatic cisterns are opened, and the optic nerves, chiasm, internal carotid artery (ICA), III cranial nerve, and tumor are exposed.

6.2.4.1.3 Lateral Approaches

The most important lateral approach to the third ventricle is the *subtemporal approach*. The surgical route is created by retracting the base of the temporal lobe superiorly, the vein of Labbè is identified and preserved, and the tentorium is opened behind the course of the trochlear nerve. The third ventricle is opened through an incision between the internal carotid artery and the oculomotor nerve.

The *transpetrosal approach*, which includes complete mastoidectomy and sigmoid sinus skeletonization down to the jugular bulb, is rarely performed, exclusively for giant lesions such as craniopharyngiomas [13].

6.2.4.1.4 Surgery of the Posterior Part of the Third Ventricle

Different surgical approaches have each been outlined in terms of their advantages and disadvantages. These approaches are almost the same as those used for pineal region tumors: the *posterior interhemispheric transcallosal approach, the occipital interhemispheric transtentorial approach, and the supracerebellar infratentorial approach.*

6.2.4.2 Lateral Ventricle Approaches

Tumors located in the lateral ventricles are generally approached via a *transcortical* route that is planned preoperatively, considering the shortest trajectory needed to reach the ventricular space and avoid eloquent areas. Midline lesions are approached via an *interhemispheric transcallosal approach* (see third-ventricle approaches).

6.2.5 Sellar Region Tumors

Tumors of the sellar and parasellar regions represent 10% of all primary CNS pediatric tumors [14]. The majority are craniopharyngiomas (90%), followed by pituitary adenomas and Rathke cleft cysts. In the case of intrasellar tumors, endoscopic transsphenoidal approaches are usually the best choice for managing most of these lesions (the diaphragma sella separates the tumor from suprasellar vasculonervous structures). A prerequisite for this procedure is pneumatization of the sphenoid sinus, which allows for the identification of anatomical landmarks essential for safe operation [15]. Therefore, in children younger than 4–6 years, this approach may not be feasible. In nonspecialized centers, the assistance of an ENT surgeon may often be needed. Open microsurgical approaches are necessary for lesions that extend suprasellar or laterally, with adhesion to the ICA or hypothalamus or with inferior displacement of the optic chiasm. These approaches are similar to those used to access the anterior cranial fossa and the anterolateral part of the III ventricle (e.g., *pterional approach, subtemporal approach, unilateral or bilateral subfrontal approach, anterior interhemispheric approach, and interhemispheric transcallosal approach*) [5].

6.2.6 Convexity of Supratentorial Tumors

Supratentorial tumors are common in infants and very young children (younger than 2 years of age). In older children, infratentorial tumors are predominant. These lesions are epilepsy-related; therefore, the role of surgery is both oncologic and seizure control. When an acceptable functional outcome can be achieved, the microsurgery goal should be gross total resection (GTR), which improves the 5-year progression-free survival (PFS) rate and overall survival (OS) [16]. Patient positioning and incisions depend on the tumor location; craniotomy is performed on the basis of surgical planning through the shortest and safest (without vessel lesions or eloquent area injuries) surgical *transcortical or transsulcal* trajectory. Considering the trans-sulcal approach, the opening of a sulcus allows for minimal resection of white matter and brain retraction but requires careful dissection of vascular structures; it is preferable for tumors located in eloquent areas [5, 17].

6.2.7 Spinal Cord Tumors

Spinal cord tumors in children are primarily intramedullary and account for less than 10% of pediatric CNS tumors [18]. The mass effect and/or neoplastic infiltration can lead to significant neurological symptoms, including sensory–motor and sphincteric deficits. The most represented neoplastic lesions are astrocytomas (usually low grade), ependymomas, gangliogliomas, and hemangioblastomas. These tumors are usually approached through a posterior route by performing laminotomy or laminectomy. The patient position is prone, and a horseshoe headrest is used for thoracic and lumbosacral tumors, while transfixion cranial pins are necessary for cervical lesions. The incision is linear and medial on the basis of the tumor location, the paravertebral muscles are dissected from the vertebral spinous processes and laminae, and a laminotomy is performed. After dural opening, the spinal cord incision is usually performed via a posterior median sulcus approach, splitting the dorsal columns. Another safe entry zone is the *posterolateral sulcus approach*, which is used for tumors located laterally [19]. Intraoperative monitoring is mandatory for spinal cord surgery.

6.3 The Role of Neuroendoscopy in the Management of Brain Tumors

Transventricular neuroendoscopy is a surgical technique that allows access and visualization of the ventricular system through a burr hole, with minimal disruption of normal tissue. This technique is useful in the treatment of several pathologies, such as obstructive and complex hydrocephalus and intra/paraventricular tumors and cysts, and often avoids the implantation of extracranial shunts or more invasive craniotomic approaches.

It is especially useful in lesions that obstruct the CSF pathway, which can lead to hydrocephalus. Endoscopic third ventriculostomy (ETV) is the most widely used neuroendoscopic procedure (Fig. 6.2). By establishing communication between the anterior part of the third ventricle and the interpeduncular cistern, any kind of obstructive hydrocephalus, in which obstacles to CSF flow are present between the mid-third ventricle and the peripontine cisterns, can be treated. Neuroendoscopy can be considered an important adjunct in the management of intraventricular brain tumors [20]. In the case of pineal region tumors, the role of neuroendoscopy is so important that it has been proposed as part of a therapeutic protocol [21]. Patients admitted with pineal region tumors and hydrocephalus should undergo neuroendoscopy with the aims of CSF sampling (for tumor markers and cytology), inspection of intra-

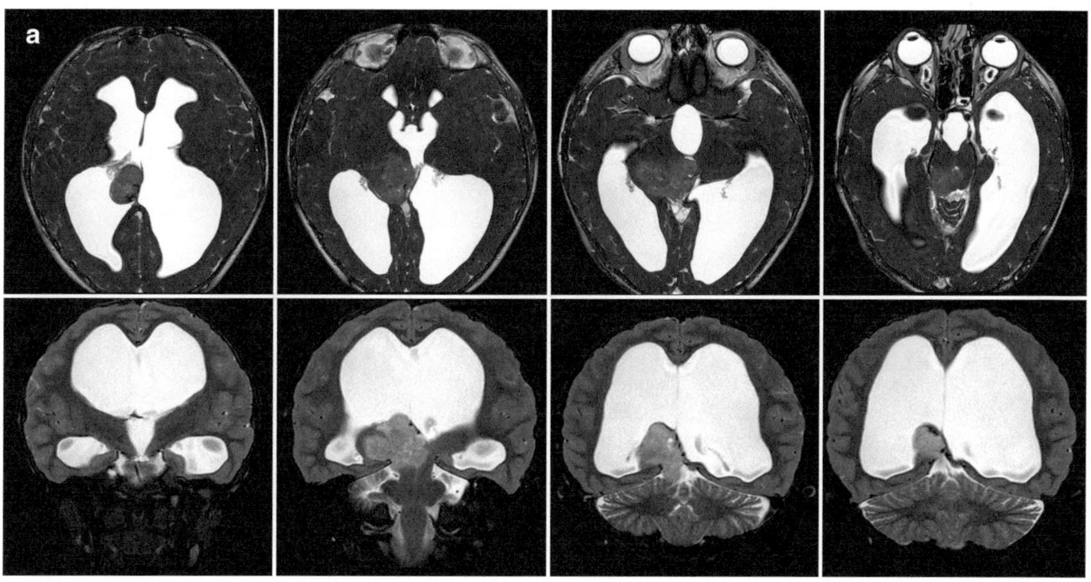

Fig. 6.2 A 10-year-old male patient. Headache, vomiting, papilledema at fundoscopy. MRI (**a**) Right thalamomesencephalic tumor with associated obstructive triventricular hydrocephalus. The decision was made to perform urgent endoscopic third ventriculostomy and tumor biopsy. (**b**) Identification of the right foramen of Monro, right anterior septal vein, right thalamostriate vein, and choroid plexus. (**c**) Identification of the floor of the III ventricle, which is perforated with Decq forceps (**d** and **e**) until a large pulsatile stomy is obtained. (**f**). Identification of the already opened interventricular septum. (**h–j**) Identification of the tumor mass; subependymal biopsy of the same mass was performed. Histology revealed a low-grade glioma. The patient underwent microsurgery with subtotal removal of the tumor

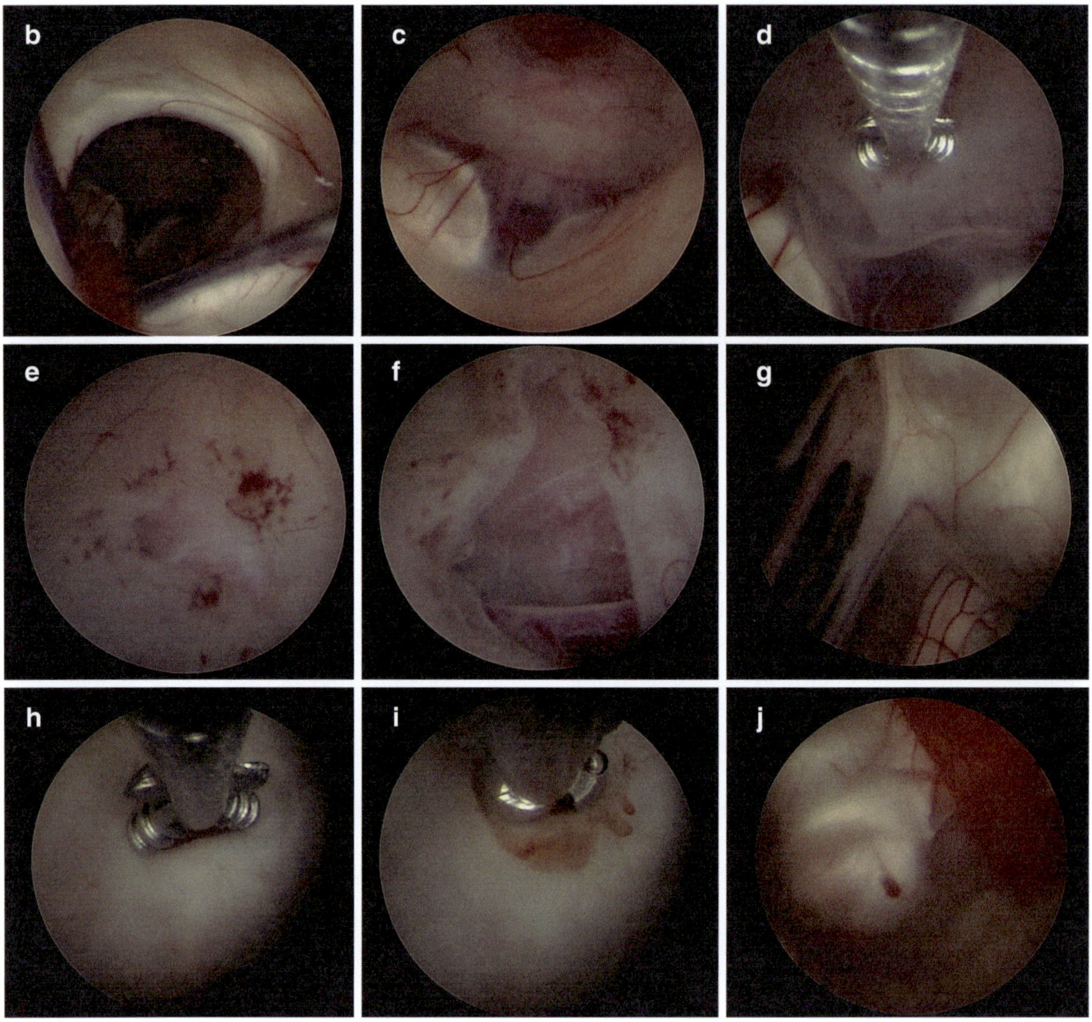

Fig. 6.2 (continued)

ventricular cavities to detect gross intraventricular metastatic nodules not visible on neuroimaging, and tumor biopsy and ETV to relieve hydrocephalus. Further treatments, such as open surgery, tumor removal, radiotherapy, and chemotherapy, will be scheduled accordingly. In the case of some midbrain tumors, such as tectal tumors, which usually present indolent oncological behavior but obstruct the aqueduct, ETV, which relieves the associated hydrocephalus, is the only treatment needed.

Biopsy and fenestration of cystic tumors are other common neuroendoscopic procedures in oncological patients. For intraventricular tumors, neuroendoscopic biopsy offers some theoretical advantages compared with stereotactic "blind" needle biopsy, such as clear visibility, the possibility of selecting a specific point for the biopsy, and the opportunity to examine the biopsy site and verify that there is no active bleeding [22]. Therefore, endoscopic biopsy can be considered the procedure of choice to biopsy intraventricular tumors. Moreover, the neuroendoscopic approach can also be used to biopsy deep-seated paraventricular tumors that do not violate the ependyma, as described by Oertel_ et_al. [23] in adult patients and by our group in pediatric patients [24]. This technique consists of inserting a biopsy needle through the operative channel of the endoscope and puncturing the ependyma with the biopsy needle under direct vision. A concern with endoscopic biopsy is sampling error: a multicentric study confirmed the effectiveness of endoscopic biopsies [22].

In cystic tumors or mixed solid-cystic tumors, such as some intraventricular craniopharyngiomas and optic pathway gliomas (OPGs), endoscopic marsupialization of the cyst into the ventricular system and/or into the subarachnoid space (ventricolocysto-cisternostomy) can relieve the mass effect of the tumor on the surrounding structures, such as the chiasm and optic nerves, and can reestablish the CSF pathway to cure the eventually associated hydrocephalus. This procedure can be performed on an emergency basis in case of rapid loss of sight to decompress the optic pathway. The remaining solid portion can be removed via a microsurgical technique or can be irradiated accordingly with oncological protocols. At the end of the procedure, a transcystic multiple-hole catheter, reaching the lateral ventricle rostrally and the basal cistern caudally, can be left in situ to prevent the re-closure of the cyst [25]. This is especially useful in case of relapsing tumors.

In pediatric patients, OPGs often present as large tumors projecting into the third ventricle, causing obstruction of the foramen of Monro and hydrocephalus. Radical resection of these tumors is not indicated because of chiasmatic and/or hypothalamic infiltration. Neuroendoscopy may be useful for these tumors (at first presentation but, in some cases, at the time of progression) because, with a minimally invasive approach, the upper pole of the tumor can be debulked, obtaining tissue for molecular and histological diagnosis and restoring CSF pathways. This procedure may obviate the need for a more invasive craniotomic approach and avoid or delay the need for a ventriculo-peritoneal shunt [26].

Intraventricular neuroendoscopy may also be useful for attempting total or "near total" removal of selected intraventricular tumors. In 2004, Teo and Nakai reviewed the characteristics of tumors for endoscopic consideration: moderate to low vascularity, soft consistency, diameter less than 2 cm, associated hydrocephalus, histologically low grade, and being situated in the lateral or third ventricle [27]. The recent availability of modern tools, such as endoscopic ultrasonic surgical aspirators (Sonoca, Söring-GmbH, Quickborn, Germany) and Thullium LASER (Revo-Lix Jr, LISA Laser Germany), may expand the spectrum of intracranial pathologies that can be treated by modern neuroendoscopic means: tumors larger than 2 cm, with high vascularity (such as choroid plexus tumors) and calcific tumors, may be considered [28–30].

Finally, endoscopy is a useful aid to microsurgery in any type of tumor surgery, with the aim of enhancing the surgeon's view by increasing illumination, magnification, and angle of view (endoscope-assisted microsurgery) [31].

6.4 Stereotactic and Robot-Guided Biopsy

Although surgical excision is almost always the gold standard of treatment, performing it with an acceptable risk rate is not always feasible. Hence, there is a need for biopsies that, through a minimally invasive approach, allow for obtaining a histological diagnosis, guiding subsequent therapy even for deep lesions or those located in eloquent areas, and treating conditions associated with the neoplasm, such as hydrocephalus [32].

In the case of superficial lesions near or within the cerebral cortex or when it is necessary to biopsy the leptomeninges, open biopsy through a small craniotomy centered on the lesion is the treatment of choice. In most cases, neuronavigation is used to determine the precise location of the lesion, enabling a smaller craniotomy.

Stereotactic biopsies are minimally invasive procedures that employ a thin needle to access deep-seated lesions while avoiding eloquent areas. The entry point, tumor biopsy site, and trajectory are determined during preoperative planning on the basis of radiological images. The method of reaching the target during the procedure has evolved over time.

The pioneers in using devices capable of reaching inside the skull in animal models were Clarke and Horsley at the beginning of the last century [33]. This device was a frame fixed to the bony structure of the animal's skull, enabling it to serve as a regular geometric structure for calculating coordinates to reach the target. Human applications began in the 1940s when Spiegel and Wycis used a stereotactic frame very similar to Clarke and Horsley's to perform thalamotomies in patients with movement disorders [34]. Throughout the last century, as neuroimaging technology has advanced rapidly from pneumoencephalography to CT and MRI, the surgical technique involving the frame has remained unchanged [35, 36]. Only at the end of the last century, with the invention of neuronavigation, was an alternative system introduced that could reach the desired point without requiring a stereotactic frame, thereby reducing patient discomfort during the frame fixation procedure prior to radiological exams and shortening the overall procedural duration [37].

Neuronavigation is a tool enabling three-dimensional reconstruction of digital neuroanatomical images (CT or MRI) of the brain. It synchronizes these images with the patient's actual brain shape and visualizes the relationship between anatomical structures and the positions of various surgical instruments, such as the biopsy needle used in frameless systems [38]. In such systems, after all the components are attached to the patient's skull, the surgeon manually inserts the biopsy needle along the planned trajectory guided by the neuronavigator until the target is reached. Despite the high precision of navigation, this system involves multiple surgeon-dependent steps, which could affect procedure accuracy and precision, especially for very small or deep lesions [39].

This challenge has been more recently addressed with the introduction of robotic technology. These systems, whether floor-based, such as ROSA (Zimmer Biomet, Warsaw, IN, USA) and Neuromate (Renishaw, New Mills, UK) [40], or fixed to the head holder and coupled to a navigation system, such as Stealth Autoguide (Medtronic, Minneapolis, MN, USA) [41], automatically position surgical instruments according to the trajectory set, thereby avoiding the multiple steps required by previous systems (Fig. 6.3). However, being shared-control technologies, they can be monitored and adjusted by the operator at each stage [42].

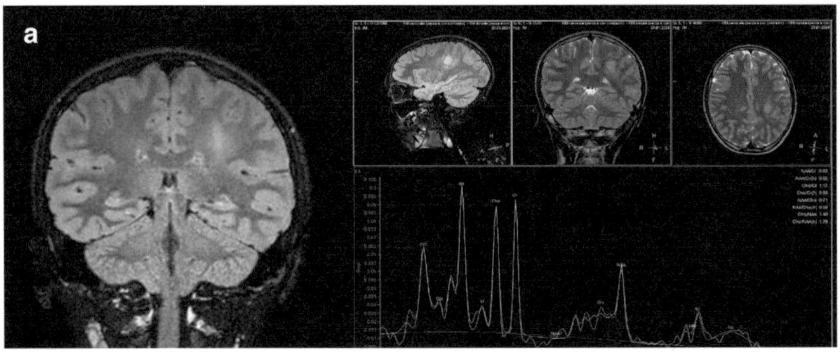

Fig. 6.3 15-year-old male patient. Subacute onset of right brachio-crural hemiparesis. On neuroimaging, (**a**) area of abnormal signal at the level of the supratrigonal deep white matter and left posterior corona radiata with extension to the deep white matter of the postcentral gyrus, superior parietal lobule and precentral gyrus, posterolateral thalamus, and posterior lenticulo-capsular region. The absence of abnormal postcontrastographic impregnation. On spectroscopy: presence of myoinositol, choline elevation with N-acetylaspartate deflection and lactate peak. After 1 month, motor deficits worsened. New brain MRI (**b**) revealed an increased area of altered signals with a further increase in choline and a reduction in N-acetylaspartate, resulting from neural depletion, on spectroscopy. We opted for a robot-assisted, neuronavigated biopsy after careful presurgical planning (yellow line in **c**) to define the anatomical relationship between the lesion and the corticospinal tract (blue line in **c**). (**d**) Postoperative CT scan. A diffuse astrocytoma with an ATRX mutation was identified via histopathology. The patient underwent radiotherapy and chemotherapy

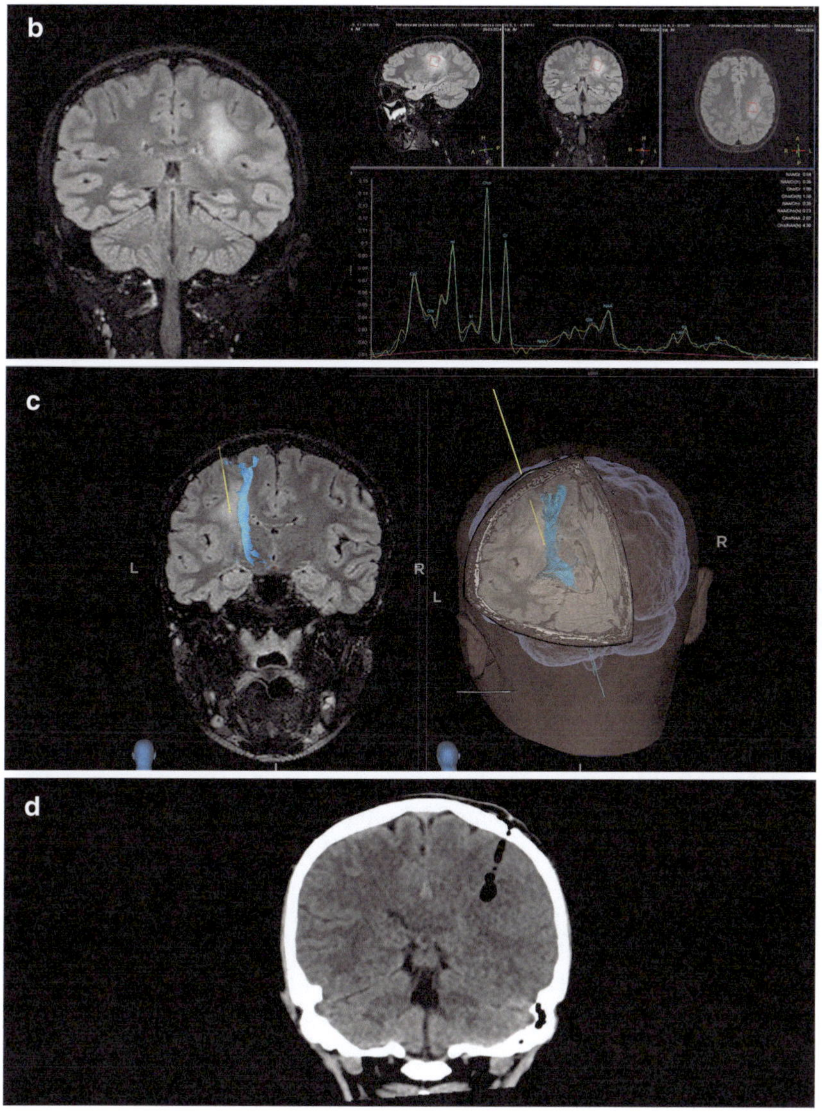

Fig. 6.3 (continued)

6.5 The Role of Laser Interstitial Thermal Therapy in Pediatric Brain Tumors

Deep-seated brain tumors pose a significant challenge, particularly in the pediatric population. Gross total surgical removal of these lesions often carries unacceptable risks of postoperative neurological deficits. MR-guided Laser Interstitial Thermal Therapy (MRgLITT) is a minimally invasive neurosurgical technique used for the treatment of drug-resistant epilepsy and brain tumors. By utilizing near-infrared light energy delivery guided by real-time MR thermometry, MRgLITT enables precise ablation of targeted brain tissues.

LITT was first introduced in the late 1980s by Bown et al. [43]. Their initial technique lacked a real-time monitoring modality, preventing precise evaluation of the ablation size and control of critical surrounding tissue, which limited the use of thermal therapy in neuro-oncology. The introduction of MR thermography has overcome this limitation by providing real-time visualization of heat diffusion and its effects on tissues.

LITT involves the stereotactic insertion of a thin fiber-optic catheter cooled with water or saline into the lesion. The catheter delivers light energy to the target tissue, which is then converted into heat, inducing cell death through time-dependent thermal damage to intracellular proteins and DNA. Cellular apoptosis is triggered when temperatures range from 46 °C to 60 °C, whereas coagulative necrosis is induced when temperatures increase to 60 °C. The degree of permanent cell damage was evaluated via the Arrhenius equation, which is visually depicted through color gradation and superimposed on the baseline image in the MRI-guided procedure. During thermal ablation, safe targets within eloquent areas are carefully identified to avoid reaching critical temperatures and causing subsequent permanent damage in these regions. Currently, two systems are commercialized for MRI-guided LITT: the Visualase™ MRI-Guided Laser Ablation System (Medtronic) and the NeuroBlate® Laser Ablation System (Monteris Medical).

In neuro-oncology, LITT was initially developed for adult brain tumors; several studies have demonstrated its efficacy in controlling residual or recurrent high-grade gliomas and metastases, especially in patients who are unsuitable for surgical intervention [44, 45].

In the pediatric population, LITT has mostly been applied in patients with epilepsy. In 2011, Jethwa et al. first reported the use of LITT in a pediatric brain tumor, thalamic PNET [46].

In 2020, Arocho-Quinones and colleagues published the largest series of pediatric brain tumors treated with LITT. In this multi-institutional study, the authors evaluated the outcomes of 86 pediatric brain tumors treated with LITT, including 76 low-grade tumors and 10 high-grade tumors, with a mean follow-up time of 14 months. The majority of low-grade tumors demonstrated a decrease in tumor volume at the last follow-up (83.1%), whereas the remaining 16.9% remained stable or increased. Conversely, LITT appeared to be less effective for high-grade lesions, where only 57.1% of high-grade lesions presented a decrease in volume at the last follow-up. These findings suggest that LITT is an effective treatment for select pediatric brain tumors, with greater efficacy and a lower risk for further surgery in low-grade lesions than in high-grade tumors [47].

MR-guided LITT has also been successfully applied to pediatric posterior fossa tumors. Mirone et al. reported promising results in treating three patients with recurrent pilocytic astrocytoma. The treatment significantly reduced the tumor volume without major complications [48].

The main advantages of LITT in pediatric brain tumors include short hospitalization, minimal use of painkillers, a low risk of permanent deficits, a very low risk of infection and wound complications, and the possibility of further surgery if needed. In contrast, surgical procedures typically require several hours and are quite expensive. Moreover, even if a needle biopsy can be performed concurrently with LITT, the limited samples obtained may interfere with the histological and molecular diagnosis. One limitation of LITT, especially in the pediatric population, is skull thickness. Indeed, both frame-based and frameless neuronavigation techniques involve rigid immobilization of the skull with pins, which requires sufficient bone thickness to prevent intracranial damage. This limits the use of LITT to patients aged 2 years or older. Pediatric pins and additional head gel rings can assist surgeons in firmly securing patients' heads. Additionally, a robotic guidance platform (Stealth AutoGuide, Medtronic) can help improve the accuracy of laser fiber placement [48].

Another advantage suggested by several authors is a better response to chemotherapy after LITT. Indeed, LITT seems to induce prolonged damage to the blood–brain barrier (BBB), increasing its permeability, as demonstrated by a postcontrast enhancement ring surrounding the lesion that appears up to 6 months after surgery. Accordingly, a recent phase II study on recurrent glioblastoma revealed greater overall survival in patients treated with LITT and low-dose doxorubicin, a BBB-impermeant chemotherapy drug, than in those receiving standard treatment, with even better results when the therapy was started later [49].

The enhanced efficacy of delayed chemotherapy can be attributed to the theory of immune stimulation of the host against the tumor. Hyperthermia, and consequently LITT, augments the body's immune response against tumors. When chemotherapy is started immediately following the procedure, it may interfere with this immune response, thereby diminishing the beneficial effects of LITT [50].

6.6 Treatment of Associated Conditions

In children, hydrocephalus is often associated with brain tumors, especially in the posterior fossa and midline tumors. The main mechanism is obstruction of cerebrospinal fluid (CSF) flow by the tumor. Hydrocephalus may be severe and life-threatening. Initial management is dictated by the clinical condition of the patient. Urgent treatment of hydrocephalus, prior to tumor removal, is indicated in unstable patients with clinical symptoms and signs of elevated intracranial hypertension (headache, vomiting, diplopia, drowsiness) and significant hydrocephalus on neuroimaging. The presence of papilledema at neuro-ophthalmologic examination further supports early management. Neurosurgeons have different options for treating hydrocephalus at this stage: the most common option is the insertion of an external ventricular drain (EVD). A catheter is inserted through a paramedian burr hole in the frontal region; the anterior horn of the lateral ventricle is incannulated according to anatomical landmarks (or with the help of neuronavigation), draining CSF in an external collecting device. EVD is a temporizing measure until tumor removal restores CSF flow. Endoscopic third ventriculostomy (ETV) is an option in cases of triventricular hydrocephalus from posterior fossa or pineal region tumors. In cases of unresectable tumors, or if hydrocephalus persists following tumor removal, permanent diversion of CSF is needed. The two main methods for permanent diversion of CSF are ETV and ventriculoperitoneal shunt (VPS). ETV, which avoids the insertion of foreign bodies (prone to mechanical failure and infection), is the preferred method when it is technically feasible. However, in very young children with hemorrhagic and metastatic tumors, the risk of failure is high. The VPS consists of a three-part device: a proximal catheter, which is inserted inside the lateral ventricle; a distal catheter, which is tunnelized subcutaneously, reaching the peritoneum where CSF can be reabsorbed; and a valve, which is interposed between them to control drainage. VPS can be used in every type of hydrocephalus but has the theoretical risk of dissemination of neoplastic cells in the peritoneum and a high rate of infective and mechanical complications, often requiring reintervention (sometimes interrupting oncological treatment).

Various pediatric CNS tumors are composed of a large cystic component. Sometimes, urgent drainage of the cyst may be required due to the unstable condition of the patient secondary to intracranial hypertension. In these cases, a catheter may be positioned in the cyst, and the fluid may be aspirated. Usually, this catheter is connected to a subcutaneous reservoir (Ommaya reservoir or Ventricular Access Device—VAD). The fluid can also be aspirated through the subcutaneous reservoir in subsequent days. In very selected cases, a subcutaneous device may be used to administer intracystic (cystic craniopharyngiomas) or intraventricular (atypical teratoid-rhabdoid tumors) medications.

Following large brain tumors and/or hydrocephalus drainage, macrocephalic children can develop subdural collections. These collections are often small in volume and self-limiting, but sometimes they exhibit a compressive effect requiring treatment. When needed, surgical intervention consists of positioning a subduroperitoneal shunt. Usually, this shunt can be removed in the following weeks, when the collections are resolved. If adjuvant treatments are needed, we prefer to treat these collections promptly to avoid any delay.

References

1. Ullrich NJ, Pomeroy SL. Pediatric brain tumors. Neurol Clin. 2003;21:897–913.
2. Cinalli G, Aguirre DT, Mirone G, et al. Surgical treatment of thalamic tumors in children. J Neurosurg Pediatr. 2018;21:247–57.
3. Scheinemann K, Bouffet E. Pediatric neuro-oncology. New York: Springer; 2015.
4. Sala F. Intraoperative neurophysiology in pediatric neurosurgery: a historical perspective. Childs Nerv Syst. 2023;39:2929–41.
5. Silva AHD, Aquilina K. Surgical approaches in pediatric neuro-oncology. Cancer Metastasis Rev. 2019;38:723–47.
6. Dolecek TA, Propp JM, Stroup NE, Kruchko C. CBTRUS statistical report: primary brain and central nervous system tumors diagnosed in the United States in 2005-2009. Neuro-Oncology. 2012;14:v1–v49.
7. Elhammady MS, Telischi FF, Morcos JJ. Retrosigmoid approach: indications, techniques, and results. Otolaryngol Clin N Am. 2012;45:375–97, ix
8. Berger MS, Edwards MS, LaMasters D, Davis RL, Wilson CB. Pediatric brain stem tumors: radiographic, pathological, and clinical correlations. Neurosurgery. 1983;12:298–302.
9. Al-Hussaini M, Sultan I, Abuirmileh N, Jaradat I, Qaddoumi I. Pineal gland tumors: experience from the SEER database. J Neuro-Oncol. 2009;94:351–8.
10. Mottolese C, Szathmari A, Ricci-Franchi AC, Gallo P, Beuriat PA, Capone G. Supracerebellar infratentorial approach for pineal region tumors: our surgical and technical considerations. Neurochirurgie. 2015;61:176–83.
11. Cinalli G, Marini A, Russo C, Spennato P, Mirone G, Ruggiero C, Quaglietta L, De' Santi MS, Covelli E. Herophilus-Galen line as a predictor of extent of resection in the occipital interhemispheric transtentorial approach to pineal tumors in children. J Neurosurg Pediatr. 2022;30:119–27.
12. Imperato A, Marini A, Spennato P, Mirone G, Cinalli G. Occipital interhemispheric transtentorial approach to a pineoblastoma in a 4-year-old child. Neurosurg Focus Video. 2021;5:V4.
13. Onorini N, Spennato P, Mirone G, Vitulli F, Solari D, Cavallo LM, Cinalli G. Surgical approaches to the third ventricle: an update. In: Di Rocco C, editor. Advances and technical standards in neurosurgery. Cham: Springer; 2023. p. 207–49.
14. Zada G, Lin N, Ojerholm E, Ramkissoon S, Laws ER. Craniopharyngioma and other cystic epithelial lesions of the sellar region: a review of clinical, imaging, and histopathological relationships. Neurosurg Focus. 2010;28:E4.
15. de Divitiis O, d'Avella E, de Notaris M, Di Somma A, De Rosa A, Solari D, Cappabianca P. The (r)evolution of anatomy. World Neurosurg. 2019;127:710–35.
16. Wisoff JH, Sanford RA, Heier LA, Sposto R, Burger PC, Yates AJ, Holmes EJ, Kun LE. Primary neurosurgery for pediatric low-grade gliomas: a prospective multi-institutional study from the children's oncology group. Neurosurgery. 2011;68:1548–55.
17. Germano IM. Transsulcal approach to mesiotemporal lesions. Anatomy, technique, and report of three cases. Neurosurg Focus. 1996;1:e4.
18. Hsu W, Jallo GI. Pediatric spinal tumors. Handb Clin Neurol. 2013;112:959–65.
19. Shimony N, Fehnel K, Abbott IR, Jallo GI. The evolution of spinal cord surgery: history, people, instruments, and results. Childs Nerv Syst. 2023;39:2687–700.
20. Kunwar S. Endoscopic adjuncts to intraventricular surgery. Neurosurg Clin N Am. 2003;14:547–57.
21. Oi S, Shibata M, Tominaga J, Honda Y, Shinoda M, Takei F, Tsugane R, Matsuzawa K, Sato O. Efficacy of neuroendoscopic procedures in minimally invasive preferential management of pineal region tumors: a prospective study. J Neurosurg. 2000;93:245–53.
22. Constantini S, Mohanty A, Zymberg S, et al. Safety and diagnostic accuracy of neuroendoscopic biopsies: an international multicenter study: clinical article. PED. 2013;11:704–9.
23. Oertel J, Keiner D. Visual-controlled endoscopic biopsy of paraventricular Intraparenchymal tumors. World Neurosurg. 2019;126:e208–18.
24. Spennato P, Ruggiero C, Mirone G, Imperato A, Parlato RS, Cinalli G. Endoscopic needle biopsy of thalamic tumors: technical note. Childs Nerv Syst. 2020;36:2835–40.
25. Locatelli D, Levi D, Rampa F, Pezzotta S, Castelnuovo P. Endoscopic approach for the treatment of relapses in cystic craniopharyngiomas. Childs Nerv Syst. 2004;20:863–7.
26. Spennato P, De Rosa A, Meccariello G, Quaglietta L, Imperato A, Scala MR, Russo C, Cinalli G. Endoscopic ultrasonic aspiration as alternative to more invasive surgery in initial management of optic pathway gliomas in children. Childs Nerv Syst. 2022;38:1281–7.
27. Teo C, Nakaji P. Neuro-oncologic applications of endoscopy. Neurosurg Clin N Am. 2004;15:89–103.
28. Cinalli G, Imperato A, Mirone G, Di Martino G, Nicosia G, Ruggiero C, Aliberti F, Spennato P. Initial experience with endoscopic ultrasonic aspirator in purely neuroendoscopic removal of intraventricular tumors. PED. 2017;19:325–32.
29. Spennato P, Onorini N, Vitulli F, Imperato A, De Martino L, Ruggiero C, Cinalli G. Endoscopic ultrasonic resection of calcified tumor of the third ventricle. Neurosurg Focus Video. 2023;8:V6.
30. Spennato P, Onorini N, Vitulli F, Cinalli MA, Di Costanzo M, Mirone G, Cinalli G. Pure endoscopic ultrasonic removal of choroid plexus papillomas of the third ventricle: technical report of two cases. Childs Nerv Syst. 2023;39:3415–20.

31. Cinalli G, Cappabianca P, De Falco R, Spennato P, Cianciulli E, Cavallo LM, Esposito F, Ruggiero C, Maggi G, De Divitiis E. Current state and future development of intracranial neuroendoscopic surgery. Expert Rev Med Devices. 2005;2:351–73.
32. Maher CO, Raffel C. Neurosurgical treatment of brain tumors in children. Pediatr Clin N Am. 2004;51:327–57.
33. Clarke RH, Horsley V. THE CLASSIC: on a method of investigating the deep ganglia and tracts of the central nervous system (cerebellum). Br Med J 1906:1799-1800. Clin Orthop Relat Res. 2007;463:3–6.
34. Spiegel EA, Wycis HT, Marks M, Lee AJ. Stereotaxic apparatus for operations on the human brain. Science. 1947;106:349–50.
35. Leksell L, Leksell D, Schwebel J. Stereotaxis and nuclear magnetic resonance. J Neurol Neurosurg Psychiatry. 1985;48:14–8.
36. Perry JH, Rosenbaum AE, Lunsford LD, Swink CA, Zorub DS. Computed tomography/guided stereotactic surgery: conception and development of a new stereotactic methodology. Neurosurgery. 1980;7:376–81.
37. Widmann G, Schullian P, Ortler M, Bale R. Frameless stereotactic targeting devices: technical features, targeting errors and clinical results. Int J Med Robot. 2012;8:1–16.
38. Spetzger U, Laborde G, Gilsbach JM. Frameless neuronavigation in modern neurosurgery. Minim Invasive Neurosurg. 1995;38:163–6.
39. Dorward NL, Alberti O, Palmer JD, Kitchen ND, Thomas DG. Accuracy of true frameless stereotaxy: in vivo measurement and laboratory phantom studies. Technical note. J Neurosurg. 1999;90:160–8.
40. Elsabeh R, Singh S, Shasho J, Saltzman Y, Abrahams JM. Cranial neurosurgical robotics. Br J Neurosurg. 2021;35:532–40.
41. Legnani FG, Franzini A, Mattei L, et al. Image-guided biopsy of intracranial lesions with a small robotic device (iSYS1): a prospective, exploratory pilot study. Oper Neurosurg (Hagerstown). 2019;17:403–12.
42. Spennato P, Di Costanzo M, Mirone G, Cicala D, De Martino L, Onorini N, Ruggiero C, Cinalli G. Image-guided biopsy of intracranial lesions in children, with a small robotic device: a case series. Childs Nerv Syst. 2024;40:1681–8.
43. Bown SG. Phototherapy in tumors. World J Surg. 1983;7:700–9.
44. Banerjee C, Snelling B, Berger MH, Shah A, Ivan ME, Komotar RJ. The role of magnetic resonance-guided laser ablation in neurooncology. Br J Neurosurg. 2015;29:192–6.
45. Chen C, Lee I, Tatsui C, Elder T, Sloan AE. Laser interstitial thermotherapy (LITT) for the treatment of tumors of the brain and spine: a brief review. J Neuro-Oncol. 2021;151:429–42.
46. Jethwa PR, Lee JH, Assina R, Keller IA, Danish SF. Treatment of a supratentorial primitive neuroectodermal tumor using magnetic resonance–guided laser-induced thermal therapy: technical note. PED. 2011;8:468–75.
47. Arocho-Quinones EV, Lew SM, Handler MH, et al. Magnetic resonance–guided stereotactic laser ablation therapy for the treatment of pediatric brain tumors: a multiinstitutional retrospective study. J Neurosurg Pediatr. 2020;26:13–21.
48. Mirone G, Cicala D, Cinalli G. Posterior Fossa laser interstitial thermal therapy in children. Neurosurg Clin N Am. 2023;34:227–37.
49. Butt OH, Zhou AY, Huang J, et al. A phase II study of laser interstitial thermal therapy combined with doxorubicin in patients with recurrent glioblastoma. Neuro-oncol Adv. 2021;3:vdab164.
50. Spacca B, Di Maurizio M, Grandoni M, Tempesti S, Genitori L. Laser interstitial thermal therapy (LITT) for pediatric patients affected by intracranial tumors. Front Neurol. 2023;14:1120286.

Principles of Radiation Oncology

7

Sabina Vennarini, Chiara Valentini, Qi Wang, and Chi Lin

The field of pediatric neuro-oncology has undergone profound changes over the last few decades, driven by technological advancements and a growing understanding of the unique challenges faced by young patients. The earliest forms of radiotherapy, such as two-dimensional (2D) radiation therapy, were limited in their precision and posed significant risks to developing brain tissues. The evolution of these technologies reflects an ongoing commitment to not only curing pediatric brain tumors but also preserving the quality of life for survivors.

S. Vennarini (✉)
Pediatric Radiotherapy Unit, Fondazione IRCCS Istituto Nazionale Tumori, Milan, Italy
e-mail: sabina.vennarini@istitutotumori.it.it

C. Valentini
Department of Radiotherapy and Radiation Oncology, Faculty of Medicine, University Hospital Carl Gustav Carus, Technische Universität Dresden, Klinik für Strahlentherapie und Radioonkologie, Dresden, Germany
e-mail: chiara.valentini@ukdd.de

Q. Wang
Department II of Head & Neck Radiation Oncology, Pediatric Tumor Radiotherapy Group, Shandong Cancer Hospital, Jinan City, China

Oncology Committee, Shandong Society for Neuroscience, Jinan City, China

Standing Committee Member, Tumor Radiotherapy Committee, Shandong Pain Medicine Association, Jinan City, China

Shandong Cancer Hospital and Institute, Shandong First Medical University and Shandong Academy of Medical Sciences, Jinan City, China
e-mail: qiwang@tmu.edu.cn

C. Lin
Department of Radiation Oncology, University of Nebraska Medical Center, Omaha, NE, USA

7.1 Early Approaches and the Limitations of 2D Radiotherapy

The earliest forms of radiotherapy, such as two-dimensional (2D) radiation therapy, were limited in their precision and posed significant risks to developing brain tissues. Broad radiation fields were employed to ensure tumor coverage, often resulting in substantial exposure to surrounding healthy tissues. This imprecision led to severe side effects, including neurocognitive decline, hearing loss, and endocrine dysfunction, particularly when critical structures like the cochlea or pituitary gland were affected [1–3]. For example, in medulloblastoma treatment, craniospinal irradiation with 2D techniques exposed large areas of the brain and spine, resulting in long-term deficits that profoundly impacted the lives of survivors [4, 5].

Despite these challenges, 2D radiotherapy laid the foundation for subsequent advances. It highlighted the need for more sophisticated imaging and radiation delivery methods to improve the

A. Mastronuzzi, A. Carai (eds.), *Navigating Pediatric Brain Tumors*,
https://doi.org/10.1007/978-3-032-18992-9_7

therapeutic ratio—maximizing tumor control while minimizing harm to normal tissues. This imperative drove the development of three-dimensional conformal radiation therapy (3D-CRT), which marked a significant step forward.

7.2 3D Conformal Radiation Therapy (3D-CRT): A New Standard

The introduction of 3D-CRT revolutionized pediatric radiotherapy by enabling radiation beams to be shaped to match the three-dimensional contours of tumors. By integrating advanced imaging techniques, 3D-CRT reduced radiation exposure to adjacent healthy tissues compared to the broad-field methods of 2D radiotherapy [6]. This improvement was particularly impactful in treating tumors near sensitive areas of the brain, such as medulloblastomas, ependymomas, and low-grade gliomas.

For medulloblastoma, 3D-CRT allowed for more precise targeting of the posterior fossa and craniospinal axis, sparing vital structures like the cochlea and reducing the risk of hearing loss. A study by Paulino et al. demonstrated that 3D-CRT plans could significantly lower radiation exposure to the cochlea compared to 2D methods, illustrating the potential of this technique to mitigate treatment-related side effects [1, 2]. However, challenges remained. For example, despite reductions in overall radiation dose, studies like those by Mulhern et al. showed that high doses to parietotemporal and occipitotemporal regions during posterior fossa boosts could still impair neurocognitive outcomes, underscoring the need for further refinements [7].

In the case of ependymomas, which are often located near the brainstem, 3D-CRT provided greater control in sparing critical structures. By contouring radiation fields more precisely, the technique reduced the likelihood of motor and cognitive deficits that were previously common with 2D approaches [8]. Similarly, for low-grade gliomas, 3D-CRT minimized damage to the optic nerves and hypothalamus, reducing the risk of visual impairment and hormonal imbalances—key considerations when treating young patients with developing systems.

7.3 Intensity-Modulated Radiation Therapy (IMRT): Greater Precision and Flexibility

Building on the success of 3D-CRT, intensity-modulated radiation therapy (IMRT) introduced an unprecedented level of control over radiation dose distribution. By modulating the intensity of radiation beams, IMRT allowed for highly conformal dose delivery, sparing surrounding healthy tissues even in tumors located near critical structures like the hippocampus or optic pathways. This advancement significantly reduced the risk of long-term side effects, such as cognitive deficits and endocrine dysfunction, particularly in pediatric patients where even minor damage can have profound developmental implications [9].

IMRT's ability to sculpt radiation doses was especially beneficial in complex cases where tumors were situated near multiple vital structures. However, as a photon-based technique, IMRT still carried a risk of low-dose radiation exposure to healthy tissues, highlighting the need for even more precise methods.

7.4 Volumetric Modulated Arc Therapy (VMAT): Enhanced Efficiency

A further evolution of IMRT, volumetric-modulated arc therapy (VMAT), introduced continuous radiation delivery along a 360-degree arc, optimizing dose distribution while significantly reducing treatment times. This efficiency is particularly advantageous in pediatric settings, where children may require sedation to remain still during sessions [10]. By delivering treatment more quickly and effectively, VMAT reduced the burden on patients and their families, making it a preferred choice for complex dose distributions in pediatric neuro-oncology. Moreover, there has been ongoing debate regarding the use of IMRT techniques in pediatric cases due to concerns about a potential increase in radiation-induced secondary malignancies. IMRT plans often require a greater number of monitor units (MU) and longer treatment delivery times compared to conventional radiotherapy techniques, which can lead to increased low-dose radiation exposure to normal tissues. In contrast, VMAT techniques may theoretically reduce this risk, as VMAT plans generally involve fewer MU and shorter treatment times than fixed-field IMRT [11]. An additional advantage of VMAT is the capability to treat the entire target volume without the need for matching field junctions, which are required in conventional radiotherapy techniques. This eliminates the risk of junction overdosage, which can increase the likelihood of radiation myelitis, as well as the risk of underdosage, which could compromise treatment efficacy [12].

7.5 Tomotherapy: A Personalized Approach

Tomotherapy brought a novel integration of image-guided intensity-modulated radiation therapy (IMRT) that integrates computed tomography (CT) imaging with helical radiation delivery. It uses a specialized device that combines a linear accelerator with a CT scanner, allowing for precise targeting of tumors while minimizing radiation exposure to surrounding healthy tissues.

The unique feature of tomotherapy is its ability to deliver radiation in a spiral (helical) pattern as the machine rotates around the patient. Additionally, daily CT imaging helps account for anatomical changes during the course of treatment, ensuring accurate dose delivery and reducing the risk of damage to normal tissues [13].

In pediatric patients, who may experience shifts in tumor position or normal tissue anatomy due to growth or weight fluctuations, this adaptability proved invaluable. Tomotherapy's precise targeting made it particularly effective for craniospinal irradiation and tumors near sensitive central nervous system (CNS) structures [14, 15].

Tomotherapy, while highly effective, is a resource-intensive technique that demands specialized expertise and meticulous planning to fully harness its benefits while minimizing potential risks. It proves especially valuable in treating tumors located near critical structures, such as those in the brain or spine, where precision is paramount and conventional methods may result in significant collateral damage. Despite its advantages, the technique's complexity necessitates access to specialized equipment and skilled professionals.

7.6 Proton Beam Therapy: Redefining Precision

The therapeutic application of proton beams—and charged particles in general—is primarily driven by their unique depth-dose profile, which is characterized by the Bragg peak. Unlike photons, protons deposit most of their energy at a specific depth, thereby minimizing damage to healthy tissues surrounding the tumor. To treat larger target volumes, beams of varying energies are combined to create what is known as the Spread-Out Bragg Peak (SOBP), ensuring the prescribed dose is delivered uniformly across the tumor. This approach is particularly advantageous for treating deep-seated tumors located near organs at risk (OAR), where the precise dose distribution of charged particle beams can spare nearby healthy structures. The reduced radiation exposure to normal tissues is especially critical in pediatric patients, who face a higher risk of long-term complications, such as late morbidity and secondary cancers [7, 16–19]. As a rule, the integral dose delivered to the patient will be two to three times lower with protons when compared to X-rays delivered by intensity modulated radiation therapy (IMRT) [20].

Some limitations of proton therapy, such as neutron exposure—particularly pronounced with passive scattering systems—were previously a major concern due to the high biological effectiveness of neutrons. However, the advent and widespread adoption of pencil beam scanning (PBS), a more advanced and efficient delivery method, has significantly mitigated this issue. PBS has reduced neutron contamination by two to three orders of magnitude compared to passive scattering systems, greatly alleviating concerns about neutron exposure in pediatric patients. Today, the neutron background from PBS is comparable to the levels produced during photon irradiation with energies exceeding 10 MV. Nevertheless, when collimation is used, proton interactions with the collimator can still generate additional neutrons. While this contribution should not be overlooked, it remains significantly lower than the levels observed with passive scattering techniques [21].

Proton therapy has shown particular promise in treating medulloblastomas, ependymomas, high-grade gliomas, and germinoma [22–24]. Despite its benefits, the high cost and limited availability of proton therapy remain significant barriers to its widespread adoption. Ongoing efforts aim to expand access and further investigate its long-term benefits and risks, particularly in pediatric populations [25, 26].

7.7 Balancing Efficacy with Quality of Life

The evolution of radiotherapy techniques has significantly reduced the risk of long-term side effects, but the challenge of balancing tumor control with quality-of-life preservation persists. Innovations such as IMRT, VMAT, tomotherapy, and proton therapy have minimized these risks, but the potential for cognitive deficits, hormonal imbalances, and secondary malignancies remains a concern. Comprehensive follow-up care, including neurocognitive testing, endocrine evaluations, and psychosocial support, is critical to addressing the sequelae of radiation treatment [27].

Research into neuroprotective agents and personalized rehabilitation programs continues to evolve, offering hope for improved survivorship outcomes. Advances in imaging, artificial intelligence, and the integration of genomic and molecular data into treatment planning promise to further refine radiotherapy, ushering in an era of personalized care.

7.8 The Future of Pediatric Neuro-Oncology

The journey of pediatric radiotherapy—from the early days of broad-field techniques to the precision of modern methods—reflects the relentless pursuit of better outcomes for young patients. As research continues to explore the integration of radiotherapy with immunotherapies, targeted molecular treatments, and advanced imaging, the future of pediatric neuro-oncology is poised for even greater innovation. Each step forward brings us closer to achieving the dual goals of effective tumor control and preserving the potential for a full and meaningful life for every child treated.

7.9 Indications for Radiation Therapy in Pediatric Neuro-Oncology

Radiation therapy is often employed as part of the multidisciplinary treatment of pediatric brain and spine tumors. Indications for its use include, but are not limited to, the following:

7.9.1 Malignant Brain Tumors

- *Medulloblastoma:* One of the most common malignant brain tumors in children, medulloblastomas often require postoperative radiation therapy. Radiation is indicated following surgical resection and, in some cases, after chemotherapy. It is primarily used to treat the primary tumor site and areas at high risk for microscopic disease spread, such as the whole craniospinal axis.
- *Ependymomas:* both after complete tumor resection and in presence tumor rest, postoperative radiation therapy is indicated to prevent recurrence. Infratentorial tumors invade the spinal canal frequently and, therefore, are often only partially resected and require precise planning to avoid damage to the spinal cord and surrounding structures.

- *Gliomas:* For high-grade gliomas, such as glioblastomas or diffuse intrinsic pontine gliomas (DIPG), radiation is an essential part of the treatment plan, especially when surgical resection is not feasible. The goal is to control the tumor locally and extend survival, though the prognosis for DIPG remains poor despite radiation.
- *ATRT (Atypical Teratoid Tumor):* Radiation therapy plays a central role in the management of ATRT due to the tumor's aggressive nature. It is usually indicated after surgery, particularly when the tumor cannot be fully resected, or if there is residual disease postoperatively. Radiation therapy is also an essential part of treatment when ATRT is metastatic, or if there are high-risk features such as tumor spread to the cerebrospinal fluid (CSF). However, the use of radiation in very young children, especially those under the age of 3, is approached with caution due to the significant risks of neurodevelopmental delays and long-term cognitive deficits. In these cases, radiation is reserved for instances where other treatment modalities are not sufficient to control disease progression.

7.9.2 Non-malignant Tumors

- *Craniopharyngiomas:* These benign tumors often cause significant symptoms due to their proximity to critical structures such as the optic nerves, hypothalamus, and pituitary gland. Surgical resection is challenging, and radiation therapy is often used postoperatively to prevent recurrence.
- *Pineal Tumors:* Tumors such as germinomas or teratomas in the pineal region may require radiation, particularly if surgery or chemotherapy is not fully effective. Radiation is typically used to target the tumor and any involved structures to prevent relapse.

7.9.3 Spinal Cord Tumors

- *Ependymomas:* Both after complete tumor resection and in presence tumor rest, postoperative radiation therapy is indicated to prevent recurrence. Tumors located in critical spinal cord regions often require precise planning to avoid damage to the spinal cord and surrounding structures.
- *Neurofibromas:* In patients with neurofibromatosis type 1 (NF1), radiation therapy may be considered in cases of inoperable or recurrent tumors. However, due to the risk of radiation-induced malignancy in NF1 patients, radiation is used cautiously.

7.9.4 Relapsed or Refractory Tumors

In cases of recurrent tumors, radiation therapy may be used as a salvage treatment. Tumors like medulloblastomas or gliomas that have relapsed after initial treatment with chemotherapy or surgery may require a second course of radiation therapy to control disease progression.

7.9.5 Palliative Treatment

In cases where the tumor is no longer amenable to curative treatment, radiation therapy can be used for palliation to alleviate symptoms such as pain, swelling, or obstructive hydrocephalus.

7.10 Radiation Dose and Volume Considerations

The treatment of pediatric brain and spinal cord tumors with radiation therapy is a highly intricate process that requires careful calculation of both the radiation dose and the target volume. Pediatric patients are particularly sensitive to radiation due to their developing tissues, which makes precision critical in minimizing long-term toxicity while effectively treating the tumor. Different types of brain and spinal cord tumors have distinct radiation therapy needs based on their biological behavior, location, and ability to spread. Below are radiation dose and volume considerations for a wider range of pediatric brain and spine tumor entities.

1. *Medulloblastoma*
   - *Dose:* Medulloblastoma is one of the most common malignant brain tumors in children, and radiation therapy plays a central role in its treatment. After surgical resection, the typical radiation dose to the posterior fossa is *54–55.8 Gy* in daily fractions of *1.8–2.0 Gy*. For high-risk patients or those with metastasis, *craniospinal irradiation (CSI)* is often used, delivering doses ranging from *23.4 to 36 Gy* to the entire craniospinal axis, with an additional boost to the posterior fossa. In the case of medulloblastomas with distant metastases, the radiation dose may be escalated, particularly to the brain and spinal cord.
   - *Volume:* The clinical target volume (CTV) includes not only the visible tumor bed but also the regions at risk for microscopic disease spread. For CSI, the CTV encompasses the entire craniospinal axis, including the brain, spinal cord, and the areas that have a potential for microscopic disease, particularly in high-risk cases.
2. *Gliomas (including DIPG and High-Grade Gliomas)*
   - *Dose:* Radiation therapy is a key component of treatment for high-grade gliomas, including glioblastomas and diffuse intrinsic pontine gliomas (DIPG). The typical radiation dose for glioblastomas is *54–60 Gy* delivered to the resected tumor bed, while in the case of DIPG, the dose may be slightly higher, up to *60 Gy*, despite the poor prognosis. In cases of gliomas that are not surgically resectable, radiation may be used as the primary treatment. For low-grade gliomas, the dose is generally around *45–50 Gy*, but the approach is more conservative.
   - *Volume:* For gliomas, the CTV includes the tumor bed, and additional margins are added to account for potential microscopic spread. In the case of DIPG, radiation is typically directed to the entire brainstem, with some cases also involving the spinal cord if there is concern for spread. In high-grade gliomas, an extensive margin around the tumor bed is included to ensure full coverage of the potential microscopic disease.
3. *ATRT*
   - *Dose*: The typical radiation dose for ATRT is 54–60 Gy to the gross tumor volume (GTV), delivered in daily fractions of 1.8–2.0 Gy. If the disease has metastasized or there is concern for spread to the spinal cord or other areas of the central nervous system, craniospinal irradiation (CSI) is often used. The dose for CSI typically ranges from 23.4 to 36 Gy, and additional boosts may be administered to the tumor bed to treat areas of known disease involvement. For infants and very young children, the dose may be adjusted to minimize radiation exposure to developing tissues, as these patients are particularly vulnerable to the long-term side effects of radiation therapy.
   - *Volume*: the clinical target volume (CTV) must include the GTV as well as regions at high risk for microscopic disease spread. The CTV often extends beyond the visible tumor bed, as ATRT has a tendency to infiltrate surrounding tissues. In cases where the tumor has disseminated via the CSF or metastasized, the CTV may extend to include the entire craniospinal axis. The planning target volume (PTV) accounts for patient movement and set-up variations, ensuring that the tumor and surrounding tissues are accurately irradiated.
4. *Craniopharyngiomas*
   - *Dose:* Craniopharyngiomas are benign but locally invasive tumors that often require radiation therapy after incomplete surgical resection. The typical dose for craniopharyngiomas is *45–50 Gy* to the tumor bed. In some cases, an additional boost of *5–10 Gy* may be used for areas where there is residual tumor after surgery, particularly if the tumor is located near critical structures such as the optic chiasm.
   - *Volume:* The CTV includes the gross tumor volume (GTV) as seen on preoperative imaging, with an added margin to account for microscopic disease. Due to the location of these tumors, the surrounding struc-

tures such as the optic nerves and pituitary gland should be carefully spared, and radiation planning must take into account the proximity of these critical structures.

5. *Pineal Tumors (e.g., Germinomas)*
   - *Dose:* For pineal tumors such as germinomas, the radiation dose typically ranges from *30 to 36 Gy* to the tumor site following surgery. In cases of metastasis or high-risk disease, a more aggressive approach may involve treating the whole ventricular system, particularly for tumors with disseminated cells.
   - *Volume:* The CTV includes the primary tumor site, with additional radiation to any involved structures such as the pineal region and surrounding ventricles. When there is dissemination to the cerebrospinal fluid (CSF) pathways, the CTV may extend to include the entire craniospinal axis in high-risk cases. The precise location of the tumor within the pineal region requires careful attention to avoid radiation exposure to surrounding critical structures like the brainstem and optic pathways.
6. *Ependymomas*
   - *Dose:* Ependymomas, common tumors in the pediatric spinal cord, require radiation to the tumor bed following surgical resection, especially if the tumor is incompletely removed. The radiation dose is typically *54–60 Gy* to the gross tumor bed, depending on the tumor's location. For spinal ependymomas, the dose is usually *45–54 Gy* to the tumor bed. For cranial ependymomas, the dose may be slightly higher, depending on the size and location of the tumor.
   - *Volume:* The CTV for ependymomas includes the visible tumor bed and an additional margin for the microscopic disease. In cases of spinal cord tumors, the radiation volume typically includes the entire spinal cord, often extending several centimeters above and below the resection site. For cranial ependymomas, the tumor bed and surrounding areas at high risk of microscopic disease are included in the CTV.
7. *Neurofibromas (Neurofibromatosis Type 1)*
   - *Dose:* Neurofibromas in children, especially in those with neurofibromatosis type 1 (NF1), are typically benign, but when they become inoperable or symptomatic, radiation may be considered. The dose is generally *50–54 Gy*, depending on the location and size of the tumor. Given the increased risk of radiation-induced malignancy in NF1 patients, the use of radiation is carefully considered and employed only in selected cases.
   - *Volume:* The radiation volume is usually limited to the tumor and any surrounding structures that may harbor microscopic disease. Given the inherent risks of radiation in NF1 patients, the radiation oncologist will carefully delineate the tumor bed and ensure that healthy tissues receive as little radiation as possible.
8. *Pediatric Brain Metastases*
   - *Dose:* Pediatric brain metastases, though rare, are treated with radiation therapy when they are accessible. The dose is typically around *30–40 Gy* for the whole brain, with a boost to the metastatic site if needed. Whole-brain radiation therapy (WBRT) may be employed if multiple lesions are present.
   - *Volume:* The CTV for pediatric brain metastases includes the entire brain if WBRT is used, or a more focused volume if the metastasis is solitary. A more focused approach may involve stereotactic radiosurgery (SRS) to treat the specific metastatic lesions with precision, reducing the dose to surrounding healthy tissues.

References

1. Paulino AC, Mahajan A, Ye R, Grosshans DR, Fatih Okcu M, Su J, et al. Ototoxicity and cochlear sparing in children with medulloblastoma: proton vs. photon radiotherapy. Radiother Oncol. 2018;128(1):128–32.
2. Paulino AC, Narayana A, Mohideen MN, Jeswani S. Posterior fossa boost in medulloblastoma: an analysis of dose to surrounding structures using 3-dimensional (conformal) radiotherapy. Int J Radiat Oncol. 2000;46(2):281–6.

3. Merchant TE, Happersett L, Finlay JL, Leibel SA. Preliminary results of conformal radiation therapy formedulloblastoma. Neuro-Oncology. 1999;1(3):177–87.
4. Danoff BF, Cowchock FS, Marquette C, Mulgrew L, Kramer S. Assessment of the long-term effects of primary radiation. Therapy for brain tumors in children. Cancer. 1982;49(8):1580–6.
5. Grosu AL, Feldmann HJ, Albrecht C, Kneschaurek P, Wehrmann R, Groß MW, et al. Dreidimensionale Bestrahlungsplanung bei Hirntumoren. Strahlenther Onkol. 1998;174(1):7–13.
6. Purdy JA. Advances in three-dimensional treatment planning and conformal dose delivery. Semin Oncol. 1997;24(6):655–71.
7. Mulhern RK, Palmer SL, Merchant TE, Wallace D, Kocak M, Brouwers P, et al. Neurocognitive consequences of risk-adapted therapy for childhood medulloblastoma. J Clin Oncol. 2005;23(24):5511–9.
8. Merchant TE, Zhu Y, Thompson SJ, Sontag MR, Heideman RL, Kun LE. Preliminary results from a phase II trail of conforml radiation therapy for pediatric patients with localised low-grade astrocytoma and ependymoma. Int J Radiat Oncol. 2002;52(2):325–32.
9. Khan Faiz M, Gibbons JP. The physics of radiation therapy. 5th ed. Lippincott Williams & Wilkins; 2014.
10. Nguyen M, Dang T, Deegan L, Henry K, Jones S, Pullar A, et al. Modified volumetric modulated arc therapy technique with reduced planning and treatment time for CRANIOSPINAL irradiation utilising two isocentres. J Med Radiat Sci. 2022;69(3):357–66.
11. Teoh M, Clark CH, Wood K, Whitaker S, Nisbet A. Volumetric modulated arc therapy: a review of current literature and clinical use in practice. Br J Radiol. 2011;84(1007):967–96.
12. Lee YK, Brooks CJ, Bedford JL, Warrington AP, Saran FH. Development and evaluation of multiple Isocentric volumetric modulated arc therapy technique for craniospinal axis radiotherapy planning. Int J Radiat Oncol. 2012;82(2):1006–12.
13. Mackie TR, Holmes T, Swerdloff S, Reckwerdt P, Deasy JO, Yang J, et al. Tomotherapy: a new concept for the delivery of dynamic conformal radiotherapy. Med Phys. 1993;20(6):1709–19.
14. Sun Y, Liu G, Chen W, Chen T, Liu P, Zeng Q, et al. Dosimetric comparisons of craniospinal axis irradiation using helical tomotherapy, volume-modulated arc therapy and intensity-modulated radiotherapy for medulloblastoma. Transl Cancer Res. 2019;8(1):191–202.
15. Turcas A, Kelly SM, Clementel E, Cernea D. Tomotherapy for cranio-spinal irradiation. Clin Transl Radiat Oncol. 2023 Jan;38:96–103.
16. Loeffler JS, Durante M. Charged particle therapy—optimization, challenges and future directions. Nat Rev Clin Oncol. 2013;10(7):411–24.
17. Kahalley LS, Ris MD, Grosshans DR, Okcu MF, Paulino AC, Chintagumpala M, et al. Comparing intelligence quotient change after treatment with proton versus photon radiation therapy for pediatric brain tumors. J Clin Oncol. 2016;34(10):1043–9.
18. Lassaletta Á, Morales JS, Valenzuela PL, Esteso B, Kahalley LS, Mabbott DJ, et al. Neurocognitive outcomes in pediatric brain tumors after treatment with proton versus photon radiation: a systematic review and meta-analysis. World J Pediatr. 2023;19(8):727–40.
19. Child AE, Warren EA, Grosshans DR, Paulino AC, Okcu MF, Ris MD, et al. Long-term cognitive and academic outcomes among pediatric brain tumor survivors treated with proton versus photon radiotherapy. Pediatr Blood Cancer. 2021;68(9):e29125.
20. Lomax AJ, Bortfeld T, Goitein G, Debus J, Dykstra C, Tercier PA, et al. A treatment planning intercomparison of proton and intensity modulated photon radiotherapy. Radiother Oncol. 1999;51(3):257–71.
21. Hua C, Mascia AE, Seravalli E, Lomax AJ, Seiersen K, Ulin K. Advances in radiotherapy technology for pediatric cancer patients and roles of medical physicists: COG and SIOP Europe perspectives. Pediatr Blood Cancer. 2021;68(S2):e28344.
22. Merchant TE, Mulhern RK, Krasin MJ, Kun LE, Williams T, Li C, et al. Preliminary results from a phase II trial of conformal radiation therapy and evaluation of radiation-related CNS effects for pediatric patients with localized ependymoma. J Clin Oncol. 2004;22(15):3156–62.
23. Patteson BE, Baliga S, Bajaj BVM, MacDonald SM, Yeap BY, Gallotto SL, et al. Clinical outcomes in a large pediatric cohort of patients with ependymoma treated with proton radiotherapy. Neuro-Oncology. 2021;23(1):156–66.
24. Correia D, Terribilini D, Zepter S, Pica A, Bizzocchi N, Volken W, et al. Whole-ventricular irradiation for intracranial germ cell tumors: Dosimetric comparison of pencil beam scanned protons, intensity-modulated radiotherapy and volumetric-modulated arc therapy. Clin Transl Radiat Oncol. 2019;15:53–61.
25. Ige T, Lewis P, Shelley C, Pistenmaa D, Coleman CN, Aggarwal A, et al. Understanding the challenges of delivering radiotherapy in low- and middle-income countries in Africa. J Cancer Policy. 2023;35:100372.
26. Peterson RK, King TZ. A systematic review of pediatric neuropsychological outcomes with proton *versus* photon radiation therapy: a call for equity in access to treatment. J Int Neuropsychol Soc. 2023;29(8):798–811.
27. Tallen G, Resch A, Calaminus G, Wiener A, Leiss U, Pletschko T, et al. Strategies to improve the quality of survival for childhood brain tumour survivors. Eur J Paediatr Neurol. 2015;19(6):619–39.

Principles of Medical Treatment

8

Marta Perez-Somarriba, Serafin Castellano, Felisa Vázquez-Gómez, and Alvaro Lassaletta

8.1 Introduction

Central nervous system (CNS) tumors are the most common solid tumors in childhood. Despite major improvements in treatment and cure rates, childhood cancer incidence tends to increase with time worldwide. To date, more than 400,000 children and adolescents under the age of 20 are diagnosed with cancer per year. Five year overall survival accounts for 75–80% in most of the high-income countries, but still for less than 30% in low- and middle-income ones.

The management of children and adolescents with brain tumors requires a multidisciplinary approach which should be provided in specialty units that include pediatric neurosurgeons, pediatric neuro-oncologists, neuroradiologists, radiation oncologists, pathologists, and other pediatric specialists such as neurologists, endocrinologists, neuropsychologists, neurorehabilitation therapists, dieticians, speech and language therapists depending on tumor type and areas involved [1].

Treatment will depend on tumor type, staging, and age at diagnosis and is based on surgery, radiation therapy, chemotherapy, and/or targeted therapies and other novel agents, which have been progressively incorporated into different treatment strategies [2].

Chemotherapy has been used as adjuvant or neoadjuvant therapy to surgery and radiotherapy for the management of pediatric brain tumors in the last decades.

Although chemosensitivity has been demonstrated in many pediatric brain tumors, failure or inactiveness of chemotherapy has been also commonly described in the clinic and clinical trials [3].

In order to address this issue, different schedules of administration and routes have been explored.

High-dose chemotherapy with autologous hematopoietic stem-cell rescue has been used successfully in infants and children diagnosed with recurrent/refractory or poor-prognosis embryonal tumors and CNS germ cell tumors (GCTs) [4].

Metronomic chemotherapy defined as low-dose, continuous, and long-lasting oral chemotherapy has been also used in this setting with some promising results using single agents or different drugs in combination [5].

Some of these failures might be attributed to the blood-brain barrier (BBB), limiting the penetration of systemically administered chemotherapeutics into the brain. The administration of chemotherapy directly through intrathecal or

M. Perez-Somarriba · S. Castellano · F. Vázquez-Gómez · A. Lassaletta (✉)
Pediatric Neuro-Oncology Unit, Hospital Infantil Universitario Niño Jesús, Madrid, Spain
e-mail: marta.perezsomarriba@salud.madrid.org; serafin.castellano@salud.madrid.org; felisa.vazquez@salud.madrid.org; alvaro.lassaletta@salud.madrid.org

A. Mastronuzzi, A. Carai (eds.), *Navigating Pediatric Brain Tumors*,
https://doi.org/10.1007/978-3-032-18992-9_8

intraventricular infusions has been also used to overcome the BBB.

However, despite these strategies, brain tumors remain the leading cause of death among children and adolescents diagnosed with cancer.

Advances in diagnosis in the last years have identified multiple molecular pathways upregulated in these tumors potentially targetable. Additionally, novel routes of drug administration are being explored to overcome the barriers, improve drug penetration, and improve outcomes.

This chapter aims to review the most frequently used chemotherapies used in children and adolescents diagnosed with brain tumors, the different routes of administration, and some novel strategies currently under development.

Blood-Brain Barrier and Tumor Microenvironment

The blood-brain barrier (BBB) is a complex membrane composed of endothelial cells supported by vascular pericytes and astrocytes that protect and maintain homeostasis within the brain [6]. These structures create tight junctions to restrict paracellular movement and favor transcellular movement functioning as a transport and metabolic barrier [3, 7]. Small, lipophilic molecules are allowed to diffuse into the brain, whereas larger hydrophilic molecules are restricted and will require transport mechanisms. The expression of transport proteins and efflux transporters in the BBB may block the efficacy of some therapies. Brain tumors cause a lack of tight junction integrity increasing the permeability of the BBB to some therapeutic agents [8].

Research on investigating tumor microenvironment has been limited so far. More recently, unveiling the mechanisms involved on cell proliferation and migration and the interaction with their environment has aroused the interest of researchers.

A better understanding of tumor microenvironment may help to develop better treatment strategies in the future [8].

For a therapeutic intervention to be effective, chemotherapy must be capable of crossing the BBB and penetrating the brain parenchyma and tumor environment [8, 9].

Novel strategies to optimize drug penetration and increase BBB permeability under investigation will be discussed in this chapter (Fig. 8.1).

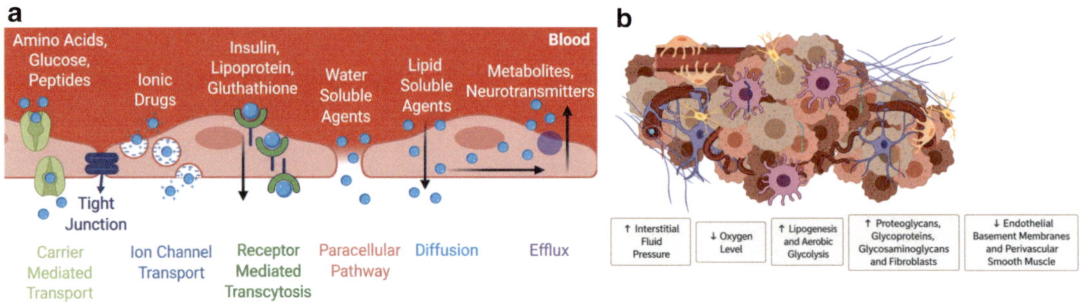

Fig. 8.1 (**a**) Transport systems of the blood-brain barrier. (**b**) Structural and mechanical characteristics of the tumor microenvironment impeding drug penetration. (Adapted from Patel et al., *Pediatric Blood Cancer. 2021*; https://doi.org/10.1002/pbc.28983 [8])

8.2 Chemotherapy Agents in Pediatric Neuro-Oncology

8.2.1 Alkylating Agents

Alkylating agents are a class of chemotherapy drugs that work by adding alkyl groups to DNA [10]. This process, known as alkylation, involves the transfer of an alkyl group from the drug to the DNA molecule within the cancer cells [10]. The alkylation typically targets the DNA's guanine base at the N7 position. By forming covalent bonds with the DNA, these agents induce several types of damage, including cross-links, strand breaks, and abnormal base pairing.

The use of alkylating agents started after World War I, when the use of sulfur mustard or "mustard gas" was widespread among the trenches as chemical warfare. During the 1940s, a similar compound, the nitrogen mustards, started to be studied at Yale University, and its anti-tumoral activity became known by 1946 [11].

Alkylating agents can be classified into several subgroups based on their chemical structure and specific mechanism of action:

8.2.1.1 Classical Alkylating Agents

8.2.1.1.1 Nitrogen Mustards

These drugs contain the bis (2-chloroethyl) amino, responsible of the alkylator effect. In pediatric neuro-oncology, the two most used drugs are cyclophosphamide and ifosfamide. They are among the earliest alkylating agents developed and are widely used in various cancers.

Cyclophosphamide is a prodrug, meaning it needs to be metabolized in the liver to become active [12]. After systemic absorption, cyclophosphamide is converted to the active metabolites 4-hydroxycyclophosphamide and aldophosphamide, which in turn is metabolized into the inactive compound carboxycyclophosphamide by the enzyme aldehyde dehydrogenase. The bone marrow stem cells are usually enriched with aldehyde dehydrogenase, so they are usually less prone to get damaged by cyclophosphamide due to quick conversion into its inactive metabolite [13]. This makes cyclophosphamide one of the chemotherapy drugs less harmful to the marrow. Afterward, aldophosphamide gets converted into two more compounds, phosphoramide mustard (the main responsible for the alkylating effect) and acrolein, which is responsible for one of the main toxicities of cyclophosphamide, hemorrhagic cystitis. Mesna can inactivate acrolein by conforming a compound with it, and it is used to prevent hemorrhagic cystitis [13, 14]. Cyclophosphamide when given at high doses can cause also cardiotoxicity. This drug is included regularly in medulloblastoma protocols [15]. Also, different oral metronomic therapies include cyclophosphamide as it can also be given orally, including some protocols for treating low-grade glioma [15–17].

Ifosfamide is another alkylating agent similar to cyclophosphamide and also requires metabolic activation in the liver. One of its most important side effects is ifosfamide-induced encephalopathy, probably caused by one of its metabolites, chloroacetaldehyde [18]. For preventing and treating encephalopathy, which can range from mild to severe, methylene blue (an oxidation-reduction agent) is usually given [18]. Ifosfamide can also cause neuropathy, as well as myelosuppression, hemorrhagic cystitis, alopecia, nausea, and vomiting [17]. In pediatric neuro-oncology, ifosfamide is given in the treatment of atypical teratoid rhabdoid tumors as well as germ-cell tumors [19–21].

8.2.1.1.2 Nitrosoureas

The name of the compound refers to the presence of a nitroso group and a urea. This group includes carmustine and lomustine, two drugs with good crossing of the blood-brain barrier due to being highly lipophilic, making them effective for treating brain tumors.

Lomustine (also known as CCNU, which stands for 1-(2-chloroethyl)-3-cyclohexyl-1-nitrosourea) is the most used drug of this group in pediatric neuro-oncology, and it is given orally. The biological effect of lomustine is secondary to the production of the chloroethyl carbenium ions in vivo as lomustine does not need activation.

Due to its high lipophilicity, it can cause delayed myelosuppression, thus lomustine is usually given in cycles of 6–8 week intervals. It is included in protocols for medulloblastoma, low-grade glioma, and high-grade glioma [22–24].

8.2.1.2 Alkylating-Like Agents

8.2.1.2.1 Platinum-Based Compounds

Although these drugs are not considered true alkylating agents due to not having an alkyl group, they form similar cross-links with DNA and are often grouped with alkylating agents due to their mechanism of action [25]. These drugs include cisplatin and carboplatin.

Cisplatin was the first drug of this group to be developed. Historically known as "Peyrone's salt," it was first synthesized after an experiment with *E. coli* bacteria showed cisplatin to be responsible for cell division arrest [25]. It is associated with severe side effects, including nephrotoxicity (due to accumulation in the nephron proximal tubule, which can be prevented by amifostine) [26], peripheral neurotoxicity (especially peripheral neuropathy, secondary to inhibition of a sodium-hydrogen ion transporter present in the peripheral nervous system cells) [25], ototoxicity (due to damage to the stria vascularis of the inner ear [27], which can be reduced by the use of sodium thiosulfate or acetylcysteine injections) [28], nausea, vomiting, and myelosuppression. Cisplatin is included in many brain tumor protocols in children and adolescents [29, 30].

Carboplatin is an analog of cisplatin but has different toxicity and a generally more amenable profile of side effects. It reduces nephrotoxicity as well as ototoxicity, while it is normally more myelosuppressive. Carboplatin may be administered concomitantly with radiotherapy in patients with high-risk Group 3 medulloblastoma; it is also included in the treatment of atypical teratoid rhabdoid tumors and low-grade glioma; and due to its myelosuppressive effect, it is one of the drugs usually used in conditioning regimens for high-dose chemotherapy with autologous rescue [4, 31–33].

8.2.1.3 Non-classical Alkylating Agents

8.2.1.3.1 Procarbazine

Procarbazine methylates guanine at the O6 position of guanine instead of alkylating the N7 position [34]. Although clinically in use since the end of the 1960s, procarbazine exact mechanism is not really known. Procarbazine is included in the low-grade glioma regimen TPCV (with thioguanine, lomustine, and vincristine) [24], as well as in the 8-in-1 regimen given in a variety of brain tumors (i.e., medulloblastoma and low-grade glioma) and in high-grade gliomas in the relapse setting [34, 35]. Some side effects include pancytopenia, nausea, and vomiting. Patients must avoid tyramine-containing foods (cured or fermented foods such as aged cheese, soy sauce, salami) to prevent hypertensive crises because procarbazine is a weak MAO inhibitor in the gastrointestinal system.

8.2.1.3.2 Triazenes

These drugs contain the group N3H3 and include dacarbazine (also used in the 8-in-1 chemotherapy regimen) and temozolomide. *Temozolomide* is an oral alkylating agent that works as a prodrug that at physiological pH converts to its active form, 3-methyl-(triazen-1-yl) imidazole-4-carboxamide (MTIC), which then converts into monomethylhydrazine and 5-aminoimidazole-4-carboxamide (AIC) [34]. Then, temozolomide can alkylate and methylate guanine at its N7 and O6 sites. However, some tumors defend from this damage by the expression of the DNA-repair enzyme O6-alkylguanine DNA alkyltransferase (AGT), which is encoded by the O6-methylguanine-DNA methyltransferase or MGMT gene. Thus, the presence of AGT correlates with a poor response to temozolomide, while the silencing of the MGMT gene can make the tumor more responsive to this drug. Temozolomide is the main chemotherapy agent used for high-grade gliomas [35] and it is also part of some oral metronomic regimens [36–39].

8.2.1.3.3 Ethyleneimines or Aziridines

These drugs contain the C2H5N group. Among them, *thiotepa* is an example. This drug, highly myeloablative, is currently only used in pediatric neuro-oncology as part of conditioning regimens in high-dose chemotherapy protocols [40].

8.2.2 Topoisomerase Inhibitors

Topoisomerases are enzymes that work by repairing changes in the topological state of the DNA, such as torsions and linkings [41]. By repairing these alterations, topoisomerases can prevent damage to the cell, allowing it to keep growing and dividing. There are two types of topoisomerases—type I topoisomerase, which induces single-strand breaks in the DNA to relieve torsional stress during DNA replication and transcription, and type II topoisomerase, which induces double-strand breaks [41]. Thus, by inhibition of these enzymes, cancer-induced changes are not repaired and the cancer cell is able to enter in apoptosis.

8.2.2.1 Topoisomerase I Inhibitors

These drugs are also called camptothecin derivatives, as camptothecin was the first drug of the group to be discovered.

Irinotecan, also called CPT-11, is one of the camptothecin derivatives. Irinotecan is converted to its active form, SN-38, which stabilizes the DNA-topoisomerase I complex leading to its deactivation, causing DNA breaks and inducing cell death. One of the most important side effects is diarrhea, which can be life-threatening. There are multiple proposed mechanisms for this, including metabolism by glucuronidation of SN-38 into SN-38G, which can be converted back in the intestinal lumen into SN-38 by bacterial beta-glucuronidase and thus accumulate in the gut, leading to secretory diarrhea [42]. This exaggerated intestinal secretion which is cholinergic in origin can be managed acutely with atropine and loperamide (especially diarrhea with delayed onset) and prophylactically with antibiotics targeted to intestinal bacterial flora such as cefixime. Irinotecan can also cause nausea, vomiting, and neutropenia. This drug is commonly given in the relapse setting of embryonal brain tumors such as medulloblastoma or CNS-neuroblastoma as part of different regimens, such as TEMIRI (with temozolomide) and BIT (with bevacizumab and temozolomide) [43]. It has also been used in low-grade gliomas, especially optic pathway gliomas with altered vision, together with bevacizumab [44, 45].

Topotecan stabilizes the DNA-topoisomerase I complex, preventing the replication and transcription of DNA and leading to cancer cell apoptosis, and has similar side-effect profile to irinotecan. It can be given intravenously, orally, or intrathecally, and it is normally used in relapsed embryonal brain tumors.

8.2.2.2 Topoisomerase II Inhibitors

Anthracyclines are derived from the *Streptomyces* bacterium. The primary mechanisms of action include DNA intercalation (inserting themselves between DNA base pairs, disrupting the DNA structure), direct topoisomerase II inhibition, and free radical formation [46]. Anthracyclines generate free radicals through redox cycling. These free radicals induce oxidative damage to cellular components, including DNA, proteins, and cell membranes, and this oxidative stress is thought to underlie one of its most important adverse effects: cumulative cardiotoxicity [47]. Some cardioprotective treatments have been used in clinical trials, among them dexrazoxane, a chelating drug [48]. Anthracyclines represent one of the most used chemotherapy drugs in medical oncology, and since the discovery of daunorubicin, similar drugs have been developed for reducing side-effects by doing some modifications to its molecule, such as doxorubicin, mitoxantrone, and idarubicin. However, in pediatric neuro-oncology, the use of anthracyclines is reduced to rhabdoid tumors which are theorized to benefit from its use [20].

Etoposide is a semisynthetic derivative of podophyllotoxin, extracted from the plant *Podophyllum peltatum* [49]. It inhibits topoisomerase II, an enzyme crucial for DNA strand separation during replication. By inhibiting this enzyme, etoposide causes DNA breaks, leading to apoptosis of cancer cells. Etoposide needs to be given intravenously slowly since it can lower blood pressure during administration. Other common side effects include myelosuppression, nausea, vomiting, alopecia, and mucositis. There is also a described risk of secondary leukemia with long-term use [50]. Etoposide is used for treating a variety of child brain tumors, such as medulloblastoma [32], ependymoma [51], embryonal tumors [52], low-grade glioma [53], germ-cell tumors [54] and in some conditioning regimens for high-dose chemotherapy [21].

8.2.3 Vinca Alkaloids

Vinca alkaloids are a class of chemotherapy drugs derived from the periwinkle plant (*Catharanthus roseus*, formerly known as *Vinca rosea*) [55]. These drugs work by inhibiting the formation of microtubules, which are essential components of the cell's cytoskeleton and are crucial for cell division. By binding to tubulin, a protein that makes up microtubules, vinca alkaloids prevent the polymerization and assembly of microtubules, thereby halting mitosis at the metaphase stage and leading to cell death.

Vinca alkaloids are widely used in pediatric neuro-oncology, mostly vincristine and vinblastine, but also vinorelbine has been used in the treatment of gliomas.

Vincristine was the first drug approved of this group in 1963. Common side effects include neurotoxicity (peripheral neuropathy) [56], myelosuppression, alopecia, constipation, ptosis, Syndrome of Inappropriate Antidiuretic Hormone secretion (SIADH) [57], and jaw pain. Neurotoxicity, more frequent in adolescents, is dose-limiting and can be severe, thus making people with a family or personal background of Charcot-Marie-Tooth disease to avoid the use of this drug [58]. It is also lethal if given intrathecally by accident, causing massive encephalopathy and spinal [55] demyelination [59]. Vincristine is usually administered as part of the treatment of low-grade glioma, medulloblastoma, embryonal tumors, and ependymoma [60, 61].

Vinblastine was the first isolated drug of this group, although it was approved for use after vincristine, and it is also derived from the periwinkle plant. It causes less neurotoxicity compared to vincristine, although there is more bone marrow suppression. It is used both as monotherapy and in combination regimens for the treatment of low-grade gliomas [62].

The efficacy of *vinorelbine* in pediatric and adult brain tumors was described in 1998 [63].

This treatment has been used for treating low-grade gliomas and also in some regimes for high-grade gliomas in combination with other treatments [64, 65].

8.2.4 Antimetabolites

Antimetabolites, as the name implies, are drugs that impair the use of a metabolite. The two most common antimetabolites used in pediatric neuro-oncology are methotrexate and thioguanine.

Methotrexate is a folate antagonist that inhibits the enzyme dihydrofolate reductase [58]. This enzyme is necessary for the synthesis of tetrahydrofolate, which is required for the synthesis of purines and thymidylate, essential components of DNA. By blocking this synthesis, methotrexate halts cell replication, particularly in rapidly dividing cells. Common side effects include myelosuppression, mucositis, hepatic toxicity, nephrotoxicity, and pulmonary toxicity. Chronic use can lead to liver damage and fibrosis. In pediatric neuro-oncology, it is usually given in embryonal tumors such as medulloblastoma and ATRT, as part of high intensity protocols, usually during a four-hour infusion period [52].

Thioguanine is another antimetabolite, which works as an analogue of guanine, thus impairing the normal metabolism of DNA synthesis. In pediatric neuro-oncology, its use is restricted to the TPCV regimen for treating low-grade gliomas associated with procarbazine, lomustine, and vincristine [24] (Table 8.1).

8.2.4.1 Chemotherapy Routes

Apart from conventional chemotherapy strategies for chemotherapy administration, different schedules are used to deliver therapeutic agents into the brain.

Table 8.1 Chemotherapy agents and main toxicities described

Drug	Family	Toxicities	Administration
Cyclophosphamide	Classical alkylating agent: Nitrogen mustards	Hemorrhagic cystitis, cardiotoxicity (high doses), nausea, vomiting	IV, oral
Ifosfamide	Classical alkylating agent: Nitrogen mustards	Hemorrhagic cystitis, cardiotoxicity (high doses), nausea, vomiting, alopecia, myelosuppression	IV
Lomustine	Classical alkylating agent: Nitrosoureas	Delayed myelosuppression, nausea, vomiting	Oral
Cisplatin	Alkylating-like agent: Platinum agent	Ototoxicity, neurotoxicity, nephrotoxicity, nausea, vomiting, myelosuppression	IV
Carboplatin	Alkylating-like agent: Platinum agent	Myelosuppression, nausea, vomiting., ototoxicity, hypersensitivity reactions	IV
Procarbazine	Non-classical alkylating agent	Myelosuppression, nausea, vomiting, hypertensive crisis with tyramine-containing foods.	Oral
Temozolomide	Non-classical alkylating agent: Triazenes	Idiosyncratic trombopenia, nausea, vomiting	Oral
Thiotepa	Non-classical alkylating agent: Aziridines	Myelosuppresion, nausea, vomiting, alopecia, dermatitis	IV
Irinotecan	Topoisomerase I inhibitor	Secretory diarrhea, nausea, vomiting, neutropenia	IV
Topotecan	Topoisomerase I inhibitor	Nausea, vomiting and neutropenia	IV, IT, oral
Doxorubicin	Topoisomerase II inhibitor: Non-intercalating agent	Cardiotoxicity, nausea, vomiting	IV
Etoposide	Topoisomerase II inhibitor: Intercalating agent	Low blood pressure during administration, myelosuppression, nausea, vomiting, alopecia, and mucositis	IV, IT, oral
Vincristine	Vinca alkaloids	Neurotoxicity, myelosuppression, alopecia, constipation, ptosis, SIADH, and jaw pain	IV
Vinblastine	Vinca alkaloids	Neurotoxicity, myelosuppression, alopecia, constipation, ptosis, SIADH, and jaw pain	IV
Methotrexate	Antimetabolites	Myelosuppression, mucositis, hepatic toxicity, nephrotoxicity, pulmonary toxicity	IV, IT, oral
Thioguanine	Antimetabolites	Nausea, vomiting	Oral

8.2.4.1.1 High-Dose Chemotherapy

Autologous hematopoietic progenitor cell transplantation allows us to use such high doses of chemotherapy that, under normal conditions, would cause irreversible bone marrow myelosuppression. High-dose chemotherapy (HDCT) followed by autologous stem cell rescue (SCR) has shown efficacy and may improve long-term survival in children diagnosed with some recurrent and chemosensitive brain tumors [66–68].

HDCT is more intensive than standard chemotherapy and may be more effective in destroying tumor cells as well as preventing recurrences.

Also relevant is its use as an alternative to radiation therapy [69, 70] which not only can be very effective in the treatment of CNS tumors but can also have serious side effects, especially in young children.

HDCT with SCR is a complex procedure that involves several steps:

1. Stem cell collection: Before high-dose chemotherapy is given, stem cells are collected from the child's blood or bone marrow. These stem cells (CD34+) are immature cells that can become mature blood cells.

2. High-dose chemotherapy: The child then receives high doses of chemotherapies, depending on the regimen used.
3. Stem cell rescue: After high-dose chemotherapy is finished, the child's collected stem cells are infused back into his/her body. These stem cells help replenish a child's blood cell count.

HDCT with SCR can cause several serious side effects, including infections, bleeding, pulmonary hypertension, mucositis, etc. Therefore, this procedure should be performed in centers with great experience and the possibility of providing continuous support to patients.

Success rates of high-dose chemotherapy with stem cell rescue for CNS tumors vary by tumor type, child age, and other factors. Phase I and II studies of HDCT have been published to find the optimal combination of chemotherapeutic agents and their doses in these children [4, 71]. These regimens have succeeded remarkably in infants with medulloblastoma [4] and in other embryonal tumors in order to avoid radiation in young children [72–74].

8.2.4.1.2 Metronomic Chemotherapy

Metronomic chemotherapy is defined as a treatment regimen involving the administration of chemotherapy drugs at low doses at frequent intervals. This approach has been investigated as a potential treatment for a variety of pediatric patient tumors, including CNS tumors [5, 75, 76].

Traditional treatment options for CNS tumors include surgery, radiation therapy, and conventional and high-dose chemotherapy. However, these treatments are often limited by the toxicity and ability of tumors to develop resistance to these therapies.

This treatment route offers a new, potentially less toxic, and sometimes effective treatment strategy for these tumors, as demonstrated in some clinical trials and/or publications, which have evaluated the safety and efficacy of metronomic chemotherapy for the treatment of various CNS tumors, especially relevant to its role in medulloblastoma [77–79].

Recently, very promising results have been published proving the efficacy of MC in medulloblastoma relapse [77]. This translates into the need for further research to determine the long-term efficacy of this approach and to identify the CNS tumors that are most likely to benefit from this treatment.

Mechanisms of Action of Metronomic Chemotherapy

Metronomic chemotherapy is thought to work through a variety of mechanisms, including [80]:

- *Inhibition of angiogenesis:* Growing tumors require an adequate blood supply to obtain nutrients and oxygen. Metronomic chemotherapy can inhibit the formation of new blood vessels—angiogenesis—with very relevant action against endothelial cells, which makes it difficult for the tumor to grow and spread [81, 82].
- *Immune Response Enhancement:* Metronomic chemotherapy may enhance the body's immune response to cancer, for example, with depletion of regulatory T cells [83].
- *Direct cytotoxic effect on cancer stem cells (Fig. 8.2).*

Metronomic chemotherapy (MC) has several potential advantages over conventional chemotherapy [76, 86, 87] including:

- Lower toxicity: Metronomic chemotherapy is given at lower doses than conventional chemotherapy, which can reduce side effects. Serious renal, hepatic, and hematological side effects are rare.
- Efficacy against drug-resistant tumors: Metronomic chemotherapy may be effective against tumors that have developed resistance to conventional chemotherapy drugs.
- Comfort: MC is taken orally, which means fewer hospital visits and, therefore, a higher quality of life.
- Wide availability: Lower costs, wide availability, and reduced need for hospitalization due to MC represent additional advantages for use in countries with limited resources.

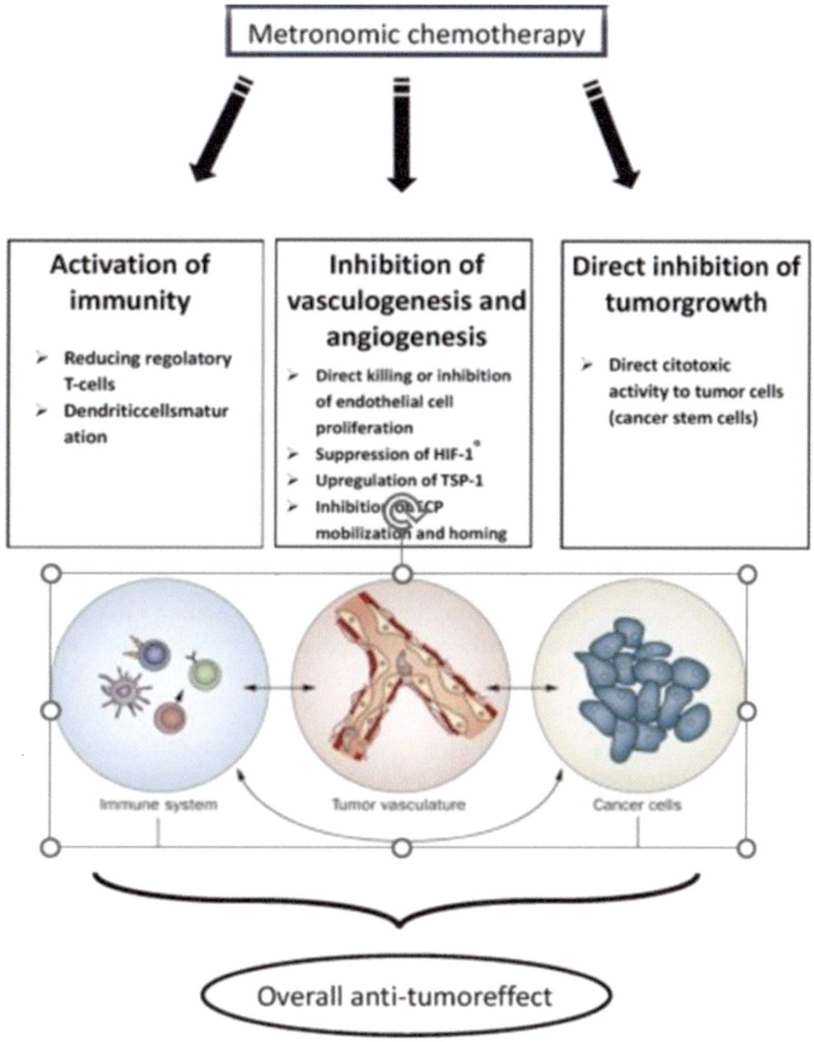

Fig. 8.2 Mechanisms of action of metronomic chemotherapy [80–85]

– Individualized approach: The best drugs and dosing schedule will depend on the specific type of tumor and the child's condition. MC may even be used in combination with surgery, radiation therapy, or other therapies [88].

In summary, metronomic treatment represents a valid strategy as maintenance or adjuvant therapy, as well as second or more lines of treatment in case of advanced/relapsed or refractory disease. Its use should be individualized according to the clinical situation and age of the patient, as well as the histology of the tumor and whether it is feasible by including patients in clinical trials (NCT01356290).

8.2.4.1.3 Intrathecal/Intraventricular Chemotherapy

The administration of chemotherapeutic agents directly into the cerebrospinal fluid (CSF) via injections into the spinal canal (intrathecal) or into the ventricular system with intraventricular devices such as the Ommaya reservoir is thought to overcome the limited distribution of anticancer drugs and their active metabolites into the CNS and to reduce systemic toxicity [6, 8].

This chemotherapy route has been incorporated into different protocols to intensify treatment in infants or as part of treatment schedules in refractory or relapse patients with CNS dissemination or periventricular nodules.

Many agents have been used for a variety of brain tumors. Intrathecal/intraventricular methotrexate has been incorporated into the treatment for some medulloblastomas in infants or ATRT protocols [6, 8, 89, 90].

Some early-phase trials have evaluated the safety and preliminary efficacy of etoposide in embryonal tumors and ependymoma [89]. Intrathecal/Intraventricular cytarabine and topotecan are also part of the current first-line treatment for some embryonal tumors such as ATRT or ETMR, and some trials that are currently ongoing are investigating their combination with other metronomic antiangiogenic agents in relapsed medulloblastoma, ATRT, and ependymoma [5, 91–93].

The safety profile reported using intraventricular devices to administer conventional chemotherapies also opens new opportunities for novel therapies currently under investigation for pediatric brain tumors such as CAR-T cells in pediatric brain tumors [94–97].

8.2.4.1.4 Intracystic Treatments

The use of intracystic treatments opened a new treatment opportunity for cystic craniopharyngiomas.

The agents administered aim to destroy the secretive properties of the epithelial cell and to induce cyst shrinkage and the subsequent adhesion of the cyst wall. Multiple radioisotopes and bleomycin were used in the past. However, in the last decade, the use of alpha-interferon replaced those previous agents due to its better toxicity profile [98].

As this drug is no longer available internationally, peg-interferon has been recently used providing a valid alternative to its non-pegylated counterpart [99].

Although this strategy has shown the potential of delaying or even avoiding more aggressive treatments in some cases, its long-term benefit is still unclear [100].

8.2.4.1.5 New Drug Delivery Strategies

In order to optimize drug penetrance through the BBB, research is currently exploring other strategies [9].

(a) *Nanoparticles*. Nanoparticles can be created from different materials (e.g., lipids, polymers, metals) that can be used as drug carriers [3, 6].

 Drugs that are not likely to cross the BBB could be adapted or packed into liposomes to make them more lipophilic. Additionally, nanomedicine can also be used for targeted therapy where nanoparticles can be equipped with specific proteins to target the tumor [9].

(b) *Focused ultrasound (FUS)*. FUS can provide reversible BBB disruption to enhance permeability by concentrating acoustic energy to a focal point. The addition of microbubbles has helped to focus the effect of FUS on the vessel walls [6]. This BBB disruption provides a window to increase drug penetration into the brain. Additionally, drug pharmacokinetics and tumor vascularity may also affect the penetration and efficacy of the drug delivered [9, 101, 102]. Some early-phase trials are currently ongoing with different drugs in different brain tumors to explore their safety and preliminary efficacy (NCT05630209, NCT05615623, NCT05762419).

(c) *Convention-enhanced delivery (CED)*. CED involves placing a catheter connected to an external infusion pump into the brain, which allows for the direct delivery of therapeutic agents into target tissues via an established pressure gradient. The local infusion ensures a higher therapeutic concentration in the brain parenchyma with less systemic toxicity [8, 9].

Although these methods are promising, they have not led to a significant improvement in drug delivery for most malignant primary brain tumors yet. Further research in the future may be needed to determine their role [9].

8.2.4.2 Targeted Therapies in Pediatric Brain Tumors

Advances in the diagnosis of childhood tumors have expanded the knowledge about genetic and epigenetic characteristics of pediatric brain tumors. Moreover, methylation array and next-generation DNA and RNA tumor sequencing have been incorporated into the last World Health Organization classification of brain tumors [103]. These techniques have highlighted the heterogeneity of tumor types and subtypes identifying different potential epigenetic and genetic targets [7, 104, 105].

With increasing knowledge of the molecular pathways upregulated in brain tumors in children, several agents have been developed in this context. However, the long-term benefit, how to maintain a lasting response over time, and how long to maintain these treatments are some questions still unresolved. Early-phase and phase 3 trials are currently ongoing testing multiple targeted therapies in children and adolescents with brain tumors to unveil the safety profile of these drugs and the benefit of incorporating them in first-line and relapse treatment protocols moving the field forward to more individualized strategies. Each tumor-type chapter will include a specific discussion on this regard.

Additionally, in recent years, multiple immunotherapies such as CAR-T cells, vaccines, or oncolytic viruses have been developed for pediatric cancer and are currently under investigation for pediatric brain tumors [97].

Immunotherapy in pediatric brain tumors will be discussed separately.

To conclude, systemic chemotherapy is one of the main treatments for brain tumors in children and adolescents. Different routes of administration and combinations have demonstrated good tolerance and responses in this setting. The incorporation of novel agents such as targeted therapies and immunotherapies, but also new routes to deliver these drugs, may provide new opportunities to improve the outcome of these patients, decreasing toxicity while improving the long-term quality of life of the survivors.

References

1. Chintagumpala M, Gajjar A. Brain tumors. Pediatr Clin N Am. 2015;62:167–78.
2. Pollack IF, Agnihotri S, Broniscer A. Childhood brain tumors: current management, biological insights, and future directions. J Neurosurg Pediatr. 2019;23:261–73.
3. Wu L, Li X, Janagam DR, et al. Overcoming the blood-brain barrier in chemotherapy treatment of pediatric brain tumors. Pharm Res. 2014;31:531–40.
4. Cohen BH, Geyer JR, Miller DC, et al. Pilot study of intensive chemotherapy with peripheral hematopoietic cell support for children less than 3 years of age with malignant brain tumors, the CCG-99703 phase I/II study. A report from the Children's Oncology Group. Pediatr Neurol. 2015;53:31–46.
5. Peyrl A, Chocholous M, Kieran MW, et al. Antiangiogenic metronomic therapy for children with recurrent embryonal brain tumors. Pediatr Blood Cancer. 2012;59:511–7.
6. Upton DH, Ung C, George SM, et al. Challenges and opportunities to penetrate the blood-brain barrier for brain cancer therapy. Theranostics. 2022;12:4734–52.
7. Malik JR, Podany AT, Khan P, et al. Chemotherapy in pediatric brain tumor and the challenge of the blood-brain barrier. Cancer Med. 2023;12:21075–96.
8. Patel JP, Spiller SE, Barker ED. Drug penetration in pediatric brain tumors: challenges and opportunities. Pediatr Blood Cancer. 2021;68:e28983.
9. Haumann R, Videira JC, Kaspers GJL, et al. Overview of current drug delivery methods across the blood-brain barrier for the treatment of primary brain tumors. CNS Drugs. 2020;34:1121–31.
10. Chiorcea-Paquim AM, Oliveira-Brett AM. Electrochemistry of chemotherapeutic alkylating agents and their interaction with DNA. J Pharm Biomed Anal. 2023;222:115036.
11. Goodman LS, Wintrobe MM, et al. Nitrogen mustard therapy; use of methyl-bis (beta-chloroethyl) amine hydrochloride and tris (beta-chloroethyl) amine hydrochloride for Hodgkin's disease, lymphosarcoma, leukemia and certain allied and miscellaneous disorders. JAMA J Am Med Assoc. 1946;132:126–32.
12. Ludeman SM. The chemistry of the metabolites of cyclophosphamide. Curr Pharm Des. 1999;5:627–43.
13. Kohn FR, Sladek NE. Aldehyde dehydrogenase activity as the basis for the relative insensitivity of murine pluripotent hematopoietic stem cells to oxazaphosphorines. Biochem Pharmacol. 1985;34:3465–71.
14. Almalag HM, Alasmari SS, Alrayes MH, et al. Incidence of hemorrhagic cystitis after cyclophosphamide therapy with or without mesna: a cohort study and comprehensive literature review. J Oncol Pharm Pract. 2021;27:340–9.
15. Friedman HS, Bigner SH, Bigner DD. Cyclophosphamide therapy of medulloblastoma: from the laboratory to the clinic and back again (and again and again). J Neuro-Oncol. 1995;24:103–8.
16. Slavc I, Mayr L, Stepien N, et al. Improved long-term survival of patients with recurrent Medulloblastoma

treated with a "MEMMAT-like" metronomic antiangiogenic approach. Cancers (Basel). 2022;14
17. Lee MJ, Ra YS, Park JB, et al. Effectiveness of novel combination chemotherapy, consisting of 5-fluorouracil, vincristine, cyclophosphamide and etoposide, in the treatment of low-grade gliomas in children. J Neuro-Oncol. 2006;80:277–84.
18. Kaijser GP, Beijnen JH, Bult A, et al. Ifosfamide metabolism and pharmacokinetics (review). Anticancer Res. 1994;14:517–31.
19. Chain G, Kalia M, Kestenbaum K, et al. A novel case of prolonged Ifosfamide encephalopathy and long-term treatment with methylene blue: a case report and review of literature. BMC Pediatr. 2022;22:76.
20. Slavc I, Chocholous M, Leiss U, et al. Atypical teratoid rhabdoid tumor: improved long-term survival with an intensive multimodal therapy and delayed radiotherapy. The Medical University of Vienna experience 1992–2012. Cancer Med. 2014;3:91–100.
21. Calaminus G, Frappaz D, Kortmann RD, et al. Outcome of patients with intracranial non-germinomatous germ cell tumors-lessons from the SIOP-CNS-GCT-96 trial. Neuro-Oncology. 2017;19:1661–72.
22. Zhang T, Zhang D, Shi F. Silico analysis of the target and possible mechanism of lomustine in the treatment of primary glioblastoma. J Mol Model. 2022;29(3)
23. Packer RJ, Sutton LN, Elterman R, et al. Outcome for children with medulloblastoma treated with radiation and cisplatin, CCNU, and vincristine chemotherapy. J Neurosurg. 1994;81:690–8.
24. Ater JL, Zhou T, Holmes E, et al. Randomized study of two chemotherapy regimens for treatment of low-grade glioma in young children: a report from the Children's Oncology Group. J Clin Oncol. 2012;30:2641–7.
25. Shah N, Dizon DS. New-generation platinum agents for solid tumors. Future Oncol. 2009;5:33–42.
26. Townsend DM, Deng M, Zhang L, et al. Metabolism of cisplatin to a nephrotoxin in proximal tubule cells. J Am Soc Nephrol. 2003;14:1–10.
27. Fisher MJ, Lange BJ, Needle MN, et al. Amifostine for children with medulloblastoma treated with cisplatin-based chemotherapy. Pediatr Blood Cancer. 2004;43:780–4.
28. Li Y, Zhang T, Song Q, et al. Cisplatin ototoxicity mechanism and antagonistic intervention strategy: a scope review. Front Cell Neurosci. 2023;17:1197051.
29. Massimino M, Spreafico F, Cefalo G, et al. High response rate to cisplatin/etoposide regimen in childhood low-grade glioma. J Clin Oncol. 2002;20:4209–16.
30. Dickey DT, Wu YJ, Muldoon LL, et al. Protection against cisplatin-induced toxicities by N-acetylcysteine and sodium thiosulfate as assessed at the molecular, cellular, and in vivo levels. J Pharmacol Exp Ther. 2005;314:1052–8.
31. Bruchim I, Goldberg A, Fishman A, et al. Carboplatin hypersensitivity: evaluation and successful desensitization protocol. Immunotherapy. 2014;6:905–12.
32. Leary SES, Packer RJ, Li Y, et al. Efficacy of carboplatin and isotretinoin in children with high-risk Medulloblastoma: a randomized clinical trial from the Children's Oncology Group. JAMA Oncol. 2021;7:1313–21.
33. Packer RJ, Ater J, Allen J, et al. Carboplatin and vincristine chemotherapy for children with newly diagnosed progressive low-grade gliomas. J Neurosurg. 1997;86:747–54.
34. Kim SH, Yoo H, Chang JH, et al. Procarbazine and CCNU chemotherapy for recurrent glioblastoma with MGMT promoter methylation. J Korean Med Sci. 2018;33:e167.
35. Pendergrass TW, Milstein JM, Geyer JR, et al. Eight drugs in one day chemotherapy for brain tumors: experience in 107 children and rationale for preradiation chemotherapy. J Clin Oncol. 1987;5:1221–31.
36. Beale P, Judson I, Moore S, et al. Effect of gastric pH on the relative oral bioavailability and pharmacokinetics of temozolomide. Cancer Chemother Pharmacol. 1999;44:389–94.
37. Jakacki RI, Cohen KJ, Buxton A, et al. Phase 2 study of concurrent radiotherapy and temozolomide followed by temozolomide and lomustine in the treatment of children with high-grade glioma: a report of the Children's Oncology Group ACNS0423 study. Neuro-Oncology. 2016;18:1442–50.
38. Grill J, Geoerger B, Gesner L, et al. Phase II study of irinotecan in combination with temozolomide (TEMIRI) in children with recurrent or refractory medulloblastoma: a joint ITCC and SIOPE brain tumor study. Neuro-Oncology. 2013;15:1236–43.
39. Dixit S, Baker L, Walmsley V, et al. Temozolomide-related idiosyncratic and other uncommon toxicities: a systematic review. Anti-Cancer Drugs. 2012;23:1099–106.
40. Kondo E, Ikeda T, Goto H, et al. Pharmacokinetics of thiotepa in high-dose regimens for autologous hematopoietic stem cell transplant in Japanese patients with pediatric tumors or adult lymphoma. Cancer Chemother Pharmacol. 2019;84:849–60.
41. Liang X, Wu Q, Luan S, et al. A comprehensive review of topoisomerase inhibitors as anticancer agents in the past decade. Eur J Med Chem. 2019;171:129–68.
42. Chamseddine AN, Ducreux M, Armand JP, et al. Intestinal bacterial beta-glucuronidase as a possible predictive biomarker of irinotecan-induced diarrhea severity. Pharmacol Ther. 2019;199:1–15.
43. Levy AS, Krailo M, Chi S, et al. Temozolomide with irinotecan versus temozolomide, irinotecan plus bevacizumab for recurrent medulloblastoma of childhood: report of a COG randomized phase II screening trial. Pediatr Blood Cancer. 2021;68:e29031.
44. Green K, Panagopoulou P, D'Arco F, et al. A nationwide evaluation of bevacizumab-based treatments

in pediatric low-grade glioma in the UK: safety, efficacy, visual morbidity, and outcomes. Neuro-Oncology. 2023;25:774–85.
45. de Marcellus C, Tauziede-Espariat A, Cuinet A, et al. The role of irinotecan-bevacizumab as rescue regimen in children with low-grade gliomas: a retrospective nationwide study in 72 patients. J Neuro-Oncol. 2022;157:355–64.
46. Marinello J, Delcuratolo M, Capranico G. Anthracyclines as topoisomerase II poisons: from early studies to new perspectives. Int J Mol Sci. 2018;19
47. McGowan JV, Chung R, Maulik A, et al. Anthracycline chemotherapy and cardiotoxicity. Cardiovasc Drugs Ther. 2017;31:63–75.
48. Cardinale D, Iacopo F, Cipolla CM. Cardiotoxicity of Anthracyclines. Front Cardiovasc Med. 2020;7:26.
49. Damayanthi Y, Lown JW. Podophyllotoxins: current status and recent developments. Curr Med Chem. 1998;5:205–52.
50. Zhang W, Gou P, Dupret JM, et al. Etoposide, an anticancer drug involved in therapy-related secondary leukemia: enzymes at play. Transl Oncol. 2021;14:101169.
51. Chamberlain MC. Recurrent intracranial ependymoma in children: salvage therapy with oral etoposide. Pediatr Neurol. 2001;24:117–21.
52. Kellie SJ, Wong CK, Pozza LD, et al. Activity of postoperative carboplatin, etoposide, and high-dose methotrexate in pediatric CNS embryonal tumors: results of a phase II study in newly diagnosed children. Med Pediatr Oncol. 2002;39:168–74.
53. Lee JH, Woo IS, Cho YY, et al. Successful treatment of intracranial germ cell tumor: report of two unusual cases and literature review. Case Rep Oncol. 2015;8:520–5.
54. Funt SA, McHugh DJ, Tsai S, et al. Four cycles of etoposide plus cisplatin for patients with good-risk advanced germ cell tumors. Oncologist. 2021;26:483–91.
55. Moudi M, Go R, Yien CY, et al. Vinca alkaloids. Int J Prev Med. 2013;4:1231–5.
56. Renbarger JL, McCammack KC, Rouse CE, et al. Effect of race on vincristine-associated neurotoxicity in pediatric acute lymphoblastic leukemia patients. Pediatr Blood Cancer. 2008;50:769–71.
57. Seetharam S, Thankamony P, Gopakumar KG, et al. Higher incidence of syndrome of inappropriate antidiuretic hormone secretion during induction chemotherapy of acute lymphoblastic leukemia in Indian children. Indian J Cancer. 2019;56:320–4.
58. Bernstock JD, Alva E, Cohen JL, et al. Treatment of pediatric high-grade central nervous system tumors with high-dose methotrexate in combination with multiagent chemotherapy: a single-institution experience. Pediatr Blood Cancer. 2020;67:e28119.
59. Alcaraz A, Rey C, Concha A, et al. Intrathecal vincristine: fatal myeloencephalopathy despite cerebrospinal fluid perfusion. J Toxicol Clin Toxicol. 2002;40:557–61.
60. Evans AE, Anderson JR, Lefkowitz-Boudreaux IB, et al. Adjuvant chemotherapy of childhood posterior fossa ependymoma: cranio-spinal irradiation with or without adjuvant CCNU, vincristine, and prednisone: a Childrens Cancer Group study. Med Pediatr Oncol. 1996;27:8–14.
61. Lefkowitz IB, Packer RJ, Siegel KR, et al. Results of treatment of children with recurrent medulloblastoma/primitive neuroectodermal tumors with lomustine, cisplatin, and vincristine. Cancer. 1990;65:412–7.
62. Lassaletta A, Scheinemann K, Zelcer SM, et al. Phase II weekly vinblastine for chemotherapy-naive children with progressive low-grade glioma: a Canadian pediatric brain tumor consortium study. J Clin Oncol. 2016;34:3537–43.
63. Hanley ML, Elion GB, Colvin OM, et al. Therapeutic efficacy of vinorelbine against pediatric and adult central nervous system tumors. Cancer Chemother Pharmacol. 1998;42:479–82.
64. Hamimed M, Gattacceca F, Andre N, et al. Pharmacokinetics of oral vinorelbine in French children with recurrent or progressive primary low-grade glioma. Br J Clin Pharmacol. 2022;88:2096–117.
65. Massimino M, Biassoni V, Miceli R, et al. Results of nimotuzumab and vinorelbine, radiation and re-irradiation for diffuse pontine glioma in childhood. J Neuro-Oncol. 2014;118:305–12.
66. Cheuk DK, Lee TL, Chiang AK, et al. Autologous hematopoietic stem cell transplantation for high-risk brain tumors in children. J Neuro-Oncol. 2008;86:337–47.
67. Panosyan EH, Ikeda AK, Chang VY, et al. High-dose chemotherapy with autologous hematopoietic stem-cell rescue for pediatric brain tumor patients: a single institution experience from UCLA. J Transp Secur. 2011;2011:740673.
68. De Giorgi U, Rosti G, Slavin S, et al. Salvage high-dose chemotherapy for children with extragonadal germ-cell tumours. Br J Cancer. 2005;93:412–7.
69. Yamada A, Kinoshita M, Kamimura S, et al. Novel strategy involving high-dose chemotherapy with stem cell rescue followed by intrathecal Topotecan maintenance therapy without whole-brain irradiation for atypical Teratoid/Rhabdoid tumors. Pediatr Hematol Oncol. 2023;40:629–42.
70. Ma Y, Lim DH, Cho H, et al. Tandem high-dose chemotherapy without Craniospinal irradiation in treatment of non-metastatic malignant brain tumors in very young children. J Korean Med Sci. 2020;35:e405.
71. Gilman AL, Jacobsen C, Bunin N, et al. Phase I study of tandem high-dose chemotherapy with autologous peripheral blood stem cell rescue for children with recurrent brain tumors: a pediatric blood and marrow transplant consortium study. Pediatr Blood Cancer. 2011;57:506–13.
72. Broniscer A, Nicolaides TP, Dunkel IJ, et al. High-dose chemotherapy with autologous stem-cell rescue in the treatment of patients with recurrent

non-cerebellar primitive neuroectodermal tumors. Pediatr Blood Cancer. 2004;42:261–7.
73. Fangusaro J, Finlay J, Sposto R, et al. Intensive chemotherapy followed by consolidative myeloablative chemotherapy with autologous hematopoietic cell rescue (AuHCR) in young children with newly diagnosed supratentorial primitive neuroectodermal tumors (sPNETs): report of the head start I and II experience. Pediatr Blood Cancer. 2008;50:312–8.
74. Dhall G, Grodman H, Ji L, et al. Outcome of children less than three years old at diagnosis with non-metastatic medulloblastoma treated with chemotherapy on the "head start" I and II protocols. Pediatr Blood Cancer. 2008;50:1169–75.
75. Andre N, Orbach D, Pasquier E. Metronomic maintenance for high-risk pediatric malignancies: one size will not fit all. Trends Cancer. 2020;6:819–28.
76. Pramanik R, Bakhshi S. Metronomic therapy in pediatric oncology: a snapshot. Pediatr Blood Cancer. 2019;66:e27811.
77. Peyrl A, Chocholous M, Sabel M, et al. Sustained survival benefit in recurrent Medulloblastoma by a metronomic antiangiogenic regimen: a nonrandomized controlled trial. JAMA Oncol. 2023;9:1688–95.
78. Winnicki C, Leblond P, Bourdeaut F, et al. Retrospective national "real life" experience of the SFCE with the metronomic MEMMAT and MEMMAT-like protocol. J Clin Med. 2023;12
79. Robison NJ, Campigotto F, Chi SN, et al. A phase II trial of a multi-agent oral antiangiogenic (metronomic) regimen in children with recurrent or progressive cancer. Pediatr Blood Cancer. 2014;61:636–42.
80. Bocci G, Kerbel RS. Pharmacokinetics of metronomic chemotherapy: a neglected but crucial aspect. Nat Rev Clin Oncol. 2016;13:659–73.
81. Natale G, Bocci G. Does metronomic chemotherapy induce tumor angiogenic dormancy? A review of available preclinical and clinical data. Cancer Lett. 2018;432:28–37.
82. Folkins C, Man S, Xu P, et al. Anticancer therapies combining antiangiogenic and tumor cell cytotoxic effects reduce the tumor stem-like cell fraction in glioma xenograft tumors. Cancer Res. 2007;67:3560–4.
83. Banissi C, Ghiringhelli F, Chen L, et al. Treg depletion with a low-dose metronomic temozolomide regimen in a rat glioma model. Cancer Immunol Immunother. 2009;58:1627–34.
84. Gnoni A, Silvestris N, Licchetta A, et al. Metronomic chemotherapy from rationale to clinical studies: a dream or reality? Crit Rev Oncol Hematol. 2015;95:46–61.
85. Pasquier E, Kavallaris M, Andre N. Metronomic chemotherapy: new rationale for new directions. Nat Rev Clin Oncol. 2010;7:455–65.
86. Pramanik R, Agarwala S, Sreenivas V, et al. Quality of life in paediatric solid tumours: a randomised study of metronomic chemotherapy versus placebo. BMJ Support Palliat Care. 2023;13:234–7.
87. Mariotto AB, Enewold L, Zhao J, et al. Medical care costs associated with cancer survivorship in the United States. Cancer Epidemiol Biomarkers Prev. 2020;29:1304–12.
88. Andre N, Carre M, Pasquier E. Metronomics: towards personalized chemotherapy? Nat Rev Clin Oncol. 2014;11:413–31.
89. Pajtler KW, Tippelt S, Siegler N, et al. Intraventricular etoposide safety and toxicity profile in children and young adults with refractory or recurrent malignant brain tumors. J Neuro-Oncol. 2016;128:463–71.
90. Fruhwald MC, Hasselblatt M, Nemes K, et al. Age and DNA methylation subgroup as potential independent risk factors for treatment stratification in children with atypical teratoid/rhabdoid tumors. Neuro-Oncology. 2020;22:1006–17.
91. Slavc I, Cohen-Pfeffer JL, Gururangan S, et al. Best practices for the use of intracerebroventricular drug delivery devices. Mol Genet Metab. 2018;124:184–8.
92. Potter SL, Berg S, Ingle AM, et al. Phase 2 clinical trial of intrathecal topotecan in children with refractory leptomeningeal leukemia: a Children's Oncology Group trial (P9962). Pediatr Blood Cancer. 2012;58:362–5.
93. Yamada A, Moritake H, Kamimura S, et al. Proposed strategy for the use of high-dose chemotherapy with stem cell rescue and intrathecal topotecan without whole-brain irradiation for infantile classic medulloblastoma. Pediatr Blood Cancer. 2014;61:2316–8.
94. Kramer K, Smith M, Souweidane MM. Safety profile of long-term intraventricular access devices in pediatric patients receiving radioimmunotherapy for central nervous system malignancies. Pediatr Blood Cancer. 2014;61:1590–2.
95. Vitanza NA, Ronsley R, Choe M, et al. Locoregional CAR T cells for children with CNS tumors: clinical procedure and catheter safety. Neoplasia. 2023;36:100870.
96. Vitanza NA, Johnson AJ, Wilson AL, et al. Locoregional infusion of HER2-specific CAR T cells in children and young adults with recurrent or refractory CNS tumors: an interim analysis. Nat Med. 2021;27:1544–52.
97. Donovan LK, Delaidelli A, Joseph SK, et al. Locoregional delivery of CAR T cells to the cerebrospinal fluid for treatment of metastatic medulloblastoma and ependymoma. Nat Med. 2020;26:720–31.
98. Bartels U, Laperriere N, Bouffet E, et al. Intracystic therapies for cystic craniopharyngioma in childhood. Front Endocrinol (Lausanne). 2012;3:39.
99. Hedrich C, Patel P, Haider L, et al. Feasibility, tolerability, and first experience of intracystic treatment with peginterferon alfa-2a in patients with cystic craniopharyngioma. Front Oncol. 2024;14
100. Kilday JP, Caldarelli M, Massimi L, et al. Intracystic interferon-alpha in pediatric craniopharyngioma patients: an international multicenter assessment

on behalf of SIOPE and ISPN. Neuro-Oncology. 2017;19:1398–407.
101. Martinez PJ, Green AL, Borden MA. Targeting diffuse midline gliomas: the promise of focused ultrasound-mediated blood-brain barrier opening. J Control Release. 2023;365:412–21.
102. Wei HJ, Upadhyayula PS, Pouliopoulos AN, et al. Focused ultrasound-mediated blood-brain barrier opening increases delivery and efficacy of etoposide for glioblastoma treatment. Int J Radiat Oncol Biol Phys. 2021;110:539–50.
103. Louis DN, Perry A, Wesseling P, et al. The 2021 WHO classification of tumors of the central nervous system: a summary. Neuro-Oncology. 2021;23:1231–51.
104. Zhou Q, Xu Y, Zhou Y, et al. Promising chemotherapy for malignant pediatric brain tumor in recent biological insights. Molecules. 2022;27
105. Skouras P, Markouli M, Strepkos D, et al. Advances on epigenetic drugs for pediatric brain tumors. Curr Neuropharmacol. 2023;21:1519–35.

Principles of Immunotherapy

9

Giada Del Baldo, Francesca Del Bufalo,
Andrea Carai, and Angela Mastronuzzi

9.1 Introduction

Pediatric brain tumors are the most common solid tumors in children [1]. The management and prognosis vary based on the histological category and molecular characteristics of the tumor, extending from a surveillance strategy following primary surgery for low-grade tumors, to intense therapeutic approaches such as chemotherapy and radiotherapy for high-grade tumors. Despite the use of aggressive multimodal treatments, brain tumors remain a significant cause of death in the pediatric population [2] and limited progress has been achieved in the treatment of pediatric brain tumors compared to other pediatric cancers [3].

Moreover, survivors frequently experience adverse effects [4], such as debilitating neurological impairments and cognitive deterioration caused by chemotherapy, radiotherapy, and surgery. Existing conventional treatments result in severe long-term toxicity, highlighting the urgent need to develop new therapeutic modalities. Immunotherapy has proven effective in both adult solid tumors and pediatric hemato-oncology, and it might also be a viable option for pediatric central nervous system (CNS) malignancies [4]. Despite this, there are still many challenges on the use of immunotherapy in pediatric CNS tumors.

The main categories of pediatric immunotherapy are immune checkpoint inhibition, therapeutic cancer vaccines, oncolytic virotherapy, chimeric antigen receptor T (CAR T).

9.2 Immune Response

The initial phase of the human immune response is the innate immune response. When phagocytes and natural killer (NK) cells bind to a pathogen through their receptors, they produce and release cytokines and chemokines that trigger inflammation. These substances can draw in naive T-cells to target and eliminate the pathogen [5]. When the innate immune system alone cannot resolve the inflammation, adaptive immunity, which involves a lymphocyte's response to a specific antigen, comes into play. Dendritic cells (DCs) serve a crucial role in linking the innate and adaptive

G. Del Baldo (✉) · F. Del Bufalo
Area of Hematology-Oncology, Cell Therapy, Gene Therapies, and Hematopoietic Transplantation, Bambino Gesù Children's Hospital, IRCCS, Rome, Italy
e-mail: giada.delbaldo@opbg.net

A. Carai
Neurosurgery Unit, IRCCS, Bambino Gesù Children's Hospital, Rome, Italy

A. Mastronuzzi
Area of Hematology-Oncology, Cell Therapy, Gene Therapies, and Hematopoietic Transplantation Bambino Gesù Children's Hospital, IRCCS, Rome, Italy

Department of Life Sciences and Public Health, Università Cattolica del Sacro Cuore, Rome, Italy

A. Mastronuzzi, A. Carai (eds.), *Navigating Pediatric Brain Tumors*,
https://doi.org/10.1007/978-3-032-18992-9_9

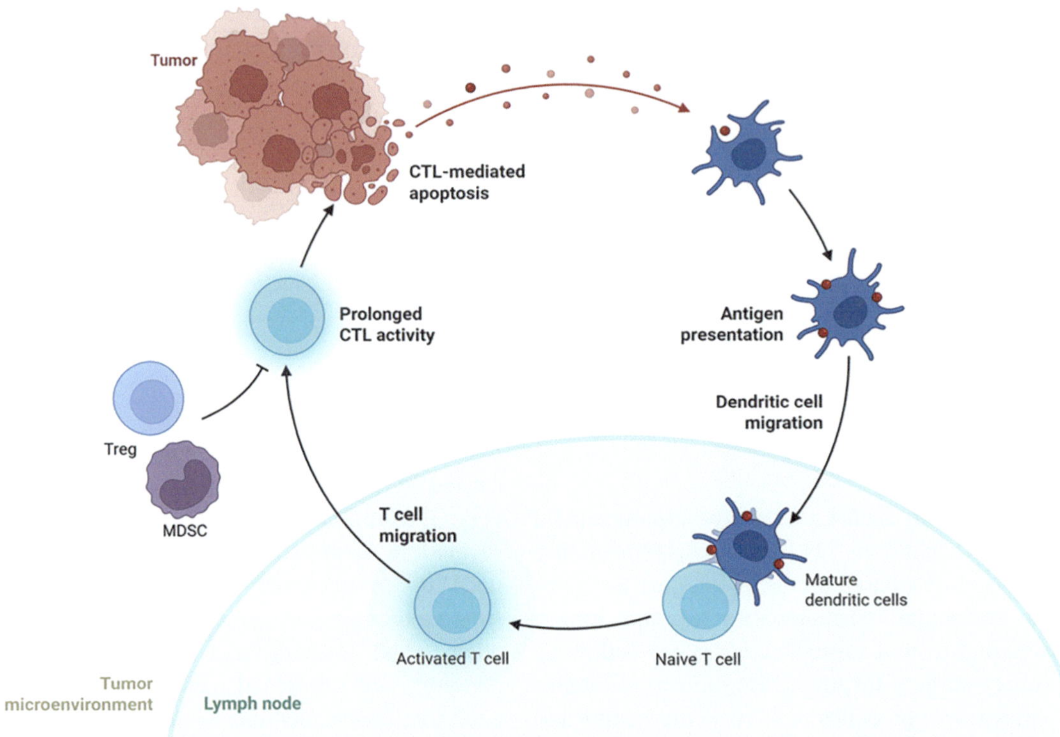

Fig. 9.1 Overview of the immune response. (Created with BioRender.com)

immune systems. They travel to the lymph nodes, where they present antigens to T-lymphocytes specific to the pathogen by displaying them on major histocompatibility complex (MHC) molecules [6–9]. When antigens are recognized, CD4+ T-cells, CD8+ T-cells, and B-cells undergo clonal expansion, producing identical clones capable of secreting monoclonal antibodies [8, 10, 11].

Tumors use various strategies to evade the immune system. This evasion is related to the tumor microenvironment (TME), as stromal cells within the tumor produce immunosuppressive factors. Tumor mechanisms include the secretion of immunosuppressive cytokines (such as transforming growth factor beta (TGF-β) and interleukin 10 (IL-10)), depletion of essential nutrients (through indoleamine 2,3-dioxygenase), recruitment of immunosuppressive cells (like regulatory T-cells, tumor-associated macrophages, and myeloid-derived suppressor cells), and expression of inhibitory molecules such as Fas ligand (FasL) or programmed death ligand 1 (PD-L1) [12]. Additionally, tumors can downregulate molecules necessary for T-cell recognition, including MHC, the antigen itself, or molecules involved in antigen processing [13] (Fig. 9.1).

9.3 Immunology in Pediatric Brain Tumors

Pediatric brain tumors are often considered immunologically “cold,” meaning they lack tumor-infiltrating T-cells [14]. This deficiency could be due to several factors: a lack of tumor antigens, insufficient antigen presentation, a failure in T-cell activation, or a deficiency in homing to the tumor site [15]. The low mutational burden typical of pediatric brain tumors may contribute to the paucity of tumor antigens, leading to fewer neoantigens available to activate T-cells [16]. The absence of infiltrating T-cells is closely connected to the TME, as it can induce downregulation of molecules necessary for T-cell recognition, further impairing T-cell infiltration.

Moreover, pediatric brain tumors may exhibit unique immunophenotypes distinct from those found in adult brain tumors, particularly regarding inflammatory and immunosuppressive TME. Adult high-grade gliomas (HGGs) are recognized for having an immunosuppressive microenvironment with significant immune cell infiltration [17]. Conversely, various immunophenotypes have been observed in pediatric cases of pilocytic astrocytoma, ependymoma, high-grade glioma, and medulloblastoma. Infiltration levels of myeloid and lymphocyte cells were notably lower in pediatric HGG and medulloblastoma compared to pilocytic astrocytoma and ependymoma [18]. Interestingly, diffuse midline glioma (DMG) has not been shown to possess either an inflammatory or an immunosuppressive TME [19, 20]. Furthermore, medulloblastoma has been found to express low levels of immune markers, with immune-stromal microenvironment patterns varying among different subtypes of the tumor, indicating distinct forms of local immunosuppression [21]. These findings suggest that immunotherapy strategies for pediatric brain tumors may need to differ from those used for adult brain tumors.

9.4 Rationale for Immunotherapy

Immunotherapy represents a promising approach for treating pediatric brain tumors due to several key factors:

1. *Unique Tumor Antigen Profile*

Pediatric brain tumors often display unique antigens that are not present in normal tissues. This distinct expression allows immunotherapies to specifically target these tumors. For example, certain gliomas express the EGFRvIII mutation, a neoantigen that immune cells can identify and attack [22]. Although pediatric tumors generally have a lower load of neoantigens compared to adult tumors, the presence of these unique targets offers opportunities for personalized immunotherapy approaches. Treatments such as cancer vaccines and T-cell receptor (TCR) therapies can be designed to specifically target these tumor antigens [23].

2. *Tumor Microenvironment*

The environment surrounding brain tumors, including pediatric variants, is often immunosuppressive. These tumors can create conditions that inhibit the immune response, such as the expression of immune checkpoint molecules like PD-L1. By targeting these checkpoints with inhibitors (e.g., anti-PD-1/PD-L1), it is possible to reactivate the immune system, enabling it to fight the tumor more effectively. Additionally, research has shown that pediatric brain tumors are infiltrated by various immune cells, including T-cells and macrophages. These cells can be reprogrammed or harnessed to attack the tumor cells, enhancing the body's natural defenses against cancer [24].

3. *Potential for Long-Lasting Remission*

One of the significant advantages of immunotherapy is its ability to provide long-term protection through the induction of immune memory. Once the immune system is trained to recognize and attack tumor cells, it can continue to monitor and prevent relapse. Clinical trials have demonstrated that immunotherapy can lead to durable responses in both adult and pediatric cancers, often lasting longer than those achieved with traditional therapies. This longevity of response is a promising aspect of immunotherapy, offering hope for sustained remission in pediatric brain tumor patients [25].

4. *Synergy with Existing Therapies*

Immunotherapy can be effectively combined with standard treatments such as surgery, radiation, and chemotherapy to enhance overall efficacy. For instance, radiation therapy can increase the expression of tumor antigens, making immunotherapy more effective. This synergistic effect helps to improve the overall treatment outcome, leveraging the strengths of each modality to combat the tumor more comprehensively. Additionally, immunotherapy can potentially overcome resistance mechanisms that limit the effectiveness of traditional therapies, offering a powerful tool in the oncological arsenal [26].

5. *Less Toxicity Compared to Conventional Treatments*

Traditional treatments for brain tumors, such as radiation and chemotherapy, are associated with significant long-term side effects, including cognitive impairment and the risk of secondary cancers. Immunotherapy, on the other hand, often has a more favorable toxicity profile. This is particularly important for the pediatric population, as reducing long-term side effects can significantly improve the quality of life for young patients. By minimizing the adverse effects associated with conventional treatments, immunotherapy provides a gentler yet effective treatment option [4].

6. *Clinical and Preclinical Evidence*

The success of immunotherapy in treating adult solid tumors and pediatric hematologic cancers provides a strong rationale for exploring these treatments in pediatric brain tumors. Encouraging results from ongoing clinical trials investigating various immunotherapeutic approaches in pediatric brain tumors further support this potential. These preliminary findings are promising, indicating that immunotherapy could become a viable and effective treatment option for these challenging cancers. As research progresses, the hope is that immunotherapy will offer new, more effective treatment strategies for pediatric brain tumor patients [27].

9.5 Application of Immunotherapy in Pediatric Brain Tumors

The different immunotherapy strategies available for pediatric brain tumors are described below (Fig. 9.2).

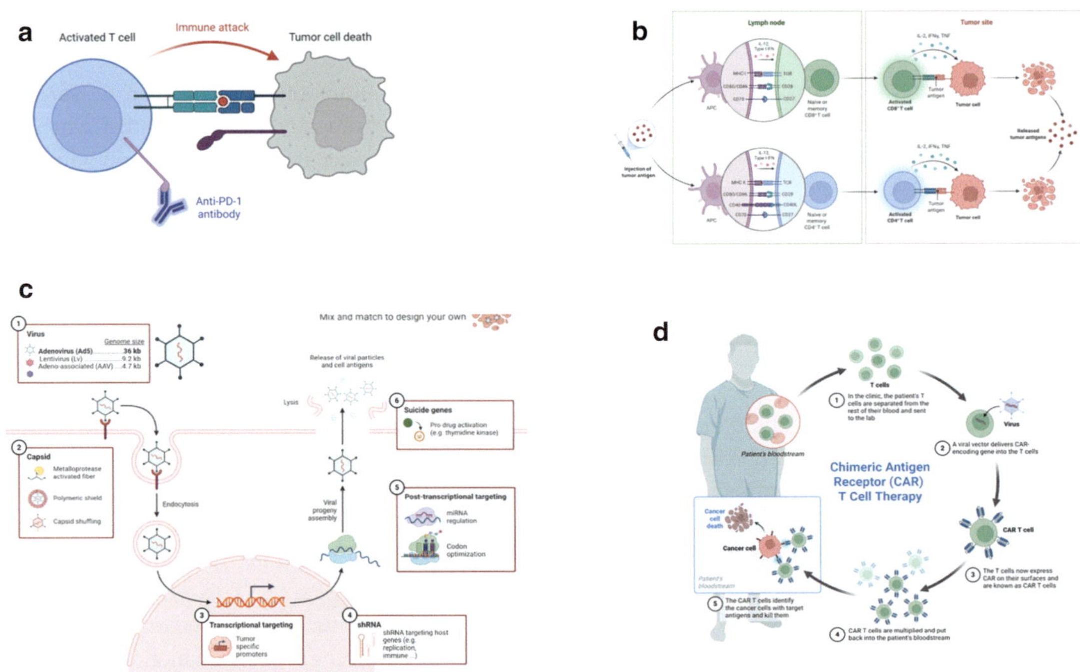

Fig. 9.2 Immunotherapy strategies for pediatric brain tumors. (**a**) Immune checkpoint inhibition; (**b**) Therapeutic cancer vaccines; (**c**) Oncolytic virotherapy; (**d**) Chimeric antigen receptor T-cell therapy. (Created with BioRender.com)

9.5.1 Immune Checkpoint Inhibition

Monoclonal antibodies targeting inhibitory molecules essential in regulating and suppressing T-cell responses [28] have been found to restore CD8+ T-cell activation within the TME. In certain cancers, these antibodies can serve as effective treatments [29, 30]. One of the pivotal discoveries was that blocking cytotoxic T lymphocyte-associated protein 4 (CTLA-4) with antibodies led to tumor shrinkage in mouse models of colon cancer and fibrosarcoma [28]. This was soon followed by the notable success of antibodies that block the checkpoints programmed death 1 (PD-1) and its primary ligand PD-L1 [31]. The effectiveness of checkpoint inhibitors in treating adult solid tumors like melanoma has been extraordinary, and in 2011, the FDA approved ipilimumab, a CTLA-4 inhibitor, for melanoma treatment [32]; since then, five additional checkpoint inhibitors have been authorized. The mutational burden of a tumor may be a critical factor in predicting the effectiveness of checkpoint inhibition for specific cancers. Patients with colon cancer and mismatch repair deficiency (and consequently a higher mutational burden) responded more effectively to PD-1 blockade with pembrolizumab compared to patients with an intact DNA damage response pathway [33]. A recent systematic review found that in cases where objective responses (ORs) were recorded, the ORs to PD-1 or PD-L1 inhibitor monotherapy were associated with tumor mutational burden across 27 human cancers. This relationship was notably strong in lung cancers, melanoma, and colorectal cancer, whereas glioblastoma (GBM) exhibited a lower mutational load (less than five coding somatic mutations per megabyte) and correspondingly lower objective responses to checkpoint inhibition [34]. In selected cases of GBM patients with DNA repair deficiencies, and then who consequently exhibit a higher tumor mutational burden, responses to checkpoint inhibitors have been observed [35, 36]. For instance, a report on two pediatric siblings with hypermutant GBM due to germline biallelic mismatch repair deficiency (bMRD) revealed that bMMRD-associated GBMs possessed a substantially elevated mutational load and a significantly greater number of predicted neoantigens compared to sporadic pediatric gliomas. Both siblings were treated with the anti-PD-1 inhibitor nivolumab and exhibited notable clinical and radiological improvements [35]. However, a recent systematic review suggested that gliomas might be a tumor subtype where clinical outcomes from checkpoint inhibition do not necessarily correlate with mutational burden [37], though it is unclear whether children were included in this analysis. Despite the uncertainty surrounding this correlation, checkpoint inhibition should still be considered when treating children with germline mutations leading to hypermutation, especially in cases of relapsed or refractory disease.

In pediatric brain tumor patients who do not have germline hypermutation syndromes, the efficacy of checkpoint inhibitors has not yet been demonstrated and many of these patients also received additional therapies, such as radiotherapy, which are known to contribute to disease stability and clinical responses. Therefore, it is crucial to avoid attributing disease response solely to novel therapies when they are administered in single-arm trials alongside conventional treatments.

9.5.2 Therapeutic Cancer Vaccines

9.5.2.1 Peptide Vaccines

Peptide cancer vaccines represent a promising treatment option for pediatric brain tumors, aiming to generate a targeted immune response against antigens specifically expressed by tumor cells. These vaccines have shown the potential to induce strong biological responses. Multiple studies have previously assessed the safety and feasibility of peptide-based vaccines in both pediatric and adult tumors [38–43]. Pollack et al. conducted three pediatric-specific studies from 2014 to 2016, exploring the use of peptide-based vaccines in recurrent low-grade gliomas, recurrent HGGs, and newly diagnosed malignant brainstem and non-brainstem gliomas [44–46].

These studies employed a consistent vaccination schedule targeting three peptide epitopes—IL-13Ra2, EphA2, and survivin—that are highly expressed in pediatric gliomas [47]. The primary objectives across these studies were to evaluate vaccine safety and T-cell responses against glioma-associated antigen (GAA) epitopes using enzyme-linked immunosorbent spot (ELISPOT) analysis. The first study, published in 2014 [46], included 26 patients with newly diagnosed malignant brainstem and non-brainstem gliomas. Of these, 12 had newly diagnosed brainstem or HGG treated with radiation and concurrent chemotherapy, while 14 had newly diagnosed brainstem gliomas treated with radiation alone. The cohort had a 50% female distribution, with ages ranging from 2.2 to 17.9 years. No dose-related toxicities or grade 3 or higher systemic toxicities were reported. Preliminary clinical outcomes, assessed via magnetic resonance imaging (MRI), revealed 19 patients with stable disease, 2 with partial responses, 1 with a minor response, 2 with prolonged disease-free status post-surgery, and 2 with progressive disease after two vaccine courses. The overall median survival was 13.3 months from diagnosis, with 12.7 months for brainstem gliomas and 25.5 months for HGGs. ELISPOT analysis showed GAA responses in 13 patients, with 10 responding to IL-13Ra2, 11 to EphA2, and 3 to survivin. In a subsequent study focused on recurrent low-grade gliomas, Pollack et al. enrolled 14 patients, excluding 2 (one for grade 3 urticaria and one due to progressive disease) [45]. The cohort had a 50% female distribution, with ages ranging from 1.9 to 19.0 years. Apart from the case of grade 3 urticaria, no other regimen-limiting toxicities were observed. MRI assessments showed that one child experienced asymptomatic pseudoprogression at 6 weeks, followed by significant tumor regression (>75% shrinkage). Three children had sustained partial responses lasting over 10, 31, and 45 months, respectively, while one had a transient response. The median progression-free survival was 9.9 months, with an overall survival rate of 100% and an average follow-up of 42 months. ELISPOT analysis showed GAA responses in all patients, including 3 to IL-13Ra2, 11 to EphA2, and 3 to survivin.

The most recent study, published in 2016, focused on pediatric patients with recurrent HGGs [44]. This study included 12 patients: 6 with glioblastoma, 5 with anaplastic astrocytoma, and 1 with malignant gliomatosis cerebri. The cohort had a 50% female distribution, with ages ranging from 2.3 to 23.3 years. No dose-limiting toxicities or grade 3 or higher toxicities were reported. MRI evaluations revealed that one child experienced symptomatic pseudoprogression, while another showed a partial response. The median progression-free survival from the start of vaccination was 4.1 months, with a median overall survival of 12.9 months. At 6 months, progression-free survival was 33%, and overall survival was 73%. ELISPOT analysis showed GAA responses in 9 patients, with 4 responding to IL-13Ra2, 9 to EphA2, and 3 to survivin.

Overall, these three studies on peptide vaccination for pediatric brain tumors have demonstrated safety, with only one case of grade 3 urticaria and no dose-limiting toxicities. They have also shown feasibility in eliciting an immunologic response, as several patients exhibited T-cell responses against GAA epitopes in ELISPOT analysis. Although these findings are promising, larger, multi-institutional studies are necessary to further evaluate the efficacy of this approach.

9.5.2.2 Dendritic Cell Vaccines

Dendritic cells (DCs) are among the most powerful antigen-presenting cells and play a crucial role in initiating immune responses and activating naïve T-cells [8, 48]. In cancer immunotherapy, DC vaccines are designed to identify tumor-specific antigens, leading to the elimination of cancer cells and the establishment of long-term immunity [8]. This strategy has gained traction in neuro-oncology, and, following encouraging results in adults using autologous dendritic cells combined with various tumor-targeting agents, dendritic cell therapy has been investigated in pediatric CNS tumors. Four studies focusing on pediatric patients employed autologous dendritic cells loaded with different forms of tumor lysate or RNA derived from surgical resections. There are four phase I trials, including those by Caruso et al. (7 patients), Ardon et al. (45 patients), Lasky et al. (3 patients), and Benitez-Ribas et al. (9 patients), which assessed the feasibility and safety of autologous dendritic cell vaccines in pediatric CNS tumor cases [49–52]. The included diagnoses varied, but the trials were generally limited to patients who had exhausted standard treatment options and had tumors with historically poor outcomes, such as recurrent HGG in 37 patients, medulloblastoma in 5 patients, ependymoma in 7 patients, and newly diagnosed diffuse intrinsic pontine glioma (DIPG) in 9 patients. Across all four studies, a total of 64 patients tolerated the treatment well, with no severe adverse events reported. Due to the small sample sizes and the primary emphasis on safety and feasibility, outcome measures such as survival rates and immune responses were variable, and the authors did not draw definitive conclusions about the efficacy of the interventions. In the largest study, which included 45 patients treated with autologous dendritic cells pulsed with tumor cell lysate, Ardon et al. reported long-term survival (over 24 months) in 6 out of 33 HGG patients, but no long-term survivors among the 5 medulloblastoma and 1 out of 4 ependymoma patients, with a median overall survival of 13.5 months [49]. In contrast, Caruso et al. found that none of the seven patients in their study exhibited a positive immune response following vaccination, raising concerns about the functionality of the adoptive immune system in these heavily pretreated patients [52]. However, Benitez-Ribas et al. observed a positive immune response in all nine patients with newly diagnosed DIPG after vaccination [50]. Overall, while pediatric studies involving autologous dendritic cells loaded with tumor lysate or RNA have demonstrated safety and feasibility in 64 pediatric patients, they have yet to show significant improvements in progression or overall survival in large, randomized trials or when compared to historical controls. The assessment of immune responses to the vaccines produced mixed results: one study reported a positive immune response, while another found no such response, indicating that further investigation is needed.

9.5.3 Oncolytic Virotherapy

Oncolytic viruses have emerged as a promising avenue in cancer immunotherapy, with the first and only FDA-approved oncolytic virus being a modified herpes virus used for the treatment of advanced melanoma [53]. The potential of oncolytic viral therapy for CNS tumors is particularly compelling due to the multiple mechanisms by which these engineered viruses can target malignant tumor cells and alter the tumor microenvironment. These mechanisms include selectively infecting tumor cells, leading to direct tumor lysis and subsequent cell death. This lysis process releases tumor-associated antigens, which can then activate the immune system to eliminate remaining tumor cells and attract lymphocytes to the tumor microenvironment, potentially enhancing the efficacy of other immunotherapies [54, 55]. However, oncolytic therapy for CNS tumors presents challenges, particularly in overcoming the blood-brain barrier to ensure adequate delivery and exposure of the therapy to the tumor. Several genetically engineered viruses, such as herpes simplex virus (HSV), adenovirus, poliovirus, and measles virus, are currently under investigation in cancer immunotherapy [27, 55].

Pediatric CNS tumors, especially HGGs and recurrent embryonal tumors, have been the focus of two completed early-phase studies evaluating the safety and feasibility of intratumoral delivery of genetically engineered oncolytic viruses. Friedman et al. reported the outcomes of a study involving 12 patients with recurrent HGGs who received a direct infusion of the modified HSV-1 G207 into the recurrent tumor tissue. The study population was 50% female, with an age range of 7–18 years. No grade 3 or 4 toxicities were observed, and the median overall survival was 12.2 months, with four patients surviving beyond 18 months [56]. In another early-phase trial, Kieran et al. investigated the use of an adenovirus genetically engineered with the tk-HSV gene in eight newly diagnosed patients who underwent second-look surgery followed by 14 days of valacyclovir treatment. The age range for this cohort was 7–17 years. This approach, considered a form of gene-mediated cytotoxic immunotherapy, was found to be generally safe, with only one case of grade 3 headache reported. Median survival was 9 months for patients in dose level 1 and 25 months for those in dose level 2 [57]. Collectively, these studies suggest that oncolytic therapy is preliminarily safe, with minimal severe adverse effects. Future directions include a larger multi-institutional clinical trial that is currently underway.

9.5.4 Chimeric Antigen Receptor T-Cell (CAR T) Therapy

Chimeric antigen receptor T-cell (CAR T) therapy has achieved remarkable success in treating relapsed or refractory B-cell acute leukemia and high-grade B-cell non-Hodgkin lymphoma (NHL) [58]. This success sparked interest in applying CAR T therapy to solid tumors, but results have not been as promising [59]. The main challenges of CAR T-cell therapy for solid tumors include the immunosuppressive and hostile TME, heterogeneous antigen expression, and rapid exhaustion of CAR T-cells [60, 61]. These limitations are even more pronounced in CNS tumors. Additionally, targeting CNS tumors presents specific challenges, such as the unique location, the presence of the blood-brain barrier (BBB), and the risk of neurotoxicity [62].

Chimeric antigen receptors were first developed by Eshhar et al. in 1989 and combine the MHC-independent antigen recognition of the ScFV portion of monoclonal antibodies with the effector functions of T cells [63]. This approach involves engineering T cells to express a chimeric molecule that fuses the variable regions of a monoclonal antibody with the cytotoxic zeta chain (ζ) of a T-cell receptor (first-generation CAR) [64]. This fusion allows targeting of various tumor-associated antigens on the surface of cancer cells and can overcome the challenges of low tumor immunogenicity due to minimal antigen levels and poor MHC presentation. CAR T-cells offer several advantages over monoclonal antibodies, including their ability to self-amplify upon activation, better tissue distribution, and enhanced immune system recruitment through cytokine release. Additionally, CAR T-cells can integrate into the memory pool, providing prolonged protection against tumor recurrence.

The design of CAR T-cells has been continuously improved to boost their effectiveness. Second- and third-generation CARs incorporate one or two co-stimulatory domains, such as CD28 and/or 4-1BB, to promote T-cell expansion, cytotoxic function, and persistence. Fourth-generation CARs, also known as TRUCKs (T-cells redirected for universal cytokine-mediated killing), expand on second-generation designs by incorporating an inducible transgene, like interleukin-12 (IL-12), to enhance the antitumor response. The fifth generation of CARs introduces a new approach by adding a truncated cytoplasmic receptor and a binding site for transcription factors like STAT3/5 to second-generation structures [65].

The main target antigens against brain tumors that have been studied are epidermal growth factor receptor variant III (EGFRvIII), human epidermal growth factor receptor 2 (HER2), interleukin 13 receptor alpha 2 subunit (IL13R 2), EGFR806, Ephrin type-A receptor (Epha2), B7-H3, and disganglioside-GD2.

IL-13Rα2, a high-affinity receptor for IL-13, is present in over 75% of GBM cases and has limited expression in normal tissues, making it a useful target for CAR T-cell therapy [66]. EGFRvIII, a mutated form of the EGFR protein found in GBM but absent in normal tissue, is a key oncogenic driver promoting tumor progression and genomic instability, making it a prime target for therapy [60]. HER2 is expressed in about 80% of GBM cases and promotes cell growth and survival through its tyrosine kinase activity [67]. Epha2 is overexpressed in many cancers, including GBM, contributing to tumor cell proliferation and invasion [68]. B7-H3, a member of the B7 family involved in immune checkpoint signaling, is linked to immune evasion and tumor growth, with expression in various CNS tumors [69]. Disialoganglioside GD2 serves as a promising target for other CNS cancers like medulloblastoma and diffuse midline glioma [70–73].

A summary of the main clinical trials available in pediatric patients and the results of published data are summarized in Tables 9.1 and 9.2.

Despite these challenges, several strategies are being developed to enhance the effectiveness of CAR T-cell therapy in pediatric brain tumors:

Targeting Multiple Antigens: To overcome antigenic heterogeneity, researchers are engineering CAR T-cells to target multiple tumor-associated antigens simultaneously. Vitanza's team has launched a new trial that will test CAR T-cells that target four different molecules found predominantly on brain and spinal tumors, reducing the likelihood of tumor escape due to loss of antigen expression [74].

Local Delivery: Intracerebral or intraventricular delivery of CAR T-cells is being explored to bypass the BBB and deliver the cells directly to the tumor site. This method can increase the concentration of CAR T-cells in the tumor bed and enhance antitumor activity while reducing systemic toxicity [75].

Armoring CAR T-Cells: To combat the immunosuppressive TME, CAR T-cells can be genetically modified to secrete cytokines like IL-12 or express dominant-negative receptors that block inhibitory signals from the tumor microenvironment. These "armored" CAR T-cells are better equipped to resist suppression and maintain their antitumor functions [76].

Combination Therapies: CAR T-cell therapy is increasingly being investigated in combination

Table 9.1 GD2 CAR T-cells clinical trial in pediatric patients and young adults

Study number	Antigen target	Disease	Site	Status
NCT05298995	GD2	Recurrent and refractory pediatric and young adults brain tumors	Bambino Gesù Hospital and Research Institute, Rome	Recruiting
NCT06221553	B7H3 IL-7Ra	DMG	Chulalongkorn University	Recruiting
NCT04099797	C7R-GD2.CART	Diffuse Intrinsic Pontine Glioma High Grade Glioma Embryonal Tumor Ependymal tumor	Baylor College of Medicine	Recruiting
NCT04510051	IL13Ralpha2	Recurrent and refractory pediatric brain tumors	City of Hope Medical Center	Recruiting
NCT03170141	Antigen-specific IgT cells	GBM	Shenzhen Geno-Immune Medical Institute	Enrolling by invitation
NCT03500991	HER2	Recurrent and refractory pediatric brain tumors	Seattle Children's Hospital	Active, not recruiting
NCT03638167	EGFR806	Recurrent and refractory pediatric brain tumors	Seattle Children's Hospital	Completed
NCT04185038	B7-H3	Recurrent and refractory pediatric brain tumors	Seattle Children's Hospital	Recruiting
NCT04196413	GD2	DMG	Stanford University	Recruiting
NCT01109095	HER.CAR CMV-specific CTLs	GBM	Baylor College of Medicine	Completed
NCT05768880	B7-H3, EGFR806, HER2, And IL13-Zetakine (Quad)	DMG Recurrent and refractory CNS Tumor	Seattle Children's Hospital	Active, not recruiting
NCT07087002	GPC2	Medulloblastoma	Stanford University	Recruiting
NCT06946680	IL-8 Receptor-modified CD70 CAR T	HGG	University of Florida	Recruiting

Table 9.2 Clinical data published on pediatrics patients affected by CNS tumors

Study number	NCT03500991	NCT04196413	NCT04185038	NCT04196413	NCT04099797
Author years	Vitanza et al. (2021)	Majzner et al. (2022)	Vitanza et al. (2024)	Monje et al. (2024)	Lin et al. (2024)
Number of patients	3 (children, young adults)	4 (children, young adults)	3 (children, young adults)	11 (children, young adults)	11 (children, young adults)
Brain tumors	1 Anaplastic astrocytoma 2 Eependymoma	DMG	DMG	DMG	HGG
Antigen target	HER2	GD2	B7H3	GD2	C7R-GD2
Construct	Second generation	Second generation	Second generation	Second generation	Second generation
Route of administration	Locoregional	Intravenously and locoregional for patients who exhibited clinical benefit	Locoregional	Intravenously and locoregional for patients who exhibited clinical benefit	Intravenously
Response		Three of four patients exhibited clinical and radiological improvement.	PR: 1 patient (6%) SD: 15 patients (83%) PD: 2 patients (11%)	Nine out of 11 patients demonstrated neurological benefit. Four patients demonstrated major volumetric tumor reductions. One patient exhibited a complete response ongoing for over 30 months since enrolment	Patients experienced temporary improvement from baseline neurologic deficits. Partial responses by iRANO criteria were observed in two of seven (29%) patients
Toxicity	No associated dose-limiting toxic effects.	CRS and TIAN (reversible in all cases). No DLT	1 DLT	Three patients experienced dose-limiting CRS on DL2. All patients exhibited TIAN (reversible in all cases)	No DLT

with other treatments, such as immune checkpoint inhibitors, radiation therapy, and chemotherapy. These combination approaches aim to enhance CAR T-cell persistence, overcome TME resistance, and improve clinical outcomes.

Novel CAR Designs: Ongoing research is focusing on the development of next-generation CARs. Fifth-generation CARs are being designed to include intracellular domains that recruit transcription factors, such as STAT3/5, which enhance T-cell activation and proliferation. These innovations aim to improve the durability and potency of CAR T-cells in the challenging CNS environment [65].

CAR T-cell therapy in brain tumors can lead to three types of toxicity: cytokine release syndrome (CRS), immune effector cell-associated neurotoxicity syndrome (ICANS), and tumor inflammation-associated neurotoxicity (TIAN).

Cytokine release syndrome is the most common and potentially severe toxicity associated with CAR T-cell therapy. CRS occurs when CAR T-cells become hyperactivated upon encountering tumor cells, releasing large amounts of pro-inflammatory cytokines, such as interleukin-6 (IL-6), IL-1, and interferon-gamma (IFN-γ). This hyperactivation triggers a systemic inflammatory response that can lead to high fever, hypotension, organ dysfunction, and, in severe cases, multi-organ failure. The severity of CRS can vary from mild, flu-like symptoms to life-threatening conditions, requiring intensive care and immunosuppressive treatment [77].

ICANS is another critical adverse effect of CAR T-cell therapy, particularly in brain tumors. ICANS manifests as a wide range of neurological symptoms, including headache, confusion, seizures, speech impairment, delirium, and, in severe cases, coma or cerebral edema. The underlying mechanism of neurotoxicity is not fully understood, but it is believed to result from the excessive inflammation caused by CAR T-cells crossing the BBB and directly affecting the CNS [78].

TIAN often indicates neuronal dysfunction resulting from localized inflammation and/or temporary edema caused by this inflammation. Unlike the widespread cerebral edema seen in ICANS, the edema in TIAN can lead to shifts in brain tissue that obstruct CSF flow, increase intracranial pressure, and potentially result in herniation. However, TIAN can also occur without edema, as direct neural dysfunction can arise from intense neural–immune interactions and the action of inflammatory signaling molecules like cytokines. Within the framework of TIAN, two distinct categories of neurotoxicity were described. Type 1 TIAN primarily encompasses neurological symptoms and signs resulting from mechanical factors, such as increased intracranial pressure due to edema constrained by the skull. In contrast, type 2 TIAN mainly signifies localized neural dysfunction. Differentiating between these two categories is crucial for effective clinical management; however, since the underlying mechanisms can be interconnected, a unified grading system is utilized [79].

CAR T-cell therapy holds great potential for treating pediatric brain tumors, offering hope for patients with otherwise poor prognoses. While significant challenges remain, ongoing research and clinical trials are rapidly advancing the field. With continued innovation, CAR T-cell therapy may one day become a viable and effective treatment option for children with brain tumors, providing a new frontier in pediatric cancer care.

9.6 Conclusions

Immunotherapy represents a promising frontier in the treatment of pediatric brain tumors, which historically have been challenging to manage due to their aggressive nature and the complexities of the central nervous system. As we continue to explore various immunotherapeutic approaches, including CAR T-cell therapy, immune checkpoint inhibitors, and therapeutic vaccines, there is growing evidence of their potential to improve outcomes for young patients.

Despite the challenges, such as the unique tumor microenvironment, antigen heterogeneity, and the risks of neurotoxicity, recent advancements are encouraging. Innovative strategies, such as the development of next-generation CAR T-cells and combination therapies, are being actively researched to enhance efficacy while minimizing adverse effects.

The integration of immunotherapy into standard treatment regimens holds the potential not only to prolong survival but also to improve the quality of life for children affected by brain tumors. Ongoing clinical trials and research efforts are critical to better understand the mechanisms of action, optimize treatment protocols, and identify biomarkers that can predict responses to therapy.

References

1. Siegel RL, Miller KD, Jemal A. Cancer statistics, 2018. CA Cancer J Clin. 2018;68(1):7–30.
2. Mochizuki AY, Frost IM, Mastrodimos MB, Plant AS, Wang AC, Moore TB, et al. Precision medicine in pediatric neurooncology: a review. ACS Chem Neurosci. 2018;9(1):11–28.
3. Smith MA, Altekruse SF, Adamson PC, Reaman GH, Seibel NL. Declining childhood and adolescent cancer mortality. Cancer. 2014;120(16):2497–506.
4. Capitini CM, Otto M, DeSantes KB, Sondel PM. Immunotherapy in pediatric malignancies: cur-

rent status and future perspectives. Future Oncol. 2014;10(9):1659–78.
5. Janeway CA, Medzhitov R. Innate immune recognition. Annu Rev Immunol. 2002;20:197–216.
6. Janeway CA Jr, Travers P, Walport M, Shlomchik MJ Jr, et al. Immunobiology. 5th ed. Garland Science; 2001.
7. Palucka K, Banchereau J. Cancer immunotherapy via dendritic cells. Nat Rev Cancer. 2012;12(4):265–77.
8. Constantino J, Gomes C, Falcão A, Neves BM, Cruz MT. Dendritic cell-based immunotherapy: a basic review and recent advances. Immunol Res. 2017;65(4):798–810.
9. Martinek J, Wu TC, Cadena D, Banchereau J, Palucka K. Interplay between dendritic cells and cancer cells. Int Rev Cell Mol Biol. 2019;348:179–215.
10. Coussens LM, Zitvogel L, Palucka AK. Neutralizing tumor-promoting chronic inflammation: a magic bullet? Science. 2013;339(6117):286–91.
11. Huang H, Sikora MJ, Islam S, Chowdhury RR, Chien YH, Scriba TJ, et al. Select sequencing of clonally expanded CD8+ T cells reveals limits to clonal expansion. Proc Natl Acad Sci USA. 2019;116(18):8995–9001.
12. Dutoit V, Migliorini D, Dietrich PY, Walker PR. Immunotherapy of malignant tumors in the brain: how different from other sites? Front Oncol. 2016;6:256.
13. Pitt JM, Marabelle A, Eggermont A, Soria JC, Kroemer G, Zitvogel L. Targeting the tumor microenvironment: removing obstruction to anticancer immune responses and immunotherapy. Ann Oncol. 2016;27(8):1482–92.
14. Mackay A, Burford A, Molinari V, Jones DTW, Izquierdo E, Brouwer-Visser J, et al. Molecular, pathological, radiological, and immune profiling of non-brainstem pediatric high-grade glioma from the HERBY phase II randomized trial. Cancer Cell. 2018;33(5):829–842.e5.
15. Bonaventura P, Shekarian T, Alcazer V, Valladeau-Guilemond J, Valsesia-Wittmann S, Amigorena S, et al. Cold tumors: a therapeutic challenge for immunotherapy. Front Immunol. 2019;10:168.
16. Gubin MM, Schreiber RD. CANCER. The odds of immunotherapy success. Science. 2015;350(6257):158–9.
17. Glass R, Synowitz M. CNS macrophages and peripheral myeloid cells in brain tumours. Acta Neuropathol. 2014;128(3):347–62.
18. Griesinger AM, Birks DK, Donson AM, Amani V, Hoffman LM, Waziri A, et al. Characterization of distinct immunophenotypes across pediatric brain tumor types. J Immunol. 2013;191(9):4880–8.
19. Lieberman NAP, DeGolier K, Kovar HM, Davis A, Hoglund V, Stevens J, et al. Characterization of the immune microenvironment of diffuse intrinsic pontine glioma: implications for development of immunotherapy. Neuro-Oncology. 2019;21(1):83–94.
20. Lin GL, Nagaraja S, Filbin MG, Suvà ML, Vogel H, Monje M. Non-inflammatory tumor microenvironment of diffuse intrinsic pontine glioma. Acta Neuropathol Commun. 2018;6(1):51.
21. Bockmayr M, Mohme M, Klauschen F, Winkler B, Budczies J, Rutkowski S, et al. Subgroup-specific immune and stromal microenvironment in medulloblastoma. Onco Targets Ther. 2018;7(9):e1462430.
22. Sampson JH, Archer GE, Mitchell DA, Heimberger AB, Bigner DD. Tumor-specific immunotherapy targeting the EGFRvIII mutation in patients with malignant glioma. Semin Immunol. 2008;20(5):267–75.
23. Therapeutic cancer vaccines: advancements, challenges and prospects – PMC [Internet]. Available on https://www.ncbi.nlm.nih.gov/pmc/articles/PMC10716479/
24. Yao B, Delaidelli A, Vogel H, Sorensen PH. Pediatric brain tumours: lessons from the immune microenvironment. Curr Oncol. 2023;30(5):5024–46.
25. Gupta SL, Basu S, Soni V, Jaiswal RK. Immunotherapy: an alternative promising therapeutic approach against cancers. Mol Biol Rep. 2022;49(10):9903–13.
26. Wang Y, Deng W, Li N, Neri S, Sharma A, Jiang W, et al. Combining immunotherapy and radiotherapy for cancer treatment: current challenges and future directions. Front Pharmacol. 2018;9:185.
27. Foster JB, Madsen PJ, Hegde M, Ahmed N, Cole KA, Maris JM, et al. Immunotherapy for pediatric brain tumors: past and present. Neuro-oncol. 2019;21(10):1226–38.
28. Leach DR, Krummel MF, Allison JP. Enhancement of antitumor immunity by CTLA-4 blockade. Science. 1996;271(5256):1734–6.
29. Wolchok JD, Chiarion-Sileni V, Gonzalez R, Rutkowski P. Overall survival with combined nivolumab and ipilimumab in advanced melanoma. N Engl J Med. 2018;18
30. Motzer RJ, Tannir NM, McDermott DF, Arén Frontera O, Melichar B, Choueiri TK, et al. Nivolumab plus Ipilimumab versus Sunitinib in advanced renal-cell carcinoma. N Engl J Med. 2018;378(14):1277–90.
31. Iwai Y, Ishida M, Tanaka Y, Okazaki T, Honjo T, Minato N. Involvement of PD-L1 on tumor cells in the escape from host immune system and tumor immunotherapy by PD-L1 blockade. Proc Natl Acad Sci USA. 2002;99(19):12293–7.
32. Administration USF and D. FDA approves new treatment for a type of late-stage skin cancer [Internet]. Available on: https://www.prnewswire.com/news-releases/fda-approves-new-treatment-for-a-type-of-late-stage-skin-cancer-118656794.html
33. Le DT, Uram JN, Wang H, Bartlett BR, Kemberling H, Eyring AD, et al. PD-1 blockade in tumors with mismatch-repair deficiency. N Engl J Med. 2015;372(26):2509–20.
34. Yarchoan M, Hopkins A, Jaffee EM. Tumor mutational burden and response rate to PD-1 inhibition. N Engl J Med. 2017;377(25):2500–1.
35. Bouffet E, Larouche V, Campbell BB, Merico D, de Borja R, Aronson M, et al. Immune checkpoint inhibition for Hypermutant glioblastoma multiforme

resulting from germline Biallelic mismatch repair deficiency. J Clin Oncol. 2016;34(19):2206–11.
36. Johanns TM, Miller CA, Dorward IG, Tsien C, Chang E, Perry A, et al. Immunogenomics of hypermutated glioblastoma: a patient with germline POLE deficiency treated with checkpoint blockade immunotherapy. Cancer Discov. 2016;6(11):1230–6.
37. Samstein RM, Lee CH, Shoushtari AN, Hellmann MD, Shen R, Janjigian YY, et al. Tumor mutational load predicts survival after immunotherapy across multiple cancer types. Nat Genet. 2019;51(2):202–6.
38. Okada H, Kalinski P, Ueda R, Hoji A, Kohanbash G, Donegan TE, et al. Induction of CD8+ T-cell responses against novel glioma-associated antigen peptides and clinical activity by vaccinations with {alpha}-type 1 polarized dendritic cells and polyinosinic-polycytidylic acid stabilized by lysine and carboxymethylcellulose in patients with recurrent malignant glioma. J Clin Oncol. 2011;29(3):330–6.
39. Sampson JH, Heimberger AB, Archer GE, Aldape KD, Friedman AH, Friedman HS, et al. Immunologic escape after prolonged progression-free survival with epidermal growth factor receptor variant III peptide vaccination in patients with newly diagnosed glioblastoma. J Clin Oncol. 2010;28(31):4722–9.
40. Wheeler CJ, Black KL, Liu G, Mazer M, Zhang X-x, Pepkowitz S, et al. Vaccination elicits correlated immune and clinical responses in glioblastoma multiforme patients. Cancer Res. 2008;68(14):5955–64.
41. Yamanaka R, Homma J, Yajima N, Tsuchiya N, Sano M, Kobayashi T, et al. Clinical evaluation of dendritic cell vaccination for patients with recurrent glioma: results of a clinical phase I/II trial. Clin Cancer Res. 2005;11(11):4160–7.
42. Yamanaka R, Abe T, Yajima N, Tsuchiya N, Homma J, Kobayashi T, et al. Vaccination of recurrent glioma patients with tumour lysate-pulsed dendritic cells elicits immune responses: results of a clinical phase I/II trial. Br J Cancer. 2003;89(7):1172–9.
43. Yu JS, Liu G, Ying H, Yong WH, Black KL, Wheeler CJ. Vaccination with tumor lysate-pulsed dendritic cells elicits antigen-specific, cytotoxic T-cells in patients with malignant glioma. Cancer Res. 2004;64(14):4973–9.
44. Pollack IF, Jakacki RI, Butterfield LH, Hamilton RL, Panigrahy A, Normolle DP, et al. Antigen-specific immunoreactivity and clinical outcome following vaccination with glioma-associated antigen peptides in children with recurrent high-grade gliomas: results of a pilot study. J Neuro-Oncol. 2016;130(3):517–27.
45. Pollack IF, Jakacki RI, Butterfield LH, Hamilton RL, Panigrahy A, Normolle DP, et al. Immune responses and outcome after vaccination with glioma-associated antigen peptides and poly-ICLC in a pilot study for pediatric recurrent low-grade gliomas. Neuro-Oncology. 2016;18(8):1157–68.
46. Pollack IF, Jakacki RI, Butterfield LH, Hamilton RL, Panigrahy A, Potter DM, et al. Antigen-specific immune responses and clinical outcome after vaccination with glioma-associated antigen peptides and polyinosinic-polycytidylic acid stabilized by lysine and carboxymethylcellulose in children with newly diagnosed malignant brainstem and nonbrainstem gliomas. J Clin Oncol. 2014;32(19):2050–8.
47. Okada H, Low KL, Kohanbash G, McDonald HA, Hamilton RL, Pollack IF. Expression of glioma-associated antigens in pediatric brain stem and non-brain stem gliomas. J Neuro-Oncol. 2008;88(3):245–50.
48. Rossi M, Young JW. Human dendritic cells: potent antigen-presenting cells at the crossroads of innate and adaptive immunity. J Immunol. 2005;175(3):1373–81.
49. Ardon H, De Vleeschouwer S, Van Calenbergh F, Claes L, Kramm CM, Rutkowski S, et al. Adjuvant dendritic cell-based tumour vaccination for children with malignant brain tumours. Pediatr Blood Cancer. 2010;54(4):519–25.
50. Benitez-Ribas D, Cabezón R, Flórez-Grau G, Molero MC, Puerta P, Guillen A, et al. Immune response generated with the administration of autologous dendritic cells pulsed with an allogenic tumoral cell-lines lysate in patients with newly diagnosed diffuse intrinsic pontine glioma. Front Oncol. 2018;8:127.
51. Lasky JL, Panosyan EH, Plant A, Davidson T, Yong WH, Prins RM, et al. Autologous tumor lysate-pulsed dendritic cell immunotherapy for pediatric patients with newly diagnosed or recurrent high-grade gliomas. Anticancer Res. 2013;33(5):2047–56.
52. Caruso DA, Orme LM, Neale AM, Radcliff FJ, Amor GM, Maixner W, et al. Results of a phase 1 study utilizing monocyte-derived dendritic cells pulsed with tumor RNA in children and young adults with brain cancer. Neuro-Oncology. 2004;6(3):236–46.
53. Andtbacka RHI, Kaufman HL, Collichio F, Amatruda T, Senzer N, Chesney J, et al. Talimogene Laherparepvec improves durable response rate in patients with advanced melanoma. J Clin Oncol. 2015;33(25):2780–8.
54. Zeng J, Li X, Sander M, Zhang H, Yan G, Lin Y. Oncolytic viro-immunotherapy: an emerging option in the treatment of gliomas. Front Immunol. 2021;12:721830.
55. Hamid O, Hoffner B, Gasal E, Hong J, Carvajal RD. Oncolytic immunotherapy: unlocking the potential of viruses to help target cancer. Cancer Immunol Immunother. 2017;66(10):1249–64.
56. Friedman GK, Johnston JM, Bag AK, Bernstock JD, Li R, Aban I, et al. Oncolytic HSV-1 G207 Immunovirotherapy for pediatric high-grade gliomas. N Engl J Med. 2021;384(17):1613–22.
57. Kieran MW, Goumnerova L, Manley P, Chi SN, Marcus KJ, Manzanera AG, et al. Phase I study of gene-mediated cytotoxic immunotherapy with AdV-tk as adjuvant to surgery and radiation for pediatric malignant glioma and recurrent ependymoma. Neuro-Oncology. 2019;21(4):537–46.
58. Sheykhhasan M, Manoochehri H, Dama P. Use of CAR T-cell for acute lymphoblastic leukemia (ALL) treatment: a review study. Cancer Gene Ther. 2022;29(8):1080–96.

59. Dai H, Wang Y, Lu X, Han W. Chimeric antigen receptors modified T-cells for cancer therapy. J Natl Cancer Inst. 2016;108(7):djv439.
60. Akhavan D, Alizadeh D, Wang D, Weist MR, Shepphird JK, Brown CE. CAR T cells for brain tumors: lessons learned and road ahead. Immunol Rev. 2019;290(1):60–84.
61. Tormoen GW, Crittenden MR, Gough MJ. Role of the immunosuppressive microenvironment in immunotherapy. Adv Radiat Oncol. 2018;3(4):520–6.
62. Del Baldo G, Carai A, Mastronuzzi A. Chimeric antigen receptor adoptive immunotherapy in central nervous system tumors: state of the art on clinical trials, challenges, and emerging strategies to addressing them. Curr Opin Oncol. 2024;36:545.
63. Gross G, Waks T, Eshhar Z. Expression of immunoglobulin-T-cell receptor chimeric molecules as functional receptors with antibody-type specificity. Proc Natl Acad Sci USA. 1989;86(24):10024–8.
64. Eshhar Z, Waks T, GROSSt G, Schindler DG. Specific activation and targeting of cytotoxic lymphocytes through chimeric single chains consisting of antibody-binding domains and the y or C subunits of the immunoglobulin and T-cell receptors. Proc Natl Acad Sci USA. 1993;5
65. Kagoya Y, Tanaka S, Guo T, Anczurowski M, Wang CH, Saso K, et al. A novel chimeric antigen receptor containing a JAK-STAT signaling domain mediates superior antitumor effects. Nat Med. 2018;24(3):352–9.
66. Bagley SJ, Desai AS, Linette GP, June CH, O'Rourke DM. CAR T-cell therapy for glioblastoma: recent clinical advances and future challenges. Neuro-Oncology. 2018;20(11):1429–38.
67. Zhang L, Ren J, Zhang H, Cheng G, Xu Y, Yang S, et al. HER2-targeted recombinant protein immuno-caspase-6 effectively induces apoptosis in HER2-overexpressing GBM cells in vitro and in vivo. Oncol Rep. 2016;36(5):2689–96.
68. Kilian M, Bunse T, Wick W, Platten M, Bunse L. Genetically modified cellular therapies for malignant gliomas. Int J Mol Sci. 2021;22(23):12810.
69. Guo X, Chang M, Wang Y, Xing B, Ma W. B7-H3 in brain malignancies: immunology and immunotherapy. Int J Biol Sci. 2023;19(12):3762–80.
70. Ciccone R, Quintarelli C, Camera A, Pezzella M, Caruso S, Manni S, et al. GD2-targeting CAR T-cell therapy for patients with GD2+ medulloblastoma. Clin Cancer Res. 2024;30:2545.
71. Mount CW, Majzner RG, Sundaresh S, Arnold EP, Kadapakkam M, Haile S, et al. Potent antitumor efficacy of anti-GD2 CAR T cells in H3-K27M+ diffuse midline gliomas. Nat Med. 2018;24(5):572–9.
72. Majzner RG, Ramakrishna S, Yeom KW, Patel S, Chinnasamy H, Schultz LM, et al. GD2-CAR T cell therapy for H3K27M-mutated diffuse midline gliomas. Nature. 2022;603(7903):934–41.
73. de Billy E, Pellegrino M, Orlando D, Pericoli G, Ferretti R, Businaro P, et al. Dual IGF1R/IR inhibitors in combination with GD2-CAR T-cells display a potent anti-tumor activity in diffuse midline glioma H3K27M-mutant. Neuro-Oncology. 2022;24(7):1150–63.
74. Ledford H. This kids' brain cancer is incurable—but immune therapy holds promise. Nature. 2024;631(8022):715–6.
75. Brown CE, Aguilar B, Starr R, Yang X, Chang WC, Weng L, et al. Optimization of IL13Rα2-targeted chimeric antigen receptor T cells for improved anti-tumor efficacy against glioblastoma. Mol Ther. 2018;26(1):31–44.
76. Ghahri-Saremi N, Akbari B, Soltantoyeh T, Hadjati J, Ghassemi S, Mirzaei HR. Genetic modification of cytokine signaling to enhance efficacy of CAR T cell therapy in solid tumors. Front Immunol. 2021;12:738456.
77. Lee DW, Gardner R, Porter DL, Louis CU, Ahmed N, Jensen M, et al. Current concepts in the diagnosis and management of cytokine release syndrome. Blood. 2014;124(2):188–95.
78. Sterner RC, Sterner RM. Immune effector cell associated neurotoxicity syndrome in chimeric antigen receptor-T cell therapy. Front Immunol [Internet]. 2022. Available on: https://www.frontiersin.org/journals/immunology/articles/10.3389/fimmu.2022.879608/full
79. Mahdi J, Dietrich J, Straathof K, Roddie C, Scott BJ, Davidson TB, et al. Tumor inflammation-associated neurotoxicity. Nat Med. 2023;29(4):803–10.

Medulloblastoma

10

Iside Alessi, Giada Del Baldo,
Giovanna Stefania Colafati, Claudia D'Orazio,
Evelina Miele, Sabrina Rossi,
and Angela Mastronuzzi

10.1 Epidemiology

Medulloblastoma (MB) is the most common malignant pediatric brain tumor, comprising approximately 20% [1]. These malignancies present age-specific incidence peaks during the first decade of life, with a higher incidence between 3–4 years and 8–10 years of age. At diagnosis, the median age has been reported at 6 years and the male-female ratio is 1.8:1 [2, 3]. MBs account for over 60% of intracranial embryonal tumors in the pediatric population and originate from the cerebellum and peri-cerebellar structures [4]. Consequently, these tumors emerge within the anatomical confines of the posterior cranial fossa, with 75–90% of cases manifesting at the level of the cerebellar vermis, with the epicenter located dorsally to the fourth ventricle.

As the other central nervous system (CNS) tumors, MB also tends to metastasize through cerebrospinal fluid, with metastases discernible in 30% of cases at the onset of the disease, occurring most commonly intracranially and along the spinal cord, or more rarely extracranially, in bones, lungs, and lymph nodes [5, 6].

Before the 1970s, the 5-year survival rate for affected individuals was documented at 30%, with fatalities primarily attributed to tumor recurrence and leptomeningeal dissemination. Over the last three decades, substantial advancements in the diagnostic field and therapeutic approaches have brought about significant progress, improving long-term survival rate at 70–80% [7].

10.2 Clinical Presentation

The most prevalent symptoms and clinical presentations in patients affected by MB are those indicative of increased intracranial pressure (ICP) secondary to obstructive hydrocephalus: the tumor obstructs the physiological pathways for cerebrospinal fluid flow via the compression of ventricle and nearby anatomical structures.

I. Alessi · G. Del Baldo · E. Miele
Area of Hematology-Oncology, Cell Therapy, Gene Therapies, and Hematopoietic Transplantation, Bambino Gesù Children's Hospital, IRCCS, Rome, Italy
e-mail: angela.mastronuzzi@opbg.net

G. S. Colafati · C. D'Orazio
Imaging Department, Bambino Gesù Children's Hospital, IRCCS, Rome, Italy

S. Rossi
Pathology Unit, Bambino Gesù Children's Hospital, IRCCS, Rome, Italy

A. Mastronuzzi (✉)
Area of Hematology-Oncology, Cell Therapy, Gene Therapies, and Hematopoietic Transplantation Bambino Gesù Children's Hospital, IRCCS, Rome, Italy

Department of Life Sciences and Public Health, Università Cattolica del Sacro Cuore, Rome, Italy
e-mail: angela.mastronuzzi@opbg.net

A. Mastronuzzi, A. Carai (eds.), *Navigating Pediatric Brain Tumors*,
https://doi.org/10.1007/978-3-032-18992-9_10

Aligned with its relatively fast growth rate, individuals with this tumor frequently manifest symptoms evolving over a span of weeks to months. The typical symptoms progression involves an initial onset of morning headache, nausea, vomiting, irritability, anorexia, lethargy, and over time, gait abnormalities, bladder or bowel disfunction, which may be indicative of spinal metastasis [4].

In MB-affected infants, the initial presentation comprises typically intermittent vomiting, macrocephaly, and non-specific indicators of ventricular dilation, such as the so-called "sun-setting sign," which represents down-deviation of the eyes and loss of upward gaze, secondary to tectal pressure [4, 8].

As the tumor increases in size, other manifestations are associated with cerebellar involvement, exhibiting differences based on the site of the lesion. Tumors situated along the midline of the cerebellum are inclined to induce truncal ataxia; conversely, cerebellar hemispheric tumors are more frequently linked to appendicular ataxia [2]. In other cases, neck stiffness or head tilt typically suggests tonsillar involvement, thus underlining the importance of discerning lesion location in evaluating clinical signs associated with cerebellar dysfunction.

Cranial nerve engagement and consequent dysfunction may also arise, either due to brainstem infiltration or more commonly, secondary to heightened ICP, as in the case of an early manifestation characterized by abducens nerve palsy [8].

Conditions like stasis papillae can be identified as a late presentation and some patients may experience behavioral changes, including decreased academic performance, depression, and anxiety [9]. Moreover, the uncommon form of congenital MBs can be present in patients with clinical features such as hyporeactivity, reduced suction reflexes, and the presence of hydrocephalus [10].

10.3 Histology

The five histological subtypes of MB outlined in the 2007 classification have been considered in the past as prognostically significant and useful for patients stratification of clinical risks; however, new studies have shown several limitations. To enhance the precision of MB diagnosis, histological types have been integrated with genetic information, using a stratified approach. In 2016, the World Health Organization (WHO) released an updated classification of CNS tumors based on molecular characteristics, identifying four histological variants of MB: classical, desmoplastic/nodular, extensive nodularity, and large cell/anaplastic. Recently, the 2021 WHO classification has consolidated all histological subtypes into a unified category named "histologically defined MB," removing the subdivision introduced in 2016 [11, 12].

The classical variant is the most common form of MB, accounting for 72% of cases. MBs of this variant consist of solid sheets of small cells with round nuclei and high nucleus/cytoplasmatic ratio. Increased cell size and frequent mitotes and apoptosis are only focal findings [12].

The desmoplastic/nodular variant (DNMB) accounts for 15% of MBs and is less aggressive than the classic variant. Characteristics found in this histological type include the presence of pale reticulin-free nodules of neoplastic cells with neuronal differentiation embedded in an abundant neuropil, and hypercellular areas of internodular desmoplasia, i.e., pericellular collagen deposition identified via reticulin staining. The nodular areas show positivity for markers such as synaptophysin and NEU-N, low proliferative activity, and low mitotic index. Conversely, the internodular desmoplastic areas are characterized by undifferentiated elements and high Ki67 levels. The DNMB histological variant is frequently identified in lateral cerebellar areas of adolescents and adults or as a manifestation of a predisposing condition to MB called Gorlin syndrome in infants and children. Recognizing the DN variant is crucial because tumors with this morphology generally carry intermediate clinical risk and are associated with the SHH molecular subgroup [4, 12–14].

A distinctive variant of desmoplastic/nodular MB is known as MB with extensive nodularity (MBEN). This variant is typically observed in very young children, often described in patients with Gorlin syndrome, and tends to be more centrally located than conventional DN tumors. It is characterized by the presence of abundant nodules, characteristically exhibiting irregular shapes and frequently merging. A typical pattern named "streaming pattern," where linear arrangements of neurocytic cells connect nearby nodules, is also observed in this histological variant [4, 12].

The large cell anaplastic variant tumors (LC/A) constitute approximately 10% of all MBs and are highly aggressive. This variant is usually located in the cerebellar vermis. LC/A MBs exhibit either cells with large round monomorphic nuclei and prominent nucleoli (i.e., large cell phenotype) or cells with highly pleomorphic nuclei with the typical features of nuclear molding and cell wrapping (i.e., anaplastic phenotypes). Areas with these morphological characteristics may be variably represented in the same tumor. The prognosis is particularly unfavorable as suggested by the elevated mitotic and apoptotic activity along with extensive areas of necrosis. These tumors often present synaptophysin and chromogranin, frequently associated with MYC oncogene amplification [4, 14].

Immunohistochemical markers such as YAP1, GAB1, and beta-catenin are invaluable surrogates of MB molecular stratifications. A nuclear and cytoplasmic expression of YAP1 when associated with a cytoplasmic expression of GAB1 is indicative of the SHH-activated group, whereas when combined to the nuclear expression of beta-catenin, it supports the diagnosis of WNT-activated group. Notably, their expression may be focal. Based on the immunohistochemistry, it is not possible to distinguish Group 3 from Group 4 and only a diagnosis of MB non-WNT/non-SHH activated may be released. Of paramount importance is also the immunostaining for p53, as diffuse and strong p53 expression in an SHH-activated MB reliably predicts the TP53-mutated subset. Even the absence of p53 expression may result from some types of TP53 inactivating mutations, but sequencing of the gene is highly recommended in these cases [13].

10.4 Molecular Classification

Over the last decade, the advent of next-generation sequencing technologies (NGS) has markedly transformed the comprehension of the molecular mechanisms underlying MB pathogenesis, revealing a complex and highly heterogeneous disease. These studies have included comprehensive analyses of all aspects of the genome such as new oncogenes and driver mutations, providing new etiological landmarks like changes in DNA copy number, gene expression, and methylation profile [15, 16]. Recent research has increasingly focused on analyzing DNA methylation profiles in cancer cells, uncovering specific modifications that hold significant prognostic and diagnostic value for this tumor condition. These epigenetic changes provide insights into tumor behavior, potentially guiding treatment strategies, and improving patient outcomes DNA methylation, along with other mechanisms, is a key modification that regulates gene expression, playing a crucial role in differentiating the characteristics and functions of cells with identical genetic material [17]. Hypermethylation, which involves an elevated level of methylation in promoter regions, can lead to the transcriptional silencing of specific tumor suppressor genes, contributing to cancer progression. Conversely, hypomethylation, or a reduced rate of methylation, is often observed in the early stages of cancer development and is associated with the promotion of genomic instability and cellular transformation. These epigenetic changes are integral to the complex processes underlying tumorigenesis [18]. In tumors, the DNA methylation profile exhibits unique characteristics that reflect both the cell of origin and the acquired methylation changes associated with neoplasia. This distinct "fingerprint" allows for the precise identification of the tumor type, significantly enhancing diagnostic accuracy, reducing the number of inconclusive diagnoses, and enabling more detailed prognostic sub-classification. By analyzing these methylation patterns, clinicians can better understand the tumor's origin and behavior, leading to more targeted and effective treatment strategies [19].

Previously, tumor classification primarily depended on histopathological categories (such as classic, desmoplastic/nodular, MB with extensive nodularity, and large cell/anaplastic) and clinical-pathological variables like age, presence of metastases, and extent of surgical resection. However, despite uniform treatment based on these classifications, patient outcomes have shown considerable variation, underscoring the need to delve deeper into the underlying tumor biology. This variability highlights the limitations of traditional methods and the importance of integrating molecular and genetic insights to better tailor treatment and improve prognostic accuracy.

The 2016 consensus classified MB into four main molecular subgroups: WNT, SHH, Group 3, and Group 4. SHH tumors were further divided based on TP53 mutational status, distinguishing between SHH-TP53 mutant and SHH-TP53 wild-type tumors. Group 3 and Group 4 tumors were categorized together under the non-WNT/non-SHH MBs, reflecting their distinct molecular profiles but shared characteristics [20]. Recent research, leveraging expanded cohort sizes and enhanced profiling techniques, has identified variations within the original molecular subgroups of MB and delineated additional molecular subtypes. This refined molecular stratification has been incorporated into the updated WHO 2021 CNS tumor classification. Under this revised system, the four main molecular groups (WNT, SHH, Group 3, and Group 4) have been further subdivided:

WNT Subgroups: Two distinct subgroups have been identified within the WNT category.

SHH Subgroups: Four different subgroups have been classified based on additional molecular features and TP53 status.

Non-WNT/Non-SHH Subgroups: This category, encompassing Group 3 and Group 4 tumors, has been further divided into eight distinct subgroups based on methylation profiling and pathway activation.

These advances in molecular classification enhance the precision of diagnosis and prognosis and facilitate more tailored treatment approaches for MB patients [20–22].

In addition to this, the updated molecular classification has opened the way for new research aimed at investigating the distinct cellular, molecular, and neurodevelopmental characteristics of each subtype [23].

The Wingless (WNT) subgroup accounts for approximately 10–15% of all cases. These tumors typically occur in children over the age of 4 and adolescents, with a median age of 10 years old, presenting a slight female predominance [12]. The most frequently associated histological variant with this subgroup is the classic variant, observed in 90% of cases, and an excellent prognosis, with over 95% survival at 5 years, is observed in pediatric patients [4]. Studies on murine models have suggested that WNT subgroup MBs originate from progenitor stem cells, located in the lower rhombic lip of the metencephalon. Indeed, these tumors are usually found in midline locations with brainstem involvement, or the cerebellar peduncle and cerebellopontine angle (CPA) cistern. Metastasis at diagnosis are rare, occurring in only 5–10% of cases and recurrences are also uncommon [24].

The most frequently identified intra-tumoral genetic alteration, accounting for approximately 90% of cases, is the mutation of exon 3 of the *CTNNB1* gene, encoding for the β-catenin 1. This mutation results in e β-catenin 1 accumulation in the nucleus secondary to reduced cytoplasmic degradation of this protein. It is responsible for uncontrolled and constitutive activation of the WNT intracellular signaling pathway that promotes tumor proliferation due to the expression of WNT responsive genes. Wild-type WNT patients that lack the *CTNNB1* gene mutation may present alteration in the *APC* tumor suppressor gene, in charge of the degradation of β-catenin. *APC* germline mutations are characteristic in patients with Turcot syndrome type II; for this reason, deregulated WNT signaling was first identified in patients affected by this condition. Monosomy 6, the loss of one copy of chromosome 6, is also observed in 80% of cases, while other genes commonly mutated are *DDX3X* (36%) encoding RNA helicase, which regulates chromosome segregation and cell cycle progression, or *SMARCA4* (19%). Finally, somatic *TP53* mutation can be found in 15% of cases, and differently from the SHH subgroup, does not represent an unfavorable prognostic factor when associated with the WNT subgroup [4, 12, 24, 25].

Recent studies based on molecular profiling, using gene expression and methylation array data, have described two subtypes of the WNT subgroup: WNT-α (70%), primarily occurring in children, characterized by ubiquitous monosomy of chromosome 6, and WNT-β (30%), usually diagnosed in older patients and characterized by diploidy of chromosome 6 [4, 26]. This subset of patients presents a highly favorable prognosis, attributed mainly to the presence of fenestrations at the blood-brain barrier (BBB), which allow better penetration of anti-neoplastic drugs. In addition, paracrine signals stimulated by mutated β-catenin in WNT-activated MB also lead to the development of abnormal fenestrated vasculature, allowing for the accumulation of elevated levels of chemotherapy within the tumor and facilitating a strong therapeutic response. Accurate identification of WNT-activated MB tumors is crucial due to their favorable prognosis in the pediatric population, and this element guides the patient's selection in clinical trials that evaluate the impact of treatment on survival and quality of life, posing a therapy de-escalation to mitigate treatment-related morbidity [27].

A new analysis of single-cell transcriptomics in MB, conducted by Hovestadt and colleagues, has revealed distinct malignant cellular states within each subgroup. Their findings have underlined the presence of a differentiated neuronal-like state in WNT-amplified MB cells, allowing the identification of four transcriptional metaprograms with unique cellular patterns: WNT-A, linked to cell cycle activity; WNT-B, associated with protein biosynthesis and metabolism; WNT-C, reflecting neuronal differentiation; and WNT-D, characterized by the expression of early response genes and those in the WNT pathway. The evaluation of these transcriptional metaprograms has a role in the identification of tumor behavior: within the WNT subgroup of MB, a developmental hierarchy has been observed, and the tumor cells exhibiting high WNT-B and low WNT-C/WNT-D signatures present a proliferative advantage that drives the tumor progression [28].

Around 30% of MBs fall under the *SHH classification*. The SHH subset displays an equal distribution between genders and exhibits two distinct peaks in age incidence, in children under 3 years of age and adolescents above 16 years. These tumors typically originate in the cerebellar hemispheres, as opposed to the midline location observed in other subgroups, probably due to the lateral location of granule neuron precursors (GNPs), which are thought to be the cells from which this type of tumor arises. Another possible location is the cerebellar vermis, typically observed in children younger than 3 years old. Histologically, these tumors are typically associated with the DN and MBEN histological variants, although several other subtypes may be observed. SHH group MB harbor genetic mutations in the SHH signaling pathway, resulting in constitutive activation of the latter and promotion of tumor advancement. Loss of functions or deletions are commonly observed in genes like *PTCH1*, representing 43% of cases, mutated usually in children under 3 years, or SUFU, representing 10% of cases. Alterations in the SHH pathway downstream of *SMO*, such as *GLI1/GLI2* amplifications, are detectable in 9% of cases and may be associated with resistance. Of note, the mutation of *TP53*, observable in approximately 20% of childhood SHH MBs, is relevant for its prognostic implication; unlike the WNT subgroup, this mutation is associated with an unfavorable prognosis and very poor outcomes [4, 24, 26]. It is not infrequent to find germline *TP53* mutations associated with Li-Fraumeni syndrome; patients with germline or somatic *TP53* mutation have a 5-year overall survival (OS) of 41% compared to patients without this mutation who achieve 76% OS [12]. Other commonly altered genes include chromatin modifiers, transcriptional regulators, and components of signal transduction pathways. Mutations in *MLL*/COMPASS family components such as *KMT2C* (7%) and *KMT2D* (13%) are also observable [29].

Examination of methylation and transcriptional data revealed four different subtypes of SHH MB subgroup tumors: SHH-1 (β), SHH-2 (γ), SHH-3 (α), and SHH-4 (δ). The SHH α subtype is associated with a high rate of *TP53* or *ELP1* mutations, as well as *MYCN* and *GLI2* amplification, occurring in childhood (children 3–16 years old) with an extremely poor prognosis, and the SHH β tumors affect mainly infants and are often metastatic at the time of diagnosis. The SHH γ subtype is also found in infants and is associated with MB with extensive nodularity (MBEN) histology but has relatively better outcomes. The SHH-δ subtype is more frequent in adults and is characterized by *TERT* promoter mutation with a good prognosis. A recent study has outlined two variants of infant SHH MB (iSSH), denominated iSHH-I and iSHH-II, both exhibiting *PTCH1* mutation/deletion and *SUFU* alterations, mainly observed in subtype iSHH-II. The latter is associated with extended progression-free survival (PFS), even under less intense treatment regimens [4, 24, 30].

According to Hovestadt et al., three transcriptional metaprograms can be described in SHH-MB cells. Starting from the SHH-A metaprogram, it corresponds to cell proliferation activity, further subdivided into SHH-A1 (S phase) and SHH-A2 (G2M phase), while SHH-B corresponds to undifferentiated progenitors, with SHH-B1 resembling GCPs and SHH-B2 having a high level of ribosome expression. Finally, SHH-C is associated with neuronal differentiation (SHH-C1 cells display high levels of axo-dendritic transport genes, while SHH-C2 cells express several neural development markers like STMN2). A peculiar point underlined by this study, consistent with epidemiological findings, is the correlation between cellular origin and age of SHH MB. It has been observed that pediatric tumors exhibit cells resembling granule neurons, expressing high levels of NEUROD1, while adult tumors express elevated levels of MATH1 and contains cells resembling either granule neuron progenitors or a mixed population of unipolar brush cells (UBCs) and granule neurons [28, 30].

Group 3 MBs account for approximately 25% of all MBs, showing a male predominance and occurring nearly exclusively in infants and young children. They are considered the most aggressive among the four subgroups, with a five-year survival rate under 60% and poor prognosis, often influenced by high rates of metastasis at diagnosis (approximately 40–45%), large cell/anaplastic histology (40%), and/or *MYC* amplification [31]. Typically, this subgroup is located at the level of the fourth ventricle. Although the exact cell type responsible for these tumors remains uncertain, multiple studies have proposed that Prominin1-positive, lineage-negative cerebellar stem cells and granule neuron precursors (GNPs) may have the potential to undergo transformation and give rise to similar tumors [26]. Recent studies have highlighted that Group 3 tumor cells may express a metaprogram similar to undifferentiated progenitors, marked by ribosomal and translational initiation/elongation, along with the expression of MYC target genes. These cells seemed to be arrested in an undifferentiated state, suggesting the presence of mutations responsible for a stop in the neural differentiation process [28]. In contrast to SHH and WNT subgroup tumors, a singular predominant pathway defining Group 3 and Group 4 has not yet been identified. However, nearly 17% of these tumors present MYC amplification, often accompanied by *PVT1MYC* fusions and other common aberrations involving the NOTCH or TGF-β signaling pathways. Cytogenetic anomalies are also observable in this subgroup, with isochromosome 17q occurring in 40–50% of cases, considered a bad prognostic factor. Events such as loss of chromosomes 8, 10q, and 16q, as well as gain of 1q, 7, and 18, may also arise [23]. Within subgroup 3, according to Cavet al., three additional subtypes can be identified: 3α, 3β, and 3γ. Around 60% of patients under 3 years old belong to the subtype 3α; subtype 3β occurs in slightly older children and is often non-metastatic, characterized by *GFI1* oncogene activation, *OTX* amplification, and *DDX31* loss. Generally, patients belonging to these two groups have a more favorable prognosis than those in subtype 3γ, which shows isodicentric chromosome 17q and *MYC* amplification (worst prognosis) [4, 28, 29].

Group 4 is documented in 35% of cases and is the most common group, often associated with the classic histological subtype. It does not have a typical age of onset, but a peak in incidence for this group is registered during late childhood and early adolescence. These tumors show male predominance with a 3:1 sex ratio and are commonly located at the level of midline vermis. The precise cellular source of Group 4 remains uncertain but transcriptional resemblances to unipolar brush cells have been identified [24]. This group remains the least biologically understood, sharing the closest molecular similarities with Group 3 concerning the other tumors; for this reason, they have been recently incorporated in the classification Group 3/4. Group 4 MBs do not typically display recurrent defining somatic mutations, instead, they frequently exhibit chromosomal structural variations, which, in some cases, lead to *GFI1/GFI1B* activation. The most common cytogenetic abnormality is isochromosome 17q (around 80% of cases), but somatic mutations in *KDM* family members (including *KDM6A*) or amplifications of *OTX2*, *SNCAIP*, *CDK6* have also been documented, highlighting the possible role of chromatin modifier dysregulation in the molecular pathogenesis [29]. Moreover, *MYCN* amplifications and overexpression are frequently detected in this subgroup, but unlike in SHH tumors, they are not linked to worse outcomes [31]. Although frequently metastatic at diagnosis (30–40%), the prognosis in these patients is intermediate, and late relapses, with longer latency compared to other subgroups, are frequently occurring [29]. A study conducted by Cavalli and colleagues has described 3 subtypes of Group 4 MB: 4α, 4β, and 4γ. Molecular characteristics linked with these subtypes comprise *MYCN* and *CDK6* amplification in Group 4α, *SNCAIP* duplication in Group 4β, and *CDK6* amplification in Group 4γ [24, 28]. Recently, two other independent studies have identified varying numbers of subtypes within both Group 3 and Group 4. To obtain clear subtype definitions, a joint analysis of numerous Group 3/4 MBs has been recently conducted, defining eight subtypes in total. Subtype I represent the least common and includes tumors from both Group 3 and Group 4. These tumor genomes are typically characterized by the amplification of the *OTX2* oncogene and activation of *GFI1/GFI1B*. Subtypes II, III, and IV are constituted only by pure Group 3 subtypes tumors: subtypes II and III present *MYC* oncogene amplification and poor outcomes, while subtype IV, typical of younger patients with a median age of 3 years, is associated with a favorable prognosis. Regarding subtypes V, VI, and VII, they mainly consist of Group 4 MBs but may include some Group 3 tumors. Amplification of both *MYC* and *MYCN* and intermediate outcome are observable in subtype V tumors. Finally, subtype VIII is the most common and composed only of Group 4 tumors, occurring predominantly in older children with a median age of 10 years. Except for isochromosome 17q, in most cases, these malignancies present a balanced genome. Although late relapse and death may occur, the subtype VIII is associated with favorable 5-year survival rates [31].

10.5 Genetic Predisposition Syndromes

The etiology associated with MB is largely unknown. Several studies have established a correlation between different factors such as maternal nutritional intake and hematological/immune complications during gestation. Other investigations suggest a connection with viral illnesses, such as early exposure to John Cunningham (JC) virus or human cytomegalovirus (CMV) [32]. However, in many cases, these malignancies arise sporadically and about 5% of cases occur within the context of Cancer Predisposition Syndromes. The most frequently associated cancer predisposition syndromes with MB are Gorlin Syndrome, Li-Fraumeni Syndrome, and Turcot Syndrome (see chapter on Cancer Predisposition Syndromes). Recently, new syndromes, for example associated with DNA damage detection defects and repair, such as the Nijmegen breakage syndrome, have been identified [4]. The frequency of genetic predisposition varies among MB molecular subtypes, with approximately 40% of patients affected by SHH group MB, while a lower prevalence, estimated around 6–8% of *APC* germline alterations, is observed in the WNT MB subgroup. Rarely *BRCA2* or *PALB2* alterations, representing 1% prevalence, are detected in patients with Group 3 or Group 4 MB (see chapter on Cancer predisposition syndromes) [33] (Table 10.1).

Table 10.1 Correlation between molecular subgroup and genetic predisposition syndromes testing

Medulloblastoma group					
	SHH				
WNT	<3 years		>3 years		Group 3 or 4
APC germline mutations (FAP syndrome)	SUFU or PTCH1 alterations (Gorlin)	GPR161 alterations	ELP1 alterations	TP53 alterations	BRCA2 or PALB2 alterations
6–8% prevalence	11% prevalence	3.4% prevalence	14% prevalence	8% prevalence	1–2% prevalence
		SHHβ subgroup	SHHα subgroup	SHHα subgroup	
Absence of CTNNB1 alterations	LOH PTCH1 or SUFU	LOH of 1q	LOH of 9q	Chromothripsis signature	Homologous recombination repair deficiency
	All negative BRCA2 or PALB2 alterations (1–2% prevalence)				

Recently, a new heterozygous protein-truncating genetic mutation in *GPR161* has been highlighted, located on chromosome 1q24 and responsible for a new TP (tumor protein). *GPR161* is involved in embryonic development, particularly in the proliferation of cerebellar granules, and acts as a suppressor of the SHH pathway. Consequently, uncontrolled activation leads to granule progression, resulting in MB development [33]. Affected patients present with infantile SHH group MB (*TP53* wild type), exhibiting a methylation profile clustering with the SHHβ subtype as their primary clinical manifestation, with a median age of onset at 1.5 years. The frequency of germline mutation is estimated to be around 6 cases per 10,000 in the general population. Molecular analysis of the tumor has revealed that the development of SHH group MB/*TP53* wild-type has been associated with biallelic inactivation of the *GPR161* gene, most commonly by copy-neutral loss of heterozygosity of chromosome 1q, in individuals with heterozygous germline mutations in this gene, a feature notably absents in SHH group MBs with wild-type *GPR16* [33, 34].

Lastly, a new condition denominated *ELP1*-MB syndrome has been newly recognized in the WHO 5th edition of CNS tumors, especially in correlation with the SHH-α subtype MB onset. This condition is an autosomal dominant disorder resulting from germline mutations in the *ELP1* gene located at 9q31.3. *ELP1* is a tumor-suppressor gene that codes for the protein ELP1, a component of the Elongator protein complex, which is responsible for the transcription process of structural proteins and neurogenesis [34]. According to different authors, three consecutive mutations are necessary for the development of SHH group MB: heterozygous germline variant in ELP1LOF, biallelic inactivation of *ELP1* with monoallelic inactivation of *PTCH1* (loss of the short arm of chromosome 9), and biallelic inactivation of the *PTCH1*. Patients with *ELP1* mutation have a median age at diagnosis of 6 years, often with a positive family history of MBs. The desmoplastic/nodular pattern is the most common histological subtype, accounting for approximately 76% of cases. This is followed by the classic morphology, representing 18%, and the large cell/anaplastic morphology, which comprises about 6% of cases. The advantage of the integrated molecular classification of MB is also to allow suspicion and investigation of any cancer-predisposing conditions [34, 35].

10.6 Diagnosis

As an initial step in the diagnostic evaluation of MB, a comprehensive medical history and physical examination, with particular emphasis on the neurological assessment, should be performed in any patient presenting with persistent constitutional symptoms or newly developed neurological signs or symptoms. According to the SIOPE (European Society for Paediatric Oncology), the definitive diagnosis of MB is based on imaging, histopathology, molecular pathology for molecular subgrouping and cerebrospinal fluid (CSF) cytology for staging.

Computed tomography (CT) is the primary neuroimaging examination commonly utilized in patients with suspected posterior fossa neoplasms, preferentially used during emergency medicine settings due to its availability and rapid execution [35]. Typically, a CT scan in affected patients reveals a well-defined, hyperdense mass, likely attributable to the tumor's high cell density and nuclear-to-cytoplasmic ratio (Fig. 10.1a) associated hydrocephalus present in 10–20% of cases. In children with open sutures, transfontanellar ultrasound serves as a valuable diagnostic tool for the detection of hydrocephalus [4, 34].

Magnetic resonance imaging (MRI) is the gold standard examination for evaluating brain and spine neoplasms. In addition to raising suspicion of MB based on certain typical lesion characteristics, such as location and high cellularity

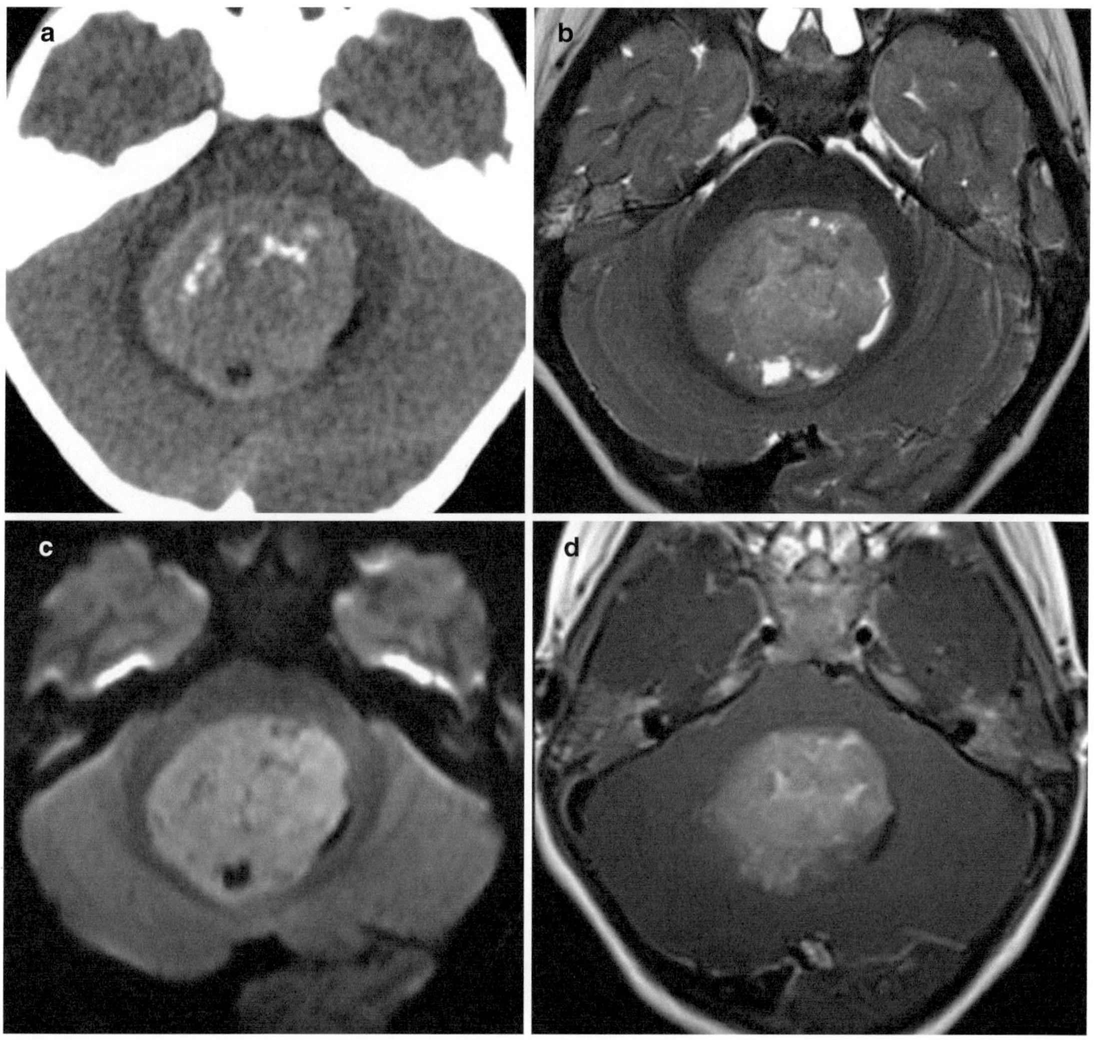

Fig. 10.1 Example of radiological findings in medulloblastoma. Expansive process of the posterior cranial fossa obliterating the IV ventricle characterized by calcifications (**a**), inhomogeneous T2 signal due to the presence of small intratumoral cysts (**b**), restricted diffusivity (**c**), and contrastographic enhancement (**d**)

on advanced sequences, MRI is essential for ruling out the presence of metastases along the neuraxis (Fig. 10.1) and also for planning surgical intervention. The tumor often exhibits heterogeneity on imaging, showing possible cysts, hemorrhage, or calcifications (Fig. 10.2) [36].

Medulloblastomas of different molecular subgroups arise from different anatomical regions of the brain and present different localizations at diagnosis [37]. SHH-subgroup MB are usually hemispheric, typically extraventricular, WNT-subgroup MB are indeed paramedian, with involvement of the foramen of Luschka, the fourth ventricle, the cisterna magna and the cerebellopontine angle cistern, Group 3 and 4 MB then occur predominantly in the midline/fourth ventricle [38]. Group 3 neoplasms generally show greater contrast enhancement than those in Group 4 [39]. The Response Assessment in Pediatric Neuro-Oncology (RAPNO) working group has

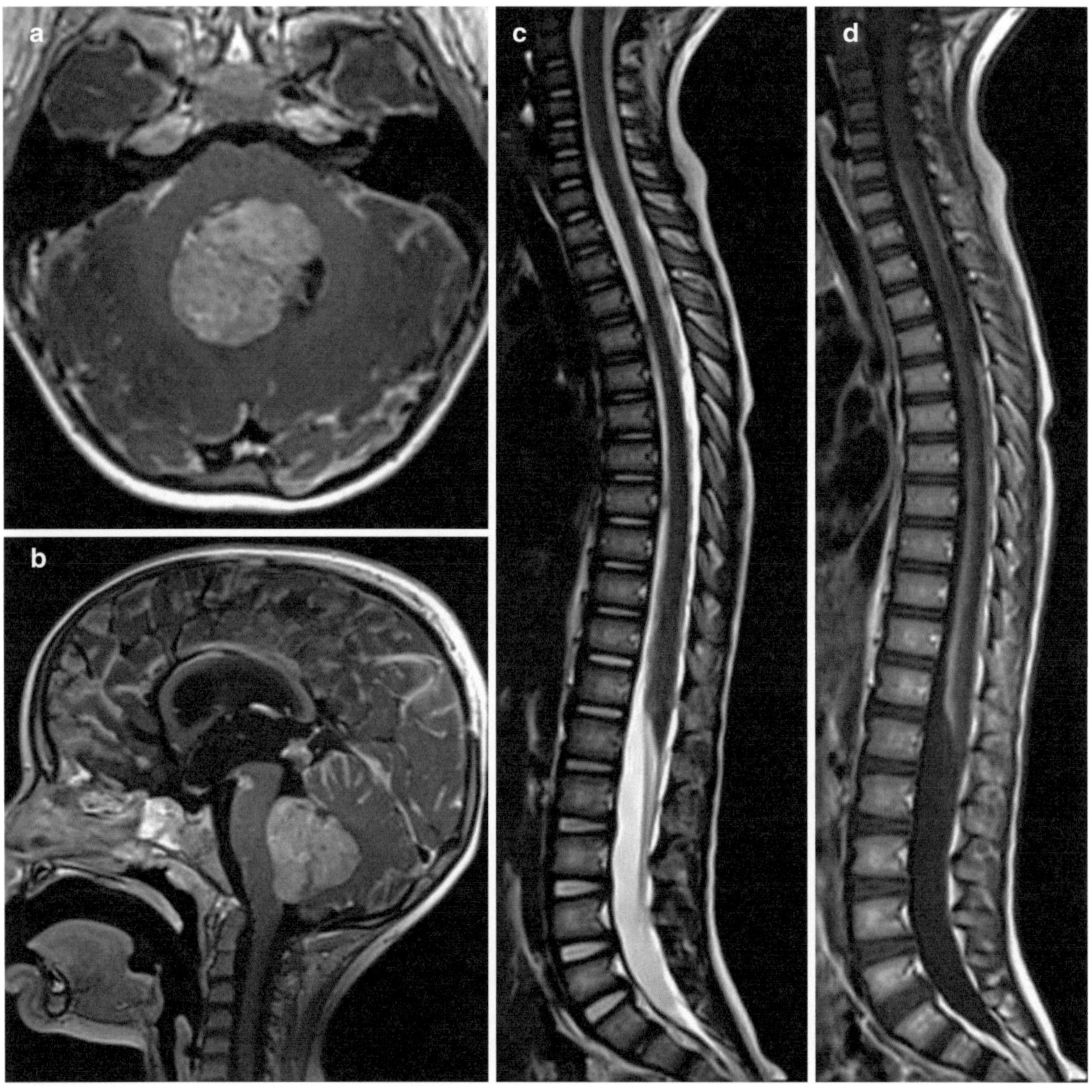

Fig. 10.2 Example of metastatic spread disease. Post-contrast axial (**a**) and sagittal (**b**) T1 images of the brain and T2 (**c**) and T1 (**d**) post-contrastographic images of the spine show diffuse nodular and linear leptomeningeal contrast enhancement due to CSF dissemination

made recommendations for response assessment in patients with MB and leptomeningeal seeding tumors [40, 41]. Diffusion-weighted imaging has excellent diagnostic accuracy for differentiating MBL from other posterior fossa tumors [32]. The high tumor cellularity of MB classically results in restricted diffusion, manifested by low ADC values (Fig. 10.2c) [42]. Magnetic resonance spectroscopy (MRS) could provide useful information about tumor metabolism, revealing features that are likely to improve preoperative diagnoses [43]. Leptomeningeal dissemination via the CSF pathway may occur and may rarely be the predominant manifestation at onset; for this reason, it is therefore important to include the examination of the neuroaxis and the use of MDC in the MRI examination protocol.

The approach for histopathological assessment of MB is accomplished through different steps. If available, samples should undergo evaluation using hematoxylin and eosin (HE) staining and a panel of immunohistochemical markers specific to central nervous system embryonal tumors, such as synaptophysin, GFAP, INI1, YAP1, GAB1, LIN28A, and beta-catenin. After the confirmation of histological diagnosis of MB, including determination of histological subtype and molecular group prediction, if possible, the molecular diagnostic panel should be done. Approaches for molecular stratification should rely on DNA methylation or transcriptomic profiling, along with DNA sequencing (e.g., CTNNB1 in WNT, TP53 sequencing in SHH MB) and specific genetic defects are evaluated by iFISH, array-based, or other methods [44].

10.7 Staging and Risk Stratification

The staging of MB relies on brain and spinal cord MRI and cerebrospinal fluid cytology obtained via lumbar puncture and conducted 14 days after surgery. If performed earlier and no malignant cells are detected, it is not necessary to repeat it [45]. Currently, the Chang staging system, introduced in 1969, remains the widely utilized staging system for the evaluation of metastasis and risk assessment. Initially, this staging system incorporated primary tumor size and local invasion (T staging) as well as the presence of metastasis at diagnosis (M staging) to predict potential outcomes. While the M staging has retained its prognostic value in clinical practice, studies conducted over the years have demonstrated that T staging may not be as reliable as prognostic indicator. Traditional risk stratification criteria for MB have been based on clinical factors such as age at diagnosis, extent of surgical excision, M staging, and histological characteristics (e.g., anaplastic or large cell features). Through these variables, it was feasible to stratify patients into risk categories, useful for outcome prediction and treatment planning. Specifically, high-risk patients exhibited one or more of the following characteristics: age under 3 years old, residual tumor size >1.5 cm^2 after resection, large cell or anaplastic histologic variants, and M1 to M4 staging, while average-risk patients did not display any of this feature [46].

In the last decade, biological and molecular discoveries have identified additional risk factors, such as *MYC* oncogene amplification and molecular subgrouping, which have revolutionized prognostic assessment, defining different risk groups.

Patients classified as *low-risk* present a survival >90%, a median age under 16 years old without other clinical risk factors, usually belonging to the WNT subgroup. A subgroup within the average-risk Group 4, particularly patients with loss of chromosome 11 and/or whole gain of chromosome 17, may also be classified as low risk and treated with reduced therapy, showing favorable prognosis during standard treatment.

The *standard-risk* MB shows more than 80% five-year survival rate, belonging to this category there are the great majority of non-metastatic non-MYCN amplified SHH patients, excepted TP53-mutated SHH forms, exhibiting a poor prognosis, regardless of the presence of metastasis. Group 3 MB without MYC amplification and MB Group 4 without loss of chromosome 11 are also stratified as medium/standard risk. MYC amplification has been considered in many cases as a predictor of unfavorable prognosis, although its significance in non-metastatic Group 3 remains uncertain.

The *high-risk* class, with 50–75% survival, includes those individuals with metastatic SHH MB, metastatic *TP53*-wild type, Group 4 metastatic tumors, or non-metastatic SHH MB with *MYCN* amplification.

Lastly, *very high-risk* patients, reporting a survival percentage less than 50%, are Group 3 with metastasis and MYC amplification along with the SHH group with TP53 mutation, typically exhibiting anaplastic morphology or association with Li-Fraumeni syndrome in pediatric patients (Table 10.2).

Differences have been underlined in risk group stratification for children under 3–5 years old, as described in Table 10.3 [47]. However, this consensus was defined before the new introduction of the eight second-generation non-WNT/non-SHH G3/4 subgroups. In recent clinical trials, SJMB03 and MB subgroups have been retrospectively analyzed by Gajjar et al., identifying a low-risk group within Group 3/4 MB, characterized by M0 and subgroup VII. A retrospective analysis of the HIT2000 and I-HIT-MED cohorts have integrated clinical parameters with new subgroups and whole chromosomal aberration WCA, improving low-risk and very high-risk stratification models for Group 3/4 subgroup VII-WCA phenotype, as well as subgroups II, III, and V [48]. Furthermore, a study conducted by Goddard et al. in a cohort of Group 4 affected patients has redefined MB Group 4 risk stratification, identifying a favorable-risk category of non-metastatic tumors with either subgroup 7 or WCA-FR, very-high-

Table 10.2 Risk stratification for children with medulloblastomas aged >5 years

Risk	Molecular characteristics	Histology	Residual disease	Metastatic disease
Low	WNT subgroup (age < 16 years), TP53 wildtype, MYC/N not amplified	Classic, Desmoplastic / Nodular	<1.5 cm^2	M0
Standard	TP53 wildtype, MYC/N not amplified (except MYCN amplified Group 4)	Classic, Desmoplastic / Nodular	Any	M0
	WNT subgroup (any age, not low risk)	Classic, Desmoplastic / Nodular	Any	M+ if <16 years; M0 if >16 years
	Non-WNT subgroups without high-risk biological features	Classic, Desmoplastic / Nodular	>1.5 cm^2	M0
High	TP53 mutated and/or MYCN amplified (except MYCN amplified Group 4)	Any	Any	Any
	Any non-WNT and WNT >16 years	Any	Any	M+
	MYC amplified	Any	Any	Any
	Any	Anaplastic/Large cell	Any	Any

Table 10.3 Risk stratification for children with medulloblastomas aged 3–5 years

Risk	Molecular characteristics	Histology	Residual disease	Metastatic disease
Low	SHH-TP53 wildtype, MYC/N not amplified	DN / MBEN	Any	M0
Standard	Non-high risk, non-WNT	Classic	Any	M0
	SHH-TP53 wildtype, MYC/N not amplified	DN / MBEN	Any	M+
High	TP53 mutated and/or MYC/N amplified	Any	Any	Any
	Non-SHH, non-WNT	Classic	Any	M+
	Any	Large cell / Anaplastic	Any	Any

risk category of metastatic tumors with WCA-HR, and high-risk category of remaining patients. Of note, in this study, it has been underlined that the previously established disease-wide risk features, such as LC/A histology and MYC amplification, have had limited prognostic relevance in Group 4 MBs. In this new prospective, future evaluations are needed to implement and update risk-tailored therapeutic approaches for favorable- risk and very-high-risk patients [49].

10.8 Treatment

The therapeutic approach to MB is multidisciplinary: standard treatment involves a combination of maximal safe surgical removal, craniospinal irradiation (CSI) tailored to the risk category, based on metastatic stage and extent of resection, and chemotherapy, typically with cyclophosphamide, lomustine, cisplatin, and vincristine combinations [50, 51].

In Table 10.4 are summarized the principal treatments based on molecular characteristics and risk stratification for both children <3–5 years old and >3–5 years old, according to SIOPE recommendations.

The initial step in managing MB involves surgery, often requiring cerebrospinal fluid diversion, typically via endoscopic third ventriculostomy preceding or following tumor removal. In cases where this procedure is inadequate, ventriculoperitoneal shunting may be necessary [4]. Surgical resection is usually done via craniotomy or craniectomy, and according to several studies, there is a correlation between resection extent and patient outcomes. Near-total resection (NTR) and gross-total resection (GTR) yield better outcomes compared to subtotal resection (STR) or biopsy. The significance of resection has been re-evaluated also in light of MB subgrouping, suggesting that there is no definitive advantage to GTR over near-total resection, especially when the risk of neurological morbidity is high with GTR [52]. A postoperative brain MRI is usually performed within 24–72 hours to accurately assess residual tumor and avoid post-surgical complications. It is not infrequent that

Table 10.4 Treatment algorithm details based on molecular characteristics and risk stratification for both children <3–5 years old and >3–5 years old, according to SIOPE recommendations

Age < 3–5 years	SHH MBEN/DMB MYC non-amplified TP53 WT		HIT SKK 2000 with intraventricular methotrexate
	Non-SHH Non-MBEN/DMB MYC amplified TP53 mutant		Head Start II Regimen A2
Age > 3–5 years	Low Risk	WNT Non-metastatic <16 y old MYCN non-amplified TP53 WT	23.4 Gy CSI + boost + PNETs chemotherapy
	Standard Risk	WNT > 16 y or with high-risk features Non-WNT Non-metastatic Non-LCA MYCN non-amplified (except Group 4) TP53 WT	23.4 Gy CSI + boost + PNETs chemotherapy
	High Risk	Non-standard risk Non-low risk	36–40 Gy CSI + boost chemotherapy e.g. SJMB 03 POG 9031 PNET5 like

children affected by tumors around the cerebellar vermis may develop a condition named posterior fossa syndrome in the postoperative period. These patients may manifest mutism, ataxia, hemiparesis, cognitive deficits, behavioral changes, cranial and bulbar nerve paralysis, and tremor. Some of these symptoms like mutism are often fully reversible within weeks, while others may persist in the form of long-term neurological impairments [4].

Radiation therapy along with chemotherapy are considered of paramount importance in MB treatment after surgical removal. The therapeutic plan for radiation typically involves its delivery to the entire cranio-spinal axis, a technique termed CSI, associated with a boost to the tumor bed and posterior cranial fossa [4]. This approach represents a major challenge in infants and young children's treatment since severe post-radiation neurological and endocrinological impairments arise in patients younger than 3 years old. As a result, trials have attempted to delay, omit, and replace this therapy. The timing and dose of radiation in older children with MBs depend on risk stratification. Initially, the treatment regimen for standard-risk patients consisted of 36 Gy of CSI with a posterior fossa boost up to 54 Gy, aimed at preventing leptomeningeal relapse and achieving a cure rate of 60%. However, the doses of cranial radiation led to significant cognitive and endocrine effects on survivors (mainly younger children 3–7 years old). With the introduction of chemotherapy into the treatment protocol, a reduction in the CSI dose to 23.4 Gy with a 54 Gy boost has been possible, resulting in nearly comparable survival outcomes. Unfortunately, further dose reduction of CSI to 18 Gy led to inferior outcomes, particularly in patients with Group 4 tumors [52, 53]. For what concerns the treatment approach for high-risk MB, there is no definitive consensus yet, but the established radiation therapy regimen involves the administration of dose ranging from 36 to 39.6 Gy to the craniospinal axis, with a boost of up to 54 Gy targeted at the primary tumor site [54].

In affected infant patients, radiation therapy is not typically used due to the risk of various long-term sequelae. Traditionally, patients were categorized as "infants" when under 3 years of age. However, different protocols are extended to patients aged 4 or older and distinctions are present among different countries. Several studies have evaluated the therapeutic options available instead of radiation. Chemotherapy assumes a fundamental role in the treatment of pediatric patients, specific approaches have relied on the use of aggressive induction chemotherapy followed by even more intensive consolidation with stem cell transplantation (HDC/ASCT), commonly employed to mitigate hematological toxicity and maintain dose intensity. Alternatively, a regimen involving intraventricular or high-dose methotrexate (MTX) has been shown to enhance survival rates. Both these approaches have been combined and evaluated in the Children's Oncology Group study ACNS0334. Infants with SHH group tumors exhibited the most favorable outcomes, whereas those with non-WNT/non-SHH tumors had inferior survival rates [30, 51, 52]. HDC/ASCT also constitutes a critical therapeutic measure in high-risk MB patients. The OS rate in non-metastatic MB patients treated with high-dose chemotherapy and autologous stem cell rescue has been estimated at around 70% [53, 54].

Innovative techniques like intensity-modulated radiation therapy (IMRT) and proton beam radiation therapy (PBRT) have been developed to selectively target tumors, reducing damage to healthy brain tissue and other organs to improve long-term neurocognitive outcomes. Novel fields of interest are represented by FLASH proton therapy, which administers proton radiation at exceptionally high dose rates along with memantine, a competitive NMDA receptor antagonist known for its neurocognitive protective effect [4, 30]. Recent studies conducted by Donovan et al. are investigating the locoregional delivery of CAR T cells presenting a target for specific MB cell surface proteins, like EPHA2, HER2, and interleukin 13. Currently, this approach has demonstrated efficacy in metastatic Group 3 mouse models. Further future investigations and strategies to enhance tumor immunogenicity will likely be necessary for the success of immunotherapy in MB [30].

10.9 Outcome and Toxicity After Treatment

One of the fundamental prognostic factors for MB is represented by the extent of surgical removal. According to several studies, there is a correlation between resection extent and patient outcomes. NTR and GTR yield better outcomes compared to STR or biopsy. The significance of resection has been re-evaluated also considering MB subgrouping, suggesting that there is no definitive advantage GTR over NTR, especially when the risk of neurological morbidity is high with GTR [52].

The type and dose of chemotherapy and radiation have resulted in numerous delayed issues, including degradation in neurocognitive functions, ototoxicity with auditory impairment, endocrine complications, psychosocial disabilities, compromised renal function, infertility, cerebrovascular complications, and second malignancies.

Surviving patients treated with CSI, especially children under 7 years old, have experienced a significant decline in 20–30 points IQ which worsens over the lifespan, degrading memory loss, and executive or attentional function, especially due to irradiation of frontal and temporal areas. It has been demonstrated that radiation produces changes in brain white matter and vasculature, with a reduction in the cerebral cortex thickness and hippocampus dimension. A reduced-dose CSI of 18.0 Gy has demonstrated an elevated cognitive function score, despite not impacting survival rates, compared to patients receiving high-dose CSI. Since dose reduction can preserve neurocognitive functions, risk stratification is crucial to minimize therapeutic burden when feasible [4, 55, 56].

In addition to this, several hormonal alterations have been documented in survivors of MB, predominantly ascribed to direct radiation-induced damage to the pituitary gland and hypothalamus. Hypothyroidism has been observed in a range of patients, varying from 8 to 60%, presenting with clinically evident thyroid hormone deficiency or elevated levels of TSH. Another common long-term side effect of therapy is auditory toxicity, evident in more than 15% of MB patients lowering the surviving patients' independence and quality of life [4, 57].

It has been demonstrated that patients undergoing radiotherapy are at risk of developing cerebrovascular adverse events; recent studies are evaluating the chemotherapy-induced-cardiotoxicity, especially in younger patients, as it may induce conditions such as pericardial effusion, left ventricular dysfunction, heart failure, arrhythmias, thrombotic events, and myocardial infarction [58]. In conclusion, radiation-induced tumors may appear many years after treatment and represent significant sequelae in long-term survivors.

Generally, patients treated with cranial irradiation greater than 50 Gy have had increased incidence of secondary tumor onset, estimated around 7% at 25 years from diagnosis, while this percentage drops to 1% for patients not treated with radiation. Among benign tumors, the most described is meningioma, while high-grade gliomas represent the most malignant secondary tumors. Other possible neoplasms include leukemia, tumors of the urinary and GI tract, thyroid tumors, and notably, cutaneous tumors [4].

Bibliography

1. Damodharan S, Puccetti D. Pediatric central nervous system tumor overview and emerging treatment considerations. Brain Sci. 2023;13(7):1106.
2. Millard NE, De Braganca KC. Medulloblastoma. J Child Neurol. 2016;31(12):1341–53. https://doi.org/10.1177/0883073815600866.
3. Northcott PA, Robinson GW, Kratz CP, Mabbott DJ, Pomeroy SL, Clifford SC, Rutkowski S, Ellison DW, Malkin D, Taylor MD, Gajjar A, Pfister SM. Medulloblastoma. Nat Rev Dis Primers. 2019;5(1):11.
4. Pizzo PA, Poplack DG, Blaney SM, Helman LJ. Pizzo and Poplack's pediatric oncology. 8th ed. Philadelphia: Lippincott Williams & Wilkins; 2020.
5. Poretti A, Meoded A, Huisman TA. Neuroimaging of pediatric posterior fossa tumors including review of the literature. J Magn Reson Imaging. 2012;35(1):32–47. https://doi.org/10.1002/jmri.22722.
6. Elsayed A, Alardati H, Al-Maghrabi J, Meliti A. Extracranial medulloblastoma with myogenic differentiation: report of a rare event. Cureus. 2023;15(11):e48301. https://doi.org/10.7759/cureus.48301.

7. Aref D, Croul S. Medulloblastoma: recurrence and metastasis. CNS Oncol. 2013;2(4):377–85.
8. Packer RJ, Cogen P, Vezina G, Rorke LB. Medulloblastoma: clinical and biologic aspects. Neuro-Oncology. 1999;1(3):232–50.
9. Gajjar A, Reaman GH, Racadio JM, Smith FO. Brain tumors in children. New York: Springer; 2018.
10. García-Espinosa P, Molina-Ayala M, Botello-Hernández E, Villareal-Garza E, Barbosa-Quintana Á. Congenital medulloblastoma presented in the neonatal period. Autops Case Rep. 2021;11:11.
11. Mengide JP, Berros MF, Turza ME, Liñares JM. Posterior fossa tumors in children: an update and new concepts. Surg Neurol Int. 2023;14:114. https://doi.org/10.25259/SNI_43_2023.
12. Orr BA. Pathology, diagnostics, and classification of medulloblastoma. Brain Pathol. 2020;30(3):664–78. https://doi.org/10.1111/bpa.12837.
13. Ellison D. Classifying the medulloblastoma: insights from morphology and molecular genetics. Neuropathol Appl Neurobiol. 2002;28(4):257–82. https://doi.org/10.1046/j.1365-2990.2002.00419.x.
14. Mahapatra S, Amsbaugh MJ. Medulloblastoma. In: StatPearls [internet]. Treasure Island (FL): StatPearls Publishing; 2024. PMID: 28613723.
15. Alharbi M, Mobark N, Bashawri Y, Abu Safieh L, Alowayn A, Aljelaify R, AlSaeed M, Almutairi A, Alqubaishi F, AlSolme E, Ahmad M, Al-Banyan A, Alotabi FE, Serrano J, Snuderl M, Al-Rashed M, Abedalthagafi M. Methylation profiling of medulloblastoma in a clinical setting permits sub-classification and reveals new outcome predictions. Front Neurol. 2020;11:167. https://doi.org/10.3389/fneur.2020.00167.
16. Northcott PA, Rutka JT, Taylor MD. Genomics of medulloblastoma: from Giemsa-banding to next-generation sequencing in 20 years. Neurosurg Focus. 2010;28(1):E6. https://doi.org/10.3171/2009.10.FOCUS09218.
17. Esteller M. Relevance of DNA methylation in the management of cancer. Lancet Oncol. 2003;4(6):351–8. https://doi.org/10.1016/s1470-2045(03)01115-x.
18. Martisova A, Holcakova J, Izadi N, Sebuyoya R, Hrstka R, Bartosik M. DNA methylation in solid tumors: functions and methods of detection. Int J Mol Sci. 2021;22(8):4247.
19. Galbraith K, Vasudevaraja V, Serrano J, Shen G, Tran I, Abdallat N, Wen M, Patel S, Movahed-Ezazi M, Faustin A, Spino-Keeton M, Roberts LG, Maloku E, Drexler SA, Liechty BL, Pisapia D, Krasnozhen-Ratush O, Rosenblum M, Shroff S, Boué DR, Davidson C, Mao Q, Suchi M, North P, Hopp A, Segura A, Jarzembowski JA, Parsons L, Johnson MD, Mobley B, Samore W, McGuone D, Gopal PP, Canoll PD, Horbinski C, Fullmer JM, Farooqui MS, Gokden M, Wadhwani NR, Richardson TE, Umphlett M, Tsankova NM, DeWitt JC, Sen C, Placantonakis DG, Pacione D, Wisoff JH, Teresa Hidalgo E, Harter D, William CM, Cordova C, Kurz SC, Barbaro M, Orringer DA, Karajannis MA, Sulman EP, Gardner SL, Zagzag D, Tsirigos A, Allen JC, Golfinos JG, Snuderl M. Clinical utility of whole-genome DNA methylation profiling as a primary molecular diagnostic assay for central nervous system tumors-a prospective study and guidelines for clinical testing. Neurooncol Adv. 2023;5(1):vdad076.
20. Haltom AR, Toll SA, Cheng D, Maegawa S, Gopalakrishnan V, Khatua S. Medulloblastoma epigenetics and the path to clinical innovation. J Neuro-Oncol. 2020;150(1):35–46.
21. Zhou Z, Zhu B, Meng Q, Zhang T, Wu Y, Yu R, Gao S. Research progress in molecular pathology markers in medulloblastoma. Explor Target Antitumor Ther. 2023;4(1):139.
22. Hicks D, Rafiee G, Schwalbe EC, Howell CI, Lindsey JC, Hill RM, Smith AJ, Adidharma P, Steel C, Richardson S, Pease L, Danilenko M, Crosier S, Joshi A, Wharton SB, Jacques TS, Pizer B, Michalski A, Williamson D, Bailey S, Clifford SC. The molecular landscape and associated clinical experience in infant medulloblastoma: prognostic significance of second-generation subtypes. Neuropathol Appl Neurobiol. 2021;47(2):236–50.
23. Louis DN, Perry A, Wesseling P, Brat DJ, Cree IA, Figarella-Branger D, Hawkins C, Ng HK, Pfister SM, Reifenberger G, Soffietti R, von Deimling A, Ellison DW. The 2021 WHO classification of tumors of the central nervous system: a summary. Neuro-Oncology. 2021;23(8):1231–51. https://doi.org/10.1093/neuonc/noab106.
24. Juraschka K, Taylor MD. Medulloblastoma in the age of molecular subgroups: a review. J Neurosurg Pediatr. 2019;24(4):353–63. https://doi.org/10.3171/2019.5.PEDS18381. PMID: 3157448
25. Roussel MF, Hatten ME. Cerebellum development and medulloblastoma. Curr Top Dev Biol. 2011;94:235–82. https://doi.org/10.1016/B978-0-12-380916-2.00008-5.
26. Wang J, Garancher A, Ramaswamy V, Wechsler-Reya RJ. Medulloblastoma: from molecular subgroups to molecular targeted therapies. Annu Rev Neurosci. 2018;41:207–32. https://doi.org/10.1146/annurev-neuro-070815-013838.
27. Alaña L, Nunes-Xavier CE, Zaldumbide L, Martin-Guerrero I, Mosteiro L, Alba-Pavón P, Villate O, García-Obregón S, González-García H, Herraiz R, Astigarraga I, Pulido R, García-Ariza M. Identification and functional analysis of a novel CTNNB1 mutation in pediatric medulloblastoma. Cancers (Basel). 2022;14(2):421. https://doi.org/10.3390/cancers14020421.
28. Slika H, Alimonti P, Raj D, Caraway C, Alomari S, Jackson EM, Tyler B. The neurodevelopmental and molecular landscape of medulloblastoma subgroups: current targets and the potential for combined therapies. Cancers (Basel). 2023;15(15):3889. https://doi.org/10.3390/cancers15153889.
29. Kumar R, Liu APY, Northcott PA. Medulloblastoma genomics in the modern molecular era. Brain

Pathol. 2020;30(3):679–90. https://doi.org/10.1111/bpa.12804.

30. Gold MP, Ong W, Masteller AM, Ghasemi DR, Galindo JA, Park NR, Huynh NC, Donde A, Pister V, Saurez RA, Vladoiu MC, Hwang GH, Eisemann T, Donovan LK, Walker AD, Benetatos J, Dufour C, Garzia L, Segal RA, Wechsler-Reya RJ, Mesirov JP, Korshunov A, Pajtler KW, Pomeroy SL, Ayrault O, Davidson SM, Cotter JA, Taylor MD, Fraenkel E. Developmental basis of SHH medulloblastoma heterogeneity. Nat Commun. 2024;15(1):270.
31. Lazow MA, Palmer JD, Fouladi M, Salloum R. Medulloblastoma in the modern era: review of contemporary trials, molecular advances, and updates in management. Neurotherapeutics. 2022;19(6):1733–51.
32. Luo Y, Zhang S, Tan W, Lin G, Zhuang Y, Zeng H. The diagnostic efficiency of quantitative diffusion weighted imaging in differentiating medulloblastoma from posterior fossa tumors: a systematic review and meta-analysis. Diagnostics (Basel). 2022;12(11):2796. https://doi.org/10.3390/diagnostics12112796. PMID: 36428860; PMCID: PMC9689934.
33. Farouk Sait S, Walsh MF, Karajannis MA. Genetic syndromes predisposing to pediatric brain tumors. Neurooncol Pract. 2021;8(4):375–90.
34. Carta R, Del Baldo G, Miele E, Po A, Besharat ZM, Nazio F, et al. Cancer predisposition syndromes and medulloblastoma in the molecular era. Front Oncologia. 2020;10:566822.
35. Quinlan A, Rizzolo D. Understanding medulloblastoma. JAAPA. 2017;30(10):30–6. https://doi.org/10.1097/01.JAA.0000524717.71084.50.
36. Colafati GS, Voicu IP, Carducci C, Miele E, Carai A, Di Loreto S, Marrazzo A, Cacchione A, Cecinati V, Tornesello A, Mastronuzzi A. MRI features as a helpful tool to predict the molecular subgroups of medulloblastoma: state of the art. Ther Adv Neurol Disord. 2018;11:1756286418775375. https://doi.org/10.1177/1756286418775375. PMID: 29977341; PMCID: PMC6024494.
37. Gibson P, Tong Y, Robinson G, Thompson MC, Currle DS, Eden C, Kranenburg TA, Hogg T, Poppleton H, Martin J, Finkelstein D, Pounds S, Weiss A, Patay Z, Scoggins M, Ogg R, Pei Y, Yang ZJ, Brun S, Lee Y, Zindy F, Lindsey JC, Taketo MM, Boop FA, Sanford RA, Gajjar A, Clifford SC, Roussel MF, McKinnon PJ, Gutmann DH, Ellison DW, Wechsler-Reya R, Gilbertson RJ. Subtypes of medulloblastoma have distinct developmental origins. Nature. 2010;468(7327):1095–9. https://doi.org/10.1038/nature09587. Epub 2010 Dec 8. PMID: 21150899; PMCID: PMC3059767.
38. Patay Z, DeSain LA, Hwang SN, Coan A, Li Y, Ellison DW. MR imaging characteristics of wingless-type-subgroup pediatric medulloblastoma. Am J Neuroradiol. 2015;36(12):2386–93. https://doi.org/10.3174/ajnr.A4495. Epub 2015 Sep 3. PMID: 26338912; PMCID: PMC4827780.
39. Perreault S, Ramaswamy V, Achrol AS, Chao K, Liu TT, Shih D, Remke M, Schubert S, Bouffet E, Fisher PG, Partap S, Vogel H, Taylor MD, Cho YJ, Yeom KW. MRI surrogates for molecular subgroups of medulloblastoma. Am J Neuroradiol. 2014;35(7):1263–9. https://doi.org/10.3174/ajnr.A3990. Epub 2014 May 15. PMID: 24831600; PMCID: PMC4819007.
40. Peng J, Zhou H, Tang O, Chang K, Wang P, Zeng X, Shen Q, Wu J, Xiao Y, Patel SH, Hu C, Jin K, Xiao B, Boxerman J, Gao X, Wen PY, Bai HX, Huang RY, Yang L. Evaluation of RAPNO criteria in medulloblastoma and other leptomeningeal seeding tumors using MRI and clinical data. Neuro-Oncology. 2020;22(10):1536–44. https://doi.org/10.1093/neuonc/noaa072. PMID: 32215549; PMCID: PMC7566367.
41. Warren KE, Vezina G, Poussaint TY, Warmuth-Metz M, Chamberlain MC, Packer RJ, Brandes AA, Reiss M, Goldman S, Fisher MJ, Pollack IF, Prados MD, Wen PY, Chang SM, Dufour C, Zurakowski D, Kortmann RD, Kieran MW. Response assessment in medulloblastoma and leptomeningeal seeding tumors: recommendations from the response assessment in pediatric neuro-oncology committee. Neuro-Oncology. 2018;20(1):13–23. https://doi.org/10.1093/neuonc/nox087. PMID: 28449033; PMCID: PMC5761545.
42. Brandão LA, Young Poussaint T. Posterior Fossa Tumors. Neuroimaging Clin N Am. 2017;27(1):1–37. https://doi.org/10.1016/j.nic.2016.08.001. PMID: 27889018.
43. Blüml S, Margol AS, Sposto R, Kennedy RJ, Robison NJ, Vali M, Hung LT, Muthugounder S, Finlay JL, Erdreich-Epstein A, Gilles FH, Judkins AR, Krieger MD, Dhall G, Nelson MD, Asgharzadeh S. Molecular subgroups of medulloblastoma identification using noninvasive magnetic resonance spectroscopy. Neuro-Oncology. 2016;18(1):126–31. https://doi.org/10.1093/neuonc/nov097. Epub 2015 Aug 8. PMID: 26254476; PMCID: PMC4677409.
44. Dangouloff-Ros V, Varlet P, Levy R, Beccaria K, Puget S, Dufour C, Boddaert N. Imaging features of medulloblastoma: conventional imaging, diffusion-weighted imaging, perfusion-weighted imaging, and spectroscopy: from general features to subtypes and characteristics. Neurochirurgie. 2021;67(1):6–13.
45. Taylor MD, Taylor RE, Ellison DW, Bailey S, Clifford SC. DNA methylation profiling of medulloblastoma allows robust subclassification and improved outcome prediction using formalin-fixed biopsies. Acta Neuropathol. 2013;125(3):359–71.
46. Khattab A, Monga DK. Turcot Syndrome. 2023 Jun 26. In: StatPearls [Internet]. Treasure Island (FL): StatPearls Publishing; 2024 Jan–.
47. European Society for Paediatric Oncology (SIOP Europe). Medulloblastoma guidelines. Available from: https://siope.eu/media/documents/escp--medulloblasto-ma.pdf. Accessed 2024 Jun 22.

48. Ramaswamy V, Remke M, Bouffet E, Bailey S, Clifford SC, Doz F, Kool M, Dufour C, Vassal G, Milde T, Witt O, von Hoff K, Pietsch T, Northcott PA, Gajjar A, Robinson GW, Padovani L, André N, Massimino M, Pizer B, Packer R, Rutkowski S, Pfister SM, Taylor MD, Pomeroy SL. Risk stratification of childhood medulloblastoma in the molecular era: the current consensus. Acta Neuropathol. 2016;131(6):821–31.
49. Mynarek M, Obrecht D, Sill M, Sturm D, Kloth-Stachnau K, Selt F, et al. Identification of low and very high-risk patients with non-WNT/non-SHH medulloblastoma by improved clinico-molecular stratification of the HIT2000 and I-HIT-MED cohorts. Acta Neuropathol. 2023;145(1):97–112. https://doi.org/10.1007/s00401-022-02522-4.
50. Goddard J, Castle J, Southworth E, Fletcher A, Crosier S, Martin-Guerrero I, García-Ariza M, Navajas A, Masliah-Planchon J, Bourdeaut F, Dufour C, Ayrault O, Goschzik T, Pietsch T, Sill M, Pfister SM, Rutkowski S, Richardson S, Hill RM, Williamson D, Bailey S, Schwalbe EC, Clifford SC, Hicks D. Molecular characterisation defines clinically-actionable heterogeneity within Group 4 medulloblastoma and improves disease risk-stratification. Acta Neuropathol. 2023;145(5):651–66.
51. Bagchi A, Dhanda SK, Dunphy P, Sioson E, Robinson GW. Molecular classification improves therapeutic options for infants and young children with medulloblastoma. J Natl Compr Cancer Netw. 2023;21(10):1097–105. https://doi.org/10.6004/jnccn.2023.7024.
52. Prados MD. Current strategies for management of medulloblastoma. Diagnostics (Basel). 2023;13(16):2622.
53. Mushtaq N, Ul Ain R, Hamid SA, Bouffet E. Evolution of systemic therapy in medulloblastoma including irradiation-sparing approaches. Diagnostics (Basel). 2023;13(24):3680.
54. Jackson K, Packer RJ. Recent advances in pediatric medulloblastoma. Curr Neurol Neurosci Rep. 2023;23(12):841–8. https://doi.org/10.1007/s11910-023-01316-9.
55. Choi JY. Medulloblastoma: current perspectives and recent advances. Brain Tumor Res Treat. 2023;11(1):28–38. https://doi.org/10.14791/btrt.2022.0046.
56. Ahn WK, Hahn SM, Yoon HI, Lee J, Park EK, Shim KW, Kim DS, Suh CO, Kim SH, Lyu CJ, Han JW. Long-term outcomes of protocol-based treatment for newly diagnosed medulloblastoma. Cancer Res Treat. 2024;56(2):652–64.
57. Partanen M, Bouffet E, Laughlin S, Strother D, Hukin J, Skocic J, Szulc-Lerch K, Mabbott DJ. Early changes in white matter predict intellectual outcome in children treated for posterior fossa tumors. Neuroimage Clin. 2018;20:697–704.
58. Fossati P, Ricardi U, Orecchia R. Pediatric medulloblastoma: toxicity of current treatment and potential role of protontherapy. Cancer Treat Rev. 2009;35(1):79–96. https://doi.org/10.1016/j.ctrv.2008.09.002.

Atypical Teratoid/Rhabdoid Tumor 11

Giacomina Megaro, Giada Del Baldo,
Sabrina Rossi, Giovanna Stefania Colafati,
Eleonora Piccirilli, Evelina Miele,
and Angela Mastronuzzi

11.1 Introduction

Atypical Teratoid/Rhabdoid Tumor (AT/RT) is a rare, highly malignant central nervous system (CNS) tumor that predominantly affects infants and young children. The incidence of AT/RT is approximately 1–2% of all pediatric brain tumors, but despite its rarity, AT/RT accounts for a significant percentage of childhood brain tumor-related deaths due to its aggressive behavior and resistance to conventional therapies. The median age at diagnosis is typically around 1–3 years, although AT/RT can occur in older children and, in rare cases, adults [1–5].

G. Megaro · G. Del Baldo · E. Miele
Area of Hematology-Oncology, Cell Therapy, Gene Therapies, and Hematopoietic Transplantation Bambino Gesù Children's Hospital, IRCCS, Rome, Italy

S. Rossi
Pathology Unit, Bambino Gesù Children's Hospital, IRCCS, Rome, Italy

G. S. Colafati · E. Piccirilli
Imaging Department, Bambino Gesù Children's Hospital, IRCCS, Rome, Italy

A. Mastronuzzi (✉)
Area of Hematology-Oncology, Cell Therapy, Gene Therapies, and Hematopoietic Transplantation Bambino Gesù Children's Hospital, IRCCS, Rome, Italy

Department of Life Sciences and Public Health, Università Cattolica del Sacro Cuore, Rome, Italy
e-mail: angela.mastronuzzi@opbg.net

The major hallmark of AT/RT is inactivation of the SMARCB1 gene (also known as INI1 or hSNF5) (Fig. 11.1), which encodes a key component of the SWI/SNF chromatin-remodeling complex. Loss of SMARCB1 function leads to widespread epigenetic changes that disrupt normal cellular processes and promote tumorigenesis. In a minority of cases, the SMARCA4 gene is also implicated, particularly in cases where SMARCB1 is intact. Loss of SMARCB1 or SMARCA4 is so characteristic of AT/RT that it is used as a diagnostic criterion, with immunohistochemical staining for SMARCB1 protein serving as a standard diagnostic tool [6–8].

The complexity of AT/RT extends beyond its genetic mutations, as recent molecular profiling studies have identified distinct subgroups within AT/RT. Four subgroups, which include AT/RT–SHH, AT/RT–TYR, AT/RT–MYC, and AT/RT–SMARCA4, are defined by unique genetic, epigenetic, and transcriptomic profiles that influence tumor behavior, prognosis, and response to therapy [8]. Understanding these subgroups has become crucial for the development of personalized treatment strategies that can improve outcomes for patients with this challenging disease.

A. Mastronuzzi, A. Carai (eds.), *Navigating Pediatric Brain Tumors*,
https://doi.org/10.1007/978-3-032-18992-9_11

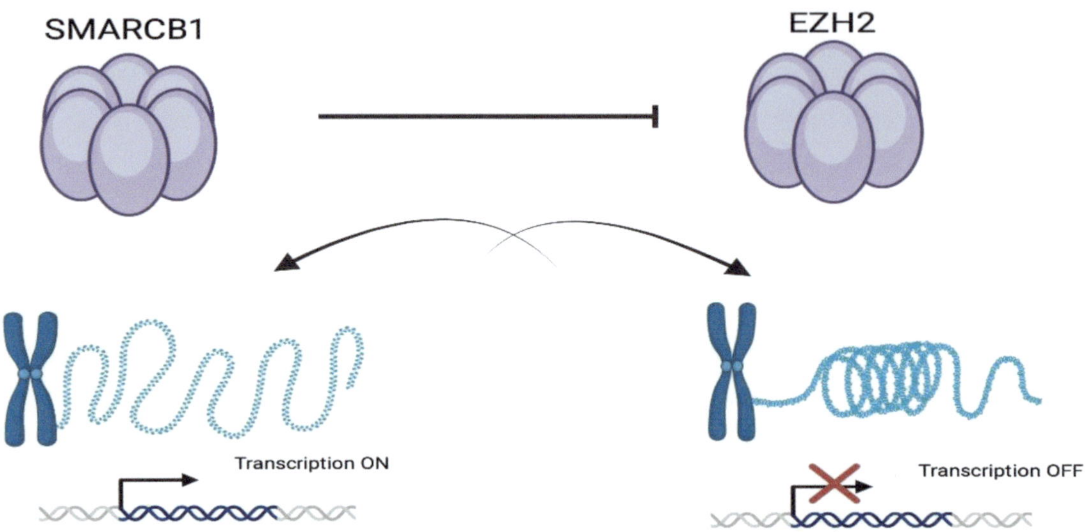

Fig. 11.1 Inactivation of the SMARCB1 gene encodes a key component of the SWI/SNF chromatin-remodeling complex. Loss of SMARCB1 function disrupts normal cellular processes and promotes tumorigenesis

11.2 Molecular and Genetic Profiling

AT/RT is a genetically heterogeneous tumor, with its molecular subgroups reflecting different pathways of oncogenesis. The four primary molecular subgroups—AT/RT–SHH, AT/RT–TYR, AT/RT–MYC, and AT/RT–SMARCA4—are each associated with distinct clinical features and prognoses, providing valuable insights to personalize therapeutic approaches [8–10] (Fig. 11.2).

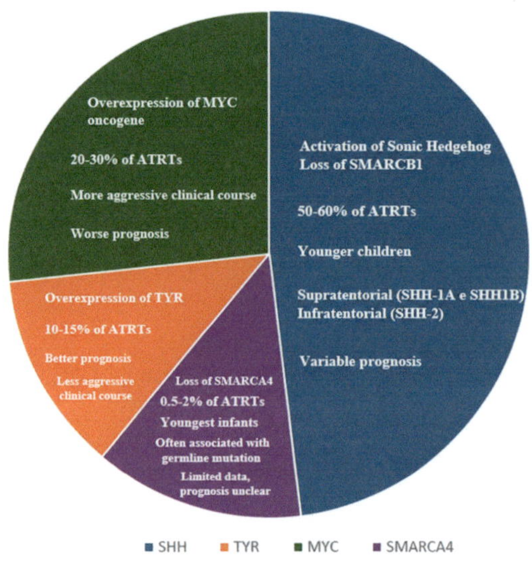

Fig. 11.2 Molecular subgroups and main features

AT/RT–SHH: This subgroup is characterized by the activation of the Sonic Hedgehog (SHH) signaling pathway, a key regulator of embryonic development, particularly in the central nervous system. Activation of the SHH in AT/RT is not typically due to the classical mutations seen in medulloblastomas but is instead a consequence of the loss of SMARCB1, which disrupts the regulation of this pathway. AT/RT–SHH is further divided into SHH-1A, SHH-1B, and SHH-2 subgroups, each with unique genetic profiles and clinical presentations. SHH-1A tumors are often located in the supratentorial region and seen in younger children, while SHH-1B tumors, also supratentorial, tend to affect older children. SHH-2 tumors are typically infratentorial and present in younger patients. The role of SHH pathway in neurodevelopment is reflected in the gene expression patterns of these tumors, with different subsets showing varying levels of expression of CNS development genes such as GSX1, FOXG1, and NEUROD6.

AT/RT–TYR: This subgroup is defined by the overexpression of tyrosinase (TYR) and other melanocytic lineage markers, suggesting a neural crest origin for these tumors. AT/RT–TYR is associated with a relatively better prognosis compared to the other subgroups, possibly due to its distinct cellular origin and the potential for targeted therapies that exploit the melanocytic differentiation. The presence of TYR and other melanocytic markers like MITF and DCT in these tumors highlights their unique biology, which is markedly different from the other AT/RT subtypes.

AT/RT–MYC: The AT/RT–MYC subgroup is defined by the overexpression of the MYC oncogene, a potent driver of cell proliferation and survival. MYC-driven AT/RTs are among the most aggressive, with poor prognosis due to MYC's role in promoting rapid cell growth and resistance to apoptosis. The involvement of MYC pathway in AT/RT highlights the need for novel therapeutic strategies targeting MYC or its downstream effectors. MYC-driven tumors often have a more complex karyotype, including multiple chromosomal abnormalities, which further complicates treatment and contributes to the aggressive nature of this subgroup.

Atypical Teratoid/Rhabdoid Tumor ATRT-SMARCA4 accounts for approximately 0.5–2% of all ATRT cases, making it the rarest molecular subgroup. Because of its low frequency, there is still limited knowledge about its biological and clinical characteristics. Clinically, these tumors are more commonly diagnosed in very young children and are frequently associated with inherited germline mutations. In contrast, their radiological and histopathological features remain poorly defined. The genetic alterations typical of the ATRT-SMARCA4 subgroup mainly involve point mutations or focal deletions. Similar to ATRT-MYC tumors, they also exhibit a hypomethylated genomic profile. In addition, these tumors show increased expression of several molecules and growth-related factors, including EPHA5, ROCK1, and FGF10.

11.3 Rhabdoid Tumor Predisposition Syndromes (RTPS)

A critical aspect of AT/RT that links it to a broader category of malignancies is its association with Rhabdoid Tumor Predisposition Syndrome (RTPS). RTPS is a genetic condition characterized by a predisposition to developing rhabdoid tumors in multiple organs, including the brain (as AT/RT), kidneys (as malignant rhabdoid tumors of the kidney, MRTK), and soft tissues. This syndrome is most often associated with germline mutations in the SMARCB1 gene, although mutations in SMARCA4 are also implicated in a smaller subset of cases [11, 12] (Fig. 11.3).

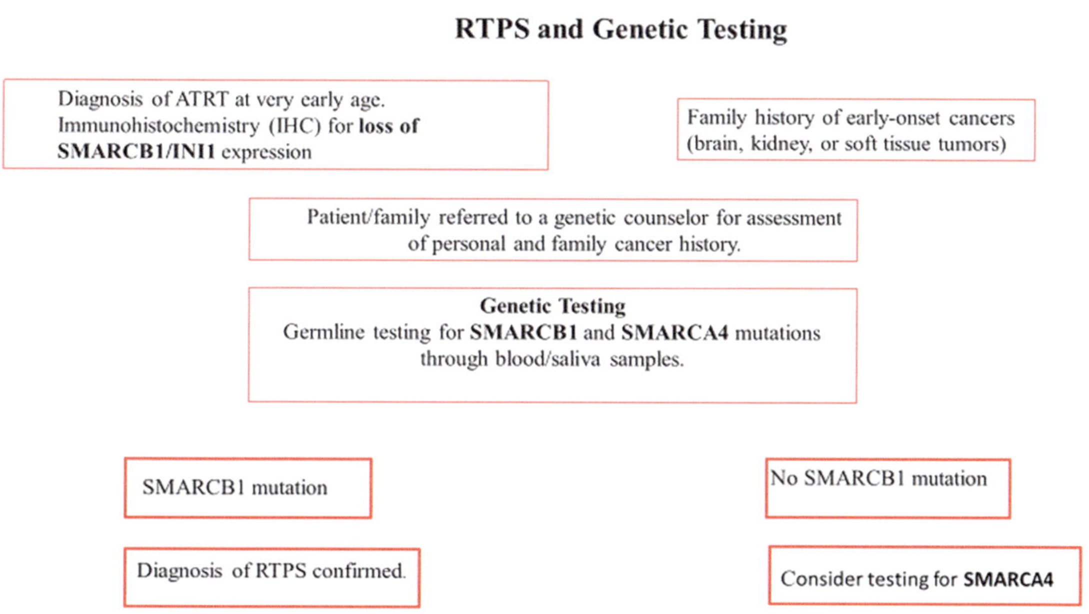

Fig. 11.3 Steps for diagnosing Rhabdoid Tumor Predisposition Syndrome

Children with RTPS often present with AT/RT at a very early age, and because of the hereditary nature of the syndrome, these patients may develop multiple rhabdoid tumors, either simultaneously or sequentially, in multiple organ systems. The diagnosis of RTPS has significant implications for family members, as they may also carry germline mutations in SMARCB1 or SMARCA4, necessitating genetic counseling and potential surveillance for early tumor detection [11–13].

The presence of germline SMARCB1 mutations in RTPS underscores the importance of genetic testing in children diagnosed with AT/RT, particularly those diagnosed at a very early age or those with a family history of rhabdoid tumors. Early identification of RTPS allows for a more comprehensive management approach, including regular surveillance for other potential tumors and consideration of prophylactic interventions [13].

11.4 Clinical and Histopathological Features

AT/RT presents with a wide range of clinical symptoms that vary depending on the tumor's location within the CNS. Given the young age of most patients, symptoms are often nonspecific and may include irritability, vomiting, and changes in behavior, which can delay diagnosis. Specific neurological signs and symptoms typically arise as the tumor grows and exerts pressure on surrounding brain structures [1, 3, 14].

Supratentorial AT/RTs: These tumors, common in the SHH-1A and SHH-1B subgroups, are located in the cerebral hemispheres and often present with symptoms of increased intracranial pressure, such as headaches, vomiting, and lethargy. Seizures are also common, reflecting the involvement of cortical regions. Focal neurological deficits, including hemiparesis or visual disturbances, can occur depending on the tumor's exact location [15].

Infratentorial AT/RTs: Commonly associated with the SHH-2 and TYR subgroups, these tumors typically arise in the cerebellum or brainstem, leading to symptoms of cerebellar dysfunction such as ataxia, dysmetria, and nystagmus. Brainstem involvement can result in cranial nerve palsies, dysphagia, and respiratory difficulties, making these tumors particularly dangerous due to their potential to affect vital functions [16, 17].

At the histological level, rhabdoid cells—large cells characterized by eccentric nuclei, prominent nucleoli, and abundant eosinophilic cytoplasm—are only one of the cellular components that may be observed in AT/RT, and their presence is not mandatory for diagnosis. More commonly, tumors also display areas composed of small undifferentiated cells, frequently associated with a spindle-cell mesenchymal component. AT/RTs are typically highly proliferative neoplasms, often showing numerous mitotic figures and areas of necrosis [2, 18].

AT/RTs are considered polyphenotypic tumors because they can express markers belonging to different cellular lineages, including EMA, SMA, GFAP, synaptophysin, and cytokeratins, reflecting their heterogeneous cellular differentiation. In particular, the AT/RT–TYR subgroup may express melanocytic markers such as tyrosinase and MITF, underlining the distinct biological profile of this subgroup. Immunohistochemical evaluation of SMARCB1/INI1 plays a fundamental diagnostic role, as loss of INI1 expression is detected in nearly all AT/RT cases. Conversely, loss of BRG1 expression in tumors with AT/RT histological features and preserved INI1 staining is indicative of the rare SMARCA4-deficient variants of AT/RT [19–21].

11.5 Molecular Pathways and Experimental Models

The pathogenesis of AT/RT is closely linked to disruptions of several key molecular pathways, particularly the SHH and Notch pathways. The SHH pathway, which is crucial for normal CNS development, is aberrantly activated in AT/RT due to the loss of SMARCB1. This dysregulation leads to uncontrolled cell proliferation and tumor growth. The Notch signaling pathway, another critical regulator of neural development, has also been implicated in AT/RT, particularly in the context of SMARCB1 deficiency, where it may contribute to the maintenance of an undifferentiated, proliferative state in tumor cells [22–24].

Experimental models have been invaluable in studying AT/RT, particularly genetically engineered mouse models (GEMMs) and patient-derived xenografts (PDXs). GEMMs that recapitulate the loss of SMARCB1 in neural progenitor cells have been instrumental in elucidating the molecular mechanisms driving AT/RT. These models allow the study of tumor initiation and progression in a controlled environment, providing insights into the cellular origins of AT/RT and the role of the tumor microenvironment in supporting tumor growth [25].

PDX models, in which human AT/RT tumors are implanted into immunocompromised mice, offer a complementary approach to GEMMs by allowing the testing of novel therapeutic agents and studying tumor-stroma interactions in vivo. These models are particularly valuable for preclinical drug development, as they closely mimic the human disease, allowing for the assessment of treatment efficacy in a context that closely resembles the clinical scenario [26].

The development and refinement of these models continue to be crucial for advancing our understanding of AT/RT and for the identification of new therapeutic targets. Future research efforts will likely focus on developing models that better capture the heterogeneity of AT/RT, including the distinct molecular subgroups, to facilitate the development of subgroup-specific therapies.

11.6 Diagnostic Imaging and Biomarkers

Like all pediatric brain tumors, neuroimaging is the cornerstone of the diagnosis and follow-up of AT/RTs. They can arise anywhere in the CNS; although the most common location is infratentorial compartment (52%), they can also be found in the cerebral hemispheres (39%), pineal region (5%) and spinal cord (2%). Rarely, AT/RTs can also originate from cranial nerves (5%) [27]. Tumor location may partially correlate with molecular subgroup, as ATRT-TYR tumors are more frequently infratentorial, whereas ATRT-MYC lesions are more commonly supratentorial.

Although magnetic resonance imaging (MRI) MR is the key modality, regardless of acute clinical presentation, CT is usually performed first in the diagnostic workup of brain lesions, showing a hyperdense solid lesion with possible calcifications and hemorrhage [28] In infratentorial AT/RT, hydrocephalus was not as common as in medulloblastomas [29].

At MRI, the appearance of AT/RTs is that of tumors with a predominantly solid component showing T2 iso to hypointensity and reduced diffusivity in keeping with their hypercellular nature, surrounded by little or no vasogenic edema. Hemorrhagic components can be found in up to 45% of tumors [30] If present, cysts are usually eccentrically located. AT/RTs are variably enhancing, and contrast enhancement of the solid component can be faint and limited to certain portions of the mass. The "wavy band-like rim" surrounding a central area of necrosis has been reported as a "typical" enhancement pattern (Fig. 11.4) [30]. Diffusion-weighted imaging (DWI) and apparent diffusion coefficient (ADC) maps are particularly useful in differentiating AT/RTs from lower-grade pediatric tumors because of the markedly restricted diffusion associated with high tumor cellularity.

Leptomeningeal dissemination is present in 20–30% of patients at clinical presentation [28]. Spinal MRI and cerebrospinal fluid (CSF) cytology are essential components of staging, given the strong propensity of AT/RTs for CSF dissemination.

Imaging of the entire neuraxis is therefore mandatory at both diagnosis and follow-up.

Due to the rarity of these tumors, the findings at advanced MRI techniques, such as perfusion MRI and magnetic resonance spectroscopy (MRS), are relatively scarce.

Elevated choline and decreased N-acetylaspartate (NAA) at MRS, broadly indicative of high cell turnover and malignancy, are

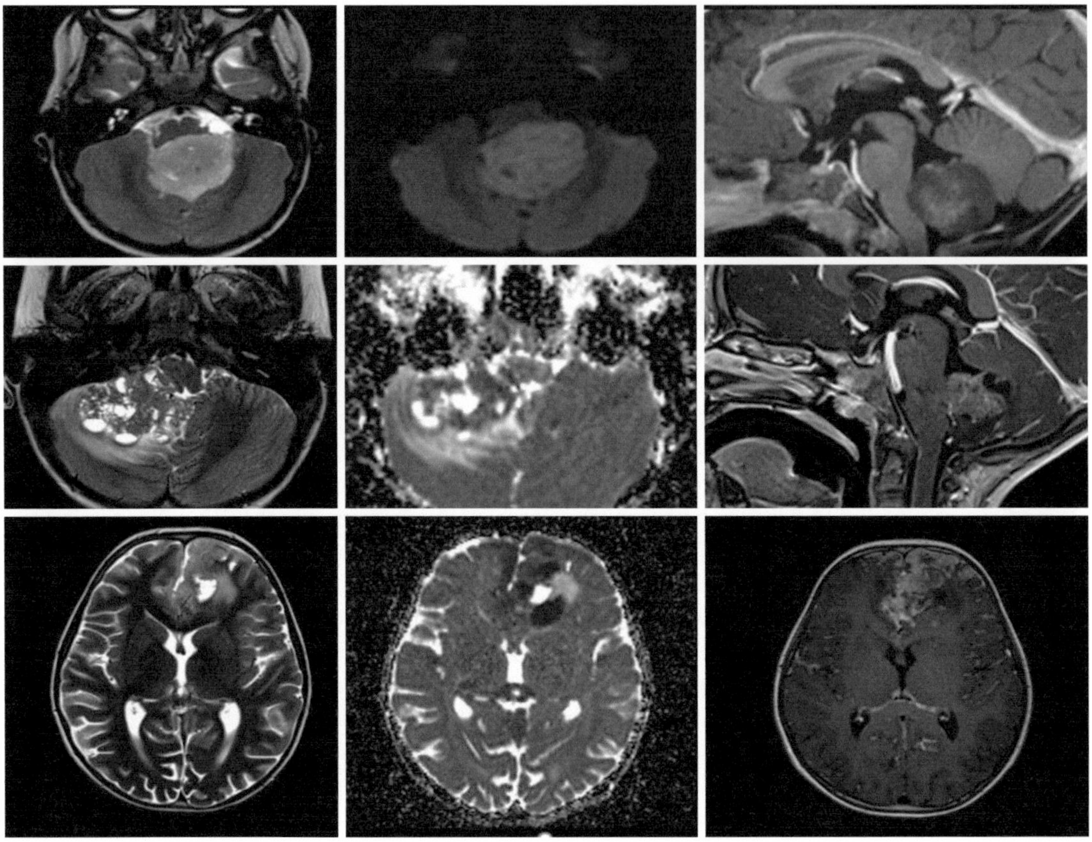

Fig. 11.4 MRI features of AT/RT on T2-weighted, DWI, and post-contrast T1 sequences of three different patients. Upper row: 1-year-old female child with a solid lesion centered in the IV ventricle, showing low signal on T2 weighted images and hyperintensity on DWI (b1000). Contrast enhancement was faint and limited to a smaller portion of the lesion. No surrounding edema is noted. Middle row: 3-year-old female child with a voluminous lesion centered in the caudal IV ventricle, the right ponto-cerebellar angle and infiltrating the posterior aspect of the medulla oblongata. The lesion looks mainly solid, with the small cystic components located mostly at the periphery. Contrast enhancement is inhomogeneous but more intense and extensive as compared to the previous patient. Lower row: 5-year-old male child with supratentorial AT/RT of the left frontal lobe. The lesion is hypercellular with little edema and a small, central area of necrosis. The "wavy band-like rim" pattern of enhancement can be recognized. Diffuse leptomeningeal enhancement in the cerebral sulci bilaterally can also be appreciated

quite nonspecific, as they can be commonly encountered in other WHO grade 4 tumors.

MRI features such as tumor location, peritumoral edema, peripheral cysts, diffusion restriction, and contrast enhancement vary across the 3 molecular subgroups of AT/RT [31].

Hopefully, the refinement of radiomics will help uncover distinctive MR imaging–based phenotypes of AT/RTs, further improving the preoperative diagnosis, tumor subgroup classification, and prognosis.

In recent years, the search for non-invasive biomarkers for AT/RT has gained momentum. Circulating tumor DNA (ctDNA), which can be detected in blood or CSF, is emerging as a promising biomarker for monitoring tumor burden and detecting residual disease. The analysis of ctDNA allows for the detection of specific genetic mutations associated with AT/RT, providing a potential tool for early diagnosis, monitoring of treatment response, and detection of recurrence [32]. Notably, CSF-derived ctDNA appears to provide higher sensitivity compared with plasma samples because of the direct contact with CNS tumors.

MicroRNAs (miRNAs), small non-coding RNAs that regulate gene expression, are also being investigated as potential biomarkers for AT/RT. Specific miRNA signatures have been identified in AT/RT, with some showing promise as diagnostic tools. For example, miR-10b and miR-21, which are involved in cell proliferation and apoptosis, have been found to be upregulated in AT/RT and could serve as markers for the disease. The detection of these miRNAs in CSF offers a minimally invasive approach to monitoring disease status, potentially allowing for earlier detection of recurrence and better assessment of treatment efficacy [33]. Future integration of liquid biopsy approaches with molecular imaging and methylation profiling may significantly improve personalized management strategies for children affected by AT/RT.

11.7 Treatment Approaches

The treatment of AT/RT is challenging due to the tumor's aggressive nature and the young age of most patients, which limits the use of certain therapies. A multimodal approach that includes surgery, radiation therapy, and chemotherapy is typically employed, with the goal of achieving maximal tumor control while minimizing long-term toxicities (Fig. 11.5) [34–36].

Surgery: The primary goal of surgery in AT/RT is maximal safe resection of the tumor. However, complete resection is often difficult due to the tumor's infiltrative nature and its location in critical areas of the brain. Incomplete resection is associated with a higher risk of recurrence, highlighting the importance of achieving as extensive a resection as possible without compromising neurological function. Advances in surgical techniques, such as the use of intraoperative MRI, neuronavigation systems, and fluorescence-guided surgery, have improved the precision of tumor resection, potentially leading to better outcomes [37, 38].

Radiation Therapy: Postoperative radiation therapy is a key component of AT/RT treatment, particularly in children older than 3 years. Craniospinal irradiation (CSI) is often employed to address the high risk of metastatic spread, while focal radiation therapy may be used to target the primary tumor site. Proton beam therapy, which delivers highly targeted radiation with

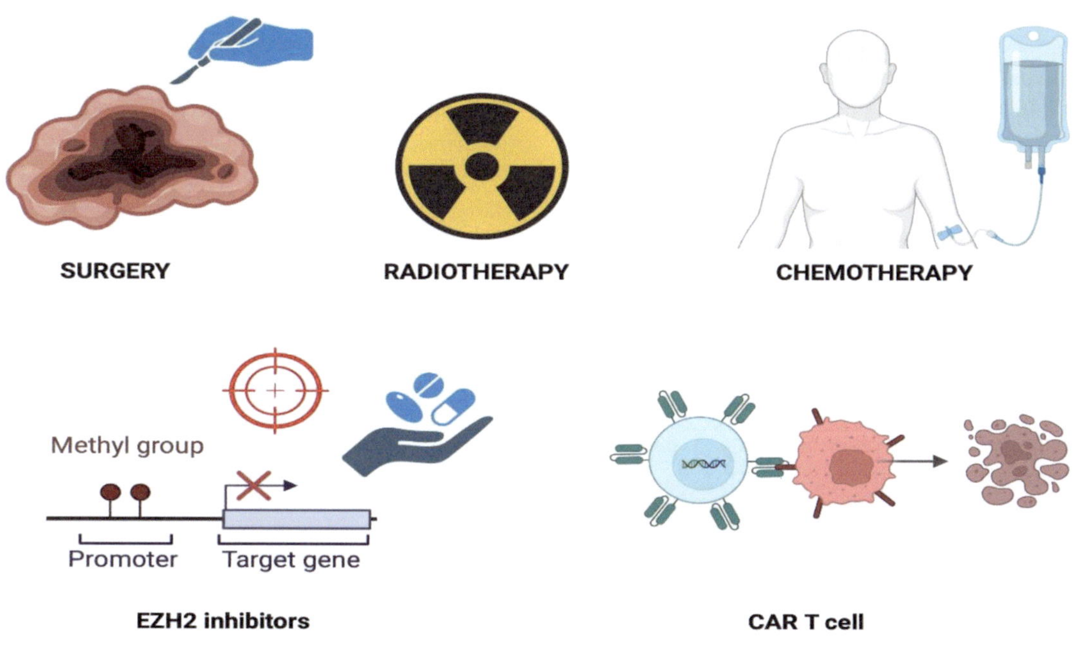

Fig. 11.5 Multimodal strategy to improve survival in AT/RT: consolidated treatments and new perspectives

reduced exposure to surrounding healthy tissues, is increasingly being used in AT/RT patients to minimize the long-term side effects of radiation, particularly in young children whose developing brains are highly sensitive to radiation damage [39–42].

Chemotherapy: Chemotherapy regimens for AT/RT are typically intense, involving high-dose chemotherapy followed by autologous stem cell rescue. Agents such as methotrexate, cisplatin, vincristine, and cyclophosphamide are commonly used in various combinations, with the goal of delivering high doses of cytotoxic drugs while allowing for bone marrow recovery. However, these regimens are associated with significant toxicity, particularly in very young children, who are at higher risk for treatment-related morbidity. The development of less toxic chemotherapy regimens, or the identification of targeted therapies that can reduce the need for intense chemotherapy, remains a critical area of research [40, 41, 43–46].

Emerging Therapies: Given the limitations of current therapies, there is significant interest in the development of targeted therapies and immunotherapies for AT/RT. One promising area of research is the use of EZH2 inhibitors, which target the histone methyltransferase EZH2, a key regulator of chromatin structure and gene expression in AT/RT. Preclinical studies have shown that EZH2 inhibitors can reduce tumor growth in AT/RT models, and early-phase clinical trials are underway to assess their efficacy in patients [41, 47].

Immune checkpoint inhibitors, which have revolutionized the treatment of many adult cancers, are also being explored in AT/RT, particularly in the context of MYC-driven tumors, where the tumor's aggressive nature may be linked to immune evasion. Additionally, CAR-T cell therapy, which involves engineering a patient's T cells to target tumor-specific antigens, is being investigated as a highly personalized treatment approach for AT/RT. The development of CAR-T cells that target specific antigens expressed by AT/RT, such as GD2 or B7-H3, could offer a new avenue for treating this deadly disease [41, 48–56].

11.8 Prognosis and Survivorship

Despite aggressive multimodal treatment, the prognosis for AT/RT remains poor, with overall survival rates generally ranging from 30% to 40%. Prognosis varies significantly depending on factors such as the tumor's molecular subgroup, the extent of resection, and the patient's age at diagnosis. For example, patients with MYC-driven tumors or those with significant residual disease after surgery typically have worse outcomes. In contrast, patients with TYR-driven tumors, which tend to have a less aggressive clinical course, may experience better long-term survival [38, 40, 41].

Long-term survivors of AT/RT often face significant challenges related to the treatment toxicity. Neurocognitive deficits are common, particularly in patients who receive craniospinal irradiation at a young age (Fig. 11.6) These deficits can affect memory, attention, processing speed, and general intellectual functioning, significantly impacting quality of life and academic performance. Survivors may also experience endocrinopathies, such as growth hormone deficiency and hypothyroidism, following cranial irradiation. Additionally, there is an increased risk of secondary malignancies due to the aggressive nature of treatment regimens, particularly in patients with RTPS, who already carry an underlying genetic predisposition to developing multiple tumors. These long-term effects emphasize the need for comprehensive survivor care plans that include neurocognitive rehabilitation, endocrine monitoring, and psychosocial support [38, 40–42].

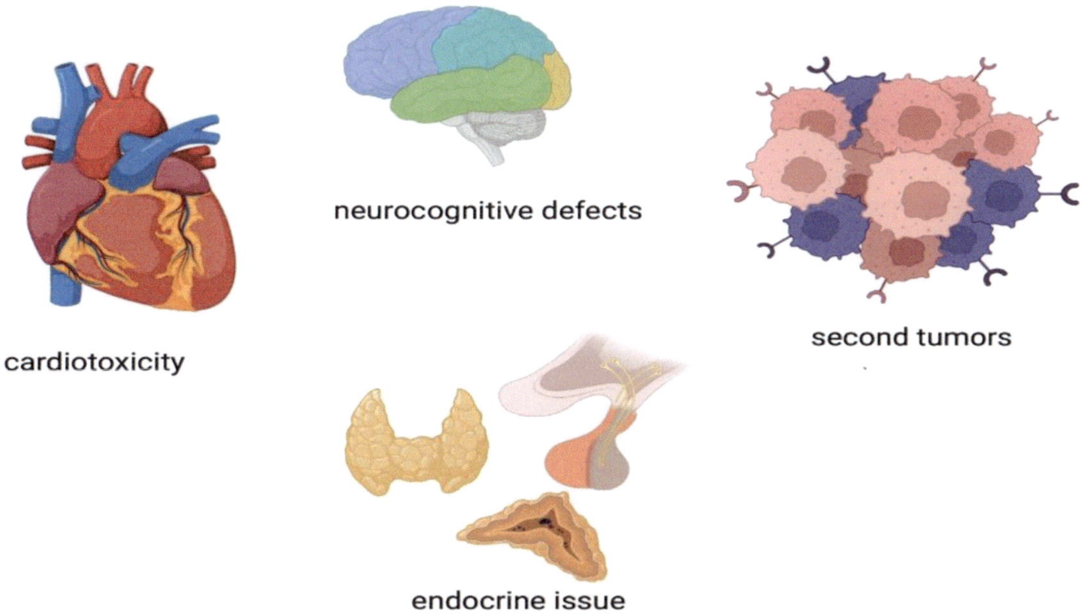

Fig. 11.6 Long-term toxicities related to craniospinal irradiation (i.e., neurocognitive defects and endocrinopathies)

11.9 Future Directions

The future of AT/RT research and treatment lies in the continued exploration of its molecular and genetic underpinnings. Advances in next-generation sequencing (NGS) and single-cell RNA sequencing are providing unprecedented insights into the cellular diversity within AT/RT tumors, revealing new potential targets for therapy. For instance, the identification of specific genetic and epigenetic alterations that drive tumorigenesis in each molecular subgroup will be critical for the development of targeted therapies that can improve outcomes with fewer side effects [41].

Collaborative efforts through international research networks are essential for advancing the understanding of AT/RT and accelerating the development of new treatments. Given the rarity of AT/RT, pooling data and resources across institutions is necessary to conduct robust clinical trials and validate new therapeutic approaches. Such collaborations will also facilitate the development of standardized treatment protocols that can be tailored to the molecular profile of each patient's tumor, potentially leading to more personalized and effective treatment strategies.

Personalized medicine approaches, which leverage the molecular and genetic characteristics of each tumor to guide treatment decisions, hold great promise for improving outcomes in AT/RT. This approach may include the use of targeted therapies, immunotherapies, and novel drug combinations that are specifically designed to target the molecular drivers of each tumor. Additionally, the integration of advanced imaging techniques and biomarkers into clinical practice will enhance the ability to monitor treatment response and detect early signs of recurrence, allowing for timely interventions that can improve survival [41].

In conclusion, AT/RT represents one of the most challenging and deadly pediatric CNS tumors. However, the growing understanding of its molecular landscape offers hope for more precise diagnostic tools and targeted therapies that could significantly improve survival rates and quality of life for affected patients. The continued dedication to research, clinical trials, and international collaboration will be essential in the fight against this devastating disease.

References

1. Packer RJ, Biegel JA, Blaney S, et al. Atypical teratoid/rhabdoid tumor of the central nervous system: report on workshop. J Pediatr Hematol Oncol. 2002;24:337–42.
2. Burger PC, Yu IT, Tihan T, et al. Atypical teratoid/rhabdoid tumor of the central nervous system; a highly malignant tumor of infancy and childhood frequently mistaken for medulloblastoma: a Pediatric Oncology Group study. Am J Surg Pathol. 1998;22:1083–92.
3. Hilden JM, Meerbaum S, burger P, et al. Central nervous system atypical teratoid/rhabdoid tumor: results of therapy in children enrolled in a registry. J Clin Oncol. 2004;22:2877–84.
4. Erdmann F, Kaatsch P, Grabow D, Spix C. German Childhood Cancer Registry - Annual Report 2019 (1980–2018). Mainz: Institute of Medical Biostatistics, Epidemiology and informatics (IMBEI) at the University Medical Center of the Johannes Gutenberg University; 2020.
5. Ostrom QT, Price M, Neff C, et al. CBTRUS statistical report: primary brain and other central nervous system tumors diagnosed in the United States in 2015–2019. Neuro-Oncology. 2022;24(Suppl 5):v1–v95. https://doi.org/10.1093/neuonc/noac202.
6. Eaton KW, Tooke LS, Wainwright LM, et al. Spectrum of SMARCB1/INI1 mutations in familial and sporadic rhabdoid tumors. Pediatric Blood Cancer. 2011;56(1):7–15. https://doi.org/10.1002/pbc22831.
7. Scheppenheim R, Fruhwald MC, Gesk S, et al. Germline nonsense mutation and somatic inactivation of SMARCA4/BRG1 in a family with rhabdoid tumor predisposition syndrome. Am J Human Genet. 2010;86(2):279–84. https://doi.org/10.1016/j.ajhg.2010.01.013.
8. Frühwald MC, Hasselblatt M, Nemes K, et al. Age and DNA methylation subgroup as potential independent risk factors for treatment stratification in children with atypical teratoid/rhabdoid tumors. Neuro-Oncology. 2020;22(7):1006–17. https://doi.org/10.1093/neuonc/noz244.
9. Bartelheim K, Sumerauer D, Behrends U, et al. Clinical and genetic features of rhabdoid tumors of the heart registered with the European Rhabdoid Registry (EU-RHAB). Cancer Genet. 2014;207(9):379–83. https://doi.org/10.1016/j.cancergen.2014.04.005.
10. Johann PD, Erkek S, Zapatka M, et al. Atypical teratoid/rhabdoid tumors are comprised of three epigenetic subgroups with distinct enhancer landscapes. Cancer Cell. 2016;29(3):379–93.
11. Eaton K, Tooke LS, Wainwright LM, et al. Spectrum of SMARCB1/INI1 mutations in familial and sporadic rhabdoid tumors. Pediatric Blood Cancer. 2010;56:7–15.
12. Schneppenheim R, Fruhwald MC, Gesk S, et al. Germline nonsense mutation and somatic inactivation of SMARCA4/BRG1 in a family with rhabdoid tumor predisposition syndrome. Am J Hum Genet. 2010;86(2):279–84.
13. Del Baldo G, Carta R, Alessi I, et al. Rhabdoid tumor predisposition syndrome: from clinica suspicion to general management. Front Oncol. 2021;11:586288. https://doi.org/10.3389/fonc.2021.586288.
14. Meyers SP, Khademian ZP, Biegel JA, et al. Primary intracranial atypical teratoid/rhabdoid tumors of infancy. Am J Neuroradiol. 2006;27:962–71.
15. Massimino M, Gandola L, Spreafico F, et al. Supratentorial primitive neuroectodermal tumors (S-PNET) in children: a prospective experience with adjuvant intensive chemiotherapy and hyperfractionated accelerated radiotherapy. Int J Radiat Oncol Biol Phys. 2006;64(4):1031–7.
16. Arslanoglu A, Aygun N, Tekhtani D, et al. Imaging findings of CNS atypical teratoid/rhabdoid tumors. AJNR Am J Neuroradiol. 2004;25(3):476–80.
17. Koral K, Gargan L, Bowers DC, et al. Imaging characteristics of atypical teratoid-rhabdoid tumor in children compared with medulloblastoma. AJR Am J Roentgenol. 2008;190(3):809–14.
18. Rorke-Adams L. Tumors. In: Gilbert-Barness E, editor. Potter's pathology of the fetus, infant and child. 2nd ed. Philadelphia, PA: Mosby-Elsevier; 2007. p. 2077–92.
19. Wharton SB, Wardle C, Ironside JW, et al. Comparative genomic hybridization and pathological findings in atypical teratoid/rhabdoid tumor of the central nervous system. Nerupathol Appl Neurobiol. 2003;29:254–61.
20. Rickert CH, Paulus W. Chromosomal imbalances detected by comparative genomic hybridization in atypical teratoid/rhabdoid tumors. Childs Nerv Syst. 2004;20:221–4.
21. Lopez-Gines C, CerdaNicolas M, Kepes J, et al. Complex rearrangement of chromosomes 6 and 11as the sole anomaly in atypical teratoid/rhabdoid tumors of the central nervous system. Cancer Genet Cytogenet. 2000;122:149–52.
22. Frühwald MC, Biegel JA, Bourdeaut F, Roberts CW, Chi SN. Atypical teratoid/rhabdoid tumors—current concepts, advances in biology, and potential future therapies. Neuro-Oncology. 2016;18(6):764–78.
23. Hasselblatt M, Nagel I, Oyen F, et al. SMARCA4-mutated atypical teratoid/rhabdoid tumors are associated with inherited germline alterations and poor prognosis. Acta Neuropathol. 2014;128(3):453–6.
24. Schneppenheim R, Frühwald MC, Gesk S, et al. Germline nonsense mutation and somatic inactivation of SMARCA4/BRG1 in a family with rhabdoid tumor predisposition syndrome. Am J Hum Genet. 2010;86(2):279–84.
25. Kim SS, Moghe M, Rait A, et al. SMARCB1 gene therapy using a novel tumor-targeted Nanomedicine enhances anti-cancer efficacy in a mouse model of atypical teratoid rhabdoid tumors. Int J Nanomedicine. 2024;19:5973–93. https://doi.org/10.2147/IJN.S458323.

26. Duan J, Wang Y. Modeling nervous system tumors with human stem cells and organoids. Cell Regen. 2023;12(1):4. https://doi.org/10.1186/s13619-022-00150-7.
27. Wykoff CC, Lam BL, Brathwaite CD, Biegel JA, McKeown CA, Rosenblum MK, Allewelt HB, Sandberg DI. Atypical teratoid/rhabdoid tumor arising from the third cranial nerve. J Neuroophthalmol. 2008;28(3):207–11.
28. Meyers SP, Khademian ZP, Biegel JA, Chuang SH, Korones DN, Zimmerman RA. Primary intracranial atypical teratoid/rhabdoid tumors of infancy and childhood: MRI features and patient outcomes. AJNR Am J Neuroradiol. 2006;27(5):962–71.
29. Koral K, Gargan L, Bowers DC, Gimi B, Timmons CF, Weprin B, Rollins NK. Imaging characteristics of atypical teratoid-rhabdoid tumor in children compared with medulloblastoma. AJR Am J Roentgenol. 2008;190(3):809–14.
30. Warmuth-Metz M, Bison B, Dannemann-Stern E, Kortmann R, Rutkowski S, Pietsch T. CT and MR imaging in atypical teratoid/rhabdoid tumors of the central nervous system. Neuroradiology. 2008;50(5):447–52.
31. Nowak J, Nemes K, Hohm A, Vandergrift LA, Hasselblatt M, Johann PD, Kool M, Frühwald MC, Warmuth-Metz M. Magnetic resonance imaging surrogates of molecular subgroups in atypical teratoid/rhabdoid tumor. Neuro-Oncology. 2018;20(12):1672–9.
32. Ronsley R, Karvonen KA, Cole B, et al. Detection of tumor-derived cell-free DNA in cerebrospinal fluid using a clinically validated targeted sequencing panel for pediatric brain tumors. J Neuro-Oncol. 2024;168(2):215–24. https://doi.org/10.1007/s11060-024-04645-y.
33. Xinke X, Hongyao Y, Junping P, et al. The identification of miRNA and mRNA expression profiles associated with pediatric atypical teratoid/rhabdoid tumor. BMC Cancer. 2022;22(1):499. https://doi.org/10.1186/s12885-022-09549-6.
34. Rorke LB, Packer R, Biegel J. Central nervous system atypical teratoid/rhabdoid tumors of infancy and childhood. J Neuro-Oncol. 1995;24:21–8.
35. Rorke LB, Packer RJ, Biegel JA. Central nervous system atypical teratoid/rhabdoid tumors of infancy and childhood: definition of an entity. J Neurosurg. 1996;85:56.
36. Burger PC, Yu IT, Tihan T, et al. Atypical teratoid/rhabdoid tumor of the central nervous system: a highly malignant tumor of infancy and childhood frequently mistaken for medulloblastoma: a Pediatric Oncology Group study. Am J Surg Pathol. 1998;22:1083.
37. Gupta NK, Godbole N, Sanmugananthan P, et al. Management of atypical teratoid/rhabdoid tumors in the pediatric population: a systematic review and meta-analysis. World Neurosurg. 2024;181:e504–15. https://doi.org/10.1016/j.wneu.2023.10.089.
38. Egiz A, Kannan S, Asl SF. The impact of surgical resection and adjuvant therapy on survival in pediatric patients with atypical teratoid/rhabdoid tumor: systematic review and pooled survival analysis. World Neurosurg. 2022;164:216–27. https://doi.org/10.1016/j.wneu.2022.04.073.
39. Chen YW, Wong TT, Ho DM, et al. Impact of radiotherapy for pediatric CNS atypical teratoid/rhabdoid tumor (single institute experience). Int J Radiat Oncol Biol Phys. 2006;64(4):1038–43.
40. Tekautz TM, Fuller CE, Blaney S, et al. Atypical teratoid/rhabdoid tumors (AT/RT): improved survival in children 3 years of age and older with radiation therapy and high-dose alkylator-based chemotherapy. J Clin Oncol. 2005;23(7):1491–9.
41. Gastberger K, Fincke VE, Mucha M, et al. Current molecular and clinical landscape of AT/RT - the link to future therapies. Cancer Manag Res. 2023;15:1369–93. https://doi.org/10.2147/CMAR.S379451.
42. Tran S, Lim PS, Bojaxhiu B, et al. Clinical outcomes and quality of life in children and adolescents with primary brain tumors treated with pencil beam scanning proton therapy. Pediatr Blood Cancer. 2020;67(12):e28465. https://doi.org/10.1002/pbc.28465.
43. Bennett J, Erker C, Lafay-Cousin L, et al. Canadian pediatric neuro-oncology standards of practice. Front Oncol. 2020;10:593192. https://doi.org/10.3389/fonc.2020.593192.
44. Bartelheim K, Nemes K, Seeringer A, et al. Improved 6-year overall survival in AT/RT - results of the registry study Rhabdoid 2007. Cancer Med. 2016;5(8):1765–75. https://doi.org/10.1002/cam4.741.
45. Reddy AT, Strother DR, Judkins AR, et al. Efficacy of high-dose chemotherapy and three-dimensional conformal radiation for atypical teratoid/rhabdoid tumor: a report from the Children's Oncology Group Trial ACNS0333. J Clin Oncol. 2020;38(11):1175–85. https://doi.org/10.1200/JCO.19.01776.
46. Zaky W, Dhall G, Ji L, et al. Intensive induction chemotherapy followed by myeloablative chemotherapy with autologous hematopoietic progenitor cell rescue for young children newly-diagnosed with central nervous system atypical teratoid/rhabdoid tumors: the Head Start III experience. Pediatr Blood Cancer. 2014;61(1):95–101. https://doi.org/10.1002/pbc.24648.
47. Ishi Y, Zhang Y, Zhang A, et al. Therapeutic targeting of EZH2 and BET BRD4 in pediatric rhabdoid tumors. Mol Cancer Ther. 2022;21(5):715–26. https://doi.org/10.1158/1535-7163.MCT-21-0646.
48. Geoerger B, Kang HJ, Yalon-Oren M, et al. Pembrolizumab in paediatric patients with advanced melanoma or a PD-L1-positive, advanced, relapsed, or refractory solid tumour or lymphoma (KEYNOTE-051): interim analysis of an open-label, single-arm, phase 1–2 trial. Lancet Oncol. 2020;21(1):121–33. https://doi.org/10.1016/S1470-2045(19)30671-0.

49. Gorsi HS, Malicki DM, Barsan V, et al. Nivolumab in the treatment of recurrent or refractory pediatric brain tumors: a single institutional experience. J Pediatr Hematol Oncol. 2019;41(4):e235–41. https://doi.org/10.1097/MPH.0000000000001339.
50. Geoerger B, Zwaan CM, Marshall LV, et al. Atezolizumab for children and young adults with previously treated solid tumours, non-Hodgkin lymphoma, and Hodgkin lymphoma (iMATRIX): a multicentre phase 1–2 study. Lancet Oncol. 2020;21(1):134–44. https://doi.org/10.1016/S1470-2045(19)30693-X.
51. Haydar D, Houke H, Chiang J, et al. Cell-surface antigen profiling of pediatric brain tumors: B7-H3 is consistently expressed and can be targeted via local or systemic CAR T-cell delivery. Neuro-Oncology. 2021;23(6):999–1011. https://doi.org/10.1093/neuonc/noaa278.
52. Rao P, Furst L, Meyran D, et al. Advances in CAR T cell immunotherapy for paediatric brain tumours. Front Oncol. 2022;12:873722. https://doi.org/10.3389/fonc.2022.873722.
53. Vitanza NA, Johnson AJ, Wilson AL, et al. Locoregional infusion of HER2-specific CAR T cells in children and young adults with recurrent or refractory CNS tumors: an interim analysis. Nat Med. 2021;27(9):1544–52. https://doi.org/10.1038/s41591-021-01404-8.
54. Theruvath J, Sotillo E, Mount CW, et al. Locoregionally administered B7-H3-targeted CAR T cells for treatment of atypical teratoid/rhabdoid tumors. Nat Med. 2020;26(5):712–9. https://doi.org/10.1038/s41591-020-0821-8.
55. Vitanza NA, Wilson AL, Huang W, et al. Intraventricular B7-H3 CAR T cells for diffuse intrinsic pontine glioma: preliminary first-in-human bioactivity and safety. Cancer Discov. 2023;13(1):114–31. https://doi.org/10.1158/2159-8290.CD-22-0750.
56. Ravanpay AC, Gust J, Johnson AJ, et al. EGFR806-CAR T cells selectively target a tumor-restricted EGFR epitope in glioblastoma. Oncotarget. 2019;10(66):7080–95. https://doi.org/10.18632/oncotarget.27389.

12 Rare CNS Embryonal, Sarcomatous Tumor and Other Rare Entity

Elisabetta Schiavello and Maura Massimino

12.1 Introduction

Central nervous system (CNS) embryonal tumors include a mainly pediatric heterogeneous group of malignant tumors composed of immature cells similar to neural progenitors. Among all CNS embryonal tumors, medulloblastoma is quite common, while other CNS embryonal tumors are very rare. Unlike medulloblastoma arising from the cerebellum or dorsal brainstem, other types can occur anywhere in the cranio-spinal axis.

The classification of rare embryonal and sarcomatous tumors of the CNS underwent several changes in the years; in fact with the contribution of an increased knowledge of the diversity and biology of these tumors and the development of a classification based on new molecular features, the term "CNS primitive neuroectodermal tumor" can be considered outdated [1]. In the fifth edition of the WHO CNS tumors classification (WHO CNS5), the diagnostic criteria of previously known histological entities have been modified and new tumor subtypes have been added [2].

Many of the tumors, which can now be classified into a specific type within the spectrum of rare CNS embryonal tumors and CNS mesenchymal, non-meningothelial tumors, had a diagnosis of "primitive neuroectodermal tumor" (PNET) over the past years. This term was introduced to classify tumors based on their morphological features as small-round-cells, malignant CNS tumors [3].

These tumors were then reclassified as supratentorial PNET (stPNET) in 2000 WHO CNS4 [4]and later, in 2007 [5], as CNS PNET WHO CNS5 [2].

More recent molecular analyses have made it clear that other tumors including high-grade glioma (HGG), ependymoma, atypical teratoid rhabdoid tumors (ATRT), and medulloblastoma have been misclassified as CNS PNETs when the diagnosis relied exclusively on histopathological evaluation.

These new molecular analyses have allowed to better outline already known tumor types and new entities such as embryonal tumor with multilayered rosettes (ETMR), which are characterized by a typical molecular alteration and a very aggressive clinical course [1].

Therefore, in 2016 WHO CNS4, the term PNET of the CNS was changed to embryonal CNS tumor, NOS [6]. The latest 2021 WHO CNS5 classification thus includes within the group of other CNS embryonal tumors the following new entities: ETMR, CNS neuroblastoma, *FOXR2*-activated (CNS NB-*FOXR2*), CNS tumors with *BCOR* internal tandem duplication (CNS *BCOR* ITD), and CNS embryonal tumor NEC/NOS [2] (Table 12.1).

E. Schiavello (✉) · M. Massimino
Pediatric Oncology Unit, Fondazione IRCCS Istituto Nazionale dei Tumori, Milan, Italy
e-mail: Elisabetta.Schiavello@istitutotumori.mi.it

A. Mastronuzzi, A. Carai (eds.), *Navigating Pediatric Brain Tumors*,
https://doi.org/10.1007/978-3-032-18992-9_12

Along with rare CNS embryonal tumors, some newly introduced CNS mesenchymal tumors of uncertain differentiation are also always addressed as *CIC*-rearranged sarcoma, primary intracranial sarcoma *DICER1*-mutant and intracranial Ewing sarcoma that will not be included in this chapter because they are usually discussed by working groups dealing with Ewing's sarcomas (Table 12.2).

Because of the recent identification and heterogeneity of these tumors, there isn't specific prospective clinical data on these entities, so they present a great challenge for both diagnosis and clinical management. Treatment is still mainly based on the historical guidelines of treating CNS PNET. Similarly, there is no standard treatment for recently emerging CNS mesenchymal tumor entities with specific molecular alterations.

Another small group of tumors characterized by *MN1* fusions has been outlined from DNA methylation analysis of retrospective CNS PNETs [1] (Table 12.3). Other cases with similar methylation profile had different histological characteristics and this group was initially called high-grade neuroepithelial tumors with *MN1* alteration (HGNET-*MN1*).

Successively it was shown how most of these tumors harboring MN1 fusion had morphologically the same characteristics of astroblastomas, and the group was renamed in the WHO CNS5 astroblastoma MN1-altered, although no WHO grade was currently assigned there are not yet prospective data on the clinical behavior of this entity. Therefore, this tumors together with sarcomatous CNS tumors are usually included as "orphan" entities in the description of rare embryonal CNS tumors.

Some recently described entities with distinct molecular features such as gene fusions involving PATZ1 [7, 8]. *BCOR/BCORL1* [9, 10] or PLAGL1 [11] have recently been described and are not included in the fifth edition of the WHO classification of CNS tumors, yet. The classification of rare embryonal and sarcomatous CNS tumors will be in continuously evolving understanding of molecular profiling.

Recently, guidelines that reflect current best standards of care, defined by the collective European experts in these tumors, have been drafted for this purpose (available at https://paedcan.ern-net.eu/the-escp-project/).

Rare CNS Embryonal Tumors

Table 12.1 Essential diagnostic criteria of rare embryonal tumors

Rare CNS embryonal tumors			
Tumor type	ETMR	CNS NB-FOXR2	CNS BCOR-ITD
Diagnostic Criteria	Embryonal tumor with abundant neuropil and true rosettes, ependymoblastoma or medulloepithelioma, and *C19*MC	Embryonal tumor with foci of neuroblastic differentiation	Solid growth pattern, uniform oval/spindle-shaped cells with round to oval nuclei, dense capillary network
		Activation of *FOXR2* by structural rearrangements and gene fusion	
			Internal tandem duplication in exon 15 of BCOR
	MIR17HG	DNA methylation in doubtful cases	
	DICER1 alteration		DNA methylation in doubtful cases
Molecular Features	LIN28 expression (IHC)	FOXR2 re-arrangement/ activation	Nuclear BCOR expression (IHC)
	C19MC amplification (90%)	1q gain (94%)	BCOR internal tandem duplication
	MIR17HG amplification (1%)		
	bi-allelic DICER1 mutation (5%)		
Sex	♀ ♂ 50%: 50%	♀ ♂ 50%: 50%	♀ ♂ 40%: 60%
Site	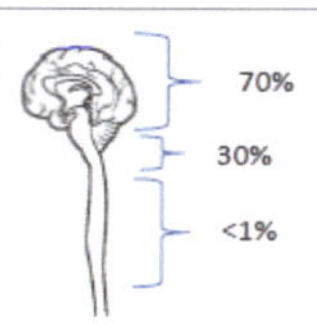	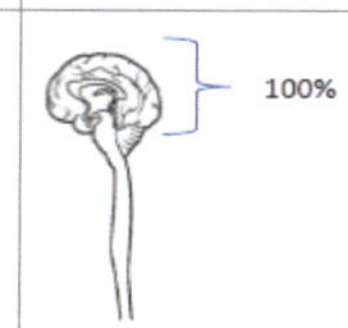	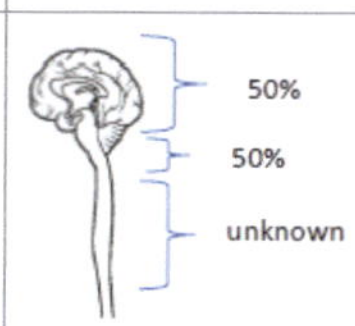
Age			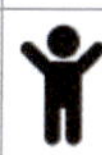
Outcome	25% 5-year OS	≥80% 5-year OS	70% 2-year OS data are lacking

12.2 Embryonal Tumor with Multilayered Rosettes (ETMR)

12.2.1 Introduction

It is a rare and aggressive disease, first introduced in the 2016 CNS WHO classification, mainly occurring in children younger than 3–5 years of age. This underestimated entity might comprise a substantial proportion of embryonal brain tumors that were previously identified as embryonal tumor with abundant neuropil and true rosettes (ETANTR), ependymoblastoma, medulloepithelioma, or PNET. In fact, a new histological category called ETANTR was first described in 2000 [12]. Improving knowledge in the molecular biology led to the finding that some rare histological entities of embryonal rosette-forming tumors such as supratentorial PNETs, including ETANTR, medulloepithelioma, and ependymoblastoma, shared a unifying molecular signature of chromosome 19 microRNA cluster (C19MC) amplification first described within a subset of CNS-PNETs with poor survival [13]and primitive transcriptome enriched for LIN28A, a pluripotency factor [14, 15]. Then, C19MC-altered ETMRs were incorporated in WHO CNS5 as a new entity. There is also a category without C19MC alterations (called ETMR not otherwise specified). Amplification of *C19MC* in ETMR is often correlated with fusion to the *TTYH1* gene in 90% of ETMR [16, 17]. In *C19MC*-negative ETMR, amplification of another microRNA cluster (*MIR17HG*) and biallelic mutations of *DICER1*, a gene encoding a critical protein that plays a fundamental role in the process of genetic regulation through microRNAs (miRNA), have been identified. Significantly, the majority of DICER1-mutant ETMRs originate from a germline mutation in DICER1, a hereditary cancer predisposition condition known as DICER1 predisposition syndrome [18–20].

12.2.2 Molecular and Immunohistochemical Features

The typical morphological structure is usually recognizable on hematoxylin-eosin sections as multi-layered rosettes consisting of embryonal cells in a pseudostratified neuroepithelium with a central round or slit-like lumen; mitotic figures are usually present. ETMRs have three different histological aspects: embryonal tumor with abundant neuropil and true rosettes, ependymoblastoma, and medulloepithelioma; they are now considered as a various pattern within a single entity, rather than distinct tumor types [21]. Molecularly these tumors are, irrespective of their morphology, very similar and characterized by a *C19MC* alteration or in rare cases by biallelic *DICER1* mutations.

These typical morfological features can be identified on histological examination on HE sections; immunohistochemical LIN28A expression can guide the diagnosis, also in small samples without typical morphological features; even if LIN28A expression is not specific and may be present in other tumor (ATRT or HGG). *C19MC* amplification can be detected by FISH, SNP (single nucleotide polymorphism)-array-based techniques, or DNA methylation array–based copy number plots generated by the Heidelberg classifier (www.molecularneuropathology.org) as part of DNA methylation data analysis. Cases with a small cluster of *C19MC* cells, which may not be detected by the methylation arrays, can be detected by FISH. Tumors without *C19MC* amplification need to be assessed for *DICER1* mutations and if present genetic counselling is recommended. There is the rare possibility of having negativity for *C19MC* amplification and *DICER1* mutation, and identification of *MIR17HG* amplification may help in defining the correct diagnosis.

12.2.3 Clinical and Radiological Characteristics

ETMR accounts for a small percentage of pediatric brain tumors. The specific incidence rates are not well established due to its rarity. This tumor is typical in very young children (median age at diagnosis: 2.5 years, range 0.5–8 years) affecting boys and girls equally [17, 18, 22, 23].

ETMR typically arises in supratentorial region, then in the posterior fossa, including the cerebellum and brainstem, but can occasionally occur in the spinal cord [17, 24–26].

From a radiological perspective, ETMR typically presents as a well-vircumscribed tumor is in general a well circumscribed tumor, at MRI has a heterogeneous signal with frequent diffusion restriction, it can be characterized as large lesion (compared to other CNS embryonal tumors) with both cystic and hemorrhagic intratumoral areas [27] (Fig. 12.1). Metastases are present at diagnosis in 15–25% of patients with ETMR, presenting as solid tumors, leptomeningeal spread, or positive cerebrospinal fluid (CSF) cytology [14, 22–25]. There is no evident correlation between histological different patterns and primary site of the tumor; however, a trend was observed for brainstem occurrence of *C19MC*—ETMR [18].

The overall prognosis for these patients is poor, primarily due to early and frequent relapses that can occur within months of diagnosis. Few patients survive for more than 4–5 years [23, 25]. Supratentorial tumor location has been identified as a positive prognostic factor in one retrospective study [22]. A worse prognosis has been associated with brainstem location and metastatic

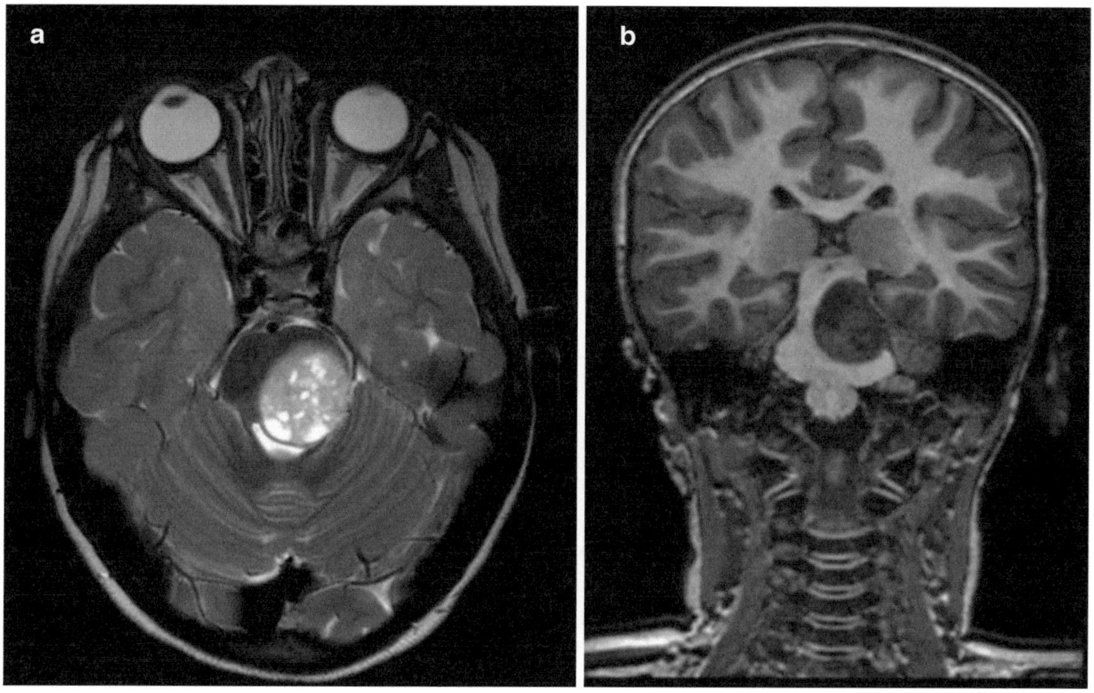

Fig. 12.1 Pontine ETMR; (**a**) axial T2 weighted; (**b**) coronal FLAIR weighted

disease at diagnosis [14, 22–25]. Metastatic spread is commonly observed during the disease course, and even extra-CNS metastases have been reported [26, 28]. Notably, the histopathological pattern of the tumor does not correlate with clinical outcome [14, 16, 24].

12.2.4 Treatment

No specific treatment for ETMR has been prospectively assessed until now. Most reported patients have been treated according to medulloblastoma or CNS PNET guidelines/trials or according to other high-risk infant CNS tumor or ATRT protocols.

Available evidence indicates that the largest resection possible has a positive prognostic effect. Complete resection has been identified as a favorable prognostic factor in two retrospective studies [24, 25]. Focused analyses of long-term survivors show that most patients underwent gross total resection as part of their treatment course [29–31].

Some reports on ETMR patients suggest that an intensive regimen may improve overall survival [22, 23, 25, 29, 30]. Regarding radiotherapy, both focal and craniospinal irradiation (CSI) have been used, and most long-term survivors have received irradiation [23, 25, 29, 30]. The tendency of ETMR to metastasize might indicate a potential benefit from CSI. However, due to the young age of the patients, this approach cannot be routinely applied. Current data on patients treated with local irradiation show comparable outcomes to those receiving CSI [23, 29, 31]. Notably, a few patients who survived longer than the observation period did not undergo irradiation after gross total resection and high-dose chemotherapy [22, 25, 29]. Some retrospective studies and meta-analysis have demonstrated the superiority of intensified chemotherapy regimen with high-dose chemotherapy, over the conventional chemotherapy approach [22, 25, 32]. The chemotherapy response rate reported is approximately 30% in ETMR retrospective studies [23].

The need of new treatment strategies that leverage genomic and preclinical data to identify specific therapeutic strategies has led to preclinical drug screening aimed at developing innovative treatment options for children with ETMR. Both in vitro and in vivo drug screenings using the patient-derived ETMR cell line BT183 and its xenograft model have revealed that ETMR is sensitive to both topotecan and doxorubicin [33]. In xenograft mice, treatment with topotecan or actinomycin D as a monotherapy resulted in a temporary reduction in tumor size and a significant extension in survival. Combining topotecan or doxorubicin with methotrexate and vincristine in multi-agent regimens further enhanced the tumor response.

Different infant brain tumor regimens are usually used in the treatment of ETMR given that there is no current standard of care. These approaches include the PNET-HR protocol, the German HIT protocols, US cooperative group protocols (CCG99703 and ACNS0334), as well as the Head Start protocols. They all similarly incorporate platinum and etoposide-based induction therapy with or without cyclophosphamide, vincristine, and high-dose methotrexate. The DFCIIRS-III for atypical teratoid rhabdoid tumor (AT/RT), however, does incorporate the use of both doxorubicin and actinomycin D into a platinum-based induction backbone [14, 17, 34] In fact, a very small cohort of patients treated with a modified IRS-III protocol showed promising results, although these patients received multiple, heterogeneous adjunct treatments. The use of intrathecal therapy in combination with focal irradiation has been also investigated, resulting in prolonged survival beyond 5 years in certain cases [29, 35].

Data on targeted or experimental therapies are very limited. In preclinical drug screening, epigenetic modifiers, mTOR inhibitors, bromodomain inhibitors, and GLI inhibitor arsenic trioxide demonstrated additional efficacy in mouse models [19, 27, 36, 37]. A small case series of patients treated with targeted radioimmunotherapy using intraventricular 131I-Omburtamab targeting B7-H3 showed potential therapeutic benefits. Two patients remained disease-free after multi-agent chemotherapy, local irradiation, and 131I-Omburtamab treatment [36].

Given the rarity and severity of this tumor, several ETMR patients have been included in molecular profiling trials to identify potential treatment targets. There is only one report in a patient with refractory ETMR who was successfully treated using a molecular profiling approach which identified the tyrosine kinase inhibitor dasatinib as a useful treatment [37].

12.3 CNS Neuroblastoma, FOXR2-Activated

12.3.1 Introduction

CNS neuroblastoma, FOXR2-activated, is a rare, grade 4 embryonal neoplasm with neuroblastic differentiation and activation of FOXR2 transcription factor.

In 2016, a new tumor type was first described characterized by chromosomal rearrangements identified through DNA methylation profiling, which leads to increased expression of the forkhead box R2 (FOXR2) gene [1]. This gene has been shown to play a role in tumorigenesis and proliferation in several cancers and a functional role in the induction of tumors. Due to the morphological resemblance of a subset of FOXR2-activated CNS-embryonal tumors to the previously described CNS neuroblastoma, the entity was classified as CNS neuroblastoma, FOXR2-activated (CNS NB-FOXR2), and it was introduced as a molecularly defined entity within the 2021 edition of the WHO CNS5.

12.3.2 Molecular and Immunohistochemical Features

The exact cellular origin is not well defined. The most frequent genetic alterations are inter- and intra-chromosomal rearrangements on the transcription factor FOXR2 gene, leading a fusion between the FOXR2 gene and some partner genes.

The morphological structure is characterized by poorly differentiated cells with palisades of embryonal cells and neuroblastic rosettes. The majority of cells express Olig2 and synaptophysin; generally without expression of GFAP and vimentin; usually the index of proliferation is high.

Detection of FOXR2 rearrangement could be complex requiring NGS sequencing or CNV analysis; DNA methylation profiling can help the correct diagnosis. CSF evaluation could detect the presence of liquoral tumor cells during the staging at diagnosis.

12.3.3 Clinical and Radiological Characteristics

This tumor occurs in childhood with a slight female preponderance but at a higher age than ETMR patients. It is a rare recently described tumor, for this reason, epidemiological data are incomplete. These tumors may represent approximately 10% of previously classified CNS-PNET.

CNS NB-FOXR2 is typically located in the supratentorial cerebral hemisphere, with frequent intraventricular location and leptomeningeal dissemination in some cases at diagnosis.

Radiologically, it appears as a well demarcated lesion with solid (with heterogeneous enhancement) and cystic components [23, 38], (Fig. 12.2).

The prognosis of CNS NB-FOXR2 is better than that of other embryonal tumors, with 5-year progression-free survival (PFS) and 5-year overall survival (OS) of 63% and 85%, respectively [39, 40].

12.3.4 Management

The mainstay of the treatment is maximal surgical resection followed by chemotherapy and/or radiation [41]. Additionally, based on retrospective reviews, CNS NB-FOXR2 tumors appear to be more chemosensitive than other tumors previously categorized under the larger "PNET" classification [23, 42, 43]. Most of the patients with CNS NB-FOXR2 reported to date have been

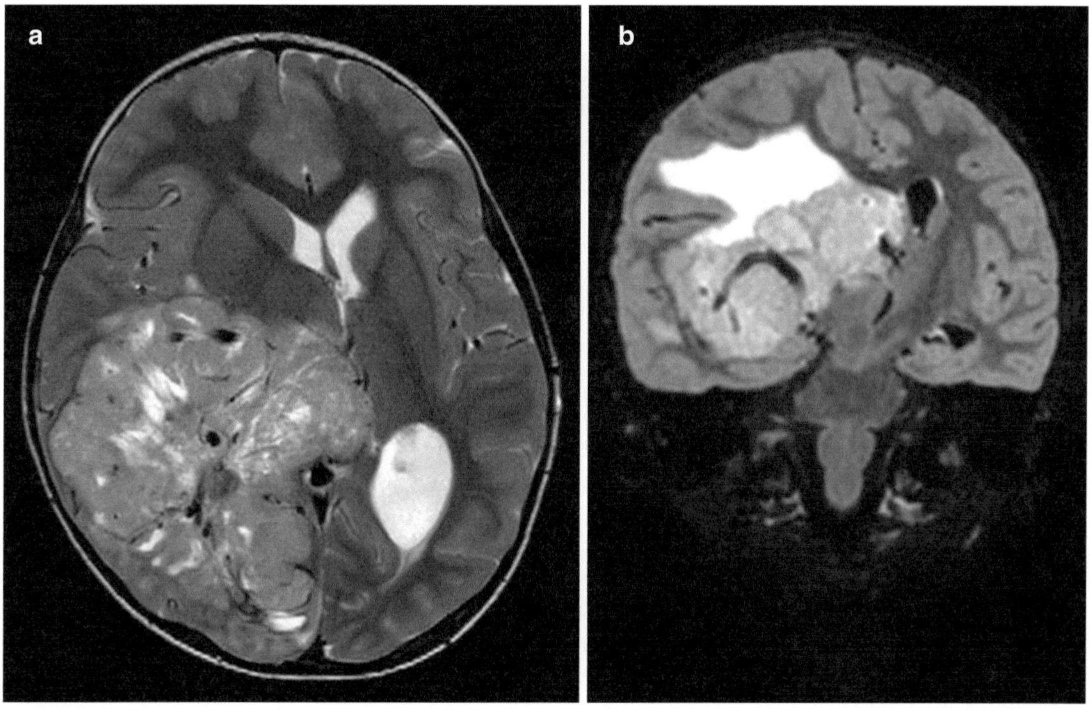

Fig. 12.2 Supratentorial CNS FOXR2 neuroblastoma; (**b**) axial T2-weighted sequence; (**b**) coronal FLAIR-weighted sequence

treated according to previous CNS PNET protocols. Retrospective studies indicate that these tumors generally have a favorable prognosis, with 5-year overall survival rates of 80% or higher. However, relapses, both local and distant, do occur, and progression-free survival rates range from 60% to 80% [23, 26]. Information regarding the prognostic significance of staging at diagnosis is scarce. Notably, among the few patients with metastatic disease, there have been several survivors, supporting the use of curative treatment for metastatic presentations.

Current evidence suggests that the highest survival rates have been observed in patients treated with upfront CSI combined with chemotherapy, as seen in previous CNS PNET studies. In one retrospective pooled analysis, patients who received local irradiation had a higher incidence of distant relapses. The study reported objective response rates of 60–70% after chemotherapy and high-dose chemotherapy, and the effective use of salvage radiotherapy in RT-naïve patients was also documented. This implies that younger patients with CNS NB-FOXR2 who are not candidates for CSI may benefit from regimens that omit radiotherapy, with local irradiation being avoided when possible [26, 44]. Overall, the number of reported cases remains very low, leading to a risk of inconsistent outcomes in future cohorts and highlighting the need for prospective registration and documentation of treatment and outcomes for CNS NB-FOXR2 patients until a dedicated prospective trial is planned.

12.4 CNS Tumor with *BCOR* Internal Tandem Duplication (ITD)

12.4.1 Introduction

In 2016, a novel molecularly defined tumor type characterized by distinct alterations in the BCL6 Corepressor (BCOR) gene was first described [1]. These tumors are marked by an internal tandem duplication (ITD) in exon 15 of the BCOR gene, which is located in the C-terminal region of the protein. BCOR is a component of the polycomb repressor complex, which plays a role in regulating gene expression related to cell differentiation, proliferation, and survival. The disruption of BCOR function due to such genetic alterations can lead to uncontrolled cell growth and tumor formation. This high-grade neuroepithelial tumor was initially named high-grade neuroepithelial tumor with BCOR alteration (HGNET-BCOR). However, in the fifth edition of the WHO classification of CNS tumors [2] it was officially designated as CNS BCOR-ITD, reflecting its distinct molecular and genetic features. Interestingly, the same BCOR ITD alteration has also been identified in clear cell sarcomas of the kidney and soft-tissue sarcomas, both of which predominantly affect young children [45]. While BCOR mutations are present in a variety of other tumor types, such as high-grade gliomas or SHH medulloblastomas, these do not qualify as CNS BCOR-ITD. Alterations other than the ITD, including point mutations and deletions within the BCOR gene, are seen in different tumor contexts but are not diagnostic of CNS BCOR-ITD [46, 47].

12.4.2 Molecular and Immunohistochemical Features

CNS BCOR-ITD tumors typically present with a solid growth pattern, consisting of uniform, oval-, or spindle-shaped cells with round to oval nuclei. A dense capillary network and focal pseudorosette formations can be seen. A key diagnostic challenge is that these tumors are frequently misdiagnosed as gliomas, ependymomas, or other embryonal tumors. This is due to their potential resemblance to glioma-like fibrillarity and the presence of relatively undifferentiated tumor cells. Additionally, while OLIG2 expression may be focally present, GFAP and synaptophysin are typically negative. The immunohistochemical detection of strong nuclear BCOR overexpression is a highly suggestive, though not entirely specific, biomarker [39, 48–50] Consequently, molecular confirmation is crucial for diagnosis. This can be achieved through techniques such as

PCR [51], targeted sequencing, or NGS. Alternatively, the presence of a characteristic DNA methylation profile can provide additional diagnostic support [2].

The BCOR ITD mutation occurs within the C-terminal domain of the BCOR protein. Interestingly, this same alteration has been observed in clear cell sarcomas of the kidney and soft-tissue sarcomas [62] suggesting a broader role of BCOR alterations in pediatric cancers.

In the first study [1], methylation profiling led to the identification of additional cases with BCOR gene alterations, such as point mutations or deletions. However, these cases, which are not diagnostic for CNS BCOR-ITD, would currently fall under the broader category of embryonal tumors, NEC. Recent research has also described tumors with BCOR or BCORL1 gene fusions involving EP300 or CREBBP as fusion partners [9, 52, 53] These tumors have been primarily morphologically classified as gliomas (both high- and low-grade), though further research is needed to clarify whether they differ clinically from CNS BCOR-ITD tumors in terms of presentation and prognosis.

12.4.3 Clinical and Radiological Characteristics

CNS tumors with BCOR-ITD have predominantly been reported in young children, with a median age of 4 years (range 7 months–22 years), but they can also be diagnosed in older children and young adults [1, 54]. These tumors have been observed in both genders and can arise at various locations throughout the CNS [39, 48, 50, 54, 55]. A characteristic feature of these tumors is their high propensity for metastasis, not only within the CNS but also to distant extracranial sites, with reports of spread to surrounding tissues (e.g., wound site seeding) [54, 56, 57]

On MRI, the tumor appears as a solid, well-defined mass, typically located in the superficial layer of the cerebral or cerebellar hemisphere. In certain instances, cystic components, intratumoral necrosis, and/or hemorrhages (visible on T2 imaging) may be observed (Fig. 12.3). The aggressive behavior of these tumors is reflected in the poor overall survival, with an approximate survival rate of 70% at 2 years and 50% at 4 years, as reported in a pooled analysis of 24 cases [54].

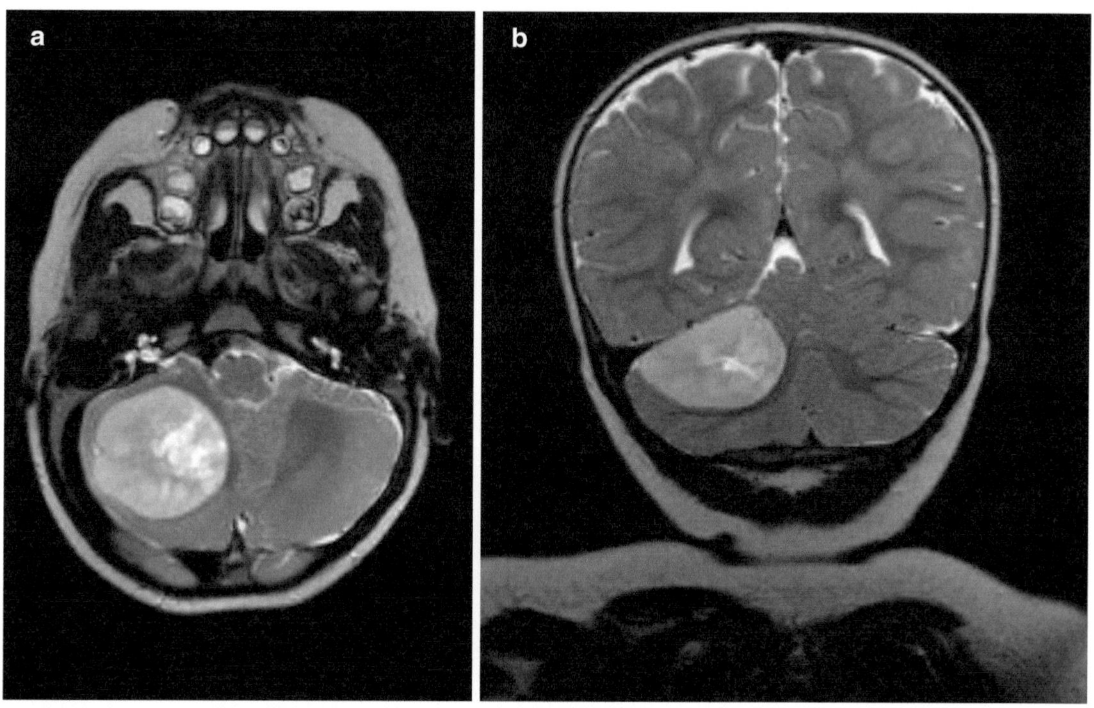

Fig. 12.3 Cerebellar BCOR ITD sarcoma; (**a**) axial T2 weighted; (**b**) coronal T2 weighted

12.4.4 Management

Regarding treatment, the data on CNS tumors with BCOR-ITD are highly heterogeneous, mainly due to frequent misdiagnoses based on the varying morphologies these tumors may exhibit. Gross total resection is considered essential for longer survival, and the majority of patients appear to benefit from irradiation and multiagent therapies [39, 55, 58]. A retrospective case series has suggested potential benefits of CSI, which may be further supported by the observed tendency for distant CNS relapses [54]. Given the aggressive clinical course and the molecular similarities to extracranial sarcomas, intensive multimodal therapies are generally recommended for these tumors, including chemotherapy regimens typically used for high-risk embryonal tumors or sarcomas.

The clinical behavior of CNS tumors with BCOR-ITD is considered highly aggressive, as indicated by early disease progression and recurrence. Although the survival prognosis is typically poor, with most cases reporting limited survival, a few long-term survivors have been documented, with survival exceeding 10 years in isolated cases [54, 57]. The tumor's high aggressiveness and molecular characteristics, which resemble those of extracranial sarcomas, justify the use of aggressive treatment regimens similar to those used for high-risk sarcoma or CNS PNET (primitive neuroectodermal tumor) cases.

In summary, CNS tumors with BCOR-ITD are biologically and clinically aggressive, with a tendency for metastasis both within the CNS and extracranially. While treatment strategies vary, a combination of surgery, irradiation, and chemotherapy is generally considered effective, with CSI possibly offering additional benefit. Given the molecular similarities to extracranial sarcomas, an aggressive, multimodal treatment approach appears warranted.

12.5 CNS Embryonal Tumors NEC/ NOS

CNS embryonal tumors NEC/NOS are subtypes arising in the CNS with embryonal features (morphology and immunohistochemistry, either lacking a signature that would classify it as a molecularly defined entity (not elsewhere classified NEC) or not susceptible to further analysis (not otherwise specified, NOS).

12.6 CNS Embryonal Tumor NEC

It refers to a CNS tumor that demonstrates embryonal morphology and immunophenotype. Although molecular analyses are successfully performed, the results do not lead to an established diagnosis according to the WHO CNS5. This tumor type encompasses very rare and poorly characterized tumor subtypes. Future studies involving larger cohorts and more detailed molecular profiling will help refine the diagnostic criteria and classification of this entity. Currently, the diagnostic criteria for NEC require the presence of an embryonal tumor in the CNS and the absence of features that would qualify it for a more specific embryonal CNS tumor diagnosis. Molecular analyses are necessary, but as of now, they do not yield a definitive classification.

The clinical behavior of NEC is highly heterogeneous, and therefore, no uniform treatment approach can be assumed. Moreover, there is a lack of focused clinical data specific to this group. Historically, patients with CNS embryonal tumors (excluding medulloblastomas and ATRTs) were treated according to protocols designed for CNS PNETs. However, due to the molecular reclassification of many tumors previously diagnosed as CNS PNET, most were reassigned to different or newly defined diagnoses [59, 60].

In a retrospective cohort of patients initially diagnosed with CNS PNET, DNA methylation analysis showed that 22% of these tumors could not be classified into any specific entity. The 5-year progression-free survival (PFS) and overall survival (OS) rates for this group were 54% and 69%, respectively [61]. This moderate prognosis is likely due to the exclusion of cases with poor prognoses, such as ETMR and high-grade gliomas, from the cohort. Further characterization of this heterogeneous group will be critical to improving clinical management.

12.7 CNS Embryonal Tumor, NOS

This entity refers to a CNS tumor with an embryonal morphology and immunophenotype, for which molecular analyses have either not been performed or were unsuccessful. It is strongly recommended to refer such cases (including available tumor tissue and molecular data) to a national or international reference center for further diagnostic evaluation. This diagnosis likely includes the entities discussed in previous sections, as well as a subset of rare, not yet well-characterized tumors (e.g., NEC). Timely molecular analysis is crucial for assigning the correct diagnosis and determining the appropriate treatment.

Currently, the diagnostic criteria for NOS are an embryonal tumor originating in the CNS, with the absence of features that would qualify it as a more specific embryonal CNS tumor, and molecular analyses that have not been successfully completed or performed. The diagnostic workup involves the exclusion of other embryonal tumor types, as well as sarcomas and malignant gliomas.

For NOS, timely molecular profiling is critical to refine the diagnosis and classify the tumor into a known entity (e.g., ETMR, CNS NB-FOXR2, CNS BCOR-ITD, or other). This will guide treatment decisions based on the specific tumor type.

In cases where NOS is diagnosed, further diagnostic evaluations should be prioritized, including referral to a national or international reference center for additional analysis.

In cases where a highly proliferative tumor is morphologically classified as a CNS embryonal tumor but molecular results are pending (temporary classification as NOS), chemotherapy may be considered. This ensures that treatment does not get delayed more than 28–40 days after surgery. A reasonable approach would be to initiate treatment with two courses of carboplatin/etoposide, as used in the SIOP HRMB protocol, although other embryonal CNS tumor protocols may also be applicable.

CNS Sarcomatous Tumors

Table 12.2 Essential diagnostic criteria of CNS sarcomatous tumors

CNS sarcomatous tumors		
Tumor type	CNS CIC	CNS DICER1
Diagnostic Criteria	Round cell, mild nuclear pleomorphism, epithelioid and/or spindle cell components, variably myxoid stroma	Spindled/pleomorphic tumor cells typically displaying eosinophilic cytoplasmic globules
	Variable CD99	IHC evidence of myogenic differentiation
	Frequent ETV4 and WT1 expression	Occasionally foci of chondroid differentiation
	CIC-fusion	DICER1 mutation
Molecular features	CD99/ETV4/WT1 expression IHC	Myogenic markers expression IHC
	CIC rearrangement	Loss of H3 pK28.me3 IHC
		DICER1 mutation
Sex	♀ ♂ 50%: 50%	♀ ♂ 50%: 50%
Site	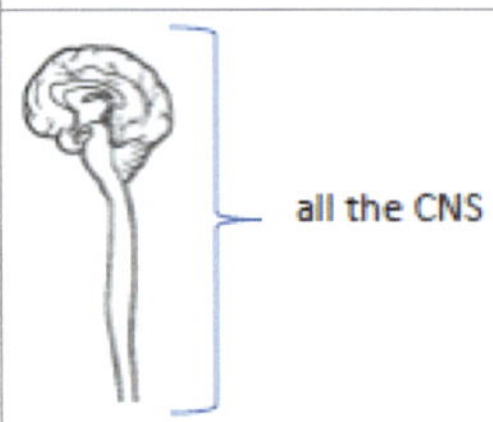	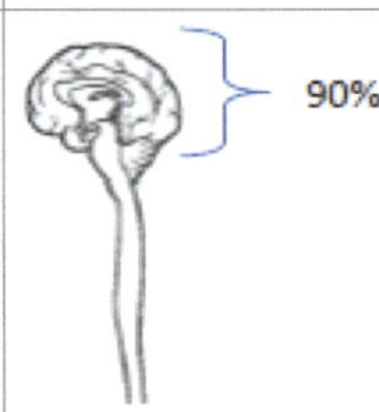
Age	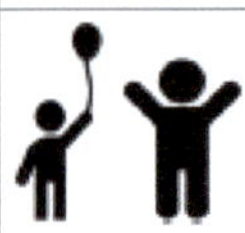	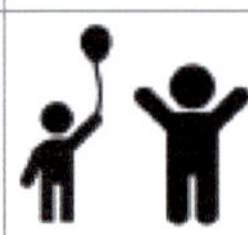
Outcome	Data are lacking	Data are lacking

12.8 Primary Intracranial Sarcoma DICER1 Mutant

12.8.1 Introduction

This is a molecularly defined entity introduced in the 2021 WHO classification that is characterized by DICER1 mutation most often biallelic, frequently accompanied by additional somatic mutations (e.g., NF1, FGFR4, NRAS, KRAS, EGFR) [62–64] Immunohistochemically, this entity presents with spindled or pleomorphic tumor cells, often expressing myogenic markers and showing loss of H3 p.K28me3 (or K27me3). Diagnosis must be confirmed through detection of pathogenic DICER1 mutations or a DNA methylation profile consistent with this tumor type.

12.8.1.1 Molecular and Immunohistochemical Features

It is composed of spindled or pleomorphic tumor cells typically displaying eosinophilic cytoplasmic globules, immunophenotypic evidence of myogenic differentiation, and occasionally foci of chondroid differentiation. These tumors are genetically defined by mutations in the DICER1 gene (either somatic or germline as part of DICER1 syndrome) and often harbor additional alterations of the mitogen-activated protein kinase (MAPK) pathway (e.g., KRAS, NF1, FGFR4, NRAS, EGFR).

Essential diagnostic criterion is the pathogenic mutations in DICER1 or a DNA methylation profile aligned with this tumor type. Immunohistochemical markers are myogenic markers, loss of H3 p.K28me3 (or K27me3), loss of ATRX, and strong p53 expression. This entity is typically negative for GFAP, OLIG2, cytokeratins, EMA, S100, SOX10, and SOX2.

Primary intracranial sarcoma, DICER1-mutant, may occur in the context of previous malignancies [62]. It is still unclear whether this is exclusively within the context of DICER1 syndrome or if other tumor predisposition syndromes, such as neurofibromatosis 1, may play a role [65]. Notably, an increased incidence of primary CNS sarcoma with DICER1 mutations has been described in a Peruvian cohort, with no evidence of recurrent germline mutations in known cancer-related genes, highlighting the potential involvement of so-far unknown tumor predisposition syndromes [63]. Clinical data are limited but suggest an aggressive disease course. Staging and follow-up should take into account the patient's tumor predisposition. Affected patients and their family members should be included in a cancer predisposition surveillance program for early detection of other potential malignancies.

12.8.1.2 Clinical and Radiological Characteristics

Primary intracranial sarcoma, DICER1-mutant, predominantly affects young children (median age 6 years; range 2–17.5 years), though cases have also been described in adults, with no gender predominance. These tumors are most commonly located in the supratentorial region but can also rarely affect the cerebellum and spine [62–64, 66] Metastatic disease at the time of presentation is rare, but both local and distant recurrences, including extra-CNS relapses, have been reported [63] (Fig. 12.4). The "sarcomatous" metastatic pattern typically involves pulmonary and bone lesions outside of the CNS. Clinical behavior is difficult to predict due to the small number of cases and short follow-up, though preliminary data suggests an aggressive disease course.

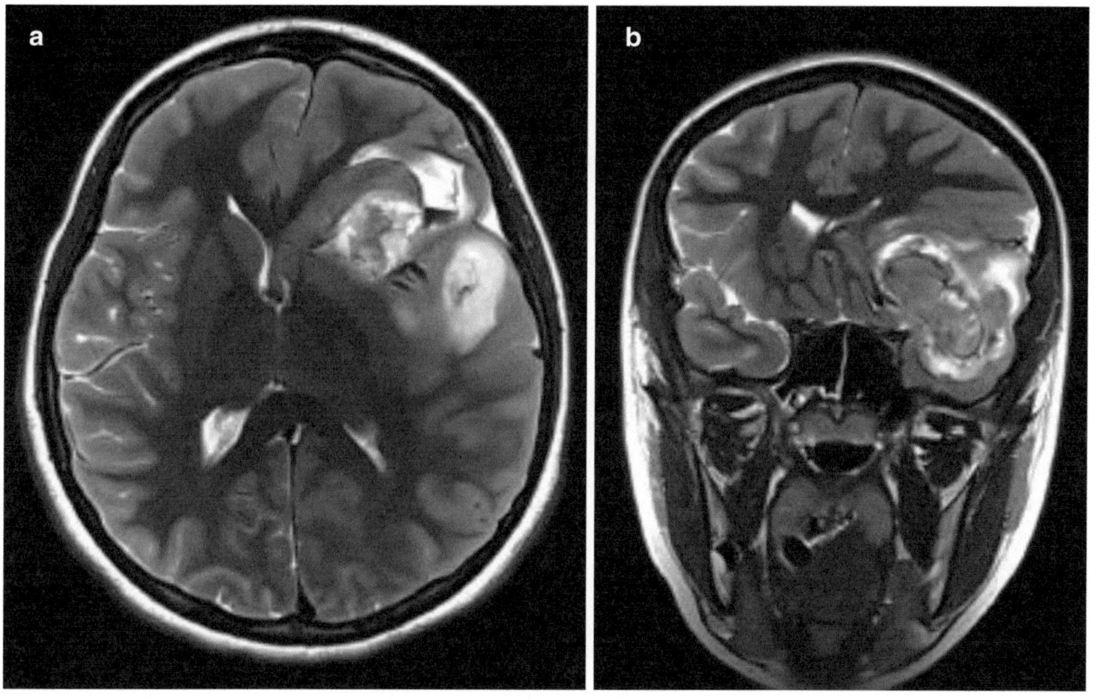

Fig. 12.4 Frontal DICER1 sarcoma; (**a**) axial T2 weighted; (**b**) coronal T2 weighted

12.8.2 Management

Most patients with primary intracranial sarcoma harboring DICER1 mutations have typically undergone surgery (usually aimed at complete resection) and radiation, with chemotherapy administered in some cases [62–64]. In the first major series [64], many of these tumors were initially diagnosed as sarcoma NOS or embryonal rhabdomyosarcoma. Detailed clinical data and follow-up are lacking, but if chemotherapy was used, patients were most likely treated according to soft tissue sarcoma protocols. A small group of patients has been treated with chemotherapy protocols that included agents used in advanced pleuropulmonary blastoma (PPB), such as ifosfamide, doxorubicin, vincristine, and dactinomycin [63].

In a large cohort of 70 patients, progression-free survival was highest in those treated with upfront surgery followed by a "sandwich" of ICE chemotherapy (ifosfamide, carboplatin, etoposide) and focal radiotherapy [63]. Given the presence of Ras pathway gene activation in DICER1-associated tumors, targeted therapies that inhibit Ras or its effector pathways (such as MAPK pathway inhibition) should be further explored in these rare tumors.

Due to the lack of standardized treatment guidelines for primary intracranial sarcoma, DICER1-mutant, available data from other DICER1-associated malignancies, such as PPB, may be informative. Complete tumor resection has strong prognostic significance, and chemotherapy is essential for any chance of cure in solid types II–III PPB. Different polychemotherapy regimens similar to those used in rhabdomyosarcoma have been utilized, including the IVA regimen (ifosfamide, vincristine, actinomycin D).

12.9 CIC-Rearranged Sarcoma

12.9.1 Introduction

CIC-rearranged sarcomas within the CNS is a high-grade, poorly differentiated sarcoma defined by CIC fusion with different gene partners. This entity was first identified in a cohort of tumors historically diagnosed as "CNS PNETs" in the first molecular classification [1] and has since been described in several individual cases and smaller series [67–69] These tumors share many features with extra-CNS sarcomas and are classified as CIC-rearranged sarcomas of the WHO CNS5. While CIC-rearranged sarcomas typically present as malignant soft tissue tumors outside the CNS, most cases involve a CIC::DUX4 fusion [70, 71]. In contrast, many CNS tumors exhibit CIC::NUTM1 fusions [2, 72] with recent reports also describing ATXN1::DUX4 and ATXN1::NUTM1 fusions in CNS primitive tumors [73, 74]. Initially classified as "Ewing sarcoma family tumors," CIC-rearranged sarcomas are now recognized as distinct from Ewing sarcoma, exhibiting clear differences in both their biology and clinical behavior [75–77]

12.9.2 Molecular and Immunohistochemical Features

Within the CNS, the clinic pathological and radiological data remains scarce in the literature, limited to small series [10]. CIC-fused CNS tumors seem to present particularities compared to their soft tissue counterparts in terms of phenotype glioneuronal characteristics. A CIC-rearranged sarcoma, independently from location, contains an oncogenic gene fusion of CIC transcriptional repressor with different partners (most often DUX4; but also FOXO4, LEUTX, NUTM1, NUTM2A). It remains unclear whether these different fusion variants represent a single entity. Histologically, these tumors closely resemble their extra-CNS counterparts, characterized by diffuse sheets of undifferentiated, round cells. Focal lobular arrangements, often separated by thin fibrous septa, as well as a minor spindle or epithelioid cell component, are frequently observed. The tumor cells are relatively uniform, but moderate nuclear pleomorphism is often present. The cytoplasm is eosinophilic, and necrosis is common, with brisk mitotic activity. Immunohistochemically, patchy expression of

CD99, as well as frequent expression of ETV4 and WT1, is often observed. Diagnostic criteria include evidence of a CIC gene fusion, histology showing a predominant round cell phenotype with mild nuclear pleomorphism, and immunohistochemical staining for CD99, ETV4, and WT1. A DNA methylation profile consistent with CIC-rearranged sarcoma further supports the diagnosis.

12.9.3 Clinical and Radiological Characteristics

These entity affects children and young adults (median age 8 years), with 70% of patients being found in the pediatric age group [1, 67, 73, 78] No gender predisposition is reported in the literature. Most CIC sarcomas of the CNS occur in supratentorial sites (85% of reported tumors), whereas spinal and posterior fossa presentation accounts for 10% and 5% of reported cases, respectively. This entity may present recurrent imaging features; these are characterized by large intra-axial tumors with frequent meningeal contact, marked perituMoral edema, intense contrast enhancement, hemorrhagic foci, diffusion restriction, and high perfusion.

Because of the age of onset, morphology, and pluriphenotypic immunoprofile, the main differential diagnosis is with AT/RT and rhabdoid tumors, which are easily ruled out by a retained expression of INI1 at immunohistochemistry.

12.9.4 Management

Treatment strategies for CNS cases have mainly followed protocols used for peripheral soft tissue sarcomas and embryonal CNS tumors, including multiagent systemic therapies, surgery, and irradiation. Reports on CNS CIC-rearranged sarcoma suggest that some patients have achieved remission, with many surviving after upfront irradiation [10, 39, 67, 68, 79, 80].

Due to the limited published data and the evolving understanding of tumor biology and treatment response, treatment strategies for CIC-rearranged sarcomas of the CNS remain largely based on general principles rather than specific protocols. The lack of established treatment guidelines underscores the importance of involving an advisory group, on a national/international level, when determining the best approach for individual patients.

Further Rare CNS Tumor Entity

Table 12.3 Essential diagnostic criteria of CNS astroblastoma, MN1-altered

Rare CNS tumor entity	
Tumor type	Astroblastoma MN1-altered
Diagnostic criteria	Cuboidal cells arranged in perivascular pseudorosettes
	Positive for glial markers: GFAP; OLIG2
	No WHO grade assigned
	MN1 fusion
Molecular features	MN1 fusion (FISH/RNA sequencing) with BEND2 or CXXC5 as fusion partners
Sex	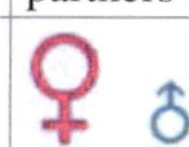 80%: 20%
Site	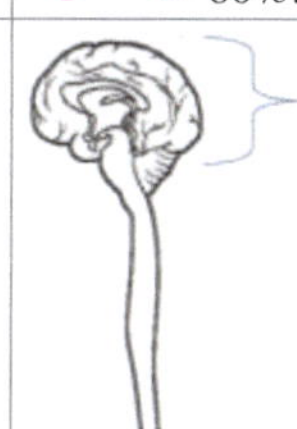
Age	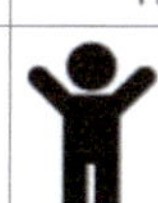
Outcome	Favorable, relapse after many years

12.10 Astroblastoma, MN1-Altered

12.10.1 Introduction

CNS tumors with MN1::BEND2/CXXC5 fusion were first identified through large-scale analyses, primarily involving tumors diagnosed as astroblastomas based on histopathological criteria. In the WHO CNS5, these tumors are referred to as "astroblastoma, MN1-altered" [2]. It is important to note that tumors with other histologic diagnoses may also carry these alterations, and not all tumors with astroblastoma-like features will necessarily harbor MN1 alterations. Therefore, this novel entity is defined by a common molecular feature: a gene fusion involving the MN1 gene with either BEND2 or CXXC5 as fusion partners. More recently, cases of astroblastomas with EWSR1::BEND2 gene fusions have been described, further expanding the molecular landscape of this tumor entity [81]. These gene fusions are mutually exclusive with hallmark alterations that define other tumor entities, such as gliomas with IDH1 or BRAF mutations and ependymomas with ZFTA (RELA) fusions [82]. Molecular analyses of astroblastoma cohorts have demonstrated that these tumors represent only a subset of all tumors originally diagnosed as astroblastomas, as many of the other cases do not harbor MN1 alterations [83]. Earlier clinical analyses of astroblastoma patient cohorts, which did not account for molecular diagnoses, may not be representative of the entity "astroblastoma, MN1-altered."

12.10.2 Molecular and Immunohistochemical Features

This is a rare, well-delineated glioma composed of cuboidal or elongated cells arranged in perivascular pseudorosettes, with prominent perivascular sclerosis and MN1 alterations [84]. No WHO grade has been assigned to this tumor. The tumor must be a glial neoplasm with astroblastic perivascular pseudorosettes and an MN1 alteration. For unresolved lesions, a DNA methylation profile consistent with astroblastoma, MN1-altered, is required. It should be recognized that some tumors diagnosed as astroblastoma, MN1-altered, based on DNA methylation may not exhibit clear histopathological features of astroblastoma, necessitating further investigation to determine their relationship to astroblastomas, MN1-altered [85]. Immunohistochemically, the tumor cells are positive for the glial markers GFAP and OLIG2. EMA expression is present in a cytoplasmic or membranous pattern, with some cases showing dot-like staining, raising the differential diagnosis of ependymoma. Mutations in IDH1 and BRAF or ZFTA (RELA) fusions are mutually exclusive with MN1 alterations and rule out the diagnosis of astroblastoma, MN1-altered [8, 86]. The MN1 fusion must be confirmed by FISH or RNA sequencing. It remains to be determined whether tumors with other fusions, such as EWSR1::BEND2, belong to this entity.

12.10.3 Clinical and Radiological Characteristics

Astroblastoma, MN1-altered, arises predominantly in older children and adults, with a median age of 13.5 years (range 2–40), and exhibits a clear gender preponderance, with over 80% of cases occurring in females. Most tumors arise in the supratentorial region and are well demarcated with both solid and cystic components (Fig. 12.5). Clinically, these tumors show a high tendency to recur, with approximately two-thirds of cases recurring, often many years after the initial diagnosis. Tumor recurrences are mostly local, although metastatic recurrences have also been reported. Despite this, overall survival appears favorable (median overall survival of 15 years), though up to 30% of patients may eventually succumb to the disease, generally after a prolonged course. Notably, a study has suggested a more favorable prognosis for astroblastomas compared to other primary CNS tumors, such as ependymomas or CNS PNETs [87].

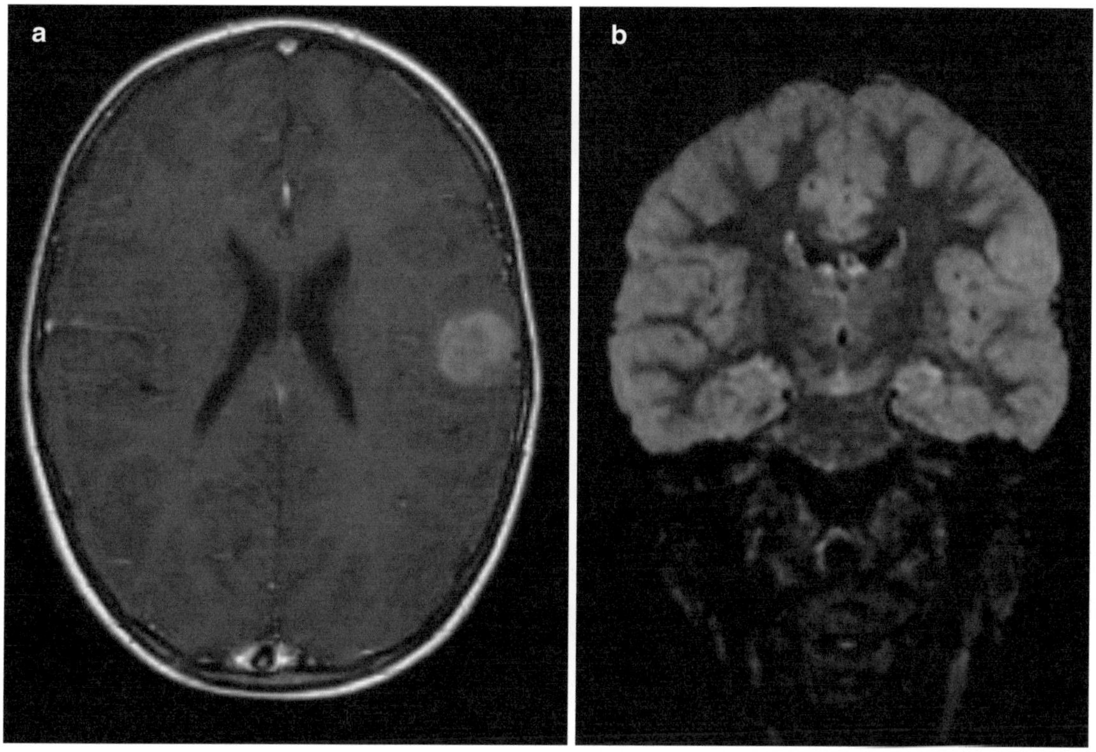

Fig. 12.5 cortical-subcortical frontal astroblastoma MN1 altered; (**a**) axial post-contrast T1 weighted; (**b**) coronal FLAIR weighted

12.10.4 Management

Most patients have been treated with surgical resection, and gross total resection is possible in more than half of cases. The extent of resection is potentially linked to improved outcomes. Post-surgery, many patients receive focal radiotherapy, with some also receiving chemotherapy based on regimens used for CNS PNETs or temozolomide-based such as Stupp regimen [88].

Treatment for metastatic disease may include CSI. Interestingly, some patients without gross total resection may not experience recurrence, even though treatment details for these cases were not available. However, irradiated tumors may still recur, indicating a subgroup with higher aggressiveness. Astroblastomas, MN1-altered, appear to have a high propensity for local relapse, although some may be cured by tumor resection alone [8, 59, 89, 90].

References

1. Sturm D, Orr BA, Toprak UH, Hovestadt V, Jones DTW, Capper D, Sill M, Buchhalter I, Northcott PA, Leis I, Ryzhova M, Koelsche C, Pfaff E, Allen SJ, Balasubramanian G, Worst BC, Pajtler KW, Brabetz S, Johann PD, Sahm F, Reimand J, Mackay A, Carvalho DM, Remke M, Phillips JJ, Perry A, Cowdrey C, Drissi R, Fouladi M, Giangaspero F, Łastowska M, Grajkowska W, Scheurlen W, Pietsch T, Hagel C, Gojo J, Lötsch D, Berger W, Slavc I, Haberler C, Jouvet A, Holm S, Hofer S, Prinz M, Keohane C, Fried I, Mawrin C, Scheie D, Mobley BC, Schniederjan MJ, Santi M, Buccoliero AM, Dahiya S, Kramm CM, von Bueren AO, von Hoff K, Rutkowski S, Herold-Mende C, Frühwald MC, Milde T, Hasselblatt M, Wesseling P, Rößler J, Schüller U, Ebinger M, Schittenhelm J, Frank S, Grobholz R, Vajtai I, Hans V, Schneppenheim R, Zitterbart K, Collins VP, Aronica E, Varlet P, Puget S, Dufour C, Grill J, Figarella-Branger D, Wolter M, Schuhmann MU, Shalaby T, Grotzer M, van Meter T, Monoranu CM, Felsberg J, Reifenberger G, Snuderl M, Forrester LA, Koster J, Versteeg R, Volckmann R, van Sluis P,

Wolf S, Mikkelsen T, Gajjar A, Aldape K, Moore AS, Taylor MD, Jones C, Jabado N, Karajannis MA, Eils R, Schlesner M, Lichter P, von Deimling A, Pfister SM, Ellison DW, Korshunov A, Kool M. New brain tumor entities emerge from molecular classification of CNS-PNETs. Cell. 2016;164(5):1060–72. https://doi.org/10.1016/j.cell.2016.01.015. PMID: 26919435; PMCID: PMC5139621.

2. Louis DN, Perry A, Wesseling P, Brat DJ, Cree IA, Figarella-Branger D, Hawkins C, Ng HK, Pfister SM, Reifenberger G, Soffietti R, von Deimling A, Ellison DW. The 2021 WHO classification of tumors of the central nervous system: a summary. Neuro-Oncology. 2021;23(8):1231–51. https://doi.org/10.1093/neuonc/noab106. PMID: 34185076; PMCID: PMC832801.
3. Rorke LB, Trojanowski JQ, Lee VM, Zimmerman RA, Sutton LN, Biegel JA, Goldwein JW, Packer RJ. Primitive neuroectodermal tumors of the central nervous system. Brain Pathol. 1997;7(2):765–84. https://doi.org/10.1111/j.1750-3639.1997.tb01063.x. PMID: 9161728; PMCID: PMC8098595.
4. Kleihues P, Louis DN, Scheithauer BW, Rorke LB, Reifenberger G, Burger PC, Cavenee WK. The WHO classification of tumors of the nervous system. J Neuropathol Exp Neurol. 2002;61(3):215–25; discussion 226–9. https://doi.org/10.1093/jnen/61.3.215. PMID: 11895036.
5. Louis DN, Ohgaki H, Wiestler OD, Cavenee WK, Burger PC, Jouvet A, Scheithauer BW, Kleihues P. The 2007 WHO classification of tumours of the central nervous system. Acta Neuropathol. 2007;114(2):97–109. https://doi.org/10.1007/s00401-007-0243-4. Epub 2007 Jul 6. Erratum in: Acta Neuropathol. 2007 Nov;114(5):547. PMID: 17618441; PMCID: PMC1929165.
6. Louis DN, Perry A, Reifenberger G, von Deimling A, Figarella-Branger D, Cavenee WK, Ohgaki H, Wiestler OD, Kleihues P, Ellison DW. The 2016 World Health Organization classification of tumors of the central nervous system: a summary. Acta Neuropathol. 2016;131(6):803–20. https://doi.org/10.1007/s00401-016-1545-1. Epub 2016 May 9. PMID: 27157931.
7. Alhalabi KT, Stichel D, Sievers P, Peterziel H, Sommerkamp AC, Sturm D, Wittmann A, Sill M, Jäger N, Beck P, Pajtler KW, Snuderl M, Jour G, Delorenzo M, Martin AM, Levy A, Dalvi N, Hansford JR, Gottardo NG, Uro-Coste E, Maurage CA, Godfraind C, Vandenbos F, Pietsch T, Kramm C, Filippidou M, Kattamis A, Jones C, Øra I, Mikkelsen TS, Zapotocky M, Sumerauer D, Scheie D, McCabe M, Wesseling P, Tops BBJ, Kranendonk MEG, Karajannis MA, Bouvier N, Papaemmanuil E, Dohmen H, Acker T, von Hoff K, Schmid S, Miele E, Filipski K, Kitanovski L, Krskova L, Gojo J, Haberler C, Alvaro F, Ecker J, Selt F, Milde T, Witt O, Oehme I, Kool M, von Deimling A, Korshunov A, Pfister SM, Sahm F, Jones DTW. PATZ1 fusions define a novel molecularly distinct neuroepithelial tumor entity with a broad histological spectrum. Acta Neuropathol. 2021;142(5):841–57. https://doi.org/10.1007/s00401-021-02354-8. Epub 2021 Aug 21. PMID: 34417833; PMCID: PMC8500868.
8. Rossi S, Barresi S, Colafati GS, Genovese S, Tancredi C, Costabile V, Patrizi S, Giovannoni I, Asioli S, Poliani PL, Gardiman MP, Cardoni A, Del Baldo G, Antonelli M, Gianno F, Piccirilli E, Catino G, Martucci L, Quacquarini D, Toni F, Melchionda F, Viscardi E, Zucchelli M, Dal Pos S, Gatti E, Liserre R, Schiavello E, Diomedi-Camassei F, Carai A, Mastronuzzi A, Gessi M, Giannini C, Novelli A, Onetti Muda A, Miele E, Alesi V, Alaggio R. PATZ1-rearranged tumors of the central nervous system: characterization of a pediatric series of seven cases. Mod Pathol. 2024;37(2):100387. https://doi.org/10.1016/j.modpat.2023.100387. Epub 2023 Nov 23. PMID: 38007157.
9. Pisapia DJ, Ohara K, Bareja R, Wilkes DC, Hissong E, Croyle JA, Kim JH, Saab J, MacDonald TY, Beg S, O'Reilly C, Kudman S, Rubin MA, Elemento O, Sboner A, Greenfield J, Mosquera JM. Fusions involving BCOR and CREBBP are rare events in infiltrating glioma. Acta Neuropathol Commun. 2020;8(1):80. https://doi.org/10.1186/s40478-020-00951-4. PMID: 32493417; PMCID: PMC7271411.
10. Tauziède-Espariat A, Uro-Coste E, Sievers P, Nicaise Y, Mariet C, Siegfried A, Pierron G, Guillemot D, Benzakoun J, Pallud J, Roques M, Bonneville F, Larrieu-Ciron D, Chaynes P, Saffroy R, Hamelin J, Hasty L, Métais A, Chrétien F, Kool M, Gojo J, Varlet P, RENOCLIP-LOC. CNS tumor with EP300::BCOR fusion: discussing its prevalence in adult population. Acta Neuropathol Commun. 2023;11(1):26. https://doi.org/10.1186/s40478-023-01523-y. PMID: 36782314; PMCID: PMC9926824.
11. Tauziède-Espariat A, Siegfried A, Nicaise Y, Dghayem D, Laprie A, Lubrano V, Richard P, Gauchotte G, Malczuk J, Klein O, Hasty L, Métais A, Chrétien F, Dangouloff-Ros V, Boddaert N, Sahm F, Sievers P, Varlet P, Uro-Coste E, RENOCLIP-LOC. PLAG1 fusions extend the spectrum of PLAG(L)-altered CNS tumors. Acta Neuropathol. 2023;146(6):841–4. https://doi.org/10.1007/s00401-023-02643-4. Epub 2023 Oct 23. PMID: 37870637; PMCID: PMC10627894.
12. Eberhart CG, Brat DJ, Cohen KJ, Burger PC. Pediatric neuroblastic brain tumors containing abundant neuropil and true rosettes. Pediatr Dev Pathol. 2000;3(4):346–52. https://doi.org/10.1007/s100249910049. PMID: 10890250.
13. Li M, Lee KF, Lu Y, Clarke I, Shih D, Eberhart C, Collins VP, Van Meter T, Picard D, Zhou L, Boutros PC, Modena P, Liang ML, Scherer SW, Bouffet E, Rutka JT, Pomeroy SL, Lau CC, Taylor MD, Gajjar A, Dirks PB, Hawkins CE, Huang A. Frequent amplification of a chr19q13.41 microRNA polycistron in aggressive primitive neuroectodermal brain tumors. Cancer Cell. 2009;16(6):533–46. https://doi.org/10.1016/j.ccr.2009.10.025. Erratum in: Cancer

Cell. 2010 Apr 13;17(4):413. PMID: 19962671; PMCID: PMC3431561.

14. Spence T, Sin-Chan P, Picard D, Barszczyk M, Hoss K, Lu M, Kim SK, Ra YS, Nakamura H, Fangusaro J, Hwang E, Kiehna E, Toledano H, Wang Y, Shi Q, Johnston D, Michaud J, La Spina M, Buccoliero AM, Adamek D, Camelo-Piragua S, Peter Collins V, Jones C, Kabbara N, Jurdi N, Varlet P, Perry A, Scharnhorst D, Fan X, Muraszko KM, Eberhart CG, Ng HK, Gururangan S, Van Meter T, Remke M, Lafay-Cousin L, Chan JA, Sirachainan N, Pomeroy SL, Clifford SC, Gajjar A, Shago M, Halliday W, Taylor MD, Grundy R, Lau CC, Phillips J, Bouffet E, Dirks PB, Hawkins CE, Huang A. CNS-PNETs with C19MC amplification and/or LIN28 expression comprise a distinct histogenetic diagnostic and therapeutic entity. Acta Neuropathol. 2014;128(2):291–303. https://doi.org/10.1007/s00401-014-1291-1. Epub 2014 May 20. PMID: 24839957; PMCID: PMC4159569.
15. Korshunov A, Remke M, Gessi M, Ryzhova M, Hielscher T, Witt H, Tobias V, Buccoliero AM, Sardi I, Gardiman MP, Bonnin J, Scheithauer B, Kulozik AE, Witt O, Mork S, von Deimling A, Wiestler OD, Giangaspero F, Rosenblum M, Pietsch T, Lichter P, Pfister SM. Focal genomic amplification at 19q13.42 comprises a powerful diagnostic marker for embryonal tumors with ependymoblastic rosettes. Acta Neuropathol. 2010;120(2):253–60. https://doi.org/10.1007/s00401-010-0688-8. Epub 2010 Apr 21. PMID: 20407781.
16. Lambo S, von Hoff K, Korshunov A, Pfister SM, Kool M. ETMR: a tumor entity in its infancy. Acta Neuropathol. 2020;140(3):249–66. https://doi.org/10.1007/s00401-020-02182-2. Epub 2020 Jun 29. PMID: 32601913; PMCID: PMC7423804.
17. Kleinman CL, Gerges N, Papillon-Cavanagh S, Sin-Chan P, Pramatarova A, Quang DA, Adoue V, Busche S, Caron M, Djambazian H, Bemmo A, Fontebasso AM, Spence T, Schwartzentruber J, Albrecht S, Hauser P, Garami M, Klekner A, Bognar L, Montes JL, Staffa A, Montpetit A, Berube P, Zakrzewska M, Zakrzewski K, Liberski PP, Dong Z, Siegel PM, Duchaine T, Perotti C, Fleming A, Faury D, Remke M, Gallo M, Dirks P, Taylor MD, Sladek R, Pastinen T, Chan JA, Huang A, Majewski J, Jabado N. Fusion of TTYH1 with the C19MC microRNA cluster drives expression of a brain-specific DNMT3B isoform in the embryonal brain tumor ETMR. Nat Genet. 2014;46(1):39–44. https://doi.org/10.1038/ng.2849. Epub 2013 Dec 8. PMID: 24316981.
18. Lambo S, Gröbner SN, Rausch T, Waszak SM, Schmidt C, Gorthi A, Romero JC, Mauermann M, Brabetz S, Krausert S, Buchhalter I, Koster J, Zwijnenburg DA, Sill M, Hübner JM, Mack N, Schwalm B, Ryzhova M, Hovestadt V, Papillon-Cavanagh S, Chan JA, Landgraf P, Ho B, Milde T, Witt O, Ecker J, Sahm F, Sumerauer D, Ellison DW, Orr BA, Darabi A, Haberler C, Figarella-Branger D, Wesseling P, Schittenhelm J, Remke M, Taylor MD, Gil-da-Costa MJ, Łastowska M, Grajkowska W, Hasselblatt M, Hauser P, Pietsch T, Uro-Coste E, Bourdeaut F, Masliah-Planchon J, Rigau V, Alexandrescu S, Wolf S, Li XN, Schüller U, Snuderl M, Karajannis MA, Giangaspero F, Jabado N, von Deimling A, Jones DTW, Korbel JO, von Hoff K, Lichter P, Huang A, Bishop AJR, Pfister SM, Korshunov A, Kool M. The molecular landscape of ETMR at diagnosis and relapse. Nature. 2019;576(7786):274–80. https://doi.org/10.1038/s41586-019-1815-x. Epub 2019 Dec 4. PMID: 31802000; PMCID: PMC6908757.
19. Uro-Coste E, Masliah-Planchon J, Siegfried A, Blanluet M, Lambo S, Kool M, Roujeau T, Boetto S, Palenzuela G, Bertozzi AI, Gambart M, Coupier I, Oliver-Petit I, Golmard L, Julia S, Savagner F, Mohand-Oumoussa B, Tauziede-Espariat A, Delisle MB, Figarella-Branger D, Bourdeaut F, Rigau V. ETMR-like infantile cerebellar embryonal tumors in the extended morphologic spectrum of DICER1-related tumors. Acta Neuropathol. 2019;137(1):175–7. https://doi.org/10.1007/s00401-018-1935-7. Epub 2018 Nov 16. PMID: 30446821.
20. Campos Mármol MC, Aguado M, Ramón Y, Cajal T, Gallardo A, Catasús L, Gonzalez A, Méndez JE, Lasa A, Arumi M, Gallego Rubio O, Serra JB, Muñoz Hernandez F, von Deimling A, Kommoss FKF, Espinosa I. Non-C19MC-altered embryonal tumor with multilayered rosettes in a young woman with DICER1 syndrome: case report and review of the literature. Pathologica. 2024;116(3):170–5. https://doi.org/10.32074/1591-951X-970. PMID: 38979591; PMCID: PMC11447652
21. Korshunov A, Jakobiec FA, Eberhart CG, Hovestadt V, Capper D, Jones DT, Sturm D, Stagner AM, Edward DP, Eagle RC, Proia AD, Koch A, Ryzhova M, Ektova A, Schüller U, Zheludkova O, Lichter P, von Deimling A, Pfister SM, Kool M. Comparative integrated molecular analysis of intraocular medulloepitheliomas and central nervous system embryonal tumors with multilayered rosettes confirms that they are distinct nosologic entities. Neuropathology. 2015;35(6):538–44. https://doi.org/10.1111/neup.12227. Epub 2015 Jul 16. PMID: 26183384.
22. Juhnke BO, Gessi M, Gerber NU, Friedrich C, Mynarek M, von Bueren AO, Haberler C, Schüller U, Kortmann RD, Timmermann B, Bison B, Warmuth-Metz M, Kwiecien R, Pfister SM, Spix C, Pietsch T, Kool M, Rutkowski S, von Hoff K. Treatment of embryonal tumors with multilayered rosettes with carboplatin/etoposide induction and high-dose chemotherapy within the prospective P-HIT trial. Neuro-Oncology. 2022;24(1):127–37. https://doi.org/10.1093/neuonc/noab100. PMID: 33908610; PMCID: PMC8730753.
23. von Hoff K, Haberler C, Schmitt-Hoffner F, Schepke E, de Rojas T, Jacobs S, Zapotocky M, Sumerauer D, Perek-Polnik M, Dufour C, van Vuurden D, Slavc I, Gojo J, Pickles JC, Gerber NU, Massimino M, Gil-da-Costa MJ, Garami M, Kumirova E, Sehested A, Scheie D, Cruz O, Moreno L, Cho J, Zeller B, Bovenschen N, Grotzer M, Alderete D, Snuderl

M, Zheludkova O, Golanov A, Okonechnikov K, Mynarek M, Juhnke BO, Rutkowski S, Schüller U, Pizer B, von Zezschwitz B, Kwiecien R, Wechsung M, Konietschke F, Hwang EI, Sturm D, Pfister SM, von Deimling A, Rushing EJ, Ryzhova M, Hauser P, Łastowska M, Wesseling P, Giangaspero F, Hawkins C, Figarella-Branger D, Eberhart C, Burger P, Gessi M, Korshunov A, Jacques TS, Capper D, Pietsch T, Kool M. Therapeutic implications of improved molecular diagnostics for rare CNS embryonal tumor entities: results of an international, retrospective study. Neuro-Oncology. 2021;23(9):1597–611. https://doi.org/10.1093/neuonc/noab136. PMID: 34077956; PMCID: PMC8408859.
24. Horwitz M, Dufour C, Leblond P, Bourdeaut F, Faure-Conter C, Bertozzi AI, Delisle MB, Palenzuela G, Jouvet A, Scavarda D, Vinchon M, Padovani L, Gaudart J, Branger DF, Andre N. Embryonal tumors with multilayered rosettes in children: the SFCE experience. Childs Nerv Syst. 2016;32(2):299–305. https://doi.org/10.1007/s00381-015-2920-2. Epub 2015 Oct 5. PMID: 26438544.
25. Khan S, Solano-Paez P, Suwal T, Lu M, Al-Karmi S, Ho B, Mumal I, Shago M, Hoffman LM, Dodgshun A, Nobusawa S, Tabori U, Bartels U, Ziegler DS, Hansford JR, Ramaswamy V, Hawkins C, Dufour C, André N, Bouffet E. Huang A; rare brain tumor registry. Clinical phenotypes and prognostic features of embryonal tumours with multi-layered rosettes: a rare brain tumor registry study. Lancet Child Adolesc Health. 2021;5(11):800–13. https://doi.org/10.1016/S2352-4642(21)00245-5. Epub 2021 Sep 30. PMID: 34599879.
26. Korshunov A, Sturm D, Ryzhova M, Hovestadt V, Gessi M, Jones DT, Remke M, Northcott P, Perry A, Picard D, Rosenblum M, Antonelli M, Aronica E, Schüller U, Hasselblatt M, Woehrer A, Zheludkova O, Kumirova E, Puget S, Taylor MD, Giangaspero F, Peter Collins V, von Deimling A, Lichter P, Huang A, Pietsch T, Pfister SM, Kool M. Embryonal tumor with abundant neuropil and true rosettes (ETANTR), ependymoblastoma, and medulloepithelioma share molecular similarity and comprise a single clinicopathological entity. Acta Neuropathol. 2014;128(2):279–89. https://doi.org/10.1007/s00401-013-1228-0. Epub 2013 Dec 14. PMID: 24337497; PMCID: PMC4102829.
27. Nowak J, Seidel C, Berg F, Pietsch T, Friedrich C, von Hoff K, Rutkowski S, Warmuth-Metz M. MRI characteristics of ependymoblastoma: results from 22 centrally reviewed cases. AJNR Am J Neuroradiol. 2014;35(10):1996–2001. https://doi.org/10.3174/ajnr.A4002. Epub 2014 Jun 19. PMID: 24948504; PMCID: PMC7966246. (Horwitz et al., 2016; Juhnke et al., 2021; Khan et al., 2021; Spence et al., 2014; von Hoff et al., 2021).
28. Shah AH, Khatib Z, Niazi T. Extracranial extra-CNS spread of embryonal tumor with multilayered rosettes (ETMR): case series and systematic review. Childs Nerv Syst. 2018;34(4):649–54. https://doi.org/10.1007/s00381-017-3657-x. Epub 2017 Nov 25. PMID: 29177676.
29. Mayr L, Gojo J, Peyrl A, Azizi AA, Stepien NM, Pletschko T, Czech T, Dorfer C, Lambo S, Dieckmann K, Haberler C, Kool M, Slavc I. Potential importance of early focal radiotherapy following gross Total resection for long-term survival in children with embryonal tumors with multilayered rosettes. Front Oncol. 2020;10:584681. https://doi.org/10.3389/fonc.2020.584681. PMID: 33392079; PMCID: PMC7773839.
30. Mozes P, Hauser P, Hortobágyi T, Benyó G, Peták I, Garami M, Cserháti A, Bartyik K, Bognár L, Nagy Z, Turányi E, Hideghéty K. Evaluation of the good tumor response of embryonal tumor with abundant neuropil and true rosettes (ETANTR). J Neuro-Oncol. 2016;126(1):99–105. https://doi.org/10.1007/s11060-015-1938-3. Epub 2015 Sep 15. PMID: 26373296.
31. Jaramillo S, Grosshans DR, Philip N, Varan A, Akyüz C, McAleer MF, Mahajan A, McGovern SL. Radiation for ETMR: literature review and case series of patients treated with proton therapy. Clin Transl Radiat Oncol. 2018;15:31–7. https://doi.org/10.1016/j.ctro.2018.11.002. PMID: 30582019; PMCID: PMC6297264.
32. Alexiou GA, Stefanaki K, Vartholomatos G, Sfakianos G, Prodromou N, Moschovi M. Embryonal tumor with abundant neuropil and true rosettes: a systematic literature review and report of 2 new cases. J Child Neurol. 2013;28(12):1709–15.
33. Schmidt C, Schubert NA, Brabetz S, Mack N, Schwalm B, Chan JA, Selt F, Herold-Mende C, Witt O, Milde T, Pfister SM, Korshunov A, Kool M. Preclinical drug screen reveals topotecan, actinomycin D, and volasertib as potential new therapeutic candidates for ETMR brain tumor patients. Neuro-Oncology. 2017;19(12):1607–17. https://doi.org/10.1093/neuonc/nox093. PMID: 28482026; PMCID: PMC5716199.
34. Neumann JE, Wefers AK, Lambo S, Bianchi E, Bockstaller M, Dorostkar MM, Meister V, Schindler P, Korshunov A, von Hoff K, Nowak J, Warmuth-Metz M, Schneider MR, Renner-Müller I, Merk DJ, Shakarami M, Sharma T, Chavez L, Glass R, Chan JA, Taketo MM, Neumann P, Kool M, Schüller U. A mouse model for embryonal tumors with multilayered rosettes uncovers the therapeutic potential of sonic-hedgehog inhibitors. Nat Med. 2017;23(10):1191–22. https://doi.org/10.1038/nm.4402. Epub 2017 Sep 11. PMID: 28892064.
35. Hanson D, Hoffman LM, Nagabushan S, Goumnerova LC, Rathmann A, Vogel T, Ziegler DS, Chi S. A modified IRS-III chemotherapy regimen leads to prolonged survival in children with embryonal tumor with multilayer rosettes. Neuro-oncol Adv. 2020;2(1):vdaa120. https://doi.org/10.1093/noajnl/vdaa120. PMID: 33196040; PMCID: PMC7648589.
36. Bailey K, Pandit-Taskar N, Humm JL, Zanzonico P, Gilheeney S, Cheung NV, Kramer K. Targeted radioimmunotherapy for embryonal tumor with multilay-

ered rosettes. J Neuro-Oncol. 2019;143(1):101–6. https://doi.org/10.1007/s11060-019-03139-6. Epub 2019 Mar 16. PMID: 30879172; PMCID: PMC7416633
37. Hartman LLR, Oaxaca DM, Carcamo B, Wilson HL, Ross JA, Robles-Escajeda E, Kirken RA. Integration of a personalized molecular targeted therapy into the multimodal treatment of refractory childhood embryonal tumor with multilayered rosettes (ETMR). Case Rep Oncol. 2019;12(1):211–7. https://doi.org/10.1159/000497380. PMID: 31011318; PMCID: PMC6465683.
38. Tietze A, Mankad K, Lequin MH, Ivarsson L, Mirsky D, Jaju A, Kool M, Hoff KV, Bison B, Löbel U. Imaging characteristics of CNS neuroblastoma-*FOXR2*: a retrospective and multi-institutional description of 25 cases. AJNR Am J Neuroradiol. 2022;43(10):1476–80. https://doi.org/10.3174/ajnr.A7644. Epub 2022 Sep 22. PMID: 36137662; PMCID: PMC9575542.
39. Łastowska M, Trubicka J, Sobocińska A, Wojtas B, Niemira M, Szałkowska A, Krętowski A, Karkucińska-Więckowska A, Kaleta M, Ejmont M, Perek-Polnik M, Dembowska-Bagińska B, Grajkowska W, Matyja E. Molecular identification of CNS NB-FOXR2, CNS EFT-CIC, CNS HGNET-MN1 and CNS HGNET-BCOR pediatric brain tumors using tumor-specific signature genes. Acta Neuropathol Commun. 2020;8(1):105. https://doi.org/10.1186/s40478-020-00984-9. PMID: 32650833; PMCID: PMC7350623.
40. Holsten T, Lubieniecki F, Spohn M, Mynarek M, Bison B, Löbel U, Rutkowski S, Schüller U. Detailed clinical and histopathological description of 8 cases of molecularly defined CNS Neuroblastomas. J Neuropathol Exp Neurol. 2021;80(1):52–9. https://doi.org/10.1093/jnen/nlaa128. PMID: 33270865.
41. PDQ Pediatric Treatment Editorial Board. Childhood medulloblastoma and other central nervous system embryonal tumors treatment (PDQ®): Patient Version. 2024 Mar 1. In: PDQ Cancer Information Summaries [Internet]. Bethesda: National Cancer Institute (US); 2002. PMID: 26389401.
42. Mynarek M, von Hoff K, Pietsch T, Ottensmeier H, Warmuth-Metz M, Bison B, Pfister S, Korshunov A, Sharma T, Jaeger N, Ryzhova M, Zheludkova O, Golanov A, Rushing EJ, Hasselblatt M, Koch A, Schüller U, von Deimling A, Sahm F, Sill M, Riemenschneider MJ, Dohmen H, Monoranu CM, Sommer C, Staszewski O, Mawrin C, Schittenhelm J, Brück W, Filipski K, Hartmann C, Meinhardt M, Pietschmann K, Haberler C, Slavc I, Gerber NU, Grotzer M, Benesch M, Schlegel PG, Deinlein F, von Bueren AO, Friedrich C, Juhnke BO, Obrecht D, Fleischhack G, Kwiecien R, Faldum A, Kortmann RD, Kool M, Rutkowski S. Nonmetastatic medulloblastoma of early childhood: results from the prospective clinical trial HIT-2000 and an extended validation cohort. J Clin Oncol. 2020;38(18):2028–40. https://doi.org/10.1200/JCO.19.03057. Epub 2020 Apr 24. PMID: 32330099.
43. Upadhyaya SA, Robinson GW, Onar-Thomas A, Orr BA, Johann P, Wu G, Billups CA, Tatevossian RG, Dhanda SK, Srinivasan A, Broniscer A, Qaddoumi I, Vinitsky A, Armstrong GT, Bendel AE, Hassall T, Partap S, Fisher PG, Crawford JR, Chintagumpala M, Bouffet E, Gururangan S, Mostafavi R, Sanders RP, Klimo P Jr, Patay Z, Indelicato DJ, Nichols KE, Boop FA, Merchant TE, Kool M, Ellison DW, Gajjar A. Relevance of molecular groups in children with newly diagnosed atypical Teratoid Rhabdoid tumor: results from prospective St. Jude multi-institutional trials. Clin Cancer Res. 2021;27(10):2879–89. https://doi.org/10.1158/1078-0432.CCR-20-4731. Epub 2021 Mar 18. PMID: 33737307; PMCID: PMC8127412
44. Ashley DM, Merchant TE, Strother D, Zhou T, Duffner P, Burger PC, Miller DC, Lyon N, Bonner MJ, Msall M, Buxton A, Geyer R, Kun LE, Coleman L, Pollack IF. Induction chemotherapy and conformal radiation therapy for very young children with nonmetastatic medulloblastoma: Children's Oncology Group study P9934. J Clin Oncol. 2012;30(26):3181–6. https://doi.org/10.1200/JCO.2010.34.4341. Epub 2012 Jul 30. PMID: 22851568; PMCID: PMC3434977.
45. Wong MK, Ng CCY, Kuick CH, Aw SJ, Rajasegaran V, Lim JQ, Sudhanshi J, Loh E, Yin M, Ma J, Zhang Z, Iyer P, Loh AHP, Lian DWQ, Wang S, Goh SGH, Lim TH, Lim AST, Ng T, Goytain A, Loh AHL, Tan PH, Teh BT, Chang KTE. Clear cell sarcomas of the kidney are characterised by BCOR gene abnormalities, including exon 15 internal tandem duplications and BCOR-CCNB3 gene fusion. Histopathology. 2018;72(2):320–9. https://doi.org/10.1111/his.13366. Epub 2017 Oct 30. PMID: 28833375.
46. Mackay A, Burford A, Carvalho D, Izquierdo E, Fazal-Salom J, Taylor KR, Bjerke L, Clarke M, Vinci M, Nandhabalan M, Temelso S, Popov S, Molinari V, Raman P, Waanders AJ, Han HJ, Gupta S, Marshall L, Zacharoulis S, Vaidya S, Mandeville HC, Bridges LR, Martin AJ, Al-Sarraj S, Chandler C, Ng HK, Li X, Mu K, Trabelsi S, Brahim DH, Kisljakov AN, Konovalov DM, Moore AS, Carcaboso AM, Sunol M, de Torres C, Cruz O, Mora J, Shats LI, Stavale JN, Bidinotto LT, Reis RM, Entz-Werle N, Farrell M, Cryan J, Crimmins D, Caird J, Pears J, Monje M, Debily MA, Castel D, Grill J, Hawkins C, Nikbakht H, Jabado N, Baker SJ, Pfister SM, Jones DTW, Fouladi M, von Bueren AO, Baudis M, Resnick A, Jones C. Integrated molecular meta-analysis of 1,000 pediatric high-grade and diffuse intrinsic pontine glioma. Cancer Cell. 2017;32(4):520–537.e5. https://doi.org/10.1016/j.ccell.2017.08.017. Epub 2017 Sep 28. PMID: 28966033; PMCID: PMC5637314.
47. Northcott PA, Buchhalter I, Morrissy AS, Hovestadt V, Weischenfeldt J, Ehrenberger T, Gröbner S, Segura-Wang M, Zichner T, Rudneva VA, Warnatz HJ, Sidiropoulos N, Phillips AH, Schumacher S, Kleinheinz K, Waszak SM, Erkek S, Jones DTW, Worst BC, Kool M, Zapatka M, Jäger N, Chavez L, Hutter B, Bieg M, Paramasivam N, Heinold M, Gu Z,

Ishaque N, Jäger-Schmidt C, Imbusch CD, Jugold A, Hübschmann D, Risch T, Amstislavskiy V, Gonzalez FGR, Weber UD, Wolf S, Robinson GW, Zhou X, Wu G, Finkelstein D, Liu Y, Cavalli FMG, Luu B, Ramaswamy V, Wu X, Koster J, Ryzhova M, Cho YJ, Pomeroy SL, Herold-Mende C, Schuhmann M, Ebinger M, Liau LM, Mora J, McLendon RE, Jabado N, Kumabe T, Chuah E, Ma Y, Moore RA, Mungall AJ, Mungall KL, Thiessen N, Tse K, Wong T, Jones SJM, Witt O, Milde T, Von Deimling A, Capper D, Korshunov A, Yaspo ML, Kriwacki R, Gajjar A, Zhang J, Beroukhim R, Fraenkel E, Korbel JO, Brors B, Schlesner M, Eils R, Marra MA, Pfister SM, Taylor MD, Lichter P. The whole-genome landscape of medulloblastoma subtypes. Nature. 2017;547(7663):311–7. https://doi.org/10.1038/nature22973. PMID: 28726821; PMCID: PMC5905700.

48. Haberler C, Reiniger L, Rajnai H, Kalev O, Gelpi E, Tamesberger M, Pietsch T. Case of the month 1-2019: CNS high-grade neuroepithelial tumor with *BCOR* alteration. Clin Neuropathol. 2019;38(1):4–7. https://doi.org/10.5414/NP301162. PMID: 30526817; PMCID: PMC6350233.
49. Mardi L, Tauziède-Espariat A, Guillemot D, Pierron G, Gigant P, Mehdi L, Berthaud C, Pucelle N, Lacombe J, Hasty L, Wahler E, Chrétien F, Lechapt E, Varlet P. BCOR immunohistochemistry, but not SATB2 immunohistochemistry, is a sensitive and specific diagnostic biomarker for central nervous system tumours with BCOR internal tandem duplication. Histopathology. 2021;79(5):891–4. https://doi.org/10.1111/his.14439. Epub 2021 Sep 20. PMID: 34196010.
50. Yoshida Y, Nobusawa S, Nakata S, Nakada M, Arakawa Y, Mineharu Y, Sugita Y, Yoshioka T, Araki A, Sato Y, Takeshima H, Okada M, Nishi A, Yamazaki T, Kohashi K, Oda Y, Hirato J, Yokoo H. CNS high-grade neuroepithelial tumor with BCOR internal tandem duplication: a comparison with its counterparts in the kidney and soft tissue. Brain Pathol. 2018;28(5):710–20. https://doi.org/10.1111/bpa.12585. Epub 2017 Dec 28. PMID: 29226988; PMCID: PMC8028450.
51. Kenny C, Bausenwein S, Lazaro A, Furtwängler R, Gooskens SL, van den Heuvel EM, Vokuhl C, Leuschner I, Graf N, Gessler M, O'Sullivan MJ. Mutually exclusive BCOR internal tandem duplications and YWHAE-NUTM2 fusions in clear cell sarcoma of kidney: not the full story. J Pathol. 2016;238(5):617–20. https://doi.org/10.1002/path.4693. PMID: 27000436.
52. Torre M, Meredith DM, Dubuc A, Solomon DA, Perry A, Vasudevaraja V, Serrano J, Snuderl M, Ligon KL, Alexandrescu S. Recurrent EP300-BCOR fusions in pediatric gliomas with distinct clinicopathologic features. J Neuropathol Exp Neurol. 2019;78(4):305–14. https://doi.org/10.1093/jnen/nlz011. PMID: 30816933.
53. Tauziède-Espariat A, Pierron G, Siegfried A, Guillemot D, Uro-Coste E, Nicaise Y, Castel D, Catalaa I, Larrieu-Ciron D, Chaynes P, de Barros A, Nicolau J, Gareton A, Lechapt E, Chrétien F, Bourdeaut F, Doz F, Bouchoucha Y, Grill J, Beccaria K, Boddaert N, Saffroy R, Pagès M, Varlet P. The EP300:BCOR fusion extends the genetic alteration spectrum defining the new tumoral entity of "CNS tumors with BCOR internal tandem duplication". Acta Neuropathol Commun. 2020;8(1):178. https://doi.org/10.1186/s40478-020-01064-8. PMID: 33138864; PMCID: PMC7607816.
54. De Lima L, Sürme MB, Gessi M, Mastronuzzi A, Miele E, Tamburrini G, Massimi L. Central nervous system high-grade neuroepithelial tumor with BCOR alteration (CNS HGNET-BCOR)-case-based reviews. Childs Nerv Syst. 2020;36(8):1589–99. https://doi.org/10.1007/s00381-020-04692-6. Epub 2020 Jun 15. PMID: 32542405.
55. Ferris SP, Velazquez Vega J, Aboian M, Lee JC, Van Ziffle J, Onodera C, Grenert JP, Saunders T, Chen YY, Banerjee A, Kline CN, Gupta N, Raffel C, Samuel D, Ruiz-Diaz I, Magaki S, Wilson D, Neltner J, Al-Hajri Z, Phillips JJ, Pekmezci M, Bollen AW, Tihan T, Schniederjan M, Cha S, Perry A, Solomon DA. High-grade neuroepithelial tumor with BCOR exon 15 internal tandem duplication-a comprehensive clinical, radiographic, pathologic, and genomic analysis. Brain Pathol. 2020;30(1):46–62. https://doi.org/10.1111/bpa.12747. Epub 2019 Jun 10. PMID: 31104347; PMCID: PMC6859193
56. Kirkman MA, Pickles JC, Fairchild AR, Avery A, Pietsch T, Jacques TS, Aquilina K. Early wound site seeding in a patient with central nervous system high-grade Neuroepithelial tumor with BCOR alteration. World Neurosurg. 2018;116:279–84. https://doi.org/10.1016/j.wneu.2018.05.158. Epub 2018 May 30. PMID: 29859355.
57. Paret C, Theruvath J, Russo A, Kron B, El Malki K, Lehmann N, Wingerter A, Neu MA, Gerhold-Ay A, Wagner W, Sommer C, Pietsch T, Seidmann L, Faber J. Activation of the basal cell carcinoma pathway in a patient with CNS HGNET-BCOR diagnosis: consequences for personalized targeted therapy. Oncotarget. 2016;7(50):83378–91. https://doi.org/10.18632/oncotarget.13092. PMID: 27825128; PMCID: PMC5347776.
58. Bremer J, Kottke R, Johann PD, von Hoff K, Brazzola P, Grotzer MA, Kool M, Rushing E, Gerber NU. A single supratentorial high-grade neuroepithelial tumor with two distinct BCOR mutations, exceptionally long complete remission and survival. Pediatr Blood Cancer. 2020;67(7):e28384. https://doi.org/10.1002/pbc.28384. Epub 2020 May 8. PMID: 32383815.
59. Burford A, Mackay A, Popov S, Vinci M, Carvalho D, Clarke M, Izquierdo E, Avery A, Jacques TS, Ingram WJ, Moore AS, Frawley K, Hassall TE, Robertson T, Jones C. The ten-year evolutionary trajectory of a highly recurrent paediatric high grade neuroepithelial tumour with MN1:BEND2 fusion. Sci Rep. 2018;8(1):1032. https://doi.org/10.1038/s41598-018-19389-9. PMID: 29348602; PMCID: PMC5773598.

60. Zhang ZH, Lin MT, Chen L. Editorial: molecular advances in diagnosis and treatment of CNS tumors. Front Oncol. 2020;10:590293. https://doi.org/10.3389/fonc.2020.590293. PMID: 33102240; PMCID: PMC7546907.
61. Hwang EI, Kool M, Burger PC, Capper D, Chavez L, Brabetz S, Williams-Hughes C, Billups C, Heier L, Jaju A, Michalski J, Li Y, Leary S, Zhou T, von Deimling A, Jones DTW, Fouladi M, Pollack IF, Gajjar A, Packer RJ, Pfister SM, Olson JM. Extensive molecular and clinical heterogeneity in patients with histologically diagnosed CNS-PNET treated as a single entity: a report from the children's oncology group randomized ACNS0332 trial. J Clin Oncol. 2018;36(34):JCO2017764720. https://doi.org/10.1200/JCO.2017.76.4720. Epub ahead of print. PMID: 30332335; PMCID: PMC9153369.
62. Kamihara J, Paulson V, Breen MA, Laetsch TW, Rakheja D, Shulman DS, Schoettler ML, Clinton CM, Ward A, Reidy D, Pinches RS, Weiser DA, Mullen EA, Schienda J, Meyers PA, DuBois SG, Nowak JA, Foulkes WD, Schultz KAP, Janeway KA, Vargas SO, Church AJ. DICER1-associated central nervous system sarcoma in children: comprehensive clinicopathologic and genetic analysis of a newly described rare tumor. Mod Pathol. 2020;33(10):1910–21. https://doi.org/10.1038/s41379-020-0516-1. Epub 2020 Apr 14. PMID: 32291395.
63. Diaz Coronado RY, Mynarek M, Koelsche C, Mora Alferez P, Casavilca Zambrano S, Wachtel Aptowitzer A, Sahm F, von Deimling A, Schüller U, Spohn M, Sturm D, Pfister SM, Morales La Madrid A, Sernaque Quintana R, Sarria Bardales G, Negreiros Chinchihuara T, Ojeda Medina L, Garcia-Corrochano Medina P, Campos Sanchez DA, Ponce Farfan J, Rutkowski S, Garcia Leon JL. Primary central nervous system sarcoma with DICER1 mutation-treatment results of a novel molecular entity in pediatric Peruvian patients. Cancer. 2022;128(4):697–707. https://doi.org/10.1002/cncr.33977. Epub 2021 Oct 21. PMID: 34674226.
64. Koelsche C, Mynarek M, Schrimpf D, Bertero L, Serrano J, Sahm F, Reuss DE, Hou Y, Baumhoer D, Vokuhl C, Flucke U, Petersen I, Brück W, Rutkowski S, Zambrano SC, Garcia Leon JL, Diaz Coronado RY, Gessler M, Tirado OM, Mora J, Alonso J, Garcia Del Muro X, Esteller M, Sturm D, Ecker J, Milde T, Pfister SM, Korshunov A, Snuderl M, Mechtersheimer G, Schüller U, Jones DTW, von Deimling A. Primary intracranial spindle cell sarcoma with rhabdomyosarcoma-like features share a highly distinct methylation profile and DICER1 mutations. Acta Neuropathol. 2018;136(2):327–37. https://doi.org/10.1007/s00401-018-1871-6. Epub 2018 Jun 7. PMID: 29881993.
65. Lee JC, Villanueva-Meyer JE, Ferris SP, Sloan EA, Hofmann JW, Hattab EM, Williams BJ, Guo H, Torkildson J, Florez A, Van Ziffle J, Onodera C, Grenert JP, Cho SJ, Horvai AE, Jones DTW, Pfister SM, Koelsche C, von Deimling A, Korshunov A, Perry A, Solomon DA. Primary intracranial sarcomas with DICER1 mutation often contain prominent eosinophilic cytoplasmic globules and can occur in the setting of neurofibromatosis type 1. Acta Neuropathol. 2019;137(3):521–5. https://doi.org/10.1007/s00401--019-01960-x. Epub 2019 Jan 16. PMID: 30649606; PMCID: PMC6408274.
66. Schweizer L, Hartmann W, Koch A, Nunninger M, Thomale UW, Pennacchietti V, Tietze A, Horn D, Pajtler KW, Hirsch S, Wieland I, Deubzer H, Rossi R, Driever PH, von Hoff K, von Zezschwitz B. Evidence of neural crest cell origin of a DICER1 mutant CNS sarcoma in a child with DICER1 syndrome and NRAS-mutant neurocutaneous melanosis. Neuropathol Appl Neurobiol. 2022;48(6):e12830. https://doi.org/10.1111/nan.12830. Epub 2022 Jul 5. PMID: 35728810.
67. Bielle F, Zanello M, Guillemot D, Gil-Delgado M, Bertrand A, Boch AL, Fréneaux P, Mokhtari K. Unusual primary cerebral localization of a CIC-DUX4 translocation tumor of the Ewing sarcoma family. Acta Neuropathol. 2014;128(2):309–11. https://doi.org/10.1007/s00401-014-1312-0. Epub 2014 Jul 1. PMID: 24980961.
68. Yamada S, Muto J, De Leon JCA, Kumai T, Ito K, Murayama K, Hama N, Nakano Y, Satomi K, Arai Y, Shibata T, Inoue T, Nobusawa S, Ichimura K, Hirose Y, Abe M. Primary spinal intramedullary Ewing-like sarcoma harboring CIC-DUX4 translocation: a similar cytological appearance as its soft tissue counterpart but no lobulation in association with desmoplastic stroma. Brain Tumor Pathol. 2020;37(3):111–7. https://doi.org/10.1007/s10014-020-00366-y. Epub 2020 May 24. PMID: 32449046.
69. Donahue JE, Yakirevich E, Zhong S, Treaba DO, Lakis NS, Ali SM, de la Monte SM, Mangray S. Primary Spinal Epidural CIC-DUX4 Undifferentiated Sarcoma in a Child. Pediatr Dev Pathol. 2018;21(4):411–7. https://doi.org/10.1177/1093526617707856. Epub 2017 May 5. PMID: 28474974; PMCID: PMC5575979.
70. Kawamura-Saito M, Yamazaki Y, Kaneko K, Kawaguchi N, Kanda H, Mukai H, Gotoh T, Motoi T, Fukayama M, Aburatani H, Takizawa T, Nakamura T. Fusion between CIC and DUX4 up-regulates PEA3 family genes in Ewing-like sarcomas with t(4;19)(q35;q13) translocation. Hum Mol Genet. 2006;15(13):2125–37. https://doi.org/10.1093/hmg/ddl136. Epub 2006 May 22. PMID: 16717057.
71. Antonescu CR, Owosho AA, Zhang L, Chen S, Deniz K, Huryn JM, Kao YC, Huang SC, Singer S, Tap W, Schaefer IM, Fletcher CD. Sarcomas with CIC-rearrangements are a distinct pathologic entity with aggressive outcome: a clinicopathologic and molecular study of 115 cases. Am J Surg Pathol. 2017;41(7):941–9. https://doi.org/10.1097/PAS.0000000000000846. PMID: 28346326; PMCID: PMC5468475.
72. Le Loarer F, Pissaloux D, Watson S, Godfraind C, Galmiche-Rolland L, Silva K, Mayeur L, Italiano A,

Michot A, Pierron G, Vasiljevic A, Ranchère-Vince D, Coindre JM, Tirode F. Clinicopathologic features of CIC-NUTM1 sarcomas, a new molecular variant of the family of CIC-fused sarcomas. Am J Surg Pathol. 2019;43(2):268–76. https://doi.org/10.1097/PAS.0000000000001187. PMID: 30407212.

73. Siegfried A, Masliah-Planchon J, Roux FE, Larrieu-Ciron D, Pierron G, Nicaise Y, Gambart M, Catalaa I, Péricart S, Dubucs C, Mohand-Oumoussa B, Tirode F, Bourdeaut F, Uro-Coste E. Brain tumor with an ATXN1-NUTM1 fusion gene expands the histologic spectrum of NUTM1-rearranged neoplasia. Acta Neuropathol Commun. 2019;7(1):220. https://doi.org/10.1186/s40478-019-0870-8. PMID: 31888756; PMCID: PMC6937844.
74. Pratt D, Kumar-Sinha C, Cieślik M, Mehra R, Xiao H, Shao L, Franson A, Cantor E, Chinnaiyan AM, Mody R, Abdullaev Z, Aldape K, Quezado M, Camelo-Piragua S. A novel ATXN1-DUX4 fusion expands the spectrum of 'CIC-rearranged sarcoma' of the CNS to include non-CIC alterations. Acta Neuropathol. 2021;141(4):619–22.https://doi.org/10.1007/s00401--021-02278-3. Epub 2021 Feb 7. PMID: 33550509.
75. Inagaki T, Iwasaki S, Matsumura Y, Kawamura T, Tanaka T, Abe Y, Yamasaki A, Tsurutani Y, Yoshida A, Chikaoka Y, Nakamura K, Magoori K, Nakaki R, Osborne TF, Fukami K, Aburatani H, Kodama T, Sakai J. The FBXL10/KDM2B scaffolding protein associates with novel polycomb repressive complex-1 to regulate adipogenesis. J Biol Chem. 2015;290(7):4163–77. https://doi.org/10.1074/jbc.M114.626929. Epub 2014 Dec 22. PMID: 25533466; PMCID: PMC4326826.
76. Owosho AA, Estilo CL, Huryn JM, Zhang L, Fletcher CDM, Antonescu CR. Head and neck round cell sarcomas: a comparative clinicopathologic analysis of 2 molecular subsets: Ewing and CIC-rearranged sarcomas. Head Neck Pathol. 2017;11(4):450–9. https://doi.org/10.1007/s12105-017-0808-z. Epub 2017 Mar 23. PMID: 28337592; PMCID: PMC5796609
77. Koelsche C, Hartmann W, Schrimpf D, Stichel D, Jabar S, Ranft A, Reuss DE, Sahm F, Jones DTW, Bewerunge-Hudler M, Trautmann M, Klingebiel T, Vokuhl C, Gessler M, Wardelmann E, Petersen I, Baumhoer D, Flucke U, Antonescu C, Esteller M, Fröhling S, Kool M, Pfister SM, Mechtersheimer G, Dirksen U, von Deimling A. Array-based DNA-methylation profiling in sarcomas with small blue round cell histology provides valuable diagnostic information. Mod Pathol. 2018;31(8):1246–56. https://doi.org/10.1038/s41379-018-0045-3. Epub 2018 Mar 23. PMID: 29572501; PMCID: PMC7484949
78. Hu W, Wang J, Yuan L, Zhang X, Ji Y, Song C, Zeng J, Sun X. Case report: a unique case of pediatric central nervous system Embryonal tumor harboring the *CIC-LEUTX* fusion, germline *NBN* variant and somatic *TSC2* mutation: expanding the Spectrum of *CIC*-rearranged neoplasia. Front Oncol. 2020;10:598970. https://doi.org/10.3389/fonc.2020.598970. PMID: 33344249; PMCID: PMC7738346.
79. Yamada S, Muto J, De Leon JCA, Kumai T, Ito K, Murayama K, Hama N, Nakano Y, Satomi K, Donahue JE, Yakirevich E, Zhong S, Treaba DO, Lakis NS, Ali SM, de la Monte SM, Mangray S. Primary spinal epidural CIC-DUX4 undifferentiated sarcoma in a child. Pediatr Dev Pathol. 2018;21(4):411–7. https://doi.org/10.1177/1093526617707856. Epub 2017 May 5. PMID: 28474974; PMCID: PMC5575979.
80. Ito M, Ishikawa M, Kitajima M, Narita J, Hattori S, Endo O, Goto K. A case report of CIC-rearranged undifferentiated small round cell sarcoma in the cerebrum. Diagn Cytopathol. 2016;44(10):828–32. https://doi.org/10.1002/dc.23520. Epub 2016 Jun 21. PMID: 27324529.
81. Yamasaki K, Nakano Y, Nobusawa S, Okuhiro Y, Fukushima H, Inoue T, Murakami C, Hirato J, Kunihiro N, Matsusaka Y, Honda-Kitahara M, Ozawa T, Shiraishi K, Kohno T, Ichimura K, Hara J. Spinal cord astroblastoma with an EWSR1-BEND2 fusion classified as a high-grade neuroepithelial tumour with MN1 alteration. Neuropathol Appl Neurobiol. 2020;46(2):190–3. https://doi.org/10.1111/nan.12593. Epub 2020 Jan 8. PMID: 31863478.
82. Lehman NL, Usubalieva A, Lin T, Allen SJ, Tran QT, Mobley BC, McLendon RE, Schniederjan MJ, Georgescu MM, Couce M, Dulai MS, Raisanen JM, Al Abbadi M, Palmer CA, Hattab EM, Orr BA. Genomic analysis demonstrates that histologically-defined astroblastomas are molecularly heterogeneous and that tumors with MN1 rearrangement exhibit the most favorable prognosis. Acta Neuropathol Commun. 2019;7(1):42. https://doi.org/10.1186/s40478-019-0689-3. PMID: 30876455; PMCID: PMC6419470.
83. Wood MD, Tihan T, Perry A, Chacko G, Turner C, Pu C, Payne C, Yu A, Bannykh SI, Solomon DA. Multimodal molecular analysis of astroblastoma enables reclassification of most cases into more specific molecular entities. Brain Pathol. 2018;28(2):192–202. https://doi.org/10.1111/bpa.12561. Epub 2017 Oct 27. PMID: 28960623; PMCID: PMC5843525.
84. Chen W, Soon YY, Pratiseyo PD, Sutanto R, Hendriansyah L, Kuick CH, Chang KTE, Tan CL. Central nervous system neuroepithelial tumors with MN1-alteration: an individual patient data meta-analysis of 73 cases. Brain Tumor Pathol. 2020;37(4):145–53. https://doi.org/10.1007/s10014--020-00372-0. Epub 2020 Jun 29. PMID: 32601775.
85. Navarro R, Reitman AJ, de León GA, Goldman S, Marymont M, Tomita T. Astroblastoma in childhood: pathological and clinical analysis. Childs Nerv Syst. 2005;21(3):211–20. https://doi.org/10.1007/s00381--004-1055-7. Epub 2005 Jan 15. PMID: 15654633.
86. Smith-Cohn MA, Abdullaev Z, Aldape KD, Quezado M, Rosenblum MK, Vanderbilt CM, Rodriguez FJ, Laterra J, Eberhart CG. Molecular clarification of brainstem astroblastoma with

EWSR1-BEND2 fusion in a 38-year-old man. Free Neuropathol. 2021;2:2–16. https://doi.org/10.17879/freeneuropathology-2021-3334. PMID: 37284624; PMCID: PMC10209864.
87. Baroni LV, Rugilo C, Lubieniecki F, Sampor C, Freytes C, Nobre L, Hansford JR, Malalasekera VS, Zapotocky M, Dodgshun A, Martinez OC, La Madrid AM, Lavarino C, Suñol M, Rutkowski S, Schuller U, Bouffet E, Ramaswamy V, Alderete D. Treatment response of CNS high-grade neuroepithelial tumors with MN1 alteration. Pediatr Blood Cancer. 2020;67(12):e28627. https://doi.org/10.1002/pbc.28627. Epub 2020 Sep 22. PMID: 32959992.
88. Stupp R, Mason WP, van den Bent MJ, Weller M, Fisher B, Taphoorn MJ, Belanger K, Brandes AA, Marosi C, Bogdahn U, Curschmann J, Janzer RC, Ludwin SK, Gorlia T, Allgeier A, Lacombe D, Cairncross JG, Eisenhauer E, Mirimanoff RO. European Organisation for Research and Treatment of Cancer brain tumor and radiotherapy groups; National Cancer Institute of Canada clinical trials group. Radiotherapy plus concomitant and adjuvant temozolomide for glioblastoma. N Engl J Med. 2005;352(10):987–96. https://doi.org/10.1056/NEJMoa043330. PMID: 15758009.
89. Das S, Gupta D, Dan Charan B, Sahu S, Suri V, Garg A, Tandon V, Suri A, Sharma MC. Astroblastoma: a molecularly defined entity, its clinico-radiological & pathological analysis of eight cases and review of literature. Pathol Res Pract. 2024;263:155616. https://doi.org/10.1016/j.prp.2024.155616. Epub 2024 Oct 11. PMID: 39413458.
90. Nakano Y, Nobusawa S, Sato-Otsubo A, Nakashima T, Suzuki H, Yamasaki K, Shirakura T, Inoue T, Okuno T, Kato M, Ichimura K, Sakamoto H. TCF3::BEND2 in paediatric supratentorial tumour with carcinoma-like epithelial features classifying as MN1-altered astroblastoma by DNA methylation profiling. Neuropathol Appl Neurobiol. 2024;50(5):e13011. https://doi.org/10.1111/nan.13011. PMID: 39434489.

Ependymoma

13

Maura Massimino, Pierre Leblond,
Piergiorgio Modena, and Sabina Vennarini

13.1 Introduction

Ependymomas are a significant cause of cancer-related deaths in childhood and adolescence, with recent advancements beginning to improve outcomes. These tumors, which can occur along the entire neuroaxis, represent a spectrum of glial tumors. According to the 2021 WHO classification of central nervous system (CNS) tumors, an integrated diagnosis requires a combination of histological and molecular features as well as tumor location [1].

Most ependymomas in children and adolescents are intracranial, with a peak incidence in children under 3 years of age [2]. Approximately 70% of these tumors are located in the infratentorial region, while supratentorial locations are less common. Leptomeningeal dissemination is rare, occurring in up to 10% of cases, but its frequency increases at recurrence [3, 4].

Ependymomas in the posterior fossa are divided into two molecular groups: posterior fossa group A (PFA) and posterior fossa group B (PFB), now recognized as distinct tumor types in WHO 2021 [5, 6]. Supratentorial ependymomas are primarily characterized by fusion genes involving the ZFTA gene (formerly C11orf95) and the RELA gene, with other fusion partners also identified [7]. Supratentorial ependymomas with YAP1 gene fusions are less common and predominantly occur in young children [8–10]. Beyond these four distinct tumor types, additional molecular subgroups exist, though their clinical implications require further assessment.

Molecular classification is increasingly important for ependymoma and will be critical for patient stratification in upcoming clinical trials. Identifying vulnerabilities in these tumors could lead to more diversified treatment options. In children and adolescents, ZFTA fusion-positive and PFA ependymomas make up the majority of intracranial cases, with PFA ependymomas associated with the poorest outcomes under current standard-of-care treatments.

Unlike in adults, spinal ependymomas in children and adolescents are rare. These include spinal intramedullary ependymomas, myxopapillary ependymomas, and MYCN-amplified spinal ependymomas, the latter being a particularly aggressive subtype characterized by high-grade histological features and MYCN proto-oncogene amplification and overexpression [11, 12].

M. Massimino (✉) · S. Vennarini
Fondazione IRCCS Istituto Nazionale dei tumori, Milan, Italy
e-mail: maura.massimino@istitutotumori.mi.it

P. Leblond
Department of Pediatric Oncology, Institute of Pediatric Hematology and Oncology (IHOPe), Centre Léon Bérard, Lyon, France

P. Modena
Genetics Unit, ASST Lariana, Como General Hospital, Como, Italy

A. Mastronuzzi, A. Carai (eds.), *Navigating Pediatric Brain Tumors*,
https://doi.org/10.1007/978-3-032-18992-9_13

13.2 Diagnosis and Staging

Medical history and examination at diagnosis are commonly used for any oncological patient, including and in particular those with brain tumors:

- Complete medical history.
- Vital signs and detailed physical examination, including pubertal stage and occipital circumference in infants.
- Complete neurological examination. The most common presentation is nonspecific and related to raised intracranial pressure from obstructive hydrocephalus or more chronic symptomatology as cranial nerve palsies or ataxia in intracranial ependymomas. Children with spinal ependymomas most commonly present with pain, scoliosis, and urinary symptoms.
- Neuropsychologic, educational psychologic, and neuropedagogic evaluation.
- Otolaryngologic evaluation.
- Ophthalmology assessment.

13.2.1 Imaging

Pre- and postsurgery MRIs should be performed according to European guidelines and RAPNO recommendations [13, 14]. Presurgery MRIs are needed for staging and surgical planning, while postsurgery imaging assesses the extent of resection and potential residuals. Postsurgery imaging should ideally be done within 24–48 h [15]. Risk stratification in the SIOP Ependymoma II trial is based on resection status assessed by central imaging review [16, 17].

13.2.2 Lumbar Puncture

A lumbar puncture should be performed to assess for microscopic disease (M1) in the CSF. If not done before surgery, it should be performed 2 weeks post-resection to avoid detecting cells from the surgical intervention. Recent studies propose to have a sample of CSF at time zero to check for possible molecular marker to be followed longitudinally.

13.2.3 Molecular and Histological Features for Diagnosis and Prognosis

The 2021 WHO classification of CNS tumors requires an integrated diagnosis combining histological and molecular features along with tumor location. Collaborative studies have identified 10 tumor types of ependymomas, with 7 occurring in pediatric/young adult patients. DNA methylation-based profiling can reliably identify all molecular groups. Gene fusions can be detected by sequencing methods, RT-PCR, interphase fluorescence in situ hybridization (FISH), next-generation sequencing, and molecular inversion profiling [18–23].

Supratentorial ependymomas with ZFTA or YAP1 fusions are distinct in their demarcation from adjacent brain tissue and are mainly composed of cells with round uniform nuclei and often clear cytoplasm. Pseudorosettes are uncommon, and true ependymal rosettes are rare. These tumors typically feature a network of branching capillary blood vessels, with calcified regions and necrosis being common. ZFTA-RELA fusion ependymomas show nuclear accumulation of p65 and universal cytoplasmic expression of L1CAM, while YAP1 fusion ependymomas do not express L1CAM or nuclear p65 [24, 25].

Outcome data for ZFTA fusion-positive ependymomas vary widely, and a homozygous deletion of CDKN2A is linked to poor prognosis [26–29]. YAP1 fusions can be identified using similar techniques and, despite their often large size at diagnosis, tend to have a favorable prognosis [30].

Posterior fossa ependymomas, in contrast, are circumscribed tumors composed of uniform small cells with indistinct cytoplasmic borders and round nuclei. These often present perivascular pseudorosettes, where tumor cells radially arrange around blood vessels, while true rosettes are rare. PFA ependymomas are characterized by reduced H3 K27-trimethylation, detectable via immunohistochemistry, which can efficiently discriminate PFA versus PFB tumors [9, 31, 32].

Myxopapillary ependymomas feature radially arranged cuboidal to elongated tumor cells around hyalinized fibrovascular cores, with myxoid material accumulation around blood vessels and in microcysts. Mitotic activity is generally low in these tumors. MYCN-amplified spinal ependymomas exhibit pseudorosettes and can have papillary or pseudopapillary architecture, often displaying anaplastic features [33].

Molecular groups of ependymal tumors show varying degrees of anaplasia and have traditionally been categorized as WHO CNS grade 2 or 3. However, the utility of grading for risk stratification remains controversial due to interobserver variability. Molecularly defined ependymomas have yet to be assigned a WHO grade based on prospective clinical trial data [34, 35]. Traditional histological variants, such as papillary, clear cell, or tanycytic ependymoma, are no longer considered distinct subtypes, though some patterns, like the clear cell pattern in ZFTA fusion-positive tumors, are associated with specific ependymoma types.

For PFA ependymomas, DNA methylation profiling and immunohistochemistry for H3 K27-trimethylation loss are diagnostic. PFA ependymomas and MYCN-amplified ependymomas have the poorest clinical outcomes, with PFA ependymomas frequently exhibiting chromosome 1q gain and 6q loss, correlating with very poor outcomes [36]. Conversely, PFB ependymomas generally have a favorable prognosis unless there is incomplete surgical resection or 13q loss [31, 32].

Spinal ependymomas can also be identified through DNA methylation profiling. Myxopapillary ependymomas are typically associated with a relatively favorable prognosis, though complete resection is often challenging, and pediatric patients may experience dissemination, especially in sacrococcygeal variants [37]. Spinal myxopapillary ependymomas are classified as WHO CNS grade II. MYCN-amplified spinal ependymomas are aggressive, with early metastasis and dissemination common, and poor progression-free or overall survival despite aggressive treatment.

The approach to diagnosing ependymoma has evolved from relying solely on histopathological examination with limited prognostic significance to incorporating molecular data for a more comprehensive diagnosis. This integrated approach is relatively new, and, due to the rarity of some molecular ependymoma subtypes, there are few studies correlating integrated pathology with clinical outcomes. These studies often focus on a small series of specific molecular types. A very recent report [38] analyzed data from 2023 ependymomas classified by DNA methylation profiling. By correlating methylation data with clinical information, an integrated model was developed to predict progression-free survival. Patients with EPN-PFA, EPN-ZFTA, and EPN-MYCN tumors had the poorest outcomes, with 10-year overall survival rates of 56%, 62%, and 32%, respectively. EPN-PFA tumors with chromosome 1q gains and/or 6q losses were associated with worse survival. In supratentorial EPN-ZFTA, a combined loss of CDKN2A and B indicated a poorer prognosis, while a single loss did not. Also, 12 out of 200 EPN-ZFTA cases (6%) were located in the posterior fossa and had earlier relapse or progression compared to supratentorial tumors with combined CDKN2A/B loss. Patients with myxopapillary ependymoma and PF-subependymoma, typically considered nonaggressive, had 10-year progression-free survival rates of 59% and 65%, respectively. For predicting 5-year progression-free survival, Kaplan–Meier estimators based on molecular subtype, a support vector machine using methylation data, and an integrated model combining clinical factors, CNV data, and predicted methylation scores achieved balanced accuracies of 66%, 68%, and 73%, respectively. Excluding samples with low prediction scores increased balanced accuracies to over 80%. Overall, this extensive analysis of ependymomas provided valuable insights into molecular characteristics and their clinical implications, especially for rare and understudied subtypes and seemingly benign variants that instead exhibited higher recurrence rates than previously thought.

Importantly, the integrated diagnostic approach incorporating both histopathological and molecular data allows both to resolve difficult diagnoses and to properly account for differential diagnoses in order to pinpoint distinct newly and/or poorly characterized molecular groups, such as supratentorial gliomas carrying receptor tyrosine kinase gene fusions, BCOR alteration, and PLAGL2 alteration [39].

In summary, the classification and prognosis of ependymomas have become increasingly reliant on molecular profiling, which not only aids in accurate diagnosis and in prognostic stratification but also will confidently help in developing targeted treatment strategies.

13.3 Treatment Strategies

Various international study groups have developed treatment strategies over the past decades, involving surgery, radiotherapy, and chemotherapy.

13.3.1 Recommendations

Patients should be treated in specialized pediatric oncology centers, ideally within clinical trials such as the SIOP Ependymoma II trial. Data collection within a registry is highly recommended for ongoing research and treatment optimization.

13.3.2 Surgery

Complete surgical resection is the mainstay of treatment and the most consistent prognostic factor. In case of residual disease, further surgery may be considered.

The extent of neurosurgical resection has been consistently reported as an independent prognostic factor over the past decades [40–42]. Patients without residual disease typically have more favorable outcomes, and there is a significant difference in event-free and overall survival between those with complete versus incomplete resection. This has led to the concept of more aggressive resections and even second-look surgeries when necessary.

Initial surgical decisions depend on tumor size, vascularity, and localization relative to functional eloquent structures, which are critical for risk stratification. Utilizing technical adjuncts such as microsurgery, neuronavigation, intraoperative neurophysiological monitoring, intraoperative imaging (ultrasound or MRI), and endoscopic assistance can optimize conditions for safe yet maximal tumor resection. In emergency situations, a two-staged surgical approach might be planned, allowing for a second elective intervention with full technical support [43, 44]. When residual disease is present, comprehensive radiological assessment of the residual tumor's size, location, and its relationship to relevant anatomical structures is crucial. Ideally, patients should be treated at specialized centers by experienced neurosurgeons who frequently handle pediatric brain tumor cases.

13.3.3 Radiotherapy

Adjuvant radiotherapy is associated with increased overall survival, especially with doses above 54 Gy. Local control is also improved with high-dose RT and the addition of hypofractionated boost at the level of residual disease. Other favorable prognostic factors include age greater than 3 years, female gender, absence of disease spread, and absence of extension to the cervical cord [45, 46].

For the pediatric radiation oncologists, the role of radiotherapy in the multidisciplinary treatment of ependymomas remains a significant therapeutic challenge, given the origin of this disease in anatomically critical regions due to the presence of vital organs, such as the brainstem, and the comorbidities associated with the neoplasm itself and the multiple surgeries sometimes performed [47]. Several studies confirm as a therapeutic standard the use of adjuvant radiotherapy after first-line surgery [48]. The data published in the literature demonstrate an overall survival (OS) rate and event-free survival (EFS) rate at 5 years of 86% and 55%, respectively [49–52]. However, the optimal target volume for radiotherapy, the total dose required to achieve local control, its fractionation, and the best delivery technique remain controversial topics and subjects of great debate in clinical radiotherapy research.

13.3.3.1 Irradiation Volume

The irradiation volume has long been the most debated topic. Studies published from the early 1980s to the late 1990s seemed to suggest that the survival of patients with ependymoma could improve after craniospinal irradiation (CSI) in cases of anaplastic ependymoma and whole-brain irradiation for low-grade forms [53].

Nevertheless, the predilection of ependymoma to give leptomeningeal metastatic dissemination in the order of 20% had led to the belief that the standard could be craniospinal irradiation [54–56]. Recent data, obtained in patients evaluated with advanced imaging techniques (such as MRI), have instead shown that, both in children with low-grade and high-grade ependymoma, the most frequent mode of recurrence was local and not disseminated [57].

In a review of the literature published between 1969 and 1989, Vanuytsel et al. [58] demonstrated that the incidence of spinal recurrence was 2.7% for low-grade supratentorial lesions, 5.5% for low-grade infratentorial lesions, and 0% and 15% for anaplastic lesions, respectively, supratentorial and infratentorial. Furthermore, the development of spinal recurrence was not influenced by the extent of the irradiated volumes. In fact, for low-grade tumors, the incidence of spinal recurrences was 2.2% and 9.3%, respectively, without and with prophylactic spinal irradiation, while the corresponding percentages for anaplastic lesions were 6.7% and 9.4%.

Two more recent retrospective studies have further emphasized that, even in cases of anaplastic histology, the most frequent site of recurrence is local. In particular, the German group that used sandwich chemotherapy and craniospinal radiotherapy for the anaplastic histotype did not provide data in favor of craniospinal irradiation even for this category of prognostically unfavorable patients, as 20 out of 25 recurrences occurred locally [59]. Therefore, avoiding a treatment of dubious utility for most patients, but with well-known long-term side effects, such as craniospinal irradiation, focal irradiation has become the standard in the irradiation of intracranial ependymoma [60].

For all patients, a radiation treatment limited to the gross tumor volume (GTV) is based on the postoperative MRI and includes the tumor bed at the primary site modified to include any residuum. Reference to the initial preoperative imaging assists in defining the extent of the tumor bed and the anatomically involved tissues. The clinical target volume (CTV) includes the GTV with a margin added to treat subclinical microscopic disease. Older protocols recommended an expansion of 1 cm from the GTV to the CTV [61].to ensure local disease control, but it is still a subject of deep debate in focal irradiation to determine the appropriate margin.

A publication from the St. Jude Children's Research Hospital group showed that the margin could be reduced while maintaining optimal local disease control, with a possible reduction in long-term neurocognitive effects [62]. Currently under investigation both in the United States with the not yet published COG ACNS0831 trial, and in Europe, with the SIOP Ependymoma II, is a reduction of the expansion from the GTV of 0.5 cm up to 54 Gy with no expansion allowed and reduction to 0.2–0.3 for the CTV of the boost up to 59.4 Gy if adjacent to organs at risk [63].

13.3.3.2 Radiation Dose

Most authors reported a trend toward better survival for total radiotherapy doses over 45–50 Gy.

The reference dose for radiotherapy in patients without macroscopic residual disease varies from a minimum of 54 Gy to a total of 59.4 Gy in 30–33 daily fractions of 1.8 Gy per fraction, treating 5 days per week, with the possibility of reducing the dose to 54 Gy or less if the tumor is close to the optic chiasm or cervical spinal cord [45, 64]. Very young patients or those undergoing multiple surgeries with tumors adjacent to the brainstem are considered at higher risk of developing brainstem toxicity and hence the total dose in these patients may be reduced to 54 Gy in 30 daily fractions [65].

For patients with aninoperable residuum following standard radiotherapy doses of 54–59.4 Gy, results from the second AEIOP study suggest that a highly conformal boost of 8 Gy in two consecutive daily fractions may lead to improved tumor control with acceptable toxicity. This strategy was tested in stratum 2 of the SIOP Ependymoma II study; the protocol has just closed for clinical enrollment for this specific arm [63].

13.3.3.3 New Radiotherapy Modalities

When we talk about new modalities in radiotherapy for the treatment of ependymoma, we notably refer to proton therapy in this era. Solid clinical data published in the literature have demonstrated the role of three-dimensional conformal radiotherapy (3D-CRT) [66, 67] compared to historical conformal radiotherapy [61].

With the diffusion of intensity-modulated radiation therapy (IMRT) in the 1990s, there was a significant step forward in the treatment of ependymoma. Some authors have shown that local control rates and overall survival were equivalent to the cohorts of patients published so far and introduced two new concepts: the better sparing of healthy tissues adjacent to the target and that the site of disease recurrence occurred in the high-dose volumes delivered during the first cycle of radiotherapy [61]. Proton therapy fits into this context due to its physical characteristics, which have long been known to ensure better sparing of healthy tissues with a lower integral dose distribution compared to photon therapy. Clinically, this translates into a reduced impact on side effects, particularly in the development of late toxicities, and a lower risk of secondary carcinogenesis due to less exposure to low-intensity doses of radiosensitive healthy tissues [68, 69]. Ependymoma is certainly one of the most common indications for proton therapy due to the young age of patients at tumor onset and the location in the posterior cranial fossa in 66% of patients [70–72]. Multiple dosimetric studies comparing protons versus modern photon therapy techniques (XRT) have been published in the literature.

MacDonald SM et al. [72] demonstrated that, in a comparison among IMRT and various proton techniques (3DCPT-IMPT) for infratentorial ependymomas, there was better sparing of the cochleae, the lower portion of the temporal lobes, and the healthy cerebellum. This study already showed in 2010 a clear superiority in the dosimetric conformation of the target with the use of intensity-modulated proton therapy (IMPT) compared to 3D-conformal proton radiation (3DCPT), with an additional dosimetric advantage for the critical organs near the target for the IMPT technique.

Three years later, the same group from Boston published the first clinical results on a series of 70 patients treated with protons, with a median follow-up of 46 months. The 3-year local control (LC), progression-free survival (PFS), and overall survival (OS) were 83%, 76%, and 95%, respectively [73].

Other major proton therapy groups in Europe and America published their series with outcome and toxicity results that were always very good and comparable to the cohorts of patients treated with modern photon techniques [74–76].

In the era of modern proton therapy, the group from Essen in Germany [77] recently published their experience on 105 patients with localized intracranial ependymoma. The data were collected prospectively in the "KiProReg registry study." The median age of patients at proton irradiation was 2.8 years (range 0.9–17.0 years). The median total dose delivered was 59.4 Gy RBE (relative biological effectiveness) (range 54.0–62.0 Gy). The median follow-up time was 1.9 years, with estimated 3-year OS, local control (LC), and PFS rates of 93.7%, 74.1%, and 55.6%, respectively.

In univariable analysis, female gender and lower dose had a positive impact on OS, whereas age ≥4 years had a negative impact on OS, and PT given after progression had a negative impact on PFS. In multivariable analysis, multiple surgeries at diagnosis were associated with lower PFS.

Regarding late adverse events, new higher-grade toxicities (CTCAE ≥3°) occurred in 11 patients. The authors concluded that PT is effective and well-tolerated and that multiple surgical interventions have a negative impact on PFS.

In 2022, the largest series of clinical results was made available by the University of Florida and Harvard Medical School in Boston [78]. The median RT dose of 55.8 Gy (RBE) resulted in a 7-year LC, PFS, and OS of 77.0%, 63.8%, and 82.2%, respectively. At a median follow-up of 5 years, late toxicity was remarkably low. Specifically, these are the reported late toxicity data: over grade 2 CTCAE brainstem toxicity was 4% and occurred more often in patients who received >54 Gy RBE. Two patients (0.5%) died of brainstem necrosis. The second malignancy occurrence rate was 0.8%. In conclusion, we can say that the widespread use of proton therapy in intracranial ependymomas of the posterior cranial fossa is not without challenges. For these diseases, sources published by the American groups indicate that doses higher than 54 Gy (RBE), although rarely used, can lead to brainstem radionecrosis phenomena that deserve greater attention in protons compared to photons [79].

This last concept remains controversial to date given the data published in Europe by the French group [80] in a very recent retrospective study that compared the incidence of brainstem damage in 83 patients treated respectively: 42 with PBT, 37 with XRT, and 4 with both at median doses of 59.4 Gy (range: 53–60 Gy). The conclusions of these authors were that asymptomatic radiographic changes occurred in 4.8% of patients with ependymoma and there was no correlation with dose or technique. No symptomatic brainstem injury was identified.

In conclusion, we can affirm that proton therapy, due to its established physical-dosimetric potential and the increase in the number of facilities installed worldwide, will allow us to collect and deepen with more "mature" clinical data the benefits and potential toxicities of proton therapy in these young patients [81].

13.3.3.4 Reirradiation for Pediatric Intracranial Ependymoma

Despite aggressive multimodality treatment, at least one-third of patients with ependymoma experience disease relapse, requiring further therapy [82]. The pattern of relapse is predominantly local (60–75%), with a lower incidence of distant relapse or both modalities. The median time to relapse is between 11 and 25 months, but relapse may occur later, although with a lower incidence. Long-term survival of children with relapsed ependymoma is poor, with 5-year progression-free survival (PFS) rates ranging from 17% to 45% and 5-year overall survival (OS) rates ranging from 27% to 57% [82].

The treatment for relapses is not well defined. In the absence of prospective data, local treatment with complete surgery and adjuvant radiotherapy is considered the best strategy. Retrospective nonrandomized studies have shown the feasibility of this approach and a possible OS benefit (Table X: reirradiation studies).

Several studies have confirmed that the extent of surgical resection also at recurrence is the most important prognostic factor. Adolph et al. showed a significant survival benefit in patients who underwent gross total resection (GTR) or near total resection (NTR) compared to subtotal resection (STR), with a median OS of 71 months compared to 20.6 months and a median PFS of 25.9 months compared to 9.2 months. In addition, in the cohort studied, patients with complete or near-complete resection showed no survival benefit from the addition of postoperative radiation therapy (median OS of 70 months vs. 95 months in patients receiving postoperative RT vs. surgery alone), while radiation therapy showed a survival benefit when given after subtotal resection (median OS of 22 months vs. 7 months) [83]. The results of this study are in contrast to those showing that reirradiation is an effective treatment regardless of the extent of resection and disease burden. For example, in the case series reviewed by Bouffet et al., a significant improvement in outcome was seen in patients who received radiotherapy both at initial diagnosis and at recurrence compared to those who did not receive radiotherapy, with a 3-year OS of 81% vs. 7%, respectively [84].

13.3.3.5 Radiotherapy Technique, Dose, Volume, and Fractionation

The modalities of optimal reirradiation are not yet well defined in terms of dose, fractionation, treatment technique, and volume.

Different studies have reported conflicting data on treatment with radiosurgery. Most groups reported good local control with a high rate of disease dissemination in subsequent recurrences, without a consistent survival benefit.

In the multivariate analysis by Desroussraux J et al., treatments that included stereotactic hypofractionated reirradiation were associated with a better outcome (for OS $P = 0.030$; for PFS $P = 0.008$) than the other techniques. The explanation could be twofold: on the one hand, stereotaxis results in direct damage at the level of the vessels, inducing endothelial apoptosis, and, on the other hand, 87% of the patients who underwent stereotactic treatment had undergone complete surgical resection, so the better prognosis could be due to a lower disease burden [85]. The French multicenter study by Regnier et al. showed improved survival in patients treated with hypofractionated RT, which proved to be a safe modality with low toxicity rates [86]. However, these data contrast with the case series reported by Hoffman, in which 6 of 12 patients treated with hypofractionated re-RT developed radionecrosis [48].

A preliminary study evaluated 20 patients treated with proton beam therapy (PBT) who were reirradiated at a median dose of 50.4 Gy. The PFS at 1 and 3 years after reirradiation was 66.5% and 28.1%, respectively. The 3-year OS was 79%, comparable to the existing series of photon-treated patients. Only one patient developed grade 3 toxicity related to disease progression. Thus, the data demonstrate the safety and efficacy of proton therapy for reirradiation of intracranial ependymoma, with favorable survival outcomes and the absence of severe toxicity related to the treatment. This is critical for reducing the risk of late sequelae and minimizing the cumulative dose to surrounding critical structures such as the brainstem and spinal cord [68].

Notably, the introduction of focal radiotherapy in the treatment of ependymoma relapses resulted in improved local control rates, with a reduction in further local recurrence and a relative increase in distant recurrences. In addition, the use of CSI at the time of recurrence showed increased survival rates. Although the risk of cognitive impairment associated with CSI is significant, results obtained after the use of this technique suggest a survival benefit [84, 87].

The association of local reirradiation with CSI has been discussed in the literature. Studies by Bouffet and Merchant showed an overall survival benefit with adjuvant CSI at a dose of 36 Gy [48, 87]. Tsang et al. showed that craniospinal irradiation in patients with local recurrence reduced the incidence of distant failure after re-RT compared with focal treatment alone, particularly in patients with 1q gain [88]. Messahel et al. [89] showed that CSI was associated with a survival benefit in children older than 3 years. The French cohort study did not show a significant benefit, but the number of patients treated with CSI was very small (four patients) and did not allow to make conclusions [86]. On the other hand, in the Italian cohort study, CSI was not indicated in patients with local recurrence. However, in the case series analyzed, only 6/27 patients with local recurrence developed distant metastases [90]. Therefore, the indications for CSI should be discussed individually, taking into account the expected benefit and toxicity, especially in younger children.

With regard to the dose, the studies are very heterogeneous. Messahel et al. showed a trend toward better local control in children who received more than 45 Gy. Bouffet et al. emphasized the importance of full-dose (54–59 Gy) reirradiation [84, 89].

13.3.3.6 Toxicity

Several studies have shown that reirradiation for intracranial ependymoma is a safe treatment that correlates with low-grade acute toxicity and reduced rates of late toxicity and radionecrosis.

Merchant et al. showed that radiosurgical treatment (with a median dose of 18 Gy) was associated with significant brainstem toxicity and death [87]. Only one case of asymptomatic radionecrosis was reported in the French cohort in a patient reirradiated with radiosurgery with a cumulative BED at a maximum dose of 185.7 Gy at the level of the brainstem [86]. Gupta et al. observed three cases of radionecrosis in patients with a cumulative BED greater than 110 GyEQD2 [91].

In addition, several cases of cerebellar ataxia were observed in the French study in patients with a cumulative dose to the posterior fossa greater than 117 GyEQD2 [86]. This highlights the importance of delineating the cerebellum as a distinct organ at risk and the importance of keeping cumulative doses at the level of brain tissue below 100–110 GyEQD2 whenever possible, thresholds at which a relatively low risk (less than 10%) of developing brain necrosis has been reported in the literature [92, 93]. Given the increased risk of radionecrosis and the small benefit in terms of local control and survival, radiosurgery appears to be indicated only for reirradiation of small residual tumors.

13.3.3.7 Prognostic Factors

Factors associated with improved survival include female gender, non-anaplastic histology at recurrence, longer recurrence-free interval after initial radiotherapy, and distant-only failure after initial RT [82].

Chromosome 1q gain is a negative prognostic factor in de novo ependymoma, and the study by Tsang et al. showed that chromosome 1q gain was also associated with poorer prognosis in patients with distant failure after RT, but not in those with local recurrence after initial RT. The authors hypothesized that 1q gain has prognostic value in tumor clonogenes that have not been previously irradiated, but that its prognostic significance is lost in patients with locally recurrent ependymoma who have been previously irradiated [82].

13.3.4 Chemotherapy

Unlike surgery and radiotherapy, the role of chemotherapy in managing ependymomas remains unproven despite extensive investigation [94–97]. For more details, see Table 13.1.

Retrospective analyses of pediatric patient cohorts have not demonstrated a survival advantage with chemotherapy despite selection of patients but without randomized questions. For more details, see Table 13.2.

Two international randomized trials are currently underway to provide more definitive answers about the role of chemotherapy in ependymoma treatment:

ACNS0831 (USA) [108] and SIOP Ependymoma II (Europe): Similar to ACNS0831, this trial is evaluating the efficacy of post-irradiation chemotherapy versus observation [63].

These trials aim to clarify whether adding chemotherapy after irradiation improves outcomes compared to simply observing the patients post-irradiation if completely operated on at diagnosis.

13.3.4.1 Spinal Ependymomas

Gross-total resection is the primary therapeutic approach for patients with primary spinal cord ependymomas, achieved in more than 50% of cases. The role of adjuvant treatment in improving progression-free or overall survival remains unclear [109–116]. Consequently, decisions regarding additional treatments at primary diagnosis should be tailored to the individual patient's situation, potentially considering the molecular group. Retrospective data suggest that MYCN-amplified ependymomas may benefit from aggressive treatment regimens [11, 12]. Patients with residual myxopapillary ependymomas seem to benefit from adjuvant radiotherapy [114–117]. For spinal ependymomas associated with neurofibromatosis type 2, surveillance without intervention is recommended unless clinical signs or symptoms are observed [118, 119].

13.3.5 Treatment for Relapses

Despite advancements in genetic characterization, treatment for childhood ependymoma has largely remained static. Notably, outcomes for children and adolescents with recurrent intracranial ependymoma continue to be poor, with the

Table 13.1 Summary of literature for infants with ependymoma

Protocol (period)	Treatments	Age (months)	No. of patients	2-year PFS [%]	5-year PFS [%]	2-year OS [%]	5-year OS [%]	Reference
$CCG992_1$ (1993–1997)	Induction: 5 cycles A: VCR/CDDP/CY/VP16 or B: VCR/CBDCA/IFO/VP16 Maintenance: 8 cycles VCR/VP16/CBDCA/CY RD or PD → RT	0–36	74	38	32	82	72	[98]
Head Start (1991–2002)	Induction: 5 cycles CDDP/VCR/VP16/CY ± MTX HD-CBDCA/TTT + VP16 and PBSC RT: If <3 years RD after treatment or >3 years + ST residue after treatment or >3 years + PF	0,9–105	29	35	12	70	38	[99]
$VETOPE_C$ (1991–1995)	Induction: 4 cycles VCR/VP16/HD-CY maintenance: 3 cycles VCR + CY/VP16 + CDD P/V CR + CY/VP16 + CBDCA	<48	14	29		36		[100]
HIT87/92 Anaplastic (1987–1997)	SSK 87 Induction (for high risk only): PCB, IFO, VP16, MTX, CDDP, ARAC Maintenance: PCB + VCR, MTX + VCR RT: Systematic when reach 3 years HIT 92: Induction: CY + VCR + ITMTX,MTX + VCR + ITMTX,M TX + VCR + IT- MTX, CBDCA+VP16 + IT-MTX PD → RT	1–33	34	35	65			[101]
BB SFOP (1990–1998)	7 cycles: A: CBDCA, PCB B: VP16, CDDP C: VCR, C PD → RT	5–62	73	33		79		[95]
CCLG 9204 (1992–2003)	7 cycles: A: CBDCA, VCR B: MTX, VCR C: CY, VCR D: CDDP PD → RT	1–93	89	47	41	79	63	[96]

SJYC07 (2007–2017)	No metastatic: 4 cycles: HD-MTX/VCR/CY/CDDP RT focal Maintenance: CY/topotecan alternating with monthly erlotinib Metastatic: 4 cycles: HD-MTX/VCR/CY/CDDP + VBL 2 cycles: CY/topotecan Maintenance: CY/topotecan alternating with monthly Erlotinib	≤36	54	84	70	98	88	[102]
AIEOP (1994–2003)	Induction: 4 cycles VCR + MTXHD + CY alternate CDDP + VP16 or VEC RD or PD after treatment → RT	3–36	41		27		+	[103]

Adapted from https://siope.eu/media/documents/escp-ependymoma.pdf

ARAC cytarabine, *CBDCA* carboplatin, *CDDP* cisplatin, *CY* cyclophosphamide, *HD* high dose, *HFRT* hypofractionated radiation therapy, *IFO* ifosfamide, *ITMTX* intrathecal methotrexate, *MTX* methotrexate, *PBSC* peripheral blood stem cell rescue, *PCB* procarbazine, *RD* residual disease, *PD* progressive disease, *RT* radiotherapy, *R* randomization, *TTT* thiotepa, *VBL* vinblastine, *VCR* vincristine, *VP16* etoposide

Table 13.2 Summary of literature for children with ependymoma, including the use of chemotherapy

Protocol (period)	Treatments	Age (years)	No. of patients	2-year PFS [%]	3-year PFS [%]	5-year PFS [%]	2-year OS [%]	3-year OS [%]	5-year OS [%]	Reference
AIEOP$_{\#1}$ No residue (1993–2001)	No residue: HFRT (70.4 Gy, [2 × 1,1Gy])	3–21	46			65			82	[46]
AIEOP$_{\#1}$ Residue (1993–2001)	Residue: 2 cycles VEC (VCR, VP16, CY) HFRT (70.4 Gy [2x 1.1 Gy])	3–21	17			35			61	[104]
AIEOP $_{\#2}$ No residue and grade II (2002–2014)	RT 59,4Gy [1,8Gy]	>1	48			84			98	[46]
AIEOP$_{\#2}$ No residue and grade III (2002–2014)	RT 59,4Gy [1,8Gy] 4 cycles VEC (VCR, VP16, CY)	<21	62			62			79	[46]
AIEOP$_{\#2}$ Residue (2002–2014)	1–4 cycles VEC +/− second look surgery + 59,4Gy + 8 Gy boost (2 × 4Gy)	<21	50			53			67	[46]
HIT 88/89–91 ANAPLA ST. (1989–1997)	7 cycles: A: CBDCA, VCR B: MTX, VCR C: CY, VCR D: CDDP PD → RT	3–16	71	70			85			[59]
St Jude (1997–2007)	(if residue 7 w eeks CBDCA + VP16/ VCR + CY) RT 59.4 Gy focal systematic	1–22	153	85			94			[47]
SFCE (1996–2002)	HFRT: 60 Gy [2x 1Gy] If complete removal, 66 Gy otherwise	>5	24			54			74	[105]
CCG 9942 (1995–1999)	Chemo + RT + VCR, CY, CIS, VP16	3–21	84			57			71	[106]
HIT2000 (2001–2011)	CBDCA+VP16/ VCR + CY+/− MTX + RT [age adjusted] + adjuvant chemo if residual tumor	>1.5	296		66			84		[107]

ARAC cytarabine, *CBDCA* carboplatin, *CDDP* cisplatin, *CY* cyclophosphamide, *HD* high dose, *HFRT* hypofractionated radiation therapy, *IFO* ifosfamide, *ITMTX* intrathecal methotrexate, *MTX* methotrexate, *PBSC* peripheral blood stem cell rescue, *PCB* procarbazine, *RD* residual disease, *PD* progressive disease, *RT* radiotherapy, *R* randomization, *TTT* thiotepa, *VBL* vinblastine, *VCR* vincristine, *VP16* etoposide natural history of the disease remaining unclear. Long-term outcomes remain bleak, influenced by factors such as the extent of resection and metastatic stage. Salvage treatment will be needed for 30–40% of patients with recurrent ependymoma receiving first-line treatment. This is particularly significant when evaluating the efficacy of new therapeutic approaches through clinical trials for CNS tumors [120–123]. Given the current lack of a standardized treatment for relapsing intracranial ependymoma, adding updates to previously published experiences may contribute to shaping a common protocol with shared aims [83, 84, 87].

Local control has consistently been the primary goal of ependymoma therapy, with maximal safe surgical resection and radiation therapy being the cornerstone of initial treatment [56, 123]. Given ependymoma's relative resistance to chemotherapy, the role of chemotherapeutic agents remains uncertain. In recurrent cases, the extent of surgical resection has been shown to be prognostic, with gross total resection (GTR) associated with improved outcomes.

Apart from the resection of the relapse, whenever possible, the most described series describe reirradiation results.

The AIEOP experience described the outcome of 64/160 patients with intracranial ependymoma relapsing after homogeneous treatment delivered according to the second AIEOP protocol [90]. This series included a follow-up period of over 10 years, with relapsing patients monitored for a median of 84 months after their first relapse; 17 out of 64 patients survived following relapse. The most crucial prognostic factor was the complete surgical removal of relapses. Other factors, such as the fractionation/total dose of re-radiotherapy, tumor site and grade at diagnosis, need for shunting, age above or below 3 years, and molecular subgroup at diagnosis, did not influence outcomes. Multivariable analyses identified complete surgery, absence of symptoms at relapse, and female sex as favorable prognostic factors. Our findings underscored the necessity of a standardized retreatment protocol for relapsing patients, which could address many unresolved questions and improve prognosis. The likelihood of survival was influenced by the presence or absence of symptoms and the completeness of surgery for the recurrence, but not by the radiotherapy (RT) schedule or the inclusion of chemotherapy (CT). Females with symptomatic relapses had an inexplicably poor prognosis. There are still more questions than answers regarding salvage treatment for ependymoma. Only a homogeneous protocol with well-defined, possibly randomized questions and more refined biological details may be able to clarify this picture and improve patients' prognosis. This could include window therapy to facilitate complete resection, indications for craniospinal irradiation (CSI) in the presence of 1q gain even if the relapse is localized, reirradiation techniques for balanced tumors, adjuvant CT after RT for completely resected localized relapses and single distant metastases, and the modality and duration of follow-up in first-line and relapse trials.

The French radiotherapists launched the Pediatric Ependymoma Photons Protons and Imaging (PEPPI) study in a population of patients treated with surgery and radiation therapy in French Society of Childhood Cancer reference centers between 2000 and 2013 to assess overall survival (OS) and progression-free survival (PFS) after a first relapse. The median follow-up of the entire population of 202 patients was 105.1 months, with a 10-year OS of 68.2% and PFS of 45.5%. Among the 100 relapse cases, 68.0% were local relapses, 20.0% were metastatic, and 12.0% were combined (local and metastatic). Relapses were treated by surgery ($n = 79$) and/or reirradiation ($n = 52$) and/or chemotherapy ($n = 22$). The median follow-up after relapse was 77.8 months. The OS and PFS at 5 years were 43.1% and 16.2%, respectively. After surgery or radiation therapy of the first relapse, OS and PFS were more favorable, whereas treatments that included chemotherapy with or without focal treatment were associated with worse OS and PFS. In the multivariate analysis, stereotactic hypofractionated reirradiation after surgery was associated with a significantly better outcome (OS, $P = 0.030$; PFS, $P = 0.008$), and chemotherapy was associated with a worse outcome (OS, $P = 0.028$; PFS, $P = 0.033$). This analysis of relapse treatments within the PEPPI study determined that, irrespective of whether the relapse was localized or metastatic, treatments that included surgery and/or reirradiation had better outcomes [85].

13.3.6 Treatment at Relapse

13.3.6.1 MEMMAT

Due to the limited efficacy of cytotoxic agents or targeted therapies in patients with relapsing ependymoma, alternative approaches such as metronomic chemotherapy have been explored. Metronomic chemotherapy relies on a frequent administration of anticancer agents at relatively low minimally toxic doses with nonprolonged drug-free breaks. The first significant multidrug metronomic and antiangiogenic regimen used in patients with relapsing/refractory brain tumors consisted of continuous oral celecoxib, thalidomide, and fenofibrate, with alternating 21-day cycles of low-dose cyclophosphamide and etoposide [120]. In this study, 7/19 patients with relapsing ependymoma completed 27 weeks therapy without progression, with 2 PR and 10 SD. The results of this regimen paved the way to the formal MEMMAT phase II study using this backbone schedule completed by addition of oral fenofibrate, intravenous bevacizumab, and intraventricular chemotherapy [124]. Initially dedicated to patients with medulloblastoma, this ongoing trial was recently amended, including a specific cohort for patients with ependymoma (NCT01356290).

13.3.6.2 Axitinib/Etoposide

Axitinib is a second-generation tyrosine kinase inhibitor that selectively inhibits vascular endothelial growth factor receptors (VEGFR-1/2/3). Through this mechanism of action, axitinib may block tumoral angiogenesis, tumor growth, and metastases. Preclinical studies showed activity of axitinib especially in medulloblastomas and metronomic etoposide given as palliative care has demonstrated some tumor stabilizations in ependymoma [125, 126]. A phase I/II study of axitinib and oral metronomic etoposide will soon open for inclusions with a dedicated cohort for children and AYAs with recurrent ependymoma (NCT 06485908).

13.3.6.3 PARP Inhibitors

A study demonstrated that elevated expression of CXorf67/EZHIP (Enhancer of Zeste Homologs Inhibitory Protein), which frequently occurs in PFA ependymomas, suppresses homologous recombination (HR)-mediated DNA repair. Tumor cells with high EZHIP expression levels show increased sensitivity to poly(ADP-ribose) polymerase (PARP) inhibitors, especially when combined with radiotherapy, suggesting that combination of PARP inhibitors with radiotherapy could be an effective treatment option for PFA ependymomas [127].

13.3.6.4 mTOR/HIF1a Pathway

A study investigating angiogenic patterns and expression of hypoxia-related tissue factors in 100 cases of intracranial ependymoma showed that necrosis and high hypoxia score are frequently detectable in this tumor type [128]. Hypoxic environment is a pejorative prognostic factor in pediatric cancers, favoring tumor progression and resistance to treatments. The activation of mTor/hypoxia-inducible factor (HIF)-1α pathway can be targeted by rapamycin and irinotecan, respectively. The pediatric phase I trial combining rapamycin and irinotecan showed three stable diseases in four evaluable patients with ependymoma after two cycles [129]. The feasibility of a phase II study including patients with ependymomas is under discussion.

13.3.6.5 Arsenic Trioxide

An important study on characterization of oncogenic dependencies of ZFTA-RELA-fused ependymoma suggested that GLI2 could be a potential therapeutic vulnerability in ZFTA fusion-positive ependymomas. In this study, tumor-bearing animals were treated with arsenic trioxide (ATO), a blood–brain barrier-penetrating drug targeting GLI2, improving the survival when compared with vehicle-treated controls

[7]. These results could pave the way for a dedicated clinical study, favored by the fact that ATO is a drug already used for the treatment of childhood acute myeloid leukemia.

13.3.6.6 HER2

Two recent studies on the analysis of the ErbB receptor family and on the characterization of antibody–drug conjugate targets in central nervous system tumors showed that ependymomas often exhibit strong HER2 expression in immunochemistry, suggesting that HER2 could be a target of interest in ependymoma [130, 131]. A phase II study of dose-dense temozolomide combined with lapatinib in 50 adult patients with recurrent ependymoma demonstrated clinical activity with objective responses and prolonged disease control associated with disease-related symptom improvements. Nevertheless, these results cannot be extrapolated to pediatric population as half of the patients had spinal cord tumors [132]. In a pediatric early phase clinical trial of afatinib, only one of eight patients with ependymoma experienced partial response at cycle 2 but progressed at the subsequent assessment with a PFS of 110 days. Interestingly, this study confirmed a high expression of HER2 in all patients with ependymoma [133]. Despite the relatively disappointing results, HER2 overexpression remains an interesting target and is currently leading to testing new therapeutic approaches such as HER2-specific Chimeric Antigen Receptor (CAR) T cells (NCT 04903080), or the combination of intraventricular chemotherapy with 5-azacytidine (5-AZA) and trastuzumab Infusions (NCT04958486).

13.3.6.7 ONC201/ONC206

The small-molecule ONC201, a dopamine receptor D2 (DRD2) antagonist, demonstrates preclinical activity against gliomas through activation of the integrated stress response, inactivation of AKT and ERK, and respiratory function impairment in H3K27M cells [134]. PFA ependymomas are characterized by reduced H3 K27-trimethylation, detectable via immunohistochemistry. Unlike diffuse midline glioma for which the loss of histone trimethylation is mainly linked to the existence of a mutation of histones H3.3 or H3.1, this loss of trimethylation in PFA ependymomas is most often linked to an overexpression of EZHIP. ONC201 is currently under formal clinical investigation in patients with H3K27M diffuse midline glioma. Nevertheless, and although the mechanism leading to loss of histone trimethylation is different, patients with recurrent PFA ependymoma can have access to the molecule as part of a compassionate program in France.

ONC206, an analog of ONC201, is currently under clinical investigation in a phase I trial, including patients with recurrent ependymoma (NCT04732065).

13.3.6.8 Immunotherapy

Supratentorial ZFTA-RELA-fused ependymomas were shown to exhibit an immunosuppressive phenotype with evidence of T cell exhaustion. In this specific subgroup of ependymomas, the immune-checkpoint protein PD-L1 was expressed on both tumor and myeloid cells and its receptor, PD1, was expressed on infiltrating CD4+ and CD8+ T cells, suggesting that immune-checkpoint inhibitors such as nivolumab could have a therapeutic benefit [135]. Two other studies showed high densities of infiltrating CD8+ cytotoxic T lymphocytes in ependymomas (higher in supratentorial compared to posterior fossa ependymomas) combined with substantial expression of PD-L1 in both supratentorial and posterior fossa ependymomas, and especially in ST-EPN-RELA [136, 137]. These results were conducted in the CheckMate 908 phase 1b/2 study investigating the anti-PD1 nivolumab and the combination of nivolumab with the anti-CTLA4 ipilimumab in pediatric patients with high-grade CNS malignancies including recurrent ependymoma. In this study, nivolumab used as a single agent or in combination with ipilimumab failed to demonstrate clinical benefit relative to historical data, with an overall survival of 1.4 and 4.6 months, respectively. Moreover, baseline tumor PD-L1 expression was not associated with survival [138].

13.4 New Strategies for Aggressive Tumors

Chromosome 1q gain (1q+) PFA has poor outcomes, with most patients experiencing recurrence or death within 2 years. The incidence of 1q + at primary diagnosis in PFA is approximately 25%, and this number doubles at first recurrence. Time to disease recurrence and death is considerably shorter for children with 1q + PFA than for those with 1q wild-type (WT) PFA. There are no effective treatment strategies for children with highest-risk posterior fossa group A ependymoma (PFA) [139]. Seventy percent of children with chromosome 1q + PFA will die because of the tumor, highlighting the urgent need to develop new therapeutic strategies for this population. In a recent original study, the Foreman lab at the University of Colorado utilized 1q + PFA in vitro and in vivo models to test the efficacy of combination radiation and chemotherapy in a preclinical setting. 5-Fluorouracil (5FU) enhanced radiotherapy in 1q + PFA cell lines. Specifically, 5FU increased p53 activity mediated by the extra copy of UCK2 located on chromosome 1q in 1q + PFA. Experimental downregulation of UCK2 resulted in decreased 5FU sensitivity in 1q + PFA cells. In in vitro studies, a combination of 5FU, retinoid tretinoin (ATRA), and radiation provided the greatest reduction in cellular proliferation and the greatest increase in markers of apoptosis in 1q + PFA cell lines compared with other treatment arms. Similarly, in vivo experiments demonstrated significant enhancement of survival in mice treated with combination radiation and 5FU and ATRA. These results are the first to identify a chromosome 1q + -specific therapy approach in 1q + PFA. Existing phase I studies have already established single-agent pediatric safety and dosages of 5FU and ATRA, allowing for expedited clinical application as phase II trials for children with high-risk PFA [140].

13.5 Late Effects

It is now widely recognized that simply achieving survival is not a sufficient measure of success in treating childhood brain tumors. As a result, there is an increasing focus on evaluating the quality of survival. Effectively identifying areas where normal tissue irradiation risks are high or low is crucial in the planning process to reduce the likelihood or severity of side effects. Brain tumor patients are particularly susceptible to a broad spectrum of radiation therapy side effects, which are more pronounced in young children and exacerbated by prior tumors and treatments. These side effects can range from manageable deficits that seldom affect long-term functionality to severe and debilitating ones that lead to the loss of functional independence. In most cases of brain tumors requiring radiation therapy, the risk of treatment failure outweighs the risk of the most severe side effects. Is it necessary to adhere to radiation normal tissue tolerance guidelines when the chances of a cure are minimal? Neurovascular effects of irradiation can lead to motor, sensory, coordination, hearing, or visual deficits, which are typically due to parenchymal necrosis or infarction within the high-dose area. Key factors influencing these outcomes include the time elapsed after irradiation, the radiation dose, and the patient's age [141] but also the socioeconomic status as recently illustrated and confirmed [142, 143].

Endocrinopathies are significantly influenced by the radiation dose to the hypothalamus, which is the most vulnerable organ for pituitary function. In the absence of pre-existing deficits and at a given hypothalamic dose, the incidence of hormone deficiencies follows this order: growth hormone, thyroid hormone, glucocorticoid, and gonadotropin deficiency. Although hypothalamic obesity is sometimes considered a radiation-related endocrinopathy, comparable control groups have yet to be identified. Furthermore, diabetes insipidus does not directly result from hypothalamic–pituitary axis (HPA) irradiation at the doses used in human clinical trials. When it does occur post-irradiation, it often stems from an acquired structural deficit of the HPA due to tumor expansion or brain shift. The key research question has shifted from "at what dose does an endocrine deficiency occur or serve as a surrogate?" to "why is hormone replacement necessary?" or rather, "why do not all patients develop an endocrine deficiency given a high radiation dose?"

When assessing cognitive effects in adults or children post-irradiation, a consistent finding is that a significant proportion of patients exhibit baseline deficits and that factors other than radiation dose contribute to these effects. In children with medulloblastoma treated with radiation therapy, the late effects are clearly linked to radiation dose and volume. While age exacerbates these effects, it is increasingly evident that pre-existing conditions, including surgical morbidity, play a mitigating role. Among the most important factors are hydrocephalus and posterior fossa syndrome.

Ependymomas, the third most common brain tumors in children, pose significant clinical challenges. The European Society of Paediatric Oncology Ependymoma II program is a comprehensive international initiative aimed at assessing outcomes across different treatment protocols and enhancing diagnostic accuracy. A key development in this program is the decision to lower the age at which children with posterior fossa ependymoma receive focal irradiation from 3 years to either 18 months or 1 year. Previously, in Europe, radiotherapy was reserved for children older than three due to concerns about negative cognitive effects on the developing brain. Consequently, there is a duty to conduct longitudinal cognitive follow-up, which has been established as a critical trial outcome. Over the course of 10 years, representatives from 18 participating European countries have reached a consensus on an internationally accepted test battery for monitoring childhood ependymoma survivors. The "Core-Plus" model adopts a two-tier approach to assessment, with core tests providing a minimum dataset in resource-limited settings and additional tests allowing for comprehensive evaluation where feasible. The initial stages of the trial have highlighted the challenges and provided valuable insights. We suggest that this model could serve as a solution for future international trials involving childhood brain tumors and other conditions linked to cognitive impairment [144].

As of now, the more extensive studies on wider patient number treated for ependymoma have been performed by the researchers of St. Jude's Children Hospital. The widest first prospective study series was reported in 2004 with 88 patients with a median age of 2.85 years that had received conformal radiation therapy (CRT) at 54–59.4 Gy depending on age below or over 18 months and were evaluated at a median follow-up longer than 3 years [145, 146]. Neurocognitive testing was performed before (baseline) and 6, 12, 24, 36, 48, and 60 months after the start of CRT. Baseline testing was delayed slightly if the institution of CRT was given logistic priority. Age-appropriate tests gave well-documented reliability and validity and result in age-corrected standard scores. The testing regimen was based on patient age and the instrument selected was the one with which the child was expected to achieve the most valid performance. The patients underwent a total of 316 neurocognitive examinations to evaluate changes in intelligence quotient (IQ), memory, academic achievement, adaptive behavior, and visual-auditory learning with no statistically significant change in the measures of these features for patients who completed evaluation 24 months after the initiation of CRT (more than half of the cohort). Patients younger than 3 years at the time of CRT had a significantly lower mean IQ at the start of CRT than did patients older than 3 years (89.7 ± 2.8 vs. 98.7 ± 3.1; $P = 0.034$), but the IQ of those younger than 3 years improved over time. There was no statistically significant difference in IQ scores for patients comparing infratentorial and supratentorial tumor location. At the most recent follow-up, mean scores on all neurocognitive outcomes were within normal limits (i.e., no more than +10 points from the normative mean for the appropriate age group). These encouraging results need to be explored with longer follow-up and similar patients' age and treatments. This is one of the aims of the SIOP II Ependymoma trial [63]. The reirradiation trials need to keep in mind the risks of radionecrosis. A recent systematic review on different tumor types treated at different institutions with different techniques [147] afforded this issue. Treated cancers included ependymoma ($n = 279$ patients; 7 studies), medulloblastoma ($n = 98$ patients; 6 studies), any CNS tumors ($n = 62$ patients; 3 studies), and supratentorial high-grade gliomas

($n = 10$ patients; 1 study). The median interval between initial treatment and reirradiation was 2.3 years (range: 1.2–4.75 years). The median cumulative prescription dose in equivalent dose in 2-Gy fractions (EQD22; assuming an α/β value of 2 Gy) was 103.8 Gy (range: 55.8–141.3 Gy). Among 449 reirradiated children and adolescents/young adults (AYA), 22 (4.9%; 95% CI, 3.1–7.3%) developed brain necrosis and 14 (3.1%; 95% CI, 1.7–5.2%) developed brainstem necrosis with a weighted median follow-up of 1.6 years (range: 0.5–7.4 years). The median cumulative prescription EQD22 was 111.4 Gy (range: 55.8–141.3 Gy) for the development of any necrosis, 107.7 Gy (range: 55.8–141.3 Gy) for brain necrosis, and 112.1 Gy (range: 100.2–117 Gy) for brainstem necrosis. The median latent period between reirradiation and the development of necrosis was 5.7 months (range: 4.3–24 months). Although there were more events among children/AYA undergoing hypofractionated versus conventionally fractionated reirradiation, the differences were not statistically significant ($P = 0.46$). Existing reports suggested that in children and AYA with recurrent brain tumors, reirradiation with a total EQD22 of about 112 Gy is associated with an approximately 5–7% incidence of brain or brainstem necrosis after a median follow-up of 1.6 years. The initial course of radiation therapy was given with conventional prescription doses of ≤ 2 Gy per fraction, while the second course involved variable fractionations. A uniform approach for reporting dosimetric endpoints was therefore recommended to derive robust predictive models of late toxicities following reirradiation.

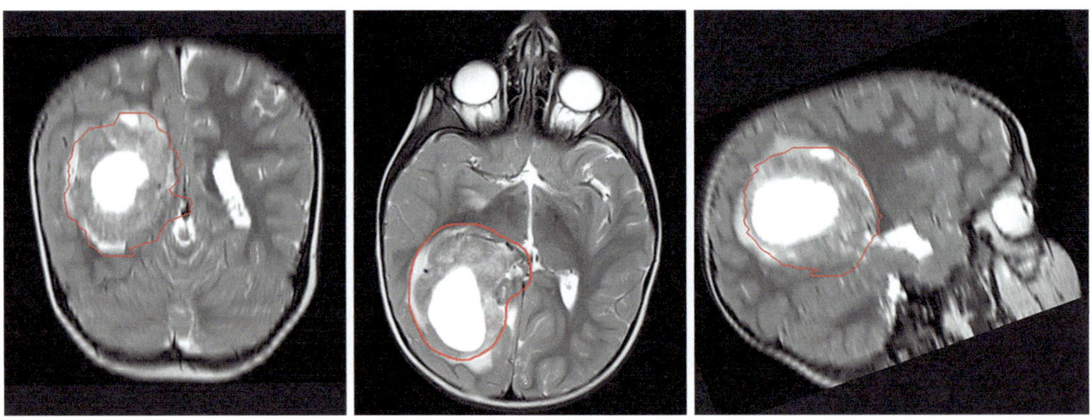

Fig. 13.1

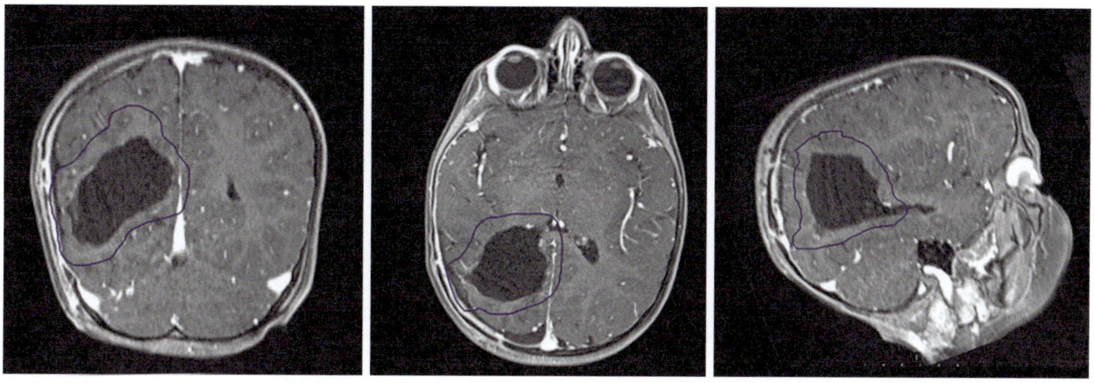

Fig. 13.2

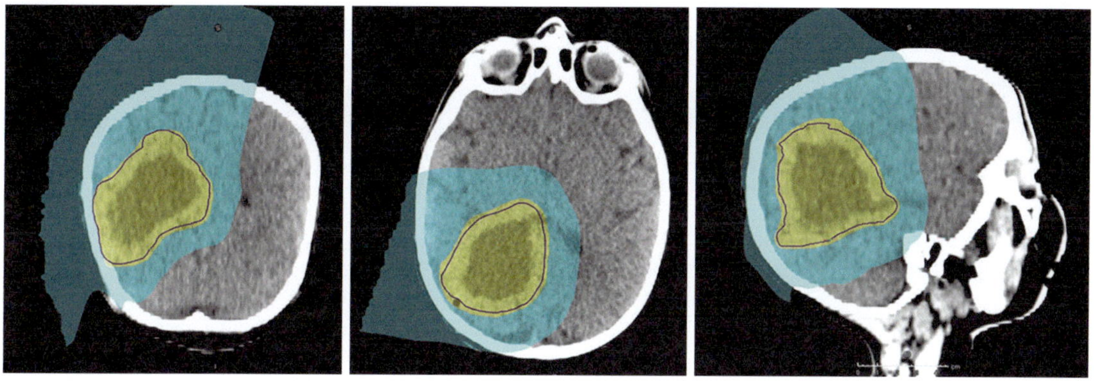

Fig. 13.3

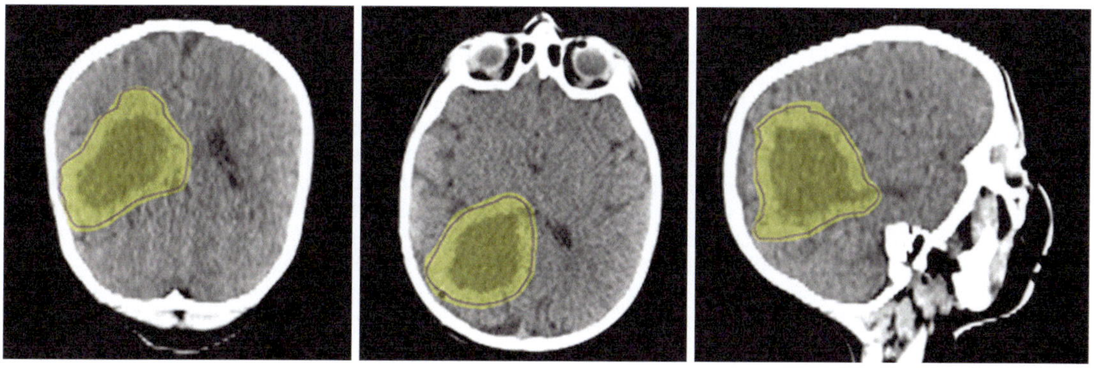

Fig. 13.4

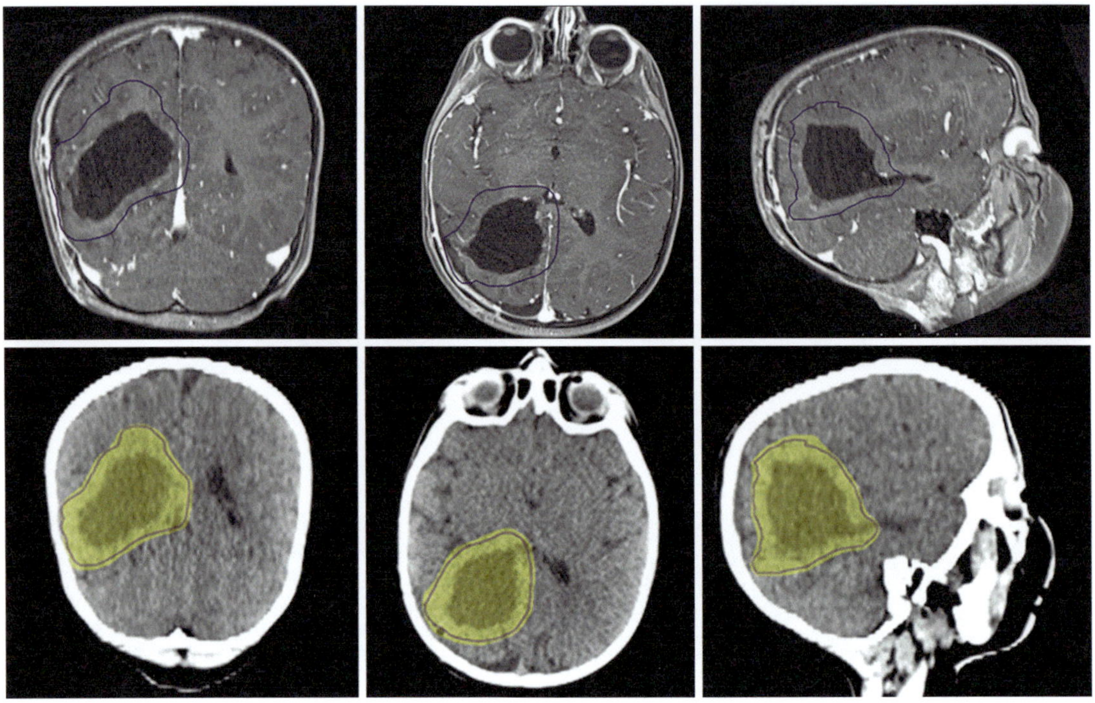

Fig. 13.5

References

1. Louis DN, Perry A, Wesseling P, Brat DJ, Cree IA, Figarella-Branger D, Hawkins C, Ng HK, Pfister SM, Reifenberger G, Soffietti R, von Deimling A, Ellison DW. The 2021 WHO classification of tumors of the central nervous system: a summary. Neuro-Oncol. 2021;23:1231–51. https://doi.org/10.1093/neuonc/noab106.
2. McGuire CS, Sainani KL, Fisher PG. Incidence patterns for ependymoma: a surveillance, epidemiology, and end results study – clinical article. J Neurosurg. 2009;110:725–9. https://doi.org/10.3171/2008.9.JNS08117.
3. Zacharoulis S, Ji L, Pollack IF, Duffner P, Geyer R, Grill J, Schild S, Jaing TH, Massimino M, Finlay J, Sposto R. Metastatic ependymoma: a multi-institutional retrospective analysis of prognostic factors. Pediatr Blood Cancer. 2008;50:231–5. https://doi.org/10.1002/pbc.2127.
4. Benesch M, Mynarek M, Witt H, Warmuth-Metz M, Pietsch T, Bison B, Pfister SM, Pajtler KW, Kool M, Schüller U, Pietschmann K, Juhnke BO, Tippelt S, Fleischhack G, Schmid I, Kramm CM, Vorwerk P, Beilken A, Classen CF, Hernáiz Driever P, Kropshofer G, Imschweiler T, Lemmer A, Kortmann RD, Rutkowski S, von Hoff K. Newly diagnosed metastatic intracranial ependymoma in children: frequency, molecular characteristics, treatment, and outcome in the prospective HIT series. Oncologist. 2019;2:e921–9. https://doi.org/10.1634/theoncologist.2018-0489.
5. Witt H, Mack SC, Ryzhova M, Bender S, Sill M, Isserlin R, Benner A, Hielscher T, Milde T, Remke M, Jones DT, Northcott PA, Garzia L, Bertrand KC, Wittmann A, Yao Y, Roberts SS, Massimi L, Van Meter T, Weiss WA, Gupta N, Grajkowska W, Lach B, Cho YJ, von Deimling A, Kulozik AE, Witt O, Bader GD, Hawkins CE, Tabori U, Guha A, Rutka JT, Lichter P, Korshunov A, Taylor MD, Pfister SM. Delineation of two clinically and molecularly distinct subgroups of posterior fossa Ependymoma. Cancer Cell. 2011;20:143–57. https://doi.org/10.1016/j.ccr.2011.07.007.
6. Pajtler KW, Witt H, Sill M, Jones DT, Hovestadt V, Kratochwil F, Wani K, Tatevossian R, Punchihewa C, Johann P, Reimand J, Warnatz HJ, Ryzhova M, Mack S, Ramaswamy V, Capper D, Schweizer L, Sieber L, Wittmann A, Huang Z, van Sluis P, Volckmann R, Koster J, Versteeg R, Fults D, Toledano H, Avigad S, Hoffman LM, Donson AM, Foreman N, Hewer E, Zitterbart K, Gilbert M, Armstrong TS, Gupta N, Allen JC, Karajannis MA, Zagzag D, Hasselblatt M, Kulozik AE, Witt O, Collins VP, von Hoff K, Rutkowski S, Pietsch T, Bader G, Yaspo ML, von Deimling A, Lichter P, Taylor MD, Gilbertson R, Ellison DW, Aldape

K, Korshunov A, Kool M, Pfister SM. Molecular classification of ependymal tumors across all CNS compartments, histopathological grades, and age groups. Cancer Cell. 2015;27:728–43. https://doi.org/10.1016/j.ccell.2015.04.002.
7. Zheng T, Ghasemi DR, Okonechnikov K, Korshunov A, Sill M, Maass KK, Goncalves B, da Silva P, Ryzhova M, Gojo J, Stichel D, Arabzade A, Kupp R, Benzel J, Taya S, Adachi T, Shiraishi R, Gerber NU, Sturm D, Ecker J, Sievers P, Selt F, Chapman R, Haberler C, Figarella-Branger D, Reifenberger G, Fleischhack G, Rutkowski S, Donson AM, Ramaswamy V, Capper D, Ellison DW, Herold-Mende CC, Schüller U, Brandner S, Driever PH, Kros JM, Snuderl M, Milde T, Grundy RG, Hoshino M, Mack SC, Gilbertson RJ, Jones DTW, Kool M, von Deimling A, Pfister SM, Sahm F, Kawauchi D, Pajtler KW. Cross-species genomics reveals oncogenic dependencies in ZFTA/C11orf95 fusion– positive supratentorial ependymomas. Cancer Discov. 2021;11(9):2230–47. https://doi.org/10.1158/2159-8290.CD-20-0963.
8. Cavalli FMG, Hübner JM, Sharma T, Luu B, Sill M, Zapotocky M, Mack SC, Witt H, Lin T, Shih DJH, Ho B, Santi M, Emery L, Hukin J, Dunham C, McLendon RE, Lipp ES, Gururangan S, Grossbach A, French P, Kros JM, van Veelen MC, Rao AAN, Giannini C, Leary S, Jung S, Faria CC, Mora J, Schüller U, Alonso MM, Chan JA, Klekner A, Chambless LB, Hwang EI, Massimino M, Eberhart CG, Karajannis MA, Lu B, Liau LM, Zollo M, Ferrucci V, Carlotti C, Tirapelli DPC, Tabori U, Bouffet E, Ryzhova M, Ellison DW, Merchant TE, Gilbert MR, Armstrong TS, Korshunov A, Pfister SM, Taylor MD, Aldape K, Pajtler KW, Kool M, Ramaswamy V. Heterogeneity within the PF-EPN-B ependymoma subgroup. Acta Neuropathol. 2018;136:227–37. https://doi.org/10.1007/s00401-018-1888-x.
9. Pajtler KW, Wen J, Sill M, Lin T, Orisme W, Tang B, Hübner JM, Ramaswamy V, Jia S, Dalton JD, Haupfear K, Rogers HA, Punchihewa C, Lee R, Easton J, Wu G, Ritzmann TA, Chapman R, Chavez L, Boop FA, Klimo P, Sabin ND, Ogg R, Mack SC, Freibaum BD, Kim HJ, Witt H, Jones DTW, Vo B, Gajjar A, Pounds S, Onar-Thomas A, Roussel MF, Zhang J, Taylor JP, Merchant TE, Grundy R, Tatevossian RG, Taylor MD, Pfister SM, Korshunov A, Kool M, Ellison DW. Molecular heterogeneity and CXorf67 alterations in posterior fossa group a (PFA) ependymomas. Acta Neuropathol. 2018;136:211–26. https://doi.org/10.1007/s00401-018-1877-0.
10. Modena P, Lualdi E, Facchinetti F, Veltman J, Reid JF, Minardi S, Janssen I, Giangaspero F, Forni M, Finocchiaro G, Genitori L, Giordano F, Riccardi R, Schoenmakers EF, Massimino M, Sozzi G. Identification of tumor-specific molecular signatures in intracranial ependymoma and association with clinical characteristics. J Clin Oncol. 2006;24:5223–33. https://doi.org/10.1200/JCO.2006.06.3701.
11. Raffeld M, Abdullaev Z, Pack SD, Xi L, Nagaraj S, Briceno N, Vera E, Pittaluga S, Lopes Abath Neto O, Quezado M, Aldape K, Armstrong TS, Gilbert M. High level MYCN amplification and distinct methylation signature define an aggressive subtype of spinal cord ependymoma. Acta Neuropathol Commun. 2020;8:101. https://doi.org/10.1186/s40478-020-00973-y.
12. Ghasemi DR, Sill M, Okonechnikov K, Korshunov A, Yip S, Schutz PW, Scheie D, Kruse A, Harter PN, Kastelan M, Wagner M, Hartmann C, Benzel J, Maass KK, Khasraw M, Sträter R, Thomas C, Paulus W, Kratz CP, Witt H, Kawauchi D, Herold-Mende C, Sahm F, Brandner S, Kool M, Jones DTW, von Deimling A, Pfister SM, Reuss DE, Pajtler KW. MYCN amplification drives an aggressive form of spinal ependymoma. Acta Neuropathol. 2019;138:1075–89. https://doi.org/10.1007/s00401-019-02056-2.
13. Warren KE, Vezina G, Poussaint TY, Warmuth-Metz M, Chamberlain MC, Packer RJ, Brandes AA, Reiss M, Goldman S, Fisher MJ, Pollack IF, Prados MD, Wen PY, Chang SM, Dufour C, Zurakowski D, Kortmann RD, Kieran MW. Response assessment in medulloblastoma and leptomeningeal seeding tumors: recommendations from the response assessment in pediatric neuro-oncology committee. Neuro-Oncology. 2018;20:13–23. https://doi.org/10.1093/neuonc/nox087.
14. Avula S, Peet A, Morana G, Morgan P, Warmuth-Metz M, Jaspan T. European Society for Paediatric Oncology (SIOPE) MRI guidelines for imaging patients with central nervous system tumours. Childs Nerv Syst. 2021;37:2497–508. https://doi.org/10.1007/s00381-021-05199-4.
15. Warmuth-Metz M, Bison B, Leykamm S. Neuroradiologic review in pediatric brain tumor studies. Clin Neuroradiol. 2009;19:263–73. https://doi.org/10.1007/s00062-009-9029-5.
16. Chang CH, Housepian EM, Herbert C. An operative staging system and a megavoltage radiotherapeutic technic for cerebellar medulloblastomas. Radiology. 1969;93:1351–9. https://doi.org/10.1148/93.6.1351.
17. Dufour C, Foulon S, Geoffray A, Masliah-Planchon J, Figarella-Branger D, Bernier-Chastagner V, Padovani L, Guerrini-Rousseau L, Faure-Conter C, Icher C, Bertozzi AI, Leblond P, Akbaraly T, Bourdeaut F, André N, Chappé C, Schneider P, De Carli E, Chastagner P, Berger C, Lejeune J, Soler C, Entz-Werlé N, Delisle MB. Metastatic medulloblastoma in childhood: Chang's classification revisited. Int J Surg Oncol. 2012:245385. https://doi.org/10.1155/2012/245385.
18. Pagès M, Pajtler KW, Puget S, Castel D, Boddaert N, Tauziède-Espariat A, Picot S, Debily MA, Kool M, Capper D, Sainte-Rose C, Chrétien F, Pfister SM, Pietsch T, Grill J, Varlet P, Andreiuolo F. Diagnostics of pediatric supratentorial RELA ependymomas: integration of information from histopathology, genetics, DNA methylation and imaging. Brain

Pathol. 2019;29:325–35. https://doi.org/10.1111/bpa.12664.
19. Fukuoka K, Kanemura Y, Shofuda T, Fukushima S, Yamashita S, Narushima D, Kato M, Honda-Kitahara M, Ichikawa H, Kohno T, Sasaki A, Hirato J, Hirose T, Komori T, Satomi K, Yoshida A, Yamasaki K, Nakano Y, Takada A, Nakamura T, Takami H, Matsushita Y, Suzuki T, Nakamura H, Makino K, Sonoda Y, Saito R, Tominaga T, Matsusaka Y, Kobayashi K, Nagane M, Furuta T, Nakada M, Narita Y, Hirose Y, Ohba S, Wada A, Shimizu K, Kurozumi K, Date I, Fukai J, Miyairi Y, Kagawa N, Kawamura A, Yoshida M, Nishida N, Wataya T, Yamaoka M, Tsuyuguchi N, Uda T, Takahashi M, Nakano Y, Akai T, Izumoto S, Nonaka M, Yoshifuji K, Kodama Y, Mano M, Ozawa T, Ramaswamy V, Taylor MD, Ushijima T, Shibui S, Yamasaki M, Arai H, Sakamoto H, Nishikawa R, Ichimura K, Japan pediatric molecular neuro-oncology group (JPMNG). Significance of molecular classification of brain tumour group standard clinical practice document ependymomas: C11orf95-RELA fusion-negative supratentorial ependymomas are a heterogeneous group of tumors. Acta Commun. 2018;6:134. https://doi.org/10.1186/s40478-018-0630-1.
20. Neumann JE, Spohn M, Obrecht D, Mynarek M, Thomas C, Hasselblatt M, Dorostkar MM, Wefers AK, Frank S, Monoranu CM, Koch A, Witt H, Kool M, Pajtler KW, Rutkowski S, Glatzel M, Schüller U. Molecular characterization of histopathological ependymoma variants. Molecular characterization of histopathological ependymoma variants. Acta Neuropathol. 2020;139:305–18. https://doi.org/10.1007/s00401-019-02090-0.
21. Jünger ST, Andreiuolo F, Mynarek M, Wohlers I, Rahmann S, Klein-Hitpass L, Dörner E, Zur Mühlen A, Velez-Char N, von Hoff K, Warmuth-Metz M, Kortmann RD, Timmermann B, von Bueren A, Rutkowski S, Pietsch T. CDKN2A deletion in supratentorial ependymoma with RELA alteration indicates a dismal prognosis: a retrospective analysis of the HIT ependymoma trial cohort. Acta Neuropathol. 2020;140:405–7. https://doi.org/10.1007/s00401-020-02169-z.
22. Gessi M, Giagnacovo M, Modena P, Elefante G, Gianno F, Buttarelli FR, Arcella A, Donofrio V, Diomedi Camassei F, Nozza P, Morra I, Massimino M, Pollo B, Giangaspero F, Antonelli M. Role of immunohistochemistry in the identification of supratentorial C11ORF95-RELA fused ependymoma in routine neuropathology. Am J Surg Pathol. 2019;43:56–63. https://doi.org/10.1097/PAS.0000000000000979.
23. Malgulwar PB, Nambirajan A, Pathak P, Faruq M, Rajeshwari M, Singh M, Suri V, Sarkar C, Sharma MC. C11orf95-RELA fusions and upregulated NF-KB signalling characterise a subset of aggressive supratentorial ependymomas that express L1CAM and nestin. J Neuro-Oncol. 2018;138:29–39. https://doi.org/10.1007/s11060-018-2767-y. Epub 2018 Jan 22. PMID: 29354850.
24. Parker M, Mohankumar KM, Punchihewa C, Weinlich R, Dalton JD, Li Y, Lee R, Tatevossian RG, Phoenix TN, Thiruvenkatam R, White E, Tang B, Orisme W, Gupta K, Rusch M, Chen X, Li Y, Nagahawhatte P, Hedlund E, Finkelstein D, Wu G, Shurtleff S, Easton J, Boggs K, Yergeau D, Vadodaria B, Mulder HL, Becksfort J, Gupta P, Huether R, Ma J, Song G, Gajjar A, Merchant T, Boop F, Smith AA, Ding L, Lu C, Ochoa K, Zhao D, Fulton RS, Fulton LL, Mardis ER, Wilson RK, Downing JR, Green DR, Zhang J, Ellison DW, Gilbertson RJ. C11orf95-RELA fusions drive oncogenic NF-κB signalling in ependymoma. Nature. 2014;506:451–5. https://doi.org/10.1038/nature13109.
25. Pietsch T, Wohlers I, Goschzik T, Dreschmann V, Denkhaus D, Dörner E, Rahmann S, Klein-Hitpass L. Supratentorial ependymomas of childhood carry C11orf95-RELA fusions leading to pathological activation of the NF-κB signaling pathway. Acta Neuropathol. 2014;127:609–11. https://doi.org/10.1007/s00401-014-1264-4.
26. Figarella-Branger D, Lechapt-Zalcman E, Tabouret E, Jünger S, de Paula AM, Bouvier C, Colin C, Jouvet A, Forest F, Andreiuolo F, Quintin-Roue I, Machet MC, Heitzmann A, Milin S, Sevestre H, Godfraind C, Labrousse F, Metellus P, Scavarda D, Pietsch T. Supratentorial clear cell ependymomas with branching capillaries demonstrate characteristic clinicopathological features and pathological activation of nuclear factor-kappaB signaling. Neuro-Oncol. 2016;18:919–27. https://doi.org/10.1093/neuonc/now025.
27. Lillard JC, Venable GT, Khan NR, Tatevossian RG, Dalton J, Vaughn BN, Klimo P. Pediatric supratentorial ependymoma: surgical, clinical, and molecular analysis. Neurosurgery. 2019;85:41–9. https://doi.org/10.1093/neuros/nyy239.
28. Witt H, Gramatzki D, Hentschel B, Pajtler KW, Felsberg J, Schackert G, Löffler M, Capper D, Sahm F, Sill M, von Deimling A, Kool M, Herrlinger U, Westphal M, Pietsch T, Reifenberger G, Pfister SM, Tonn JC, Weller M, German Glioma Network. DNA methylation-based classification of ependymomas in adulthood: implications for diagnosis and treatment. Neuro-Oncol. 2018;20:1616–24. https://doi.org/10.1093/neuonc/noy118.
29. Merchant TE, Bendel AE, Sabin ND, Burger PC, Shaw DW, Chang E, Wu S, Zhou T, Eisenstat DD, Foreman NK, Fuller CE, Anderson ET, Hukin J, Lau CC, Pollack IF, Laningham FH, Lustig RH, Armstrong FD, Handler MH, Williams-Hughes C, Kessel S, Kocak M, Ellison DW, Ramaswamy V. Conformal radiation therapy for pediatric ependymoma, chemotherapy for incompletely resected ependymoma, and observation for completely resected, supratentorial ependymoma. J Clin Oncol. 2019;37:974–83. https://doi.org/10.1200/JCO.18.01765.

30. Andreiuolo F, Varlet P, Tauziède-Espariat A, Jünger ST, Dörner E, Dreschmann V, Kuchelmeister K, Waha A, Haberler C, Slavc I, Corbacioglu S, Riemenschneider MJ, Leipold A, Rüdiger T, Körholz D, Acker T, Russo A, Faber J, Sommer C, Armbrust S, Rose M, Erdlenbruch B, Hans VH, Bernbeck B, Schneider D, Lorenzen J, Ebinger M, Handgretinger R, Neumann M, van Buiren M, Prinz M, Roganovic J, Jakovcevic A, Park SH, Grill J, Puget S, Messing-Jünger M, Reinhard H, Bergmann M, Hattingen E, Pietsch T. Childhood supratentorial ependymomas with YAP1-MAMLD1 fusion: an entity with characteristic clinical, radiological, cytogenetic and histopathological features. Brain Pathol. 2019;29:205–16. https://doi.org/10.1111/bpa.12659.
31. Panwalkar P, Clark J, Ramaswamy V, Hawes D, Yang F, Dunham C, Yip S, Hukin J, Sun Y, Schipper MJ, Chavez L, Margol A, Pekmezci M, Chung C, Banda A, Bayliss JM, Curry SJ, Santi M, Rodriguez FJ, Snuderl M, Karajannis MA, Saratsis AM, Horbinski CM, Carret AS, Wilson B, Johnston D, Lafay-Cousin L, Zelcer S, Eisenstat D, Silva M, Scheinemann K, Jabado N, McNeely PD, Kool M, Pfister SM, Taylor MD, Hawkins C, Korshunov A, Judkins AR, Venneti S. Immunohistochemical analysis of H3K27me3 demonstrates global reduction in group-A childhood posterior fossa ependymoma and is a powerful predictor of outcome. Acta Neuropathol. 2017;134:705–14. https://doi.org/10.1007/s00401-017-1752-4.
32. Bayliss J, Mukherjee P, Lu C, Jain SU, Chung C, Martinez D, Sabari B, Margol AS, Panwalkar P, Parolia A, Pekmezci M, McEachin RC, Cieslik M, Tamrazi B, Garcia BA, La Rocca G, Santi M, Lewis PW, Hawkins C, Melnick A, David Allis C, Thompson CB, Chinnaiyan AM, Judkins AR, Venneti S. Lowered H3K27me3 and DNA hypomethylation define poorly prognostic pediatric posterior fossa ependymomas. Sci Transl Med. 2016;8:366ra161. https://doi.org/10.1126/scitranslmed.aah6904.
33. Swanson AA, Raghunathan A, Jenkins RB, Messing-Jünger M, Pietsch T, Clarke MJ, Kaufmann TJ, Giannini C. Spinal cord Ependymomas with MYCN amplification show aggressive clinical behavior. J Neuropathol Exp Neurol. 2019;78:791–7. https://doi.org/10.1093/jnen/nlz064.
34. Ellison DW, Kocak M, Figarella-Branger D, Felice G, Catherine G, Pietsch T, Frappaz D, Massimino M, Grill J, Boyett JM, Grundy RG. Histopathological grading of pediatric ependymoma: reproducibility and clinical relevance in European trial cohorts. J Negat Results Biomed. 2011;10:7. https://doi.org/10.1186/1477-5751-10-7.
35. Ellison DW, Aldape KD, Capper D, Fouladi M, Gilbert MR, Gilbertson RJ, Hawkins C, Merchant TE, Pajtler K, Venneti S, Louis DN. cIMPACT-NOW update 7: advancing the molecular classification of ependymal tumors. Brain Pathol. 2020;30:863–6. https://doi.org/10.1111/bpa.12866.
36. Baroni LV, Sundaresan L, Heled A, Coltin H, Pajtler KW, Lin T, Merchant TE, McLendon R, Faria C, Buntine M, White CL, Pfister SM, Gilbert MR, Armstrong TS, Bouffet E, Kumar S, Taylor MD, Aldape KD, Ellison DW, Gottardo NG, Kool M, Korshunov A, Hansford JR, Ramaswamy V. Ultra high-risk PFA ependymoma is characterized by loss of chromosome 6q. Neuro-Oncol. 2021;23:1360–70. https://doi.org/10.1093/neuonc/noab034. PMID: 33580238; PMCID: PMC8328032.
37. Schiavello E, Biassoni V, Antonelli M, et al. Pediatric extraspinal sacrococcygeal ependymoma (ESE): an Italian AIEOP experience of six cases and literature review. Childs Nerv Syst. 2018; https://doi.org/10.1007/s00381-018-3805-y.
38. Pohl LC, Leitheiser M, Obrecht D, Schweizer L, Wefers AK, Eckhardt A, Raffeld M, Sturm D, Pajtler KW, Rutkowski S, Fukuoka K, Ichimura K, Bockmayr M, Schüller U. Molecular characteristics and improved survival prediction in a cohort of 2023 ependymomas. Acta Neuropathol. 2024;147:24. https://doi.org/10.1007/s00401-023-02674-x.
39. Tauziède-Espariat A, Beccaria K, Dangouloff-Ros V, Sievers P, Meurgey A, Pissaloux D, Appay R, Saffroy R, Grill J, Mariet C, Bourdeaut F, Hasty L, Métais A, Chrétien F, Blauwblomme T, Puget S, Boddaert N, Varlet P, RENOCLIP-LOC. A comprehensive analysis of infantile central nervous system tumors to improve distinctive criteria for infant-type hemispheric glioma versus desmoplastic infantile ganglioglioma/astrocytoma. Brain Pathol. 2023;33:e13182. https://doi.org/10.1111/bpa.13182.
40. Bouffet E, Perilongo G, Canete A, Massimino M. Intracranial ependymomas in children: a critical review of prognostic factors and a plea for cooperation. Med Pediatr Oncol. 1998;30:319–29; discussion 329-31. https://doi.org/10.1002/(sici)1096-911x(199806)30:6<319::aid-mpo1>3.0.co;2-h.
41. Cage TA, Clark AJ, Aranda D, Gupta N, Sun PP, Parsa AT, Auguste KI. A systematic review of treatment outcomes in pediatric patients with intracranial ependymomas. J Neurosurg Pediatr. 2013;11:673–81. https://doi.org/10.3171/2013.2.PEDS12345.
42. Tihan T, Zhou T, Holmes E, Burger PC, Ozuysal S, Rushing EJ. The prognostic value of histological grading of posterior fossa ependymomas in children: a children's oncology group study and a review of prognostic factors. Mod Pathol. 2008;21:165–77. https://doi.org/10.1038/modpathol.3800999.
43. Massimino M, Solero CL, Garrè ML, Biassoni V, Cama A, Genitori L, Di Rocco C, Sardi I, Viscardi E, Modena P, Potepan P, Barra S, Scarzello G, Galassi E, Giangaspero F, Antonelli M, Gandola L. Second-look surgery for ependymoma: the Italian experience. J Neurosurg Pediatr. 2011;8:246–50. https://doi.org/10.3171/2011.6.PEDS1142.
44. Pajtler KW, Mack SC, Ramaswamy V, Smith CA, Witt H, Smith A, Hansford JR, von Hoff K,

Wright KD, Hwang E, Frappaz D, Kanemura Y, Massimino M, Faure-Conter C, Modena P, Tabori U, Warren KE, Holland EC, Ichimura K, Giangaspero F, Castel D, von Deimling A, Kool M, Dirks PB, Grundy RG, Foreman NK, Gajjar A, Korshunov A, Finlay J, Gilbertson RJ, Ellison DW, Aldape KD, Merchant TE, Bouffet E, Pfister SM, Taylor MD. The current consensus on the clinical management of intracranial ependymoma and its distinct molecular variants. Acta Neuropathol. 2017;133:5–12. https://doi.org/10.1007/s00401-016-1643-0.
45. Shu HK, Sall WF, Maity A, Tochner ZA, Janss AJ, Belasco JB, Rorke-Adams LB, Phillips PC, Sutton LN, Fisher MJ. Childhood intracranial ependymoma: twenty-year experience from a single institution. Cancer. 2007;110(2):432–41. https://doi.org/10.1002/cncr.22782.
46. Massimino M, Miceli R, Giangaspero F, Boschetti L, Modena P, Antonelli M, Ferroli P, Bertin D, Pecori E, Valentini L, Biassoni V, Garrè ML, Schiavello E, Sardi I, Cama A, Viscardi E, Scarzello G, Scoccianti S, Mascarin M, Quaglietta L, Cinalli G, Diletto B, Genitori L, Peretta P, Mussano A, Buccoliero A, Calareso G, Barra S, Mastronuzzi A, Giussani C, Marras CE, Balter R, Bertolini P, Giombelli E, La Spina M, Buttarelli FR, Pollo B, Gandola L. Final results of the second prospective AIEOP protocol for pediatric intracranial ependymoma. Neuro-Oncology. 2016;18:1451–60. https://doi.org/10.1093/neuonc/now108.
47. Merchant TE, Li C, Xiong X, Kun LE, Boop FA, Sanford RA. Conformal radiotherapy after surgery for paediatric ependymoma: a prospective study. Lancet Oncol. 2009;10:258–66. https://doi.org/10.1016/s1470-2045(08)70342-5.
48. Hoffman LM, Plimpton SR, Foreman NK, Stence NV, Hankinson TC, Handler MH, Hemenway MS, Vibhakar R, Liu AK. Fractionated stereotactic radiosurgery for recurrent ependymoma in children. J Neuro-Oncol. 2014;116(1):107–11. https://doi.org/10.1007/s11060-013-1259-3.
49. Gajjar A, Packer RJ, Foreman NK, Cohen K, Haas-Kogan D, Merchant TE. Children's Oncology Group's 2013 blueprint for research: central nervous system tumors. Pediatr Blood Cancer. 2013;60(6):1022–6. https://doi.org/10.1002/pbc.24427. Epub 2012 Dec 19.
50. Paulino C, Wen BC. The significance of radiotherapy treatment duration in intracranial ependymoma. Int J Radiat Oncol Biol Phys. 2000;47(3):585–9. https://doi.org/10.1016/s0360-3016(99)00535-0.
51. Perilongo G, Massimino M, Sotti G, Belfontali T, Masiero L, Rigobello L, Garrè ML, Carli M, Lombardi F, Solero C, Sainati L, Canale V, Giangaspero F, Andreussi L, Mazza C, Madon E. Analyses of prognostic factors in a retrospective review of 92 children with ependymoma: Italian Pediatric Neuro-oncology Group. Med Pediatr Oncol. 1997;29(2):79–85. https://doi.org/10.1002/(sici)1096-911x(199708)29:2<79::aid-mpo3>3.0.co;2-o.
52. Schild SE, Nisi K, Scheithauer BW, Wong WW, Lyons MK, Schomberg PJ, Shaw EG. The results of radiotherapy for ependymomas: the Mayo Clinic experience. Int J Radiat Oncol Biol Phys. 1998;42(5):953–8. https://doi.org/10.1016/s0360-3016(98)00350-2.
53. Salazar OM, Castro-Vita H, Van Houtte P, Rubin P, Aygun C. Improved survival in cases of intracranial ependymoma after radiation therapy. Late report and recommendations. J Neurosurg. 1983;59(4):652–9. https://doi.org/10.3171/jns.1983.59.4.0652.
54. Merchant TE, Haida T, Wang MH, Finlay JL, Leibel SA. Anaplastic ependymoma: treatment of pediatric patients with or without craniospinal radiation therapy. J Neurosurg. 1997;86(6):943–9. https://doi.org/10.3171/jns.1997.86.6.0943.
55. Nazar GB, Hoffman HJ, Becker LE, Jenkin D, Humphreys RP, Hendrick EB. Infratentorial ependymomas in childhood: prognostic factors and treatment. J Neurosurg. 1990;72(3):408–17. https://doi.org/10.3171/jns.1990.72.3.0408.
56. Pollack IF, Gerszten PC, Martinez AJ, Lo KH, Shultz B, Albright AL, Janosky J, Deutsch M. Intracranial ependymomas of childhood: long-term outcome and prognostic factors. Neurosurgery. 1995;37(4):655–66; discussion 666–7.
57. Goldwein JW, Leahy JM, Packer RJ, Sutton LN, Curran WJ, Rorke LB, Schut L, Littman PS, D'angio GJ. Intracranial ependymomas in children. Int J Radiat Oncol Biol Phys. 1990;19(6):1497–502. https://doi.org/10.1016/0360-3016(90)90362-n.
58. Vanuytsel L, Brada M. The role of prophylactic spinal irradiation in localized intracranial ependymoma. Int J Radiat Oncol Biol Phys. 1991;21(3):825–30.
59. Timmermann B, Kortmann RD, Kühl J, Meisner C, Slavc I, Pietsch T, Bamberg M. Combined postoperative irradiation and chemotherapy for anaplastic ependymomas in childhood: results of the German prospective trials HIT 88/89 and HIT 91. Int J Radiat Oncol Biol Phys. 2000;46:287–95. https://doi.org/10.1016/s0360-3016(99)00414-9.
60. Chan MD, McMullen KP. Multidisciplinary management of intracranial ependymoma. Curr Probl Cancer. 2012;36(1):6–19.
61. Merchant TE, Happersett L, Finlay JL, Leibel SA. Preliminary results of conformal radiation therapy for medulloblastoma. Neuro-Oncology. 1999;1:177–87.
62. Merchant TE, Jenkins JJ, Burger PC, Sanford RA, Sherwood SH, Jones-Wallace D, Heideman RL, Thompson SJ, Helton KJ, Kun LE. Influence of tumor grade on time to progression after irradiation for localized ependymoma in children. Int J Radiat Oncol Biol Phys. 2002;53(1):5263.
63. Leblond P, Massimino M, English M, Ritzmann TA, Gandola L, Calaminus G, Thomas S, Pérol D, Gautier J, Grundy RG, Frappaz D. Toward improved diagnosis accuracy and treatment of children, ado-

lescents, and young adults with ependymoma: the international SIOP Ependymoma II protocol. Front Neurol. 2022;13:887544. https://doi.org/10.3389/fneur.2022.887544.

64. Ducassou A, Padovani L, Chaltiel L, Bolle S, Habrand J-L, Claude L, et al. Pediatric localized intracranial ependymomas: a multicenter analysis of the Societe Francaise de lutte contre les cancers de L'Enfant (SFCE) from 2000 to 2013. Int J Radiat Oncol Biol Phys. 2018;102:166e173.
65. Thorp N, Gandola L. Management of Ependymoma in children, adolescents and young adults. Clin Oncol. 2019;31:162e170.
66. Schroeder TM, Chintagumpala M, Okcu MF, Chiu JK, Teh BS, Woo SY, Paulino AC. Intensity-modulated radiation therapy in childhood ependymoma. Int J Radiat Oncol Biol Phys. 2008;71:987–93.
67. DeNunzio NJ, Yock TI. Modern radiotherapy for pediatric brain tumors. Cancers (Basel). 2020;12(6):1533. https://doi.org/10.3390/cancers12061533. PMID: 32545204 Free PMC article. Review.
68. Eaton BR, MacDonald SM, Yock TI, Tarbell NJ. Secondary malignancy risk following proton radiation therapy. Front Oncol. 2015;5:261. https://doi.org/10.3389/fonc.2015.00261. eCollection 2015.PMID: 26636040 Free PMC article. Review.
69. Smyth MD, Horn BN, Russo C, Berger MS. Intracranial ependymomas of childhood: current management strategies. Pediatr Neurosurg. 2000;33:138–50.
70. Baliga S, Yock TI. Pediatric cancer. Hematol Oncol Clin North Am. 2020;34(1):143–59. https://doi.org/10.1016/j.hoc.2019.08.021. Epub 2019 Oct 31
71. Baliga S, Yock TI. Proton beam therapy in pediatric oncology. Curr Opin Pediatr. 2019;31(1):28–34. https://doi.org/10.1097/MOP.0000000000000724. PMID: 30531222 Review.
72. MacDonald SM, Yock TI. Proton beam therapy following resection for childhood ependymoma. Childs Nerv Syst. 2010;26:285–91.
73. MacDonald SM, Sethi R, Lavally B, et al. Proton radiotherapy for pediatric central nervous system ependymoma: clinical outcomes for 70 patients. Neuro-oncol. 2013;15(11):1552–9.
74. Ares C, Albertini F, Frei-Welte M, Bolsi A, Grotzer MA, Goitein G, Weber DC. Pencil beam scanning proton therapy for pediatric intracranial ependymoma. J Neuro-Oncol. 2016;128(1):137–45. https://doi.org/10.1007/s11060-016-2090-4. Epub 2016 Mar 5.PMID: 26945580.
75. Sato M, Gunther JR, Mahajan A, Jo E, Paulino AC, Adesina AM, Jones JY, Ketonen LM, Su JM, Okcu MF, Khatua S, Dauser RC, Whitehead WE, Weinberg J, Chintagumpala MM. Progression-free survival of children with localized ependymoma treated with intensity-modulated radiation therapy or proton-beam radiation therapy. Cancer. 2017;123(13):2570–8. https://doi.org/10.1002/cncr.30623. Epub 2017 Mar 7.PMID: 28267208.
76. Indelicato DJ, Bradley JA, Rotondo RL, Nanda RH, Logie N, Sandler ES, Aldana PR, Ranalli NJ, Beier AD, Morris CG, Mendenhall NP. Outcomes following proton therapy for pediatric ependymoma. Acta Oncol. 2018;57(5):644–8. https://doi.org/10.1080/0284186X.2017.1413248. Epub 2017 Dec 14. PMID: 29239262 Clinical Trial.
77. Peters S, Merta J, Schmidt L, et al. Evaluation of dose, volume and outcome in children with localized, intracranial ependymoma treated with proton therapy within the prospective KiProReg study. Neuro-Oncology. 2022;24(7):1193–202.
78. Indelicato DJ, Ioakeim-Ioannidou M, Bradley JA, et al. Proton therapy for pediatric ependymoma: mature results from a bicentric study. Int J Radiat Oncol Biol Phys. 2021;110(3):815–20.
79. Haas-Kogan D, Indelicato D, Paganetti H, et al. National Cancer Institute workshop on proton therapy for children: considerations regarding brainstem injury. Int J Radiat Oncol Biol Phys. 2018;101(1):152–68.
80. Dalmasso C, Alapetite A, Bolle S, Goudjil F, Lusque A, Desrousseaux J, Claude L, Doyen J, Bernier-Chastagner V, Ducassou A, Sevely A, Roques M, Tensaouti F, Laprie A. Brainstem toxicity after proton or photon therapy in children and young adults with localized intracranial ependymoma: a French retrospective study. Radiother Oncol. 2024 May;194:110157.
81. Donahue BR, MacDonald SM. Protons for pediatric ependymoma: where are we now? Neuro-Oncology. 2022;24(7):1203–4.
82. Tsai JW, Manoharan N, Alexandrescu S, Zimmerman MA, Scully J, Chordas C, Clymer J, Wright KD, Filbin M, Ullrich NJ, Marcus KJ, Haas-Kogan D, Chi SN, Bandopadhayay P, Yeo KK. Outcomes after first relapse of childhood intracranial ependymoma. Pediatr Blood Cancer. 2021;68(8):e28930. https://doi.org/10.1002/pbc.28930.
83. Adolph JE, Fleischhack G, Mikasch R, Zeller J, Warmuth-Metz M, Bison B, Mynarek M, Rutkowski S, Schüller U, von Hoff K, Obrecht D, Pietsch T, Pfister SM, Pajtler KW, Witt O, Witt H, Kortmann RD, Timmermann B, Krauß J, Frühwald MC, Faldum A, Kwiecien R, Bode U, Tippelt S. Local and systemic therapy of recurrent ependymoma in children and adolescents: short- and long-term results of the E-HIT-REZ 2005 study. Neuro-Oncology. 2021;23:1012–23.
84. Bouffet E, Hawkins CE, Ballourah W, Taylor MD, Bartels UK, Schoenhoff N, Tsangaris E, Huang A, Kulkarni A, Mabbot DJ, Laperriere N, Tabori U. Survival benefit for pediatric patients with recurrent ependymoma treated with reirradiation. Survival benefit for pediatric patients with recurrent ependymoma treated with reirradiation. Int J Radiat Oncol Biol Phys. 2012;83:1541–8.

85. Desrousseaux J, Claude L, Chaltiel L, Tensaouti F, Padovani L, Bolle S, Escande A, Alapetite C, Supiot S, Bernier-Chastagner V, Huchet A, Leseur J, Truc G, Leblond P, Bertozzi AI, Ducassou A, Laprie A. Respective roles of surgery, chemotherapy, and radiation therapy for recurrent pediatric and adolescent ependymoma: a national multicentric study. Int J Radiat Oncol Biol Phys. 2023;117:404–15. https://doi.org/10.1016/j.ijrobp.2023.04.008.
86. Régnier E, Laprie A, Ducassou A, Bolle S, Supiot S, Muracciole X, Claude L, Chapet S, Coche-Dequéant B, Vigneron C, Leseur J, Bondiau PY, Habrand JL, Bernier V. Re-irradiation of locally recurrent pediatric intracranial ependymoma: experience of the French society of children's cancer. Radiother Oncol. 2019;132:1–7. https://doi.org/10.1016/j.radonc.2018.11.009.
87. Merchant TE, Boop FA, Kun LE, Sanford RA. A retrospective study of surgery and reirradiation for recurrent ependymoma. Int J Radiat Oncol Biol Phys. 2008;71:87–97. Tsang DS, Burghen E, Klimo P Jr, Boop FA, Ellison DW, Merchant TE. Outcomes after reirradiation for recurrent pediatric intracranial ependymoma. Int J Radiat Oncol Biol Phys 2018;100(2):507–15. https://doi.org/10.1016/j.ijrobp.2017.10.002.
88. Tsang DS, Murray L, Ramaswamy V, Zapotocky M, Tabori U, Bartels U, Huang A, Dirks PB, Taylor MD, Hawkins C, Bouffet E, Laperriere N. Craniospinal irradiation as part of re-irradiation for children with recurrent intracranial ependymoma. Neuro-oncol. 2019;21(4):547–57. https://doi.org/10.1093/neuonc/noy191. PMID: 30452715; PMCID: PMC6422429.
89. Messahel B, Ashley S, Saran F, Ellison D, Ironside J, Phipps K, Cox T, Chong WK, Robinson K, Picton S, Pinkerton CR, Mallucci C, Macarthur D, Jaspan T, Michalski A, Grundy RG, Children's Cancer Leukaemia Group Brain Tumour Committee. Relapsed intracranial ependymoma in children in the UK: patterns of relapse, survival and therapeutic outcome. Eur J Cancer. 2009;45(10):1815–23. https://doi.org/10.1016/j.ejca.2009.03.018.
90. Massimino M, Barretta F, Modena P, Johann P, Ferroli P, Antonelli M, Gandola L, Garrè ML, Bertin D, Mastronuzzi A, Mascarin M, Quaglietta L, Viscardi E, Sardi I, Ruggiero A, Boschetti L, Giagnacovo M, Biassoni V, Schiavello E, Chiapparini L, Erbetta A, Mussano A, Giussani C, Mura RM, Barra S, Scarzello G, Scimone G, Carai A, Giangaspero F, Buttarelli FR. Treatment and outcome of intracranial ependymoma after first relapse in the 2nd AIEOP protocol. Neuro-Oncology. 2022;24:467–79. https://doi.org/10.1093/neuonc/noab230.
91. Gupta T, Maitre M, Gupta P, Krishnatry R, Chatterjee A, Moiyadi A, Shetty P, Singh V, Chinnaswamy G, Epari S, Sahay A, Patil V, GodaSastri J. Extent of re-excision, sequence/timing of salvage re-irradiation, and disease-free interval impact upon clinical outcomes in recurrent/progressive ependymoma. J Neuro-Oncol. 2020;147(2):405–15. https://doi.org/10.1007/s11060-020-03434-793.
92. Sminia P, Mayer R. External beam radiotherapy of recurrent glioma: radiation tolerance of the human brain. Cancers (Basel). 2012;4(2):379–99. https://doi.org/10.3390/cancers4020379.
93. Minniti G, Niyazi M, Alongi F, Navarria P, Belka C. Current status and recent advances in reirradiation of glioblastoma. Radiat Oncol. 2021;16(1):36. https://doi.org/10.1186/s13014-021-01767-9.
94. Grill J, Le Deley MC, Gambarelli D, Raquin MA, Couanet D, Pierre-Kahn A, Habrand JL, Doz F, Frappaz D, Gentet JC, Edan C, Chastagner P, Kalifa C; French Society of Pediatric Oncology. Postoperative chemotherapy without irradiation for ependymoma in children under 5 years of age: a multicenter trial of the French Society of Pediatric Oncology. J Clin Oncol. 2001;19:1288–96. https://doi.org/10.1200/JCO.2001.19.5.1288.
95. Grundy RG, Wilne SA, Weston CL, Robinson K, Lashford LS, Ironside J, Cox T, Chong WK, Campbell RH, Bailey CC, Gattamaneni R, Picton S, Thorpe N, Mallucci C, English MW, Punt JA, Walker DA, Ellison DW, Machin D, Children's Cancer and Leukaemia Group (formerly UKCCSG) Brain tumour committee. Primary postoperative chemotherapy without radiotherapy for intracranial ependymoma in children: the UKCCSG/SIOP prospective study. Lancet Oncol. 2007;8:696–705. https://doi.org/10.1016/S1470-2045(07)70208-5.
96. Zacharoulis S, Levy A, Chi SN, Gardner S, Rosenblum M, Miller DC, Dunkel I, Diez B, Sposto R, Ji L, Asgharzadeh S, Hukin J, Belasco J, Dubowy R, Kellie S, Termuhlen A, Finlay J. Outcome for young children newly diagnosed with ependymoma, treated with intensive induction chemotherapy followed by myeloablative chemotherapy and autologous stem cell rescue. Pediatr Blood Cancer. 2007;49:34–40. https://doi.org/10.1002/pbc.20935.
97. Geyer J, Sposto R, Jennings M, Boyett J, Axtell R, Breiger D, Broxson E, Donahue B, Finlay J, Goldwein J, Heier L, Johnson D, Mazewski C, Miller D, Packer R, Puccetti D, Radcliffe J, Tao M, Shiminski-Maher T. Multiagent chemotherapy and deferred radiotherapy in infants with malignant brain tumors: a report from the Children's Cancer Group. J Clin Oncol. 2005;23:7621–31. https://doi.org/10.1200/JCO.2005.09.095.
98. Venkatramani R, Ji L, Lasky J, Haley K, Judkins A, Zhou S, Sposto R, Olshefski R, Garvin J, Tekautz T, Kennedy G, Rassekh SR, Moore T, Gardner S, Allen J, Shore R, Moertel C, Atlas M, Dhall G, Finlay J. Outcome of infants and young children with newly diagnosed ependymoma treated on the "Head Start" III prospective clinical trial. J Neuro-Oncol. 2013;113:285–91. https://doi.org/10.1007/s11060-013-1111-9.
99. White L, Kellie S, Gray E, Toogood I, Waters K, Lockwood L, Macfarlane S, Johnston H. Postoperative chemotherapy in children less

than 4 years of age with malignant brain tumors: promising initial response to a VETOPEC-based regimen. A study of the Australian and New Zealand Children's Cancer Study Group (ANZCCSG). J Pediatr Hematol Oncol. 1998;20:125–30. https://doi.org/10.1097/00043426-199803000-00007.
100. Timmermann B, Kortmann RD, Kühl J, Rutkowski S, Dieckmann K, Meisner C, Bamberg M. Role of radiotherapy in anaplastic ependymoma in children under age of 3 years: results of the prospective German brain tumor trials HIT-SKK 87 and 92. Radiother Oncol. 2005;77:278–85. https://doi.org/10.1016/j.radonc.2005.10.016.
101. Upadhyaya SA, Robinson GW, Onar-Thomas A, Orr BA, Billups CA, Bowers DC, Bendel AE, Hassall T, Crawford JR, Partap S, Fisher PG, Tatevossian RG, Seah T, Qaddoumi IA, Vinitsky A, Armstrong GT, Sabin ND, Tinkle CL, Klimo P, Indelicato DJ, Boop FA, Merchant TE, Ellison DW, Gajjar A. Molecular grouping and outcomes of young children with newly diagnosed ependymoma treated on the multi-institutional SJYC07 trial. Neuro-Oncology. 2019;21:1319–30. https://doi.org/10.1093/neuonc/noz069.
102. Massimino M, Gandola L, Barra S, Giangaspero F, Casali C, Potepan P, Di Rocco C, Nozza P, Collini P, Viscardi E, Bertin D, Biassoni V, Cama A, Milanaccio C, Modena P, Balter R, Tamburrini G, Peretta P, Mascarin M, Scarzello G, Fidani P, Milano GM, Sardi I, Genitori L, Garrè ML. Infant ependymoma in a 10-year AIEOP (Associazione Italiana Ematologia Oncologia Pediatrica) experience with omitted or deferred radiotherapy. Int J Radiat Oncol Biol Phys. 2011;80:807–14. https://doi.org/10.1016/j.ijrobp.2010.02.048.
103. Massimino M, Gandola L, Giangaspero F, Sandri A, Valagussa P, Perilongo G, Garrè ML, Ricardi U, Forni M, Genitori L, Scarzello G, Spreafico F, Barra S, Mascarin M, Pollo B, Gardiman M, Cama A, Navarria P, Brisigotti M, Collini P, Balter R, Fidani P, Stefanelli M, Burnelli R, Potepan P, Podda M, Sotti G, Madon E, AIEOP Pediatric Neuro-Oncology Group. Hyperfractionated radiotherapy and chemotherapy for childhood ependymoma: final results of the first prospective AIEOP (Associazione Italiana di Ematologia-Oncologia Pediatrica) study. Int J Radiat Oncol Biol Phys. 2004;58:1336–45. https://doi.org/10.1016/j.ijrobp.2003.08.030.
104. Conter C, Carrie C, Bernier V, Geoffray A, Pagnier A, Gentet JC, Lellouch-Tubiana A, Chabaud S, Frappaz D. Intracranial ependymomas in children: society of pediatric oncology experience with postoperative hyperfractionated local radiotherapy. Int J Radiat Oncol Biol Phys. 2009;74:1536–42. https://doi.org/10.1016/j.ijrobp.2008.09.051.
105. Garvin JH Jr, Selch MT, Holmes E, Berger MS, Finlay JL, Flannery A, Goldwein JW, Packer RJ, Rorke-Adams LB, Shiminski-Maher T, Sposto R, Stanley P, Tannous R, Pollack IF; Children's Oncology Group. Phase II study of pre-irradiation chemotherapy for childhood intracranial ependymoma. Children's Cancer Group protocol 9942: a report from the Children's Oncology Group. Pediatr Blood Cancer 2012 5;59:1183–1189. doi:https://doi.org/10.1002/pbc.24274.
106. Smith AA, Onar-Thomas A, Lensing S, Dalton J, Bennett J, Tatevossian RG, Bertrand K, Lindsay H, Tabori U, Owens-Pickle E, Blackburn PR, Handler MH, Chambwe N, El Khoury L, Lau C, Kunin-Batson A, Sands S, Wu S, Zhou T, Chang A, Merchant TE, Leary S, Fouladi M, Gajjar A, Pollack IF, Foreman NK, Ellison DW. Phase 3 randomized trial of post-irradiation chemotherapy in patients with newly diagnosed ependymoma, a report from the Children's Oncology Group. Neuro Oncol. 2025 Dec 19:noaf285. https://doi.org/10.1093/neuonc/noaf285. Epub ahead of print. PMID: 41423745.
107. Smith A, Onar-Thomas A, Ellison D, Owens-Pickle E, Wu S, Leary SES, Fouladi M, Merchant T, Gajjar A, Foreman N. EPEN-54. ACNS0831, Phase III randomized trial of post-radiation chemotherapy in patients with newly diagnosed ependymoma ages 1 to 21 years. Neuro Oncol. 2020;22(Suppl 3):iii318–9. https://doi.org/10.1093/neuonc/noaa222.187.
108. Benesch M, Weber-Mzell D, Gerber NU, von Hoff K, Deinlein F, Krauss J, Warmuth-Metz M, Kortmann RD, Pietsch T, Driever PH, Quehenberger F, Urban C, Rutkowski S. Ependymoma of the spinal cord in children and adolescents: a retrospective series from the HIT database. J Neurosurg Pediatr. 2010;6:137–44. https://doi.org/10.3171/2010.5.PEDS09553.
109. Abdel-Wahab M, Etuk B, Palermo J, Shirato H, Kresl J, Yapicier O, Walker G, Scheithauer BW, Shaw E, Lee C, Curran W, Thomas T, Markoe A. Spinal cord gliomas: a multi-institutional retrospective analysis. Int J Radiat Oncol Biol Phys. 2006;64:1060–71. https://doi.org/10.1016/j.ijrobp.2005.09.038.
110. Benesch M, Frappaz D, Massimino M. Spinal cord ependymomas in children and adolescents. Childs Nerv Syst. 2012;28:2017–28. https://doi.org/10.1007/s00381-012-1908-4.
111. Oh MC, Ivan ME, Sun MZ, Kaur G, Safaee M, Kim JM, Sayegh ET, Aranda D, Parsa AT. Adjuvant radiotherapy delays recurrence following subtotal resection of spinal cord ependymomas. Neuro-Oncology. 2013;15:208–15. https://doi.org/10.1093/neuonc/nos286.
112. Pędziwiatr K, Skowrońska-Gardas A, Chojnacka M. Spinal cord ependymoma in children–results of postoperative radiotherapy. Radiother Oncol. 2013;106:181–5. https://doi.org/10.1016/j.radonc.2013.02.007.
113. Agbahiwe HC, Wharam M, Batra S, Cohen K, Terezakis SA. Management of pediatric myxopapillary ependymoma: the role of adjuvant radiation. Int J Radiat Oncol Biol Phys. 2013;85(2):421–7. https://doi.org/10.1016/j.ijrobp.2012.05.001.

114. Weber DC, Wang Y, Miller R, Villà S, Zaucha R, Pica A, Poortmans P, Anacak Y, Ozygit G, Baumert B, Haller G, Preusser M, Li J. Long-term outcome of patients with spinal myxopapillary ependymoma: treatment results from the MD Anderson Cancer Center and institutions from the Rare Cancer Network. Neuro-Oncology. 2015;17:588–95. https://doi.org/10.1093/neuonc/nou293.
115. Feldman WB, Clark AJ, Safaee M, Ames CP, Parsa AT. Tumor control after surgery for spinal myxopapillary ependymomas: distinct outcomes in adults versus children: a systematic review. J Neurosurg Spine. 2013;19:471–6. https://doi.org/10.3171/2013.6.SPINE1292.
116. Pica A, Miller R, Villà S, Kadish SP, Anacak Y, Abusaris H, Ozyigit G, Baumert BG, Zaucha R, Haller G, Weber DC. The results of surgery, with or without radiotherapy, for primary spinal myxopapillary ependymoma: a retrospective study from the rare cancer network. Int J Radiat Oncol Biol Phys. 2009;74:1114–20. https://doi.org/10.1016/j.ijrobp.2008.09.034.
117. Plotkin SR, O'Donnell CC, Curry WT, Bove CM, MacCollin M, Nunes FP. Spinal ependymomas in neurofibromatosis type 2: a retrospective analysis of 55 patients. J Neurosurg Spine. 2011;14:543–7. https://doi.org/10.3171/2010.11.SPINE10350.
118. Aguilera DG, Mazewski C, Schniederjan MJ, Leong T, Boydston W, Macdonald TJ. Neurofibromatosis-2 and spinal cord ependymomas: report of two cases and review of the literature. Childs Nerv Syst. 2011;27:757–64. https://doi.org/10.1007/s00381-010-1351-3.
119. Robison NJ, Campigotto F, Chi SN, Manley PE, Turner CD, Zimmerman MA, Chordas CA, Werger AM, Allen JC, Goldman S, Rubin JB, Isakoff MS, Pan WJ, Khatib ZA, Comito MA, Bendel AE, Pietrantonio JB, Kondrat L, Hubbs SM, Neuberg DS, Kieran MW. A phase II trial of a multi-agent oral antiangiogenic (metronomic) regimen in children with recurrent or progressive cancer. Pediatr Blood Cancer. 2014;61:636–42.
120. Garvin JH Jr, Selch MT, Holmes E, Berger MS, Finlay JL, Flannery A, Goldwein JW, Packer RJ, Rorke-Adams LB, Shiminski-Maher T, Sposto R, Stanley P, Tannous R, Pollack IF, Children's Oncology Group. Phase II study of pre-irradiation chemotherapy for childhood intracranial ependymoma. Phase II study of pre-irradiation chemotherapy for childhood intracranial ependymoma. Children's Cancer Group protocol 9942: a report from the Children's Oncology Group. Pediatr Blood Cancer. 2012;59:1183–9.
121. Ferguson SD, Zhou S, Xiu J, Hashimoto Y, Sanai N, Kim L, Kesari S, de Groot J, Spetzler D, Heimberger AB. Ependymomas overexpress chemoresistance and DNA repair-related proteins. Ependymomas overexpress chemoresistance and DNA repair-related proteins. Oncotarget. 2018;9:7822–31.
122. Zacharoulis S, Ashley S, Moreno L, Gentet JC, Massimino M, Frappaz D. Treatment and outcome of children with relapsed Ependymoma: a multi-institutional retrospective analysis. Childs Nerv Syst. 2010;26:905–11.
123. Pollack IF, Gerszten PC, Martinez AJ, Lo KH, Shultz B, Albright AL, Janosky J, Deutsch M. Intracranial ependymomas of childhood: long-term outcome and prognostic factors. Intracranial ependymomas of childhood: long-term outcome and prognostic factors. Neurosurgery. 1995;37:655–66.
124. Peyrl A, Chocholous M, Sabel M, Lassaletta A, Sterba J, Leblond P, Nysom K, Torsvik I, Chi SN, Perwein T, Jones N, Holm S, Nyman P, Mörse H, Öberg A, Weiler-Wichtl L, Leiss U, Haberler C, Schmook MT, Mayr L, Dieckmann K, Kool M, Gojo J, Azizi AA, André N, Kieran M, Slavc I. Sustained survival benefit in recurrent Medulloblastoma by a metronomic antiangiogenic regimen: a nonrandomized controlled trial. JAMA Oncologia. 2023:1688–95. https://doi.org/10.1001/jamaoncol.2023.4437.
125. Pagnuzzi-Boncompagni M, Picco V, Vial V, Planas-Bielsa V, Vandenberghe A, Daubon T, Derieppe MA, Montemagno C, Durivault J, Grépin R, Martial S, Doyen J, Gavard J, Pagès G. Antiangiogenic compound Axitinib demonstrates low toxicity and antitumoral effects against medulloblastoma. Cancers (Basel). 2021;14:70. https://doi.org/10.3390/cancers14010070. PMID: 35008234
126. Fraser J, Wills L, Fardus-Reid F, Irvine L, Elliss-Brookes L, Fern L, Cameron AL, Pritchard-Jones K, Feltbower RG, Shelton J, Stiller C, McCabe MG. Oral etoposide as a single agent in childhood and young adult cancer in England: still a poorly evaluated palliative treatment. Pediatr Blood Cancer. 2021;68:e29204. https://doi.org/10.1002/pbc.29204.
127. Han J, Yu M, Bai Y, Yu J, Jin F, Li C, Zeng R, Peng J, Li A, Song X, Li H, Wu D, Li L. Elevated CXorf67 expression in PFA ependymomas suppresses DNA repair and sensitizes to PARP inhibitors. Cancer Cell. 2020;38:844–856.e7. https://doi.org/10.1016/j.ccell.2020.10.009.
128. Preusser M, Wolfsberger S, Haberler C, Breitschopf H, Czech T, Slavc I, Harris AL, Acker T, Budka H, Hainfellner JA. Vascularization and expression of hypoxia-related tissue factors in intracranial ependymoma and their impact on patient survival. Acta Neuropathol. 2005;109:211–6. https://doi.org/10.1007/s00401-004-0938-8.
129. Jannier S, Kemmel V, Sebastia Sancho C, Chammas A, Sabo AN, Pencreach E, Farace F, Chenard MP, Lhermitte B, Geoerger B, Aerts I, Frappaz D, Leblond P, André N, Ducassou S, Corradini N, Bertozzi AI, Guérin E, Vincent F, Velten M, Entz-Werle N. SFCE-RAPIRI Phase I study of rapamycin plus Irinotecan: a new way to target intra-tumor hypoxia in pediatric refractory cancers. Cancers

(Basel). 2020;12:3051. https://doi.org/10.3390/cancers12103051.
130. Coy S, Lee JS, Chan SJ, Woo T, Jones J, Alexandrescu S, Wen PY, Sorger PK, Ligon KL, Santagata S. Systematic characterization of antibody-drug conjugate targets in central nervous system tumors. Neuro-Oncology. 2024;26:458–72. https://doi.org/10.1093/neuonc/noad205.
131. Varlet P, Bouffet E, Casanova M, Giangaspero F, Antonelli M, Hargrave D, Ladenstein R, Pearson A, Hawkins C, König FB, Rüschoff J, Schmauch C, Bühnemann C, Garin-Chesa P, Schweifer N, Uttenreuther-Fischer M, Gibson N, Ittrich C, Krämer N, Solca F, Stolze B, Geoerger B. Comprehensive analysis of the ErbB receptor family in pediatric nervous system tumors and rhabdomyosarcoma. Pediatr Blood Cancer. 2022;69:e29316. https://doi.org/10.1002/pbc.29316. Epub 2021 Sep 21.
132. Gilbert MR, Yuan Y, Wu J, Mendoza T, Vera E, Omuro A, Lieberman F, Robins HI, Gerstner ER, Wu J, Wen PY, Mikkelsen T, Aldape K, Armstrong TS. A phase II study of dose-dense temozolomide and lapatinib for recurrent low-grade and anaplastic supratentorial, infratentorial, and spinal cord ependymoma. Neuro-Oncology. 2021;23:468–77. https://doi.org/10.1093/neuonc/noaa240.
133. Geoerger B, Marshall LV, Nysom K, Makin G, Bouffet E, Defachelles AS, Amoroso L, Aerts I, Leblond P, Barahona P, Van-Vlerken K, Fu E, Solca F, Lorence RM, Ziegler DS. Afatinib in paediatric patients with recurrent/refractory ErbB-dysregulated tumours: results of a phase I/expansion trial. Eur J Cancer. 2023;188:8–19. https://doi.org/10.1016/j.ejca.2023.04.007.
134. Venneti S, Kawakibi AR, Ji S, Waszak SM, Sweha SR, Mota M, Pun M, Deogharkar A, Chung C, Tarapore RS, Ramage S, Chi A, Wen PY, Arrillaga-Romany I, Batchelor TT, Butowski NA, Sumrall A, Shonka N, Harrison RA, de Groot J, Mehta M, Hall MD, Daghistani D, Cloughesy TF, Ellingson BM, Beccaria K, Varlet P, Kim MM, Umemura Y, Garton H, Franson A, Schwartz J, Jain R, Kachman M, Baum H, Burant CF, Mottl SL, Cartaxo RT, John V, Messinger D, Qin T, Peterson E, Sajjakulnukit P, Ravi K, Waugh A, Walling D, Ding Y, Xia Z, Schwendeman A, Hawes D, Yang F, Judkins AR, Wahl D, Lyssiotis CA, de la Nava D, Alonso MM, Eze A, Spitzer J, Schmidt SV, Duchatel RJ, Dun MD, Cain JE, Jiang L, Stopka SA, Baquer G, Regan MS, Filbin MG, Agar NYR, Zhao L, Kumar-Sinha C, Mody R, Chinnaiyan A, Kurokawa R, Pratt D, Yadav VN, Grill J, Kline C, Mueller S, Resnick A, Nazarian J, Allen JE, Odia Y, Gardner SL, Koschmann C. Clinical efficacy of ONC201 in H3K27M-mutant diffuse midline gliomas is driven by disruption of integrated metabolic and epigenetic pathways. Cancer Discov. 2023;13:2370–93. https://doi.org/10.1158/2159-8290.CD-23-0131.
135. Witt DA, Donson AM, Amani V, Moreira DC, Sanford B, Hoffman LM, Handler MH, Levy JMM, Jones KL, Nellan A, Foreman NK, Griesinger AM. Specific expression of PD-L1 in RELA-fusion supratentorial ependymoma: implications for PD-1-targeted therapy. Pediatr Blood Cancer. 2018;65:e26960. https://doi.org/10.1002/pbc.26960.
136. Nambirajan A, Malgulwar PB, Sharma A, Boorgula MT, Doddamani R, Singh M, Suri V, Sarkar C, Sharma MC. Clinicopathological evaluation of PD-L1 expression and cytotoxic T-lymphocyte infiltrates across intracranial molecular subgroups of ependymomas: are these tumors potential candidates for immune check-point blockade? Brain Tumor Pathol. 2019;36:152–61.
137. Nam SJ, Kim YH, Park JE, Ra YS, Khang SK, Cho YH, Kim JH, Sung CO. Tumor-infiltrating immune cell subpopulations and programmed death ligand 1 (PD-L1) expression associated with clinicopathological and prognostic parameters in ependymoma. Cancer Immunol Immunother. 2019;68:305–18.
138. Dunkel IJ, Doz F, Foreman NK, Hargrave D, Lassaletta A, André N, Hansford JR, Hassall T, Eyrich M, Gururangan S, Bartels U, Gajjar A, Howell L, Warad D, Pacius M, Tam R, Wang Y, Zhu L, Cohen K. Nivolumab with or without ipilimumab in pediatric patients with high-grade CNS malignancies: safety, efficacy, biomarker, and pharmacokinetics-CheckMate 908. Neuro-Oncology. 2023;25:1530–45. https://doi.org/10.1093/neuonc/noad031.
139. Donson AM, Bertrand KC, Riemondy KA, Gao D, Zhuang Y, Sanford B, Norris GA, Chapman RJ, Fu R, Willard N, Griesinger AM, Ribeiro de Sousa G, Amani V, Grimaldo E, Hankinson TC, Booker F, Sill M, Grundy RG, Pajtler KW, Ellison DW, Foreman NK, Ritzmann TA. Significant increase of high-risk chromosome 1q gain and 6q loss at recurrence in posterior fossa group a ependymoma: a multicenter study. Neuro-Oncology. 2023;25:1854–67.
140. Griesinger AM, Calzadilla AJ, Grimaldo E, Donson AM, Amani V, Pierce AM, Steiner J, Kargar S, Serkova NJ, Bertrand KC, Wright KD, Vibhakar R, Hankinson T, Handler M, Lindsay HB, Foreman NK, Dorris K. Development of chromosome 1q+ specific treatment for highest risk pediatric posterior fossa Ependymoma. Clin Cancer Res. 2024;30:1544–54. https://doi.org/10.1158/1078-0432.CCR-23-3156.
141. Mynarek M, Rossius A, Guiard A, Ottensmeier H, von Hoff K, Obrecht-Sturm D, Bußenius L, Friedrich C, von Bueren AO, Gerber NU, Traunwieser T, Kortmann RD, Warmuth-Metz M, Bison B, Thomale UW, Krauss J, Pietsch T, Clifford SC, Pfister SM, Sturm D, Sahm F, Tischler T, Rutkowski S. Risk factors for domain-specific neurocognitive outcome in pediatric survivors of a brain tumor in the posterior fossa – results of the HIT 2000 trial. Neuro-Oncol. 2024:noae092. https://doi.org/10.1093/neuonc/noae092. Epub ahead of print. PMID: 38835160).

142. Torres VA, Ashford JM, Wright E, Xu J, Zhang H, Merchant TE, Conklin HM. The impact of socio-economic status (SES) on cognitive outcomes following radiotherapy for pediatric brain tumors: a prospective, longitudinal trial. Neuro-Oncology. 2021;23:1173–82. https://doi.org/10.1093/neuonc/noab018.
143. Mule' TN, Hodges J, Wu S, Li Y, Ashford JM, Merchant TE, Conklin HM. Social determinants of cognitive outcomes in survivors of pediatric brain tumors treated with conformal radiation therapy. Neuro-Oncology. 2023;25:1842–51. https://doi.org/10.1093/neuonc/noad080.
144. Thomas S, Reynolds D, Morrall MCHJ, Limond J, Chevignard M, Calaminus G, Poggi G, Bennett E, Frappaz D, Slade D, Gautier J, McQuilton P, Massimino M, Grundy R. The European Society of Paediatric Oncology Ependymoma-II program Core-plus model: development and initial implementation of a cognitive test protocol for an international brain tumour trial. Eur J Paediatr Neurol. 2019;23:560–70. https://doi.org/10.1016/j.ejpn.2019.05.0094.
145. Merchant TE, Mulhern RK, Krasin MJ, Kun LE, Williams T, Li C, Xiong X, Khan RB, Lustig RH, Boop FA, Sanford RA. Preliminary results from a phase II trial of conformal radiation therapy and evaluation of radiation-related CNS effects for pediatric patients with localized ependymoma. J Clin Oncol. 2004;22:3156–62. https://doi.org/10.1200/JCO.2004.11.142.
146. Netson KL, Conklin HM, Wu S, Xiong X, Merchant TE. A 5-year investigation of children's adaptive functioning following conformal radiation therapy for localized ependymoma. Int J Radiat Oncol Biol Phys. 2012;84:217–223.e1. https://doi.org/10.1016/j.ijrobp.2011.10.043. Epub 2012 Apr 27
147. Ajithkumar T, Avanzo M, Yorke E, Tsang DS, Milano MT, Olch AJ, Merchant TE, Dieckmann K, Mahajan A, Fuji H, Paulino AC, Timmermann B, Marks LB, Bentzen SM, Jackson A, Constine LS. Brain and brain stem necrosis after Reirradiation for recurrent childhood primary central nervous system tumors: a PENTEC comprehensive review. Int J Radiat Oncol Biol Phys. 2024;119:655–68. https://doi.org/10.1016/j.ijrobp.2023.12.043.

Spinal Cord Tumors

14

Alberto Campione, Giovanna Stefania Colafati, Eleonora Piccirilli, and Andrea Carai

14.1 Introduction

Spinal tumors are rare in the pediatric population and characterized by an insidious clinical onset. Consequently, they are often associated with variable preoperative morbidity depending on the diagnostic delay and the burden of neurological deficits accumulated up to the time of surgical intervention. From a topographical perspective, they can be distinguished into primary vertebral and secondary extradural tumors, both of which are not the subject of this discussion: intradural extramedullary tumors (EMSCTs) and intramedullary tumors (IMSCTs). Based on their biological behavior, neoplastic lesions at the spinal level can also be classified as primary low-grade and high-grade, and metastatic.

A. Campione
Neurosurgery Unit, Legnano Hospital, ASST West Milan, Legnano, MI, Italy

G. S. Colafati · E. Piccirilli
Oncological Neuroradiology and Advanced Diagnostic Unit, IRCCS Bambino Gesù Children's Hospital, Rome, Italy
e-mail: gstefania.colafati@opbg.net; eleonora.piccirilli@opbg.net

A. Carai (✉)
Neurosurgery Unit, IRCCS Bambino Gesù Children's Hospital, Rome, Italy
e-mail: andrea.carai@opbg.net

14.1.1 Epidemiology

14.1.1.1 Intradural Extramedullary Tumors

EMSCTs constitute 24.6% of spinal cord tumors in children [1]. The majority comprises low-grade tumors. Despite the absence of a specific classification for spinal cord tumors, it is possible to extrapolate one from the WHO classification of central nervous system tumors, fifth edition [2], by dividing them based on histogenesis (Table 14.1).

14.1.1.2 Nerve Sheath Tumors

Sporadic nerve sheath tumors (NSTs) are exceptionally rare in the pediatric population and are rather suggestive of neurofibromatosis type 1 (neurofibromas) or NF2-related schwannomatosis [3]. Other low-grade NST—namely, perineurioma, hybrid NST, and cauda equina neuroendocrine tumor—are prevalent among adults and only anecdotally reported in children [2]. Their malignant transformation into malignant melanotic or malignant peripheral NST is rare, occurring in 5% of patients with neurofibromatosis type 1 [4], and generally occurs late in disease natural history, often following a subtotal surgical resection of a primary low-grade tumor or after radiation therapy.

A. Mastronuzzi, A. Carai (eds.), *Navigating Pediatric Brain Tumors*,
https://doi.org/10.1007/978-3-032-18992-9_14

Table 14.1 Epidemiology of pediatric spinal cord tumors

Tumor topography	Tumor histotype	Incidence among pediatric CNS tumors	Incidence among pediatric SCT	Notes
EMSCT			24.6% among pediatric SCT	
	Nerve sheath tumors	Anecdotal; malignant progression reported in 5% of NF-1 cases		
	Meningiomas		1–17% among pediatric SCT	
	Myxopapillary ependymoma			30% among pediatric spinal ependymomas 90% of pediatric lumbosacral ependymomas
	Dysembriogenetic tumor-like lesions		10–30%	
IMSCT		4%	35%	
	HGG		7.5%	
	LGG			80% among pediatric IMSCT Astrocytoma (35.4%) Ganglioglioma (26.8%), ependymomas (11.6%), and mixed gliomas (6.1%)
	Hemangioblastoma			3.3% among all-age IMSCT 1.7% among all-age EMSCT

14.1.1.3 Meningiomas

Pediatric spinal meningiomas are reported with a variable prevalence of 1–17% of all pediatric spinal tumors [1]. Unlike among adults, no sex prevalence is observed among those affected, and, as with schwannomas, this diagnosis in a child is a suspicion indicator for neurofibromatosis type 2. Generally, they are low-grade and more commonly of the psammomatous or clear cell histotype.

14.1.1.4 Myxopapillary Ependymomas

Myxopapillary ependymomas represent tumors at the boundary between formally classified extramedullary and intramedullary lesions: phylogenetically intramedullary, they are extramedullary lesions originating from cells of the filum terminale and, in the pediatric population, constitute 30% of spinal ependymomas [5] and 90% of ependymomas at the lumbosacral level.

14.1.1.5 Dysembriogenetic Tumor-Like Lesions

Within the realm of tumor-like lesions, dermoid and epidermoid tumors represent 10–30% of all pediatric spinal tumors [6]. In 30% of cases, they are associated with the presence of a dermal sinus and are often associated with other dysembryogenetic alterations within the spectrum of spinal dysraphism.

14.1.1.6 Intramedullary Tumors

IMSCT comprise 4% of intraparenchymal central nervous system (CNS) pediatric tumors and 35% of pediatric spinal cord tumors [7].

14.1.1.7 Gliomas, Glioneuronal Tumors, and Neuronal Tumors

As far as high-grade (HGG) and low-grade (LGG) glial IMSCTs are concerned, there is a paucity of data regarding the exact epidemiology due to both the rarity of the diseases and the heterogeneity of the reports in the literature. As a general consideration, a slight prevalence among males is observed [8], and an increase in tumor incidence in infants is reported, while it decreases at the end of adolescence [9, 10]. The incidence of HGG, such as anaplastic astrocytomas, glioblastomas, and PNET [9, 10], among all pediatric SCT is estimated to be 7.5%, most commonly in age groups 6–11 years (43.3%) and 12–17 years (41.2%) [11]. Most patients (80%) have LGG

[12, 13], including astrocytomas (35.4%), gangliogliomas (26.8%), ependymomas (11.6%), and mixed gliomas (6.1%). Mean age at presentation is 8.1 years, with a slight prevalence among age group 5–10 years (37%), followed by 0–5 age group (33%) [13]. While spinal ependymomas are more common in adults [14], astrocytomas are more prevalent in the pediatric population, occurring 3–4 times more frequently [15]. Further comparing the epidemiology of pediatric spinal ependymomas to those in adults, pediatric cases are significantly more aggressive: 33.3% of the total are grade 3, whereas anaplastic spinal ependymomas in adults are less than 10% [14].

14.1.1.8 Hemangioblastomas

Spinal hemangioblastomas are rare lesions, accounting for 3.3% of IMSCTs and 1.7% of EMSCTs in the general population. Fifteen percent of them are diagnosed in childhood and are associated with Von Hippel–Lindau syndrome. They are predominantly located at the dorsal level [6].

14.2 Clinical Presentation

EMSCT and IMSCT share a common clinical presentation, despite their different pathophysiology, compression in the case of EMSCT, and predominantly infiltration in the case of IMSCT. Generally, the initial symptom is back pain (48–70% of the affected), more pronounced in the segments affected by the lesion [7, 10, 16, 17]. In the differential diagnosis of tumor topography, radiating and radicular pain is more typical of extramedullary neoplasms. Sensory alterations are common (32%) but difficult to assess objectively, especially considering that young patients often are not able to describe them [10, 16, 17]. Motor and sphincter deficits tend to appear later in the natural history of spinal cord tumors, though more quickly in infiltrative tumors than in compressive ones [9, 10, 18]. They are present at diagnosis in one-third of cases and are associated with de novo kyphoscoliosis in 32% of cases [9, 16, 17]. Generally, a longer and more insidious clinical history usually correlates with low-grade tumors. Therefore, it is not surprising that the duration of symptoms is 6–20 months before a formal diagnosis in the case of benign tumors, with the notably shorter diagnostic delay in children aged under three [9], which reduces to 3–10 months in the case of malignant ones [16, 17].

As far as EMSCTs are concerned, slow-growing benign tumors allow for regional anatomical adjustments, causing various soft tissue, bony, and neural changes. Despite their size, these tumors often result in mild neural deficits and rarely cause acute symptoms. Bone erosion and thinning of vertebral bones can widen the spinal canal and intervertebral foramina. Long-standing tumors may also thin the dura and reduce extradural fat. The cerebrospinal fluid (CSF) is the first to be displaced, leading to neural thinning or atrophy adjacent to the tumor. Meningeal membranes may stretch but rarely break, even with malignant tumors. Tumors in the cervical spinal canal are typically smaller at diagnosis compared to those in the dorsal or lumbar canal, where the larger canal diameter allows tumors to grow larger before detection [19].

As for IMSCT, tumors at the cervical level typically present with neck pain that worsens at night and myelopathic signs and symptoms typically have a descending progression pattern. Motor deficits are rarely reported as such by young children, but parents might notice motor regression, a switch in hand dominance or frequent tripping. Quite characteristically, sensory abnormalities follow motor deficits and are usually unilateral, except for ependymoma where they are symmetrical [20, 21]. Thoracic spinal tumors have a more gradual onset, often being initially diagnosed as idiopathic scoliosis. Symptoms include paraspinal spasm, myelopathy, and sometimes abdominal pain. Sensory issues and bowel and bladder dysfunction occur later as the tumor extends into the conus. Conus tumors present early with bowel and bladder dysfunction, frequent urinary tract infections, and irregular bowel habits, with overt urinary tract dysfunction developing later [22]. IMSCTs are also associated with a risk of hydrocephalus. The pathophysiological mechanism underlying hydrocephalus in malignant tumors is attributed to neoplastic dissemination through the CSF pathways. Conversely, in benign tumors, the mechanism is less clear: theories suggest it may be due to increased protein concentration in the CSF, a paraneoplastic arachnoid inflammatory reaction, or, in the case of cervical lesions, the cranial extension of cervicomedullary cysts causing obstruction of the outflow from the fourth ventricle into the subarachnoid space [23]. In the absence of recent data on the epidemiology of hydrocephalus in IMSCTs, a single monocentric series from 1990 reported its incidence at clinical presentation to be 14.6% [24].

14.3 Diagnostic Workup

14.3.1 MRI-Guided Differential Diagnosis

Neuroimaging is pivotal in the diagnosis, characterization, and management of pediatric spinal tumors [25]. MRI is the cornerstone for their evaluation, both in the pre- and postoperative workup, as it allows the direct visualization of the spinal cord itself.

The primary aim is the definition of the following:

- Tumor location, extradural or intradural (intra- or extramedullary).
- Tumor extension.
- Its relationship with the spinal cord and the surrounding structures.
- Morphology.
- Intrinsic features: signal intensity, presence of blood, solid and cystic components, contrast enhancement. Standard sequences alone can give precious information on lesion biology, helping the neuroradiologist differentiate between benign tumors and more aggressive ones.
- Complications and associated features: cord compression and myelopathy (for extrinsic tumors), cord edema, syringomyelia.

Similarly to their supratentorial counterpart, when a spinal tumor is diagnosed the MRI study should not be limited to the affected region but must be extended—possibly during the same examination—to the entire CNS (i.e., whole spine and brain), not only because of the possibility of leptomeningeal dissemination but also to look for associated findings and syndromic clues.

The other imaging techniques are complementary to MRI.

Unlike supratentorial tumors where it is usually the primary imaging modality, in the diagnostic workup of spinal tumors CT has quite a limited role. Nevertheless, it is very useful to assess spine's bony structures [26].

Contribution of X-rays is marginal as well, with their use being limited to the initial assessment of children presenting with back pain or scoliosis.

14.3.2 EMSCTs

Nerve sheath tumors (Fig. 14.1) arise along the nerves' course and show avid contrast enhancement. Due to their slow growth pattern and compressive effect on surrounding structures, they tend to widen the corresponding intervertebral foramina (a finding more evident on CT, *see* Fig. 14.1d). Additionally, they can develop a dumbbell shape, where the point of greatest narrowing corresponds to the intervertebral foramen.

As well as nerve sheath tumors, spinal meningiomas (Fig. 14.2) show avid contrast enhancement. The differential diagnosis with nerve sheath tumors is necessary since nerve sheath tumors can have an extraspinal component in continuity with the corresponding intervertebral foramen (*see* Fig. 14.2d). In contrast, meningiomas are intracanalar lesions, often displaying a dural tail, and only rarely involve or proliferate through the intervertebral foramina.

Myxopapillary ependymomas envelop rather than compressing the roots of the cauda equina. In this regard, they are extra-axial neoplasms but

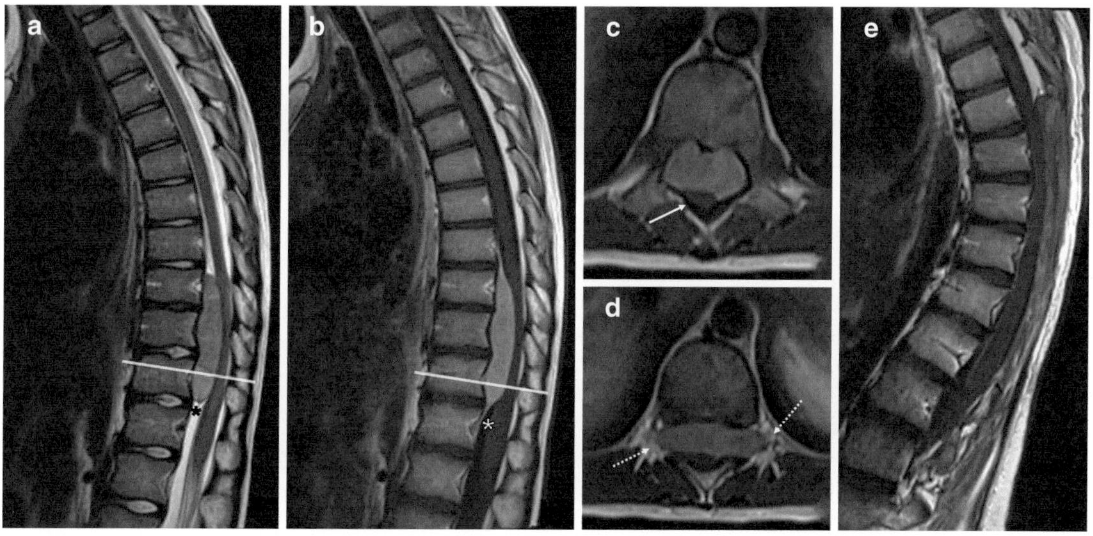

Fig. 14.1 Schwannoma. Case of a dorsal extramedullary neoplasm with topography confirmed intraoperatively as extradural. As visible in (**a**), the neoplasm is hypointense on T2 and exerts compressive effects on the spinal cord. Upon retrospective evaluation, as the dural tail in (**b**, white asterisk) is the margin of the dura mater elevated by the tumor (**a**, black asterisk). In T2 (**a**), it is evident that the tumor has rounded morphology at the ends, rather than fusiform, which would be more typical for a meningioma. Spinal cord compression is evident on the axial scan (**c**, axial plane indicated in **a**), diagnosis of schwannoma is very likely when the occupation of both foramina, enlarged by the progressive growth of the lesion, is appreciated (**d**, axial plane indicated in **b**, dashed arrows). At mid-term postoperative follow-up (**e**), evidence is visible of gross total resection with progressive kyphosis despite the use of a brace in the postoperative period

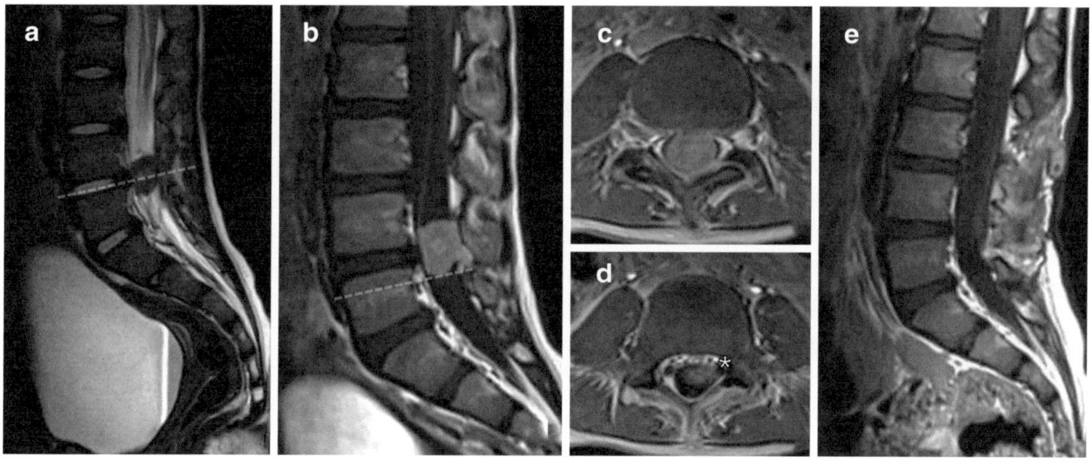

Fig. 14.2 Meningioma. Case of an intradural neoplasm at L4–5 with compression of the cauda equina, presenting initially with recurrent urinary infections and progressively worsening dysuria, consistent with the bladder distension visible in (**a**). The lesion is hypointense on T2-weighted images (**a**) and shows avid contrast enhancement (**b**); its margins are continuous with the dura mater, making meningioma the most probable differential diagnosis. The compression on the cauda equina is severe, and the nerve roots are indistinguishable on axial projection (**c**, axial plane indicated by dotted line in **a**). At the caudal pole of the lesion, infiltration of the left L5 root is noted (**d**, axial plane indicated by dotted line in **b**, white asterisk), which is not compatible with a schwannoma, as the latter would typically progress along the course of the nerve involving the respective neural foramen. (**e**) Long-term postoperative follow-up: subtotal resection (considering the L5 root infiltration) with a stable residual disease. On the clinical side, decompression of the cauda equina has resulted in an improvement in urinary retention

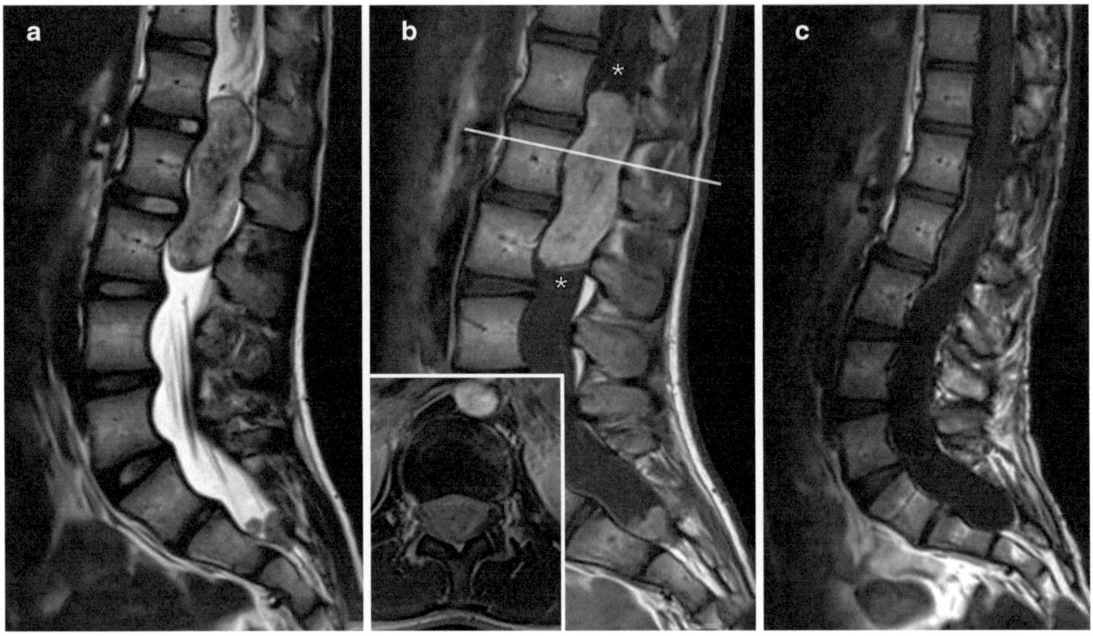

Fig. 14.3 Filum terminale ependymoma. Case of an intradural extramedullary tumor at D12-L2, hyperintense on T2-weighted sequences (**a**) and exhibiting heterogeneous contrast enhancement (**b**), with rounded ends of the lesion (**b**, white asterisks). The tumor almost completely occupies the vertebral canal (**b**, lower left inset, axial plane indicated in the figure). Histological diagnosis: myxopapillary ependymoma. (**c**) Postoperative follow-up after gross total resection

do not fit the usual "extra-axial–compressive" association. They are hyperintense on both T1- and T2-weighted sequences due to their high mucin content and exhibit heterogeneous contrast enhancement (Fig. 14.3).

Tumor-like dysembryogenetic lesions should be included in the differential diagnosis with EMSCT. A diagnostic clue could be the hyperintensity of dermoid and epidermoid on diffusion-weighted imaging (DWI). They are predominantly located in the lower thoracic and lumbar regions [27].

14.3.3 IMSCTs

Intramedullary astrocytomas are primarily located within the spinal cord. At diagnosis, the lesion typically extends over an average of four vertebral segments [28] and has an infiltrative pattern, causing a swollen appearance of the spinal cord, with indistinct margins [28, 29]. Tumor cysts and syringomyelic dilations often occur upstream and downstream of the lesion (Fig. 14.4). In cases of cervicomedullary localization, the lesion tends to extend toward the obex and the fourth ventricle, as cranial-ventral progression is limited by the decussation of the medullary pyramids and the spinal pia mater [30].

Intramedullary ependymomas show avid contrast enhancement with various patterns—homogeneous, heterogeneous, or ring-like [31]. As opposed to astrocytomas, they are distinguished by rather well-defined margins and (present in 20% of cases) hemosiderin deposits due to intralesional hemorrhages (Fig. 14.5) [31].

Gangliogliomas share radiological features with astrocytomas and ependymomas. Like astrocytomas, they tend to have eccentric intramedullary growth and are associated with peritumoral cysts. Like ependymomas, they are often

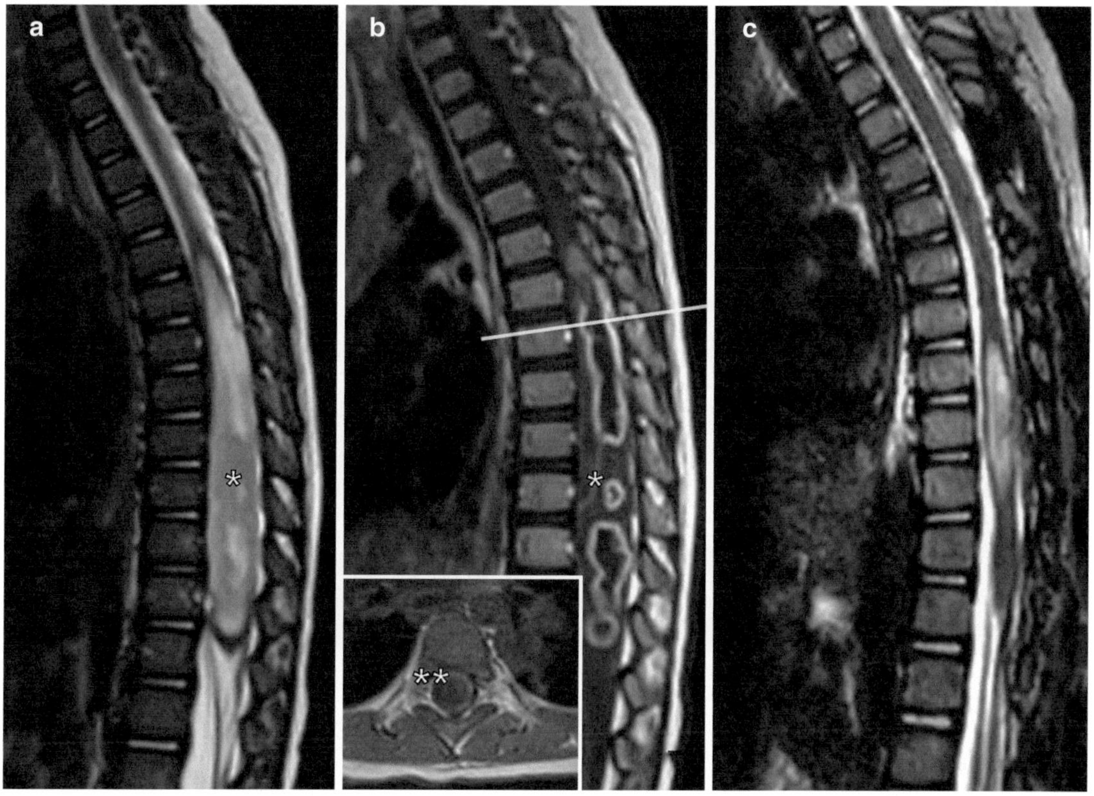

Fig. 14.4 Low-grade astrocytoma. Case of a multilevel dorsal intramedullary neoplasm causing spinal cord swelling with heterogeneous intralesional components on T2-weighted images, suggesting necrotic areas with ring contrast enhancement on T1 contrast sequences (**a**, **b**, white asterisks). In the upper component of the lesion, an axial projection (lower left inset, axial plane indicated in **b**) shows no recognizable signal of healthy spinal cord; the lesion also appears eccentric and predominantly on the right side. The surgical approach consisted of a median posterior approach with subtotal resection within functional limits, guided by intraoperative monitoring. Histological diagnosis: low-grade astrocytoma, for which adjuvant treatment was administered with long-term disease control (**c**). The laminotomy approach had the benefit of preventing de novo kyphosis (**c**)

(60%) homogeneously hyperintense on T2-weighted images and have variable contrast enhancement patterns, ranging from multifocal to nodular or even absent (15%). Compared to the other two histotypes, gangliogliomas extend over a greater number of vertebral segments—on average, eight—at the time of diagnosis [29, 32]; the anatomical location is usually cervical or cervicomedullary.

Hemangioblastomas are predominantly intramedullary and are very rare in sporadic form but have a high prevalence (38%) among patients with Von Hippel–Lindau syndrome [33]. They are located in the cervical spinal cord in 50% of cases and in the thoracic spinal cord in 30% of cases. These tumors have the typical "cyst and nodule" appearance, with contrast enhancement of the parietal nodule. The signal, and consequently the tumor tissue, becomes more heterogeneous as the lesion extends beyond 2 cm in maximum diameter [34]. Within the spinal cord, they are usually located superficially and in the posterior columns. In the differential diagnosis with more common spinal gliomas, syrinxes associated with hemangioblastomas are often disproportionately large compared to the size of the neoplastic nodule [34, 35].

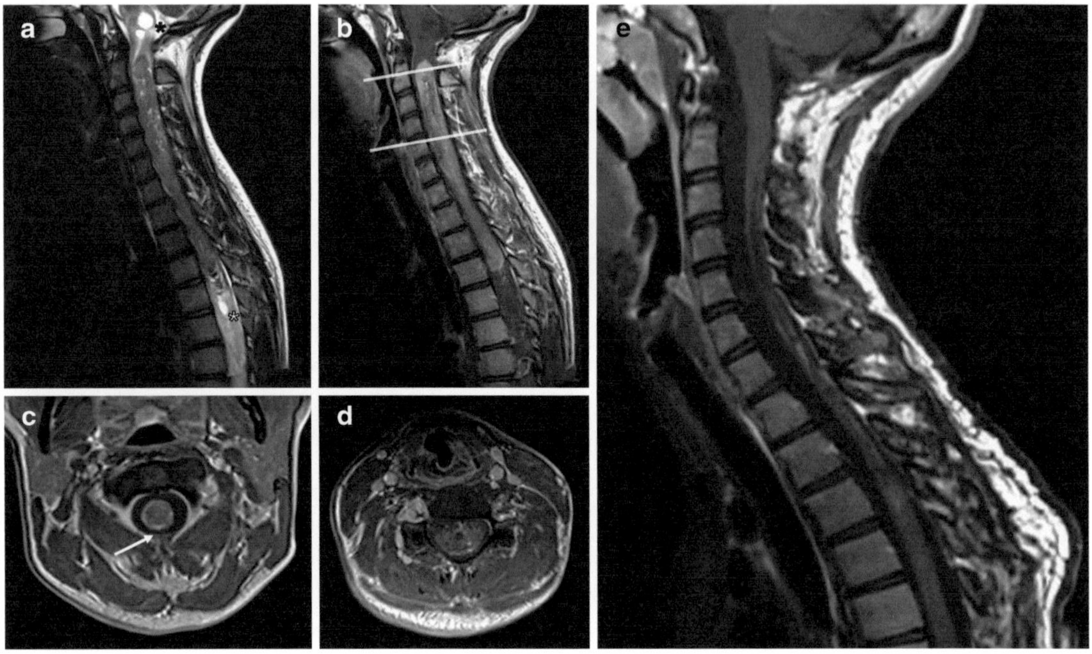

Fig. 14.5 Intramedullary ependymoma. Case of an intramedullary ependymoma C2-T3, characterized by well-defined margins with cysts at the top and bottom (**a**, asterisks) and avid contrast uptake with a heterogeneous pattern (**b**). The tumor is located centrally in the spinal cord and flattens its dorsal surface (and consequently the posterior median sulcus, **c**, arrow), as evident in image **c** (corresponding to the superior axial plane indicated in **b**). The tumor's attitude toward the surrounding spinal cord is compressive rather than infiltrative; however, due to the significant lesion size, the spinal cord is difficult to recognize at the level of the tumor's largest diameter (**d**, inferior axial plane indicated in **b**). For this reason, the surgical approach first targets the elevation and devascularization of the cranial and caudal capsule, because it is at these points that the tumor thins and its interface with the spinal cord becomes more evident (**b**). In (**e**), long-term postsurgical sagittal image: through a posterior median approach C0-T5 with laminotomy, a radical resection was achieved without permanent functional deficits

14.4 Surgical Treatment (Table 14.2)

14.4.1 EMSCTs

In general, the surgical approach to a suspected EMSCT involves complete exposure of the lesion and its dissection from the surrounding anatomical structures. Given their well-circumscribed nature, the goal is radical surgery when the tumor capsule is intact and well-defined. If there is any suspicion of spinal cord infiltration, a conservative approach with minimal morbidity is always preferred (*see* Fig. 14.2d). The chosen approach is typically a midline posterior one, extended sufficiently to fully manage the lesion. However, considering the growth curve of pediatric patients, it is crucial to avoid extensive bone removal, thus preferring laminoplasty approaches [36], or limit to unilateral removals such as hemilaminectomies [37, 38]. Indeed, aggressive bone removal is a risk factor for postoperative spinal deformities, which can also be exacerbated by postoperative motor deficits. For metameric stability, facet-sparing approaches are advisable. Once the lesion is exposed and dissected from the surrounding structures, en bloc removal is preferred for small nodules [1]. Progressive debulking is advisable for large lesions or severe spinal cord compressions to avoid spinal cord traction or increasing the risk of acute reperfusion syndromes of the spinal white matter [19].

Considering surgical technique aspects related to specific tumors, for myxopapillary ependymomas, dissection and debulking proceed simultaneously and progressively. While small lesions

Table 14.2 Pediatric spinal cord tumors: surgical strategy and technical nuances according to subtype

Tumor topography	Tumor subtype	Surgical strategy essentials	Notes
EMSCT		4Ds: de-dress, devascularize, debulk, dissect	Avoid extensive bone removal and choose laminotomy/laminoplasty instead
	Myxopapillary ependymoma	For larger lesions or those involving the conus medullaris, debulking with minimal manipulation of neural structures with the goal of functional-sparing subtotal resection	
IMSCT		Reduce disease burden and aim for maximal safe resection Morphological and functional dorsal sulcus detection and tracing prior to myelotomy	IOM-guided resection (most of all, D-wave trend is relevant)
	Astrocytoma	Resection proceeds from the tumor core to its periphery using an ultrasonic aspirator	Stop as soon as a change in tissue characteristics is visible: no cleavage plan is usually detectable
	Ependymoma	Once the dorsal wall of the tumor is exposed, blunt dissection toward its cranial or caudal pole, often characterized by a CSF cleft (a "cap") Goal is to isolate the lesion by circumferentially dissecting it through bipolar coagulation of the capillaries directed toward the tumor itself, thus progressively elevating its capsule	Capsule is usually detectable -main difference as compared to astrocytomas
	Hemangioblastoma	Peritumoral afferent arterioles targeted coagulation to obtain an orthograde flow-directed devascularization and a subsequent en bloc resection	Indocyanine green enables intraoperative angiography, effectively distinguishing arterial feeders, arterialized veins, and the tumor's draining vessels

confined to the filum terminale (FT) are candidates for en bloc gross total resection, this is not applicable for larger lesions or those involving the conus medullaris. In these cases, the tumor may fill the dural sac and envelop the cauda equina (Fig. 14.3), with nerve roots running through the tumor parenchyma sometimes without a clear dissection plane. In such cases, a debulking technique with minimal manipulation of neural structures is preferred, favoring planned subtotal or partial resection surgery, whenever significant functional impairment is anticipated in case of more extensive resection [5].

14.4.2 IMSCTs

The role of surgery in the treatment of IMSCTs has radically changed with the introduction and continuous improvement of intraoperative neurophysiological monitoring techniques. Before these technologies, the role of surgery was ancillary and predominantly diagnostic, aiming to avoid unjustified periprocedural morbidity [39, 40]. Currently, the goal of surgery in this context is not only diagnostic but also to reduce the disease burden aiming to achieve subtotal or better resection (>80% of tumor volume) [12, 39].

In pediatric low-grade IMSCTs, the extent of resection correlates with progression-free survival: a subtotal or better resection predicts a 70% event-free survival at 5 years, with no statistically significant differences between gross total resection and more conservative resections [39]. For tumors with an intact and well-defined cleavage plane relative to the surrounding spinal cord, such as ependymomas and hemangioblastomas, the surgical goal is ideally a total or near-total resection. As with EMSCTs, the most common surgical approach is a posterior midline approach aimed at exposing the lesion without extensive bone removal (Fig. 14.4) [37, 38]. Given the laxity of the ligamentum flavum in pediatric patients, multilevel laminotomies can be performed with a craniotome, and the adequacy of the exposure can be assessed with intraoperative spinal ultrasound [22]. The target for exposure and resection is the solid nodule(s), while exposure of associated cysts has to be considered on a case-to-case basis.

Once the dura mater is exposed, epidural electrodes for intraoperative D-wave monitoring should be placed before proceeding. The dura is then incised longitudinally and suspended with tack sutures. If the tumor is visible on the dorsal pial surface of the spinal cord, a pial incision can be made directly in this area to proceed with intralesional debulking. If the lesion is deeper, the posterior median sulcus must be identified, though its course may be anatomically distorted by the lesion itself. In this case, intraoperative stimulation can help identify nonresponsive areas between two contiguous zones that respond effectively to stimulation. These nonresponsive areas can be incised without causing direct damage to the posterior columns [40]. An additional visual criterion for identifying the midline is the pattern of pial capillaries, which converge into the posterior median sulcus. The midline is indicated by the invagination where vessels from both sides course ventrally. After making the midline pial incision, the posterior columns are dissected sharply until the dorsal wall of the tumor is exposed.

14.5 Astrocytomas

In planning the extent of resection, intraoperative neurophysiological monitoring plays a crucial role. The resection margins will be determined by functional limits, meaning the interface between the tumor and eloquent tracts to be preserved, to avoid the onset of permanent neurological deficits that would compromise long-term prognosis regardless. The degree of biological aggressiveness of the tumor determines the impact that maximal safe resection has on prognosis. In the case of LGG, a wider resection correlates with higher probabilities of long-term PFS; in the case of HGG, maximal safe resection increases the effectiveness of adjuvant therapies and positively correlates with overall survival [41].

Resection proceeds from the tumor core to its periphery using an ultrasonic aspirator, with the recommendation to stop as soon as a change in tissue characteristics is visible—which signals the transition from lesion to healthy spinal cord. Manipulating tumor remnants at the lesion boundary necessarily involves traction on healthy fascicles, causing mechanical distortion reflected in changes in intraoperative monitoring. The necessity of pursuing the resection of such remnants must be balanced with the goal of avoiding iatrogenic morbidity, which would compromise the survival advantage that is the aim of the surgery [42–44]. Upon completion of the resection, hemostasis is achieved through irrigation and the intermittent application of compressed hemostatic sponges with cottonoids to tamponade bleeding points. Bipolar coagulation should be avoided to prevent peri-surgical ischemia. Additionally, the application of hemostatic material that would be left in situ should be avoided, as it could later cause artifacts in MRI, complicating the interpretation of surgical results.

14.6 Ependymomas

The approach to ependymomas is essentially similar to that already described for astrocytomas. However, because ependymomas tend to grow concentrically to the spinal cord, the deviation of the posterior median sulcus from its natural anatomical position is less pronounced. Instead, the mass effect produced by the tumor may flatten the sulcus and make it less recognizable, which is why it is always advisable to use functional mapping of the posterior median sulcus. Once the dorsal wall of the tumor is exposed, blunt dissection proceeds toward its cranial or caudal pole, often characterized by a CSF cleft or cysts that separate it from healthy spinal cord tissue (Fig. 14.5) [31]. The goal is to isolate the lesion by circumferentially dissecting it through bipolar coagulation of the capillaries directed toward the tumor itself, thus progressively elevating its capsule. Cauterization of the vessels supplying the tumor must be particularly judicious ventrally, as the vascular pedicle of the tumor originates from the anterior spinal artery, and inadvertent coagulation can cause irreversible postoperative motor deficits. In the case of large tumors, to avoid excessive traction, central debulking with an ultrasonic aspirator is advisable. Considering the capsule that characterizes and separates it from the surrounding parenchyma, the goal of ependymoma surgery is a total or near-total resection. More recently, staged resection has been advocated for large volume lesions, with a first surgical procedure aiming at opening the pial surface, exposing the dorsal portion of the tumor and performing an expansion duroplasty. After about 2 weeks, dorsalization of the lesion is observed with recovery of ventral spinal cord volume, allowing a second surgical procedure to radically resect the tumor with a lower risk of functional impairment [45].

14.7 Hemangioblastomas

Hemangioblastomas typically have a well-defined peritumoral capsule that can be progressively coagulated and retracted to avoid manipulation of the spinal cord. The cystic component of hemangioblastomas often surfaces dorsally, and breaching the pial wall of such cysts allows visualization of the tumor nodule. During the coagulation of vessels, which is technically like the procedure for ependymomas, large-caliber superficial draining veins may be visualized. It is advisable to preserve these veins until the arterial devascularization of the lesion is complete. The use of intraoperative fluorescent markers provides a significant advantage in these cases. Indocyanine green enables intraoperative angiography, effectively distinguishing arterial feeders, arterialized veins, and the tumor's draining vessels [46]. This allows for targeted en bloc resection while minimizing blood loss. Takami et al. report greater efficacy of indocyanine use in tumors with a predominantly dorsal topography, and to a lesser extent, in tumors occupying the ventral part of the spinal cord [47]. It is important to note that isolating these vascular lesions temporarily interferes with the physiological vascularization of the contiguous spinal cord, leading to expected transient changes in evoked potentials during the procedure [33, 34]. Piecemeal resection is associated with sometimes copious blood loss; for this reason, some recommend preoperative embolization, although it carries the risk of iatrogenic embolism of the spinal arteries and consequent spinal cord ischemia [48].

Regardless of whether the tumor is intra- or extramedullary, closure is performed using a standard multilayer technique. This involves a watertight closure with nonresorbable heterologous dural grafts and minimizing dead spaces by carefully reapproximating the anatomical layers. The goal is to minimize the risk of CSF fistula and pseudomeningocele formation.

14.8 The Role of Intraoperative Neurophysiological Monitoring

Intraoperative neurophysiological monitoring (IONM) has significantly evolved since the last quarter of the twentieth century, starting with somatosensory-evoked potential (SSEP) monitoring in the 1970s, followed by motor-evoked potentials (MEP) in the 1980s, and the establishment of predictive criteria for deficits in 1998 [21, 49]. Improved neurological and overall outcomes have been reported in patients undergoing IMSCT surgery since 2006 [40] with the implementation of IONM, highlighting its value in surgical procedures. Developing neuroanesthetic techniques that ensure patient safety and comfort while maintaining necessary neuronal activity for reliable recordings proved challenging and remains as one of the limitations of such monitoring techniques. Even with IONM, rates of new deficits are high, with the most common new deficit being dorsal column dysfunction, affecting up to 55% of patients and characterized by diminution of proprioception and vibratory sensation [50].

Monitoring D-waves, which are upper motor potentials traveling down the spinal cord, has been found to be nearly 100% predictive for postoperative motor deficits [51]. Changes in MEP monitoring were also predictive of rehabilitation needs post-surgery [51]. Protocols for IONM are not standardized but most comprise a combination of MEP, SSEP free-running electromyography and D-wave monitoring. In a systematic review by Rijs et al., MEP showed a sensitivity of 84% and specificity of 83% for intraoperative detection of fascicle conductivity disturbances [52]. D-wave monitoring takes advantage of electrodes in the epidural space and, in comparison to MEP and SSEP, is less susceptible to interference by anesthetic agents, prompts online results of tissue manipulation and eventual current disturbances, and has higher test specificity [53]. In 2016, Verla et al. showed that IONM during IMSCT surgery predicted postoperative outcomes in all 13 reviewed studies and could improve the extent of resection, as it established a "safety boundary" by which a more aggressive tumor resection could be conducted [33, 50]. Despite the acknowledged validity of IONM, standardized guidelines for its usage in IMSCT surgery are missing, as are consensus thresholds for terminating resection in the event of IONM changes. In a consensus statement by the North American Spine Society Section of Spine Oncology, the participants agreed on halting resection following complete loss of MEP and a 50% decrease in the D-wave amplitude. In contrast, no consensus was reached in a supposed case of complete MEP loss but with preservation of D-wave amplitude. A literature review by Olmsted et al. found that declines in the D-wave amplitude <50% correlated with transient motor deficits, but a decline of higher proportion was associated with permanent damage to the corticospinal tracts [54]. Prior studies had already reported adopting a 50% threshold for stopping the resection, at least until the signal recovered [40].

14.9 Postoperative Care

14.9.1 Complications

Neuropathic pain is a frequent sequela after SCT resection, especially in the case of intramedullary tumors, with a frequency of about 50–70%. The correlation between neuropathic pain and the degree of postoperative motor disability is inconsistent, and severe pain can occur in the absence of significant neurological deficits. In this regard, hemangioblastoma carries a higher risk of postoperative neuropathic pain compared to other histotypes, which do not show significant associations in this context [55]. Nearly one-third of patients experience at least one complication within 30 days of surgery, regardless of pathology, which calls for hospital readmission. Neurological status often remains unchanged at the 90-day follow-up; improvements are reported in urinary incontinence for ependymomas and sensory changes for hemangioblastomas. However, functional independence typically decreases in the short-term postoperative period, as indicated by trends in the modified McCormick scale (MMS): 32% of worsening vs 25% of improvement [56]. At a long-term follow-up evaluation, MMS shows a trend toward neurological status stabilization or improvement: clinical improvement is reported in 27.6% of cases, stability in 54.9%, and worsening in 17.6% [45].

De novo kyphotic deformities are the most common biomechanical complications following SCT removal (*see* Figs. 14.1 and 14.5) [57, 58] and the incidence ranges between 16% and 100% [36]. Causes include, among other factors, the weakness of paravertebral muscles induced by tumor-related myelopathy and postsurgical fibrosis [59]. Cervical region and age $\leq$ 15 years are the most prominent risk factors for segmental instability [57]. The thoracolumbar region has been the most studied, with laminectomy associated with a higher risk of deformity especially if longer than three level, while laminoplasty has a protective effect. Preoperative kyphosis correlates with the persistence and worsening of kyphosis postoperatively [57, 58]. Prophylactic osteosynthesis is not recommended; however, certain risk factors are known to predispose to the progression of deformities that may require surgical intervention. These include age under 13 years, involvement of the thoracolumbar region, tumor-associated syrinx, and preoperative scoliosis [60].

A further long-term risk of EMSCT or IMSCT resection is the formation of tenacious adhesions between the spinal cord, dural substitute, and the overlying deep muscles. Practically, adhesions develop between two structures to the extent that they come into contact. This means that laminotomy and laminoplasty techniques reduce the risk of adhesions between the soft tissues and the pseudodura, even in the event of long-term bone resorption. Among synthetic dural substitutes, Gore-Tex is considered the least adhesion-inducing; however, being synthetic, it induces intense inflammation and fibrosis, unlike biological dural substitutes such as DuraGen [61].

14.9.2 Prognosis

14.9.2.1 Survival Considerations

Currently, the overall survival rate for low-grade IMSCTs is 88% at 5 years and 82% at 10 years following subtotal or better resection [39]; progression-free survival in such instances stands at 70% at 10 years [39]. High-grade IMSCTs have a completely different clinical history, characterized by an overall survival of 18% at 5 years and 12% at 10 years, with a progression-free survival of 30% at 10 years [39]. From an oncological point of view, about one-third of patients experience recurrence or progression of a residual tumor within 38 months postoperatively [39]. Although the survival benefit of resective surgery is not dramatic, it avoids the risks associated with postradiation secondary malignant tumors (18%) and radiotherapy-induced progression of low-grade IMSCT (9%) [62, 63]. Therefore, surgery is the treatment of choice for these lesions, while radiotherapy serves an adjuvant role for residual tumors.

14.9.2.2 Functional Considerations

Children under the age of three with IMSCT who are treated with subtotal or better surgery benefit from greater PFS without the need for adjuvant therapies, compared to older children [9, 39]. Three months post-surgery, 60.4% of patients remain neurologically unchanged, 15.8% improve, and 23.8% deteriorate [9, 39, 64], the latter correlating with already deficient preoperative neurological status, emphasizing the importance of early diagnosis and treatment. In the long-term follow-up (median 67 months), 40% of patients show neurological improvement compared to pre-surgery, 50% remain unchanged, and 10% worsen [64].

From a functional point of view, a surgical intervention with subtotal or better resection and free from intraoperative neurophysiological complications correlates with autonomous mobility, reported as a favorable outcome, up to 13 years after the intervention. IMSCTs located at the lower thoracic and lumbar segments are associated with a higher incidence of new-onset postoperative neurological deficits. The presence of long-standing neurological deficits at the time of surgery is a predictive factor for the absence of clinical improvements post-procedure [65]. Conversely, younger patients have a higher likelihood of recovering from deficits in the 2–6 months following surgery [65]. The most common postoperative deficit involves the posterior columns; nonetheless, the majority of patients are able to walk independently within 3 months after the surgery [66].

14.9.2.3 Adjuvant Treatments

Radiotherapy for EMSCT is indicated in cases of metastasis from malignant tumors; it does not have a role in schwannomas or meningiomas unless they are anaplastic forms. The risk of radiation-induced myelopathy increases at doses starting from 30 Gy [63] and is highest in midthoracic region, that is, the watershed area within spinal cord. As far as IMSCT are concerned, radiotherapy should be reserved for patients with high-grade tumors or with significant residual low-grade disease that cannot be further surgically addressed. In the case of IMSCT, the maximum tolerable dose of spinal radiation is approximately 5000 cGy. Tumoricidal doses can be administered to patients with astrocytomas (4500–5000 cGy in fractions of 180–200 cGy) or ependymomas (4500 cGy with the same fractionation scheme) [67]. The consideration of the indication for radiotherapy must take into account that it also negatively affects the vertebral stability of the treated segments and contributes to secondary instability in 56–71% of cases [68, 69]. Risk factors for this complication include younger age, radiation dose exceeding 20 Gy, and asymmetric irradiation work plans [59, 68, 69]. Long-term complications of radiotherapy can include post-radiation myelopathy and disruption of growth curves [62, 63, 70].

The role of chemotherapy in IMSCT is not well established. Few trials are reported in the literature, and no guidelines have been compiled due to the variability of the therapeutic regimens proposed in various centers and the small sample sizes of the studies in question. Somatic missense mutations at amino acid position 27 of the H3F3A or HIST1H3B genes are common in astrocytomas of midline structures such as the pons, thalamus, and spinal cord. These mutations define a distinct entity known as diffuse midline glioma, H3 K27M-altered (DMG-H3 K27), accounting for approximately 18–55% of intramedullary astrocytomas. They are aggressive tumors typically found in children and young adults. These gliomas are classified as WHO Grade 4, despite their microscopic appearance potentially resembling grades 2, 3, or 4 [71]. The investigational compounds imipridone, ONC201 and IDO1 inhibitor indoximod are being studied for the treatment of H3K27M-altered gliomas, both in the brain and spinal cord [72]. Ependymomas have shown responsiveness to the VEGF inhibitor bevacizumab, previously effective for vestibular schwannomas in NF-2-related schwannomatosis patients. Immunotherapy has also demonstrated efficacy in treating metastatic ependymomas. A case report by Tapia Rico et al. described a patient with myxopapillary ependymoma treated with the investigational anti-PD-1 antibody tislelizumab, resulting in disease stabilization at 18 months [73]. These findings suggest that immunotherapy may be beneficial for ependymomas, especially those with syndromic etiology [74].

14.10 Conclusions

A limited number of pathologies can cause intramedullary mass lesions in the spinal cord, with most being benign in children. The most common are astrocytoma, ganglioglioma/glial neuronal tumor, and ependymoma, which often have a slow onset and may go undiagnosed for a long time. The chapter details the presentation and diagnostic workup of these tumors, emphasizing the importance of MRI for diagnosis, especially in children with back pain, particularly at night. Initial treatment is typically surgical, with modern techniques like microsurgery and intraoperative neurophysiological monitoring improving outcomes. Understanding spinal cord anatomy and tumor effects is crucial for successful surgery. High-grade tumors may require additional therapies. Advances in surgical technology and tumor biology have led to improved management and outcomes.

References

1. Wetjen NM, Raffel C, Murphy M. Spinal extradural neoplasms and intradural extramedullary neoplasms. In: Principles and practice of pediatric neurosurgery [Internet]. 3rd ed. Stuttgart: Georg Thieme Verlag KG; 2015.
2. Louis DN, Perry A, Wesseling P, Brat DJ, Cree IA, Figarella-Branger D, et al. The 2021 WHO classification of tumors of the central nervous system: a summary. Neuro-Oncology. 2021;23(8):1231–51.
3. Plotkin SR, Messiaen L, Legius E, Pancza P, Avery RA, Blakeley JO, et al. Updated diagnostic criteria and nomenclature for neurofibromatosis type 2 and schwannomatosis: an international consensus recommendation. Genet Med. 2022;24(9):1967–77.

4. Binning M, Klimo P Jr, Gluf W, Goumnerova L. Spinal tumors in children. Neurosurg Clin N Am. 2007;18(4):631–58.
5. Teo C, Nakaji P, Symons P, Tobias V, Cohn R, Smee R. Ependymoma. Child's Nerv Syst. 2003;19:270–85.
6. Spence C, Buchanan R, Keating R. Uncommon pediatric spinal cord tumors. Tumors of the pediatric central nervous system. 1st ed. New York: Thieme; 2001. p. 464–76.
7. Jea A, Bhatia S, Ragheb J. Intramedullary spinal cord tumors. In: Surgery of the pediatric spine [Internet]. Stuttgart: Georg Thieme Verlag KG; 2008.
8. Ostrom QT, Gittleman H, Fulop J, Liu M, Blanda R, Kromer C, et al. CBTRUS statistical report: primary brain and central nervous system tumors diagnosed in the United States in 2008-2012. Neuro-Oncology. 2015;17(suppl_4):iv1–iv62.
9. Constantini S, Houten J, Miller DC, Freed D, Ozek MM, Rorke LB, et al. Intramedullary spinal cord tumors in children under the age of 3 years. J Neurosurg. 1996;85(6):1036–43.
10. Constantini S, Miller DC, Allen JC, Rorke LB, Freed D, Epstein FJ. Radical excision of intramedullary spinal cord tumors: surgical morbidity and long-term follow-up evaluation in 164 children and young adults. J Neurosurg. 2000;93(2 Suppl):183–93.
11. Nunna RS, Khalid S, Behbahani M, Mehta AI. Pediatric primary high-grade spinal glioma: a National Cancer Database analysis of current patterns in treatment and outcomes. Childs Nerv Syst. 2021;37(1):185–93.
12. Venkatesulu B. Spinal cord tumors. In: Mallick S, Giridhar P, Rath GK, editors. Evidence based practice in neuro-oncology. Springer Singapore: Singapore; 2021. p. 357–61.
13. Perwein T, Benesch M, Kandels D, Pietsch T, Schmidt R, Quehenberger F, et al. High frequency of disease progression in pediatric spinal cord low-grade glioma (LGG): management strategies and results from the German LGG study group. Neuro-Oncology. 2021;23(7):1148–62.
14. Umebayashi D, Naito K, Kurokawa R, Endo T, Mizuno M, Hoshimaru M, et al. Epidemiology and comparative analysis of outcomes of intramedullary spinal cord tumor between pediatric and adult patients. Spine (Phila Pa 1976). 2024;49(2):107–15.
15. Innocenzi G, Raco A, Cantore G, Raimondi AJ. Intramedullary astrocytomas and ependymomas in the pediatric age group: a retrospective study. Childs Nerv Syst. 1996;12(12):776–80.
16. Beer SJ, Menezes AH. Primary tumors of the spine in children. Natural history, management, and long-term follow-up. Spine (Phila Pa 1976). 1997;22(6):649–58; discussion 58-9.
17. Weinstein JN, McLain RF. Primary tumors of the spine. Spine (Phila Pa 1976). 1987;12(9):843–51.
18. Lunardi P, Licastro G, Missori P, Ferrante L, Fortuna A. Management of intramedullary tumours in children. Acta Neurochir. 1993;120:59–65.
19. Goel A. Intradural extramedullary spinal tumors. In: Di Rocco C, Pang D, Rutka JT, editors. Textbook of pediatric neurosurgery. Cham: Springer International Publishing; 2020. p. 2789–809.
20. Groves ML, Jallo GI. Intramedullary spinal cord tumors. In: Principles and practice of pediatric neurosurgery [Internet]. 3rd ed. Stuttgart: Georg Thieme Verlag KG; 2015.
21. Kothbauer KF, Deletis V, Epstein FJ. Motor-evoked potential monitoring for intramedullary spinal cord tumor surgery: correlation of clinical and neurophysiological data in a series of 100 consecutive procedures. Neurosurg Focus. 1998;4(5):E3.
22. Ammar A, Haranhalli N, Cezayirli P, Kobets AJ, Abbott R. Intramedullary tumors. In: Di Rocco C, Pang D, Rutka JT, editors. Textbook of pediatric neurosurgery. Cham: Springer International Publishing; 2020. p. 2773–88.
23. Cinalli G, Sainte-Rose C, Lellouch-Tubiana A, Sebag G, Renier D, Pierre-Kahn A. Hydrocephalus associated with intramedullary low-grade glioma. Illustrative cases and review of the literature. J Neurosurg. 1995;83(3):480–5.
24. Rifkinson-Mann S, Wisoff JH, Epstein F. The association of hydrocephalus with intramedullary spinal cord tumors: a series of 25 patients. Neurosurgery. 1990;27(5):749–54; discussion 54.
25. Marrazzo A, Cacchione A, Rossi S, Carboni A, Gandolfo C, Carai A, et al. Intradural pediatric spinal tumors: an overview from imaging to novel molecular findings. Diagnostics (Basel). 2021;11(9)
26. Colafati GS, Marrazzo A, Cirillo M, d'Angelo P, Barbuti D, Tanturri de Horatio L, et al. The pediatric spine. Semin Musculoskelet Radiol. 2021;25(1):137–54.
27. Roux A, Mercier C, Larbrisseau A, Dube LJ, Dupuis C, Del Carpio R. Intramedullary epidermoid cysts of the spinal cord. Case Rep J Neurosurg. 1992;76(3):528–33.
28. Smith JK, Lury K, Castillo M, editors. Imaging of spinal and spinal cord tumors. Semin Roentgenol. 2006;41(4):274–93.
29. Lowe GM. Magnetic resonance imaging of intramedullary spinal cord tumors. J Neuro-Oncol. 2000;47:195–210.
30. Epstein FJ, Farmer JP. Brain-stem glioma growth patterns. J Neurosurg. 1993;78(3):408–12.
31. Choi J-Y, Chang K-H, Yu IK, Kim KH, Kwon BJ, Han MH, et al. Intracranial and spinal ependymomas: review of MR images in 61 patients. Korean J Radiol. 2002;3(4):219.
32. Patel U, Pinto RS, Miller DC, Handler MS, Rorke LB, Epstein FJ, et al. MR of spinal cord ganglioglioma. Am J Neuroradiol. 1998;19(5):879–87.
33. Vougioukas VI, Gläsker S, Hubbe U, Berlis A, Omran H, Neumann HP, et al. Surgical treatment of hemangioblastomas of the central nervous system in pediatric patients. Childs Nerv Syst. 2006;22:1149–53.

34. Chu B-C, Terae S, Hida K, Furukawa M, Abe S, Miyasaka K. MR findings in spinal hemangioblastoma: correlation with symptoms and with angiographic and surgical findings. Am J Neuroradiol. 2001;22(1):206–17.
35. Baker KB, Moran CJ, Wippold FJ 2nd, Smirniotopoulos JG, Rodriguez FJ, Meyers SP, et al. MR imaging of spinal hemangioblastoma. AJR Am J Roentgenol. 2000;174(2):377–82.
36. McGirt MJ, Garces-Ambrossi GL, Parker SL, Sciubba DM, Bydon A, Wolinksy JP, et al. Short-term progressive spinal deformity following laminoplasty versus laminectomy for resection of intradural spinal tumors: analysis of 238 patients. Neurosurgery. 2010;66(5):1005–12.
37. Abbott R, Feldstein N, Wisoff JH, Epstein FJ. Osteoplastic laminotomy in children. Pediatr Neurosurg. 1992;18(3):153–6.
38. Jallo GI, Kim B-S, Epstein F. The current management of intramedullary neoplasms in children and young adults. Ann Neurosurg. 2001;1(1):1–13.
39. Constantini S, Miller DC, Allen JC, Rorke LB, Freed D, Epstein FJ. Radical excision of intramedullary spinal cord tumors: surgical morbidity and long-term follow-up evaluation in 164 children and young adults. J Neurosurg Spine. 2000;93(2):183–93.
40. Sala F, Palandri G, Basso E, Lanteri P, Deletis V, Faccioli F, et al. Motor evoked potential monitoring improves outcome after surgery for intramedullary spinal cord tumors: a historical control study. Neurosurgery. 2006;58(6):1129–43.
41. Shimony N, Fehnel K, Abbott IR, Jallo GI. The evolution of spinal cord surgery: history, people, instruments, and results. Childs Nerv Syst. 2023;39(10):2687–700.
42. Garces-Ambrossi GL, McGirt MJ, Mehta VA, Sciubba DM, Witham TF, Bydon A, et al. Factors associated with progression-free survival and long-term neurological outcome after resection of intramedullary spinal cord tumors: analysis of 101 consecutive cases. J Neurosurg Spine. 2009;11(5):591–9.
43. Jallo GI, Freed D, Epstein F. Intramedullary spinal cord tumors in children. Childs Nerv Syst. 2003;19(9):641–9.
44. McGirt MJ, Goldstein IM, Chaichana KL, Tobias ME, Kothbauer KF, Jallo GI. Extent of surgical resection of malignant astrocytomas of the spinal cord: outcome analysis of 35 patients. Neurosurgery. 2008;63(1):55–60; discussion-1.
45. Endo T, Inoue T, Mizuno M, Kurokawa R, Ito K, Ueda S, et al. Current trends in the surgical management of intramedullary tumors: a multicenter study of 1,033 patients by the Neurospinal Society of Japan. Neurospine. 2022;19(2):441–52.
46. Molina CA, Pennington Z, Ahmed AK, Westbroek E, Goodwin ML, Tamargo R, et al. Use of intraoperative indocyanine green angiography for feeder vessel ligation and En bloc resection of intramedullary hemangioblastoma. Oper Neurosurg (Hagerstown). 2019;17(6):573–9.
47. Takami T, Naito K, Yamagata T, Shimokawa N, Ohata K. Benefits and limitations of indocyanine green fluorescent image-guided surgery for spinal intramedullary tumors. Oper Neurosurg (Hagerstown). 2017;13(6):746–54.
48. Roonprapunt C, Silvera VM, Setton A, Freed D, Epstein FJ, Jallo GI. Surgical management of isolated hemangioblastomas of the spinal cord. Neurosurgery. 2001;49(2):321–7; discussion 7–8.
49. Tamaki T, Kubota S. History of the development of intraoperative spinal cord monitoring. Eur Spine J. 2007;16:140–6.
50. Verla T, Fridley JS, Khan AB, Mayer RR, Omeis I. Neuromonitoring for intramedullary spinal cord tumor surgery. World Neurosurg. 2016;95:108–16.
51. Hersh AM, Pennington Z, Lubelski D, Elsamadicy AA, Dea N, Desai A, et al. Treatment of intramedullary spinal cord tumors: a modified Delphi technique of the North American Spine Society Section of Spine Oncology. J Neurosurg Spine. 2024;40(1):1–10.
52. Rijs K, Klimek M, Scheltens-de Boer M, Biesheuvel K, Harhangi BS. Intraoperative neuromonitoring in patients with intramedullary spinal cord tumor: a systematic review, meta-analysis, and case series. World Neurosurg. 2019;125:498–510 e2.
53. Kimchi G, Knoller N, Korn A, Eyal-Mazuz Y, Sapir Y, Peled A, et al. Delayed variations in the diagnostic accuracy of intraoperative neuromonitoring in the resection of intramedullary spinal cord tumors. Neurosurg Focus. 2021;50(5):E21.
54. Olmsted ZT, Ryu B, Phayal G, Green R, Lo SL, Sciubba DM, et al. Direct wave intraoperative neuromonitoring for spinal tumor resection: a focused review. World Neurosurg X. 2023;17:100139.
55. Nakamura M, Tsuji O, Iwanami A, Tsuji T, Ishii K, Toyama Y, et al. Central neuropathic pain after surgical resection in patients with spinal intramedullary tumor. J Orthop Sci. 2012;17(4):352–7.
56. Hersh AM, Patel J, Pennington Z, Porras JL, Goldsborough E, Antar A, et al. Perioperative outcomes and survival after surgery for intramedullary spinal cord tumors: a single-institution series of 302 patients. J Neurosurg Spine. 2022;37(2):252–62.
57. Yasuoka S, Peterson HA, Laws ER Jr, MacCarty CS. Pathogenesis and prophylaxis of postlaminectomy deformity of the spine after multiple level laminectomy: difference between children and adults. Neurosurgery. 1981;9(2):145–52.
58. Yeh JS, Sgouros S, Walsh AR, Hockley AD. Spinal sagittal malalignment following surgery for primary intramedullary tumours in children. Pediatr Neurosurg. 2001;35(6):318–24.
59. Mayfield JK, Riseborough EJ, Jaffe N, Nehme ME. Spinal deformity in children treated for neuroblastoma. J Bone Joint Surg Am. 1981;63(2):183–93.
60. Yao KC, McGirt MJ, Chaichana KL, Constantini S, Jallo GI. Risk factors for progressive spinal deformity following resection of intramedullary spinal cord tumors in children: an analysis of 161 consecutive cases. J Neurosurg. 2007;107(6 Suppl):463–8.

61. Haq I, Cruz-Almeida Y, Siqueira EB, Norenberg M, Green BA, Levi AD. Postoperative fibrosis after surgical treatment of the porcine spinal cord: a comparison of dural substitutes. Invited submission from the joint section meeting on disorders of the spine and peripheral nerves, march 2004. J Neurosurg Spine. 2005;2(1):50–4.
62. Sklar CA. Growth and neuroendocrine dysfunction following therapy for childhood cancer. Pediatr Clin N Am. 1997;44(2):489–503.
63. Sundaresan N, Gutierrez F, Larsen M. Radiation myelopathy in children. Ann Neurol. 1978;4(1):47–50.
64. Lonjon M, Goh KY, Epstein FJ. Intramedullary spinal cord ependymomas in children: treatment, results and follow-up. Pediatr Neurosurg. 1998;29(4):178–83.
65. Parsa AT, Lee J, Parney IF, Weinstein P, McCormick PC, Ames C. Spinal cord and intradural-extraparenchymal spinal tumors: current best care practices and strategies. J Neuro-Oncol. 2004;69(1–3):291–318.
66. Nadkarni TD, Rekate HL. Pediatric intramedullary spinal cord tumors. Critical review of the literature. Childs Nerv Syst. 1999;15(1):17–28.
67. Kopelson G. Radiation tolerance of the spinal cord previously-damaged by tumor and operation: long term neurological improvement and time-dose-volume relationships after irradiation of intraspinal gliomas. Int J Radiat Oncol Biol Phys. 1982;8(5):925–9.
68. Katzman H, Waugh T, Berdon W. Skeletal changes following irradiation of childhood tumors. J Bone Joint Surg Am. 1969;51(5):825–42.
69. Riseborough EJ, Grabias SL, Burton RI, Jaffe N. Skeletal alterations following irradiation for Wilms' tumor: with particular reference to scoliosis and kyphosis. J Bone Joint Surg Am. 1976;58(4):526–36.
70. O'Sullivan C, Jenkin RD, Doherty MA, Hoffman HJ, Greenberg ML. Spinal cord tumors in children: long-term results of combined surgical and radiation treatment. J Neurosurg. 1994;81(4):507–12.
71. Hersh AM, Jallo GI, Shimony N. Surgical approaches to intramedullary spinal cord astrocytomas in the age of genomics. Front Oncol. 2022;12:982089.
72. Kurz SC, Tarapore R, Odia Y, Butowski NA, Koschmann CJ, Aguilera D, et al. Clinical experience of ONC201 in patients with recurrent H3 K27M-mutant spinal cord glioma. J Clin Oncol. 2020;38(15_suppl):2563.
73. Tapia Rico G, Townsend A, Price T, Patterson K. Metastatic myxopapillary ependymoma treated with immunotherapy achieving durable response. BMJ Case Rep. 2020;13(12)
74. Bryant JP, Lu VM, Govindarajan V, Perez-Roman RJ, Levi AD. Immunotherapeutic treatments for spinal and peripheral nerve tumors: a primer. Neurosurg Focus. 2022;52(2):E8.

Low-Grade Gliomas

15

Antonella Cacchione, Elisabetta Viscardi,
Bartolomeo Rossi, Alessandro Ruggi

15.1 Introduction

Pediatric low-grade gliomas (pLGGs) represent the most common central nervous system (CNS) tumors in children, accounting for approximately 30–50% of pediatric brain tumors [1]. These neoplasms are biologically and clinically distinct from their adult counterparts, exhibiting a more indolent clinical course and a markedly different molecular landscape. Over the past decade, the understanding of pLGGs has undergone a transformative evolution, driven by advances in genomics, epigenetics, and molecular pathology. This paradigm shift is firmly reflected in the 2021 World Health Organization (WHO) Classification of Tumors of the Central Nervous System [2], which introduces a refined and biologically informed framework for classifying CNS tumors.

The 2021 WHO classification marks a significant departure from previous editions by integrating histopathological features with molecular diagnostics to define tumor entities more precisely. For pediatric gliomas, particularly those classified as low-grade, this has led to a more nuanced categorization that aligns with underlying genetic drivers, such as alterations in the mitogen-activated protein kinase pathway (MAPK), including *BRAF* fusions and mutations—which are central to the biology of many pLGGs.

This chapter aims to provide a comprehensive overview of pLGGs, exploring their epidemiology, histological subtypes, molecular characteristics, clinical presentation, and current therapeutic strategies. It will also highlight how the 2021 WHO classification has reshaped diagnostic and treatment paradigms, reinforcing the importance of precision medicine in pediatric neuro-oncology.

A. Cacchione
Area of Hematology-Oncology, Cell Therapy, Gene Therapies and Hemopoietic Transplant, Bambino Gesù Children's Hospital, IRCCS, Rome, Italy
e-mail: antonella.cacchione@opbg.net

E. Viscardi (✉) · B. Rossi
Pediatric Oncology/Hematology Department, Hospital/University of Padua, Padua, Italy
e-mail: elisabetta.viscardi@unipd.it; bartolomeo.rossi_01@aopd.veneto.it

A. Ruggi
Pediatric Hematology and Oncology, IRCCS, Azienda Ospedaliero-Universitaria di Bologna, Bologna, Italy
e-mail: alessandro.ruggi@opbg.net

A. Mastronuzzi, A. Carai (eds.), *Navigating Pediatric Brain Tumors*,
https://doi.org/10.1007/978-3-032-18992-9_15

15.1.1 Definition and Classification of Pediatric LGGs

pLGGs are a group of slow-growing, WHO grade 1 and 2 glial or glioneuronal tumors (Table 15.1) that occur primarily in children and adolescents, characterized by distinct clinical behavior, histological subtypes, and frequent activation of the MAPK signaling pathway through alterations such as *BRAF* fusions or mutations.

The most frequently diagnosed subtype within this group is pilocytic astrocytoma (PA). Additional histological variants include pilomyxoid astrocytoma, pleomorphic xanthoastrocytoma (PXA), diffuse astrocytoma, ganglioglioma, dysembryoplastic neuroepithelial tumor (DNET), and subependymal giant cell astrocytoma (SEGA).

Table 15.1 Low-grade glial and glioneuronal tumors, 2021 WHO Classification of Tumors of the Central Nervous System [2]

Pediatric type diffuse low-grade gliomas	Diffuse astrocytoma, MYB- o MYBL1-altered Angiocentric glioma Polymorphous low-grade neuroepithelial tumor of the young (PLNTY) Diffuse low-grade glioma, MAPK pathway-altered
Circumscribed astrocytic gliomas	Pilocytic astrocytoma High-grade astrocytoma with piloid features (HGAP) Pleomorphic xanthoastrocytoma (PXA) Subependymal giant cell astrocytoma (SEGA) Chordoid glioma Astroblastoma, MN1-altered
Glioneuronal and neuronal tumors	Ganglioglioma Desmoplastic infantile ganglioglioma/astrocytoma (DIG/DIA) Dysembryoplastic neuroepithelial tumor (DNT) DGONC (diffuse glioneuronal tumor with oligodendroglioma-like features and nuclear clusters) Papillary glioneuronal tumor (PGNT) Rosette-forming glioneuronal tumor (RGNT) Myxoid glioneuronal tumor (MGNT) Diffuse leptomeningeal glioneuronal tumor (DLGNT) Gangliocytoma Multinodular and vacuolating neuronal tumor (MVNT) Dysplastic cerebellar gangliocytoma (Lhermitte–Duclos disease) Central neurocytoma Extraventricular neurocytoma Cerebellar liponeurocytoma

15.2 Epidemiology

pLGGs account for 30–50% of all CNS tumors in children. The annual incidence of PLGGs is estimated at 1.5 to 2.5 cases per 100,000 children under the age of 15 and the incidence's peak occurs in early childhood, particularly between ages 5 and 9 [1, 3]. There is a slight male predominance, with a male-to-female ratio ranging from 1.1:1 to 1.5:1, depending on the tumor subtype [4].

15.2.1 Associations with Genetic Syndromes

15.2.1.1 Tuberous Sclerosis Complex (TSC)

Tuberous sclerosis complex (TSC) is a rare autosomal-dominant disease caused by identifiable mutations in either the *TSC1* (hamartin) or *TSC2* (tuberin) gene in 85% of patients [5]. Patients with tuberous sclerosis have a genetic predisposition to increased activity of the mammalian target of rapamycin (mTOR) pathway. This is due to mutations in the tumor suppressor genes *TSC1* and *TSC2*, which normally function as negative regulators of mTOR signaling [6]. Because of this dysregulation, in addition to other characteristic features of the syndrome, affected individuals are at increased risk for developing subependymal giant cell astrocytomas (SEGAs). SEGAs are present in 5–20% of patients with TSC, being almost exclusively present in patients with *TSC2* variants [7]. These neoplasms commonly develop in proximity to the foramen of

Monro, with a significant risk of causing cerebrospinal fluid (CSF) [8] flow obstruction and subsequent hydrocephalus and/or typically manifesting seizures. These tumors typically exhibit a slow but progressive increase in size. Historically, standard management has involved early surgical resection. For patients in whom complete surgical excision is not feasible or carries high risk, pharmacologic therapy with mTOR inhibitors—specifically everolimus—has been approved [9].

15.2.1.2 Neurofibromatosis Type 1 (NF1)

Even though most pLGGs are sporadic, approximately 20% of them can occur in individuals with genetic predispositions for glioma development [10]. Neurofibromatosis type 1 (NF1), for example, is an autosomal-dominant condition caused by loss-of-function alterations in NF1, a negative regulator of the MAPK pathway resulting in varied central nervous system neoplasms, most commonly within the optic pathway and brainstem; patients with NF1 account for over 70% of the optic pathway/hypothalamic gliomas in children, and it is estimated that 15–20% of all children with NF1 will develop an optic pathway glioma (OPG) during early childhood [11, 12]. Tumors are thought to form with a second somatic mutation leading to inactivation of the NF1 protein. This leads to constitutive activation of RAS/RAF/MEK/ERK [11, 13]. Most studies show that the PFS and response to classic chemotherapy are superior in children with NF1-associated pLGG versus those with sporadic pLGG [14]. The pathophysiology behind these differences, despite the same histology and location, is yet unclear and assumed to be associated with the NF1 mutation.

Sporadic optic pathway and hypothalamic gliomas (OPHGs) may manifest at any age during childhood, with over 90% of cases ultimately necessitating therapeutic intervention [15]. In contrast, OPHGs associated with NF1 typically present within the first 5–6 years of life and frequently follow an indolent course that does not require active treatment [16].

15.2.2 Common Tumor Locations

The most common location of pLGGs are the optic pathway and midline structures (accounting for 35–40% of cases), followed by the cerebellum (25–30% of cases), cerebral hemispheres (20%), brainstem (10%), and spinal cord (5%) (Fig. 15.1) [17]. Affected chil-

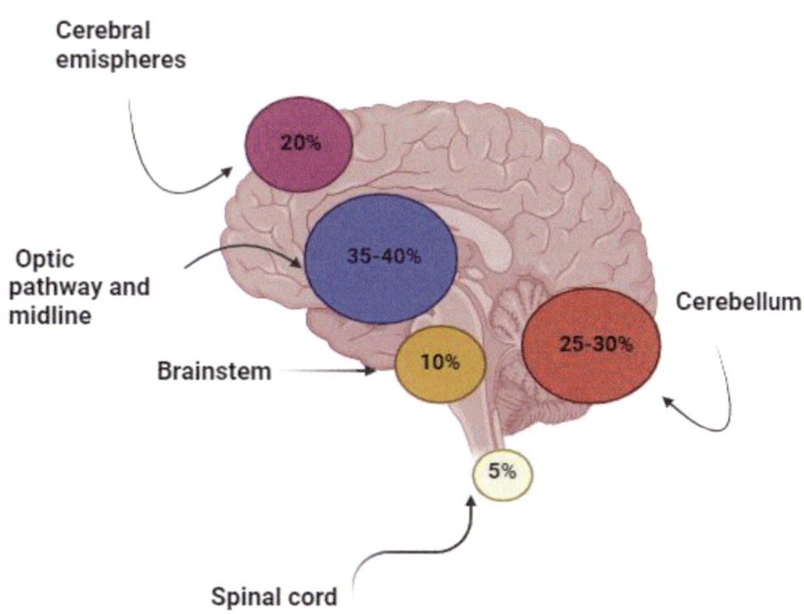

Fig. 15.1 Typical locations of pLGGs

dren are at risk of enduring chronic neurological sequelae, which may include gait ataxia, visual disturbances, ophthalmoplegia, hemiparesis, epileptic seizures, sensorineural hearing loss, cranial neuropathies, and neurocognitive impairments. The prevalence and nature of the neurological deficits that occur in children affected are closely associated with tumor localization, with approximately 30% of cases involving the infratentorial compartment and up to 73% affecting supratentorial structures [18].

15.3 Histology and Molecular Stratification

15.3.1 Overview of the 2021 WHO Classification of CNS Tumors

The 2021 WHO CNS classification for pLGGs represents a critical integration of histology and molecular biology. pLGGs near-universally upregulate the RAS-mitogen-activated protein kinase (RAS/MAPK) pathway [19]. With MAPK pathway alterations as a unifying theme and additional drivers (*MYB*, *FGFR*, *BRAF*) defining distinct entities, accurate molecular profiling is now essential for precise classification and risk stratification, selecting targeted therapies, avoiding overtreatment, optimizing quality of life. Traditional histological subtypes are now nested within these biologically defined families [2]:

1. Pediatric-type diffuse low-grade gliomas
2. Circumscribed astrocytic gliomas
3. Glioneuronal and neuronal tumors

In the 2021 WHO CNS classification, six novel pLGG entities are specifically recognized:

- Diffuse astrocytoma, *MYB/MYBL1*-altered
- PLNTY (polymorphous low-grade neuroepithelial tumor of the young)
- Diffuse low-grade glioma, MAPK-altered
- DGONC (diffuse glioneuronal tumor with oligodendroglioma-like features and nuclear clusters)
- MGT (myxoid glioneuronal tumor)
- MVNT (multinodular and vacuolating neuronal tumor)

pLGGs are characterized predominantly by glial lineage differentiation, including astrocytic, oligodendroglial, or mixed neuronal-glial phenotypes. These tumors are classified as WHO grade 1 or 2 and are distinct from their high-grade counterparts based on specific histopathological criteria—namely the absence of features such as necrosis, brisk mitotic activity, and microvascular proliferation in diffusely infiltrating lesions [20]. Histologically, pLGGs encompass several entities with characteristic microscopic features (Fig. 15.2):

- Pilocytic astrocytoma, typically exhibiting biphasic architecture and Rosenthal fibers
- Diffuse astrocytoma, with mild nuclear atypia and low cellularity
- Pleomorphic xanthoastrocytoma, noted for cytological pleomorphism and xanthomatous change
- Ganglioglioma, demonstrating dysplastic neurons intermixed with glial components
- Dysembryoplastic neuroepithelial tumor (DNET), marked by floating neurons in mucin-rich pools
- Oligodendroglioma, exhibiting perinuclear halos and a "fried egg" appearance
- Angiocentric glioma, characterized by perivascular pseudorosettes

Despite these prototypical features, considerable diagnostic overlap is documented, and morphologic similarities may exist. The complexity increases in deep midline tumors, such as those in the thalamus or brainstem, where biopsy specimens are often limited in size and may not adequately represent the full histological heterogeneity of the tumor. The integration of molecular diagnostics is therefore critical, both to refine classification and to guide clinical management (Table 15.2) [4].

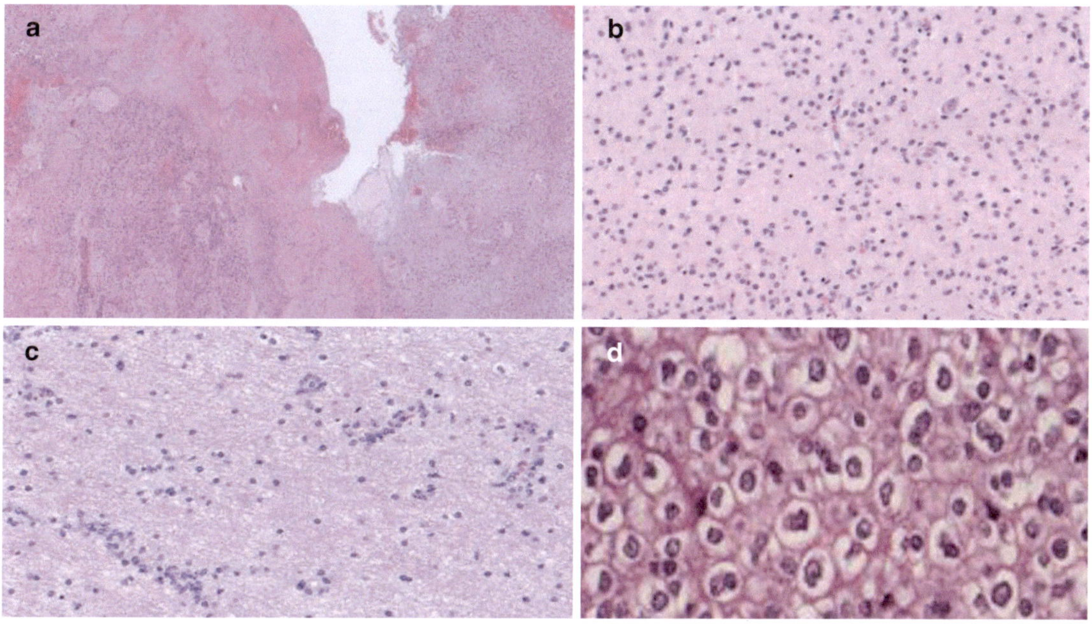

Fig. 15.2 Microscopic features of pLGGs: (**a**) pilocytic astrocytoma; (**b**) diffuse astrocytoma; (**c**) angiocentric glioma; (**d**) oligodendroglioma

Table 15.2 pLGGs' molecular biology

Tumor	Molecular features
Circumscribed astrocytic gliomas	
Pilocytic astrocytoma	*KIAA1549-BRAF* (70–80%) *FGFR1-TACC1* (3–5%) *FGFR1* mutations (3–5%) *BRAF* p.V600E (3–5%) Other *BRAF* fusions (2–5%) *CRAF* fusions (2–5%) *PTPN11* (2–5%)
Subependymal giant cell astrocytoma (SEGA)	*TSC1/TSC2* mutations (95%)
Pleomorphic xanthoastrocytoma (PXA)	*BRAF* V600E (80–90%), *NTRK* alterations (2–3%)
Chordoid glioma	*PRKCA* p.D463H mutation
Astroblastoma, MN1-altered	*MN1* gene fusions (often *MN1::BEND2*), occasional *CDKN2A* deletions, specific copy-number changes (e.g., monosomy 16)
Pediatric-type diffuse low-grade gliomas	
Diffuse astrocytoma	*BRAF* p.V600E (20–40%) *MYB* or *MYB1* rearrangements (5–10%) *KIAA1549-BRAF* (5–10%) *FGFR1* (2–5%) H3.3 p.K27M (2–5%) *IDH1* p.R132H (2–5%) Other *RTK* fusions (2–3%)

(continued)

Table 15.2 (continued)

Tumor	Molecular features
Circumscribed astrocytic gliomas	
Angiocentric glioma	*MYB-QKI* fusion
Polymorphous low-grade neuroepithelial tumor of the young (PLNTY)	*BRAF* p.V600E (30–40%) *FGFR2/3* fusions (30–40%)
Diffuse low-grade glioma, MAPK pathway-altered	MAPK pathway alterations (usually *BRAF* or *FGFR1*)
Glioneuronal and neuronal tumors	
Ganglioglioma, gangliocytoma	*BRAF* p.V600E (40–50%) *KIAA1549-BRAF* (10–15%) For gangliocytoma, no signature abnormalities
Desmoplastic infantile ganglioglioma and astrocytoma	*BRAF* pV600E/D (40–60%) *FGFR1* (5–10%) *KIAA1549-BRAF* (2–5%)
Dysembryoplastic neuroepithelial tumor (DNET)	*FGFR1-TKD* duplication (20–30%) *FGFR1* SNV (20–30%) *FGFR1-TACC1* (10–15%) *BRAF* p.V600E (5–10%) Other *RTK* fusions (5–10%)
Diffuse glioneuronal tumor with oligodendroglioma-like features and nuclear clusters	Monosomy of chromosome 14
Papillary glioneuronal tumor	*PRKCA* gene fusions (mostly *SLC44A1*::*PRKCA*) (80–90%)
Rosette-forming glioneuronal tumor	*PIK3CA* SNV (20–30%) *KIAA1549-BRAF* (20–30%) *FGFR1* mutation (20–30%)
Myxoid glioneuronal tumor	*PDGFRA* p.K385 mutation
Diffuse leptomeningeal glioneuronal tumor	MAPK pathway alterations (mostly *KIAA1549*::*BRAF*)
Multinodular and vacuolating neuronal tumor	*MAP2K1* (50–60%) *BRAF* p.V600E (5–10%) Other *BRAF* SNV (5–10%) *FGFR2* fusions (3–5%)
Dysplastic cerebellar gangliocytoma (Lhermitte–Duclos disease)	*PTEN* mutations (Cowden syndrome)
Central neurocytoma	No consistent alterations

15.3.2 Key Molecular Alterations in pLGGs

Although many pLGGs can be distinguished based on their histological features, cases with overlapping morphology are well recognized. For instance, pleomorphic xanthoastrocytoma can share histological characteristics with ganglioglioma, and dysembryoplastic neuroepithelial tumors may resemble oligodendrogliomas [21, 22]. Histopathological assessment becomes particularly challenging in deep-seated midline tumors, where only limited biopsy material is available, often lacking definitive features necessary for accurate classification. Additionally, pLGGs may exhibit morphologic similarities to gliomas more commonly seen in adults, further complicating diagnostic interpretation and treatment planning.

In the broad spectrum of molecular alterations in pLGGs, there are some that are more frequent and directly correlated as hallmark of the specific neoplasm. Aberrant activation of the MAPK signaling cascade has been recognized as a central oncogenic mechanism in the majority of pLGGs, frequently driven by a singular genetic alteration initiating gliomagenesis [19]. In sporadic pLGGs, the most prevalent molecular event involves gene fusions and point mutations affecting the oncogene *BRAF*, with the *KIAA1549::BRAF* fusion representing the most observed alteration [23], and the *BRAF* p.V600E mutation occurring in a smaller subset of cases [24]. Additional recurrent genomic events include somatic mutations in members of the fibroblast growth factor receptor (*FGFR*) family, namely *FGFR1*, *FGFR2*, and *FGFR3* [25]. Moreover, loss-of-function mutations in *NF1*, a negative regulator of the MAPK pathway, are observed either as germline mutations in patients with *BRAF* V600E mutations [26]. Elucidation of the molecular mechanisms underlying gliomagenesis has paved the way for the incorporation of targeted agents into the therapeutic landscape enhancing the subsequent main role of molecular profiling in diagnosis and treatment planning.

15.4 Clinical Presentation

pLGGs are characterized by relatively slow growth and diverse clinical presentations. Symptoms typically develop insidiously over months or years, though acute presentations occur, particularly with obstructive hydrocephalus [17]. For some patients, the lesion might also be an incidental finding on MRI [27, 28]. pLGGs symptoms can vary based on tumor location, patient age, and rate of tumor growth [17], with infants and young children having different presenting symptoms compared to older children and adolescents. The most common symptoms at presentation, irrespective of tumor location, are headache, nausea and vomiting, motor weakness, and visual disturbances [17].

15.4.1 Symptoms Based on Tumor Location

15.4.1.1 Optic Pathway Glioma (OPG)

OPGs in children often present with subtle and progressive symptoms. The most common clinical manifestations at diagnosis [29] include

- Decreased visual acuity (observed in ~40% of cases), is often unilateral or asymmetric
- Headache (23%), which may reflect increased intracranial pressure or tumor location near the hypothalamic region
- Nystagmus (approximately 20%), indicating disruption in the visual pathway or ocular motor control
- Endocrine disturbances (16.6%), including early signs of puberty or growth hormone dysregulation
- Diencephalic syndrome (13%), characterized by weight loss, failure to thrive, or emesis in young children

15.4.1.2 Sovratentorial Cortical Areas

The involvement of different cerebral cortical areas influences the specific clinical symptoms related to tumor growth. Tumors in the parietal or temporal regions, often present with drug-resistant seizures. Other common symptoms include headaches; motor deficits (e.g., hemiparesis, hyperreflexia, clonus); sensory loss; speech disturbances; memory deficits; and behavioral or personality changes, which may manifest as deterioration in school performance.

15.4.1.3 Posterior Fossa

The most common pediatric pLGGs in the posterior fossa are cerebellar pilocytic astrocytomas, brainstem gliomas, and tectal gliomas. Clinical manifestations are primarily related to increased intracranial pressure (ICP) and cerebellar dysfunction:

- *Raised ICP symptoms*: Typically include early-morning or nocturnal headaches, vomiting, and papilledema. Infants and young children may exhibit irritability, developmental delay, macrocephaly, bulging fontanelles, and failure to thrive.
- *Cerebellar dysfunction*: Often presents as ataxia, dysmetria, and nystagmus.
- *Brainstem involvement*: Brainstem gliomas can cause cranial nerve deficits (e.g., diplopia, facial weakness, hearing loss, dysphagia), gait and coordination disturbances, focal motor weakness (hemiparesis, quadriparesis), and obstructive or central apnea. Compression of the fourth ventricle or cerebral aqueduct, common with tectal gliomas, can also contribute to raised ICP [30].

An important distinction exists between diffuse intrinsic pontine gliomas (DIPG) and focal low-grade brainstem gliomas. DIPGs typically progress rapidly, presenting with severe neurological deficits, while focal low-grade tumors evolve more gradually, often initially manifesting with isolated cranial nerve dysfunction or hydrocephalus.

pLGGs of the pineal region or dorsal midbrain can cause Parinaud syndrome, characterized by impaired pupillary light reflex (with accommodation preserved), limited upward gaze ("setting-sun" sign or conjugate downward gaze), and retraction nystagmus.

15.4.1.4 Spinal Location

Rare in children, spinal pLGGs typically present with chronic, progressive back pain (worst at night and lying down), radicular pain and/or weakness, gait disturbances, weakness and sensory loss corresponding to the level of the lesion, bladder and/or bowel dysfunction, and spinal deformities (scoliosis, kyphosis). Back pain in a child should never be underestimated given it is a rather uncommon complaint in pediatrics, and MRI of the spine with contrast is essential whenever spinal involvement is suspected.

15.4.2 Common Symptoms

15.4.2.1 Seizures

Seizures are common in cortical pLGGs, especially in tumors located within the temporal, frontal, and parietal lobes [31]. Epilepsy associated with these tumors is frequently drug-resistant, making epilepsy surgery a highly effective option for achieving seizure control in eligible patients. Certain pLGG subtypes are particularly prone to seizure presentation, notably gangliogliomas and DNET [32, 33]. Seizures associated with pLGG can be focal, often providing clues about tumor location, or generalized. Diffuse astrocytomas with *MYB* or *MYBL1* alterations (WHO grade I), primarily affecting the temporal and frontal lobes, commonly present with drug-resistant epilepsy and show high rates of seizure freedom following surgical resection [34]. Additional rare entities strongly associated with epilepsy include polymorphous low-grade neuroepithelial tumors of the young (PLNTY), typically located in the temporal lobe and characterized by early-onset, drug-resistant epilepsy, as well as angiocentric gliomas (WHO grade I) and diffuse low-grade gliomas with MAPK pathway alterations [34].

15.4.2.2 Visual Disturbances

Visual disturbances vary from asymptomatic to severe impairment based on the specific location within the optic pathway. Optic pathway gliomas (OPGs) represent approximately 3–5% of all pediatric brain tumors and are especially common in NF1 patients (up to 30% of OPGs are found in patients with NF1) [35]. Given this strong association, routine ophthalmological surveillance in NF1 patients is recommended. OPGs usually present with headache, squinting, decreased vision, and visual field defects (which may hint at tumor location, such as bitemporal hemianopsia for chiasma tumors, central scotoma for post-chiasmatic tumors) [36]. There can also be proptosis, nystagmus, and esotropia. Risk factors for severe visual deficits include younger age at presentation, optic nerve atrophy, and involvement of post-chiasmatic structures.

15.4.2.3 Endocrine Dysfunction

Tumors involving hypothalamic structures frequently present with endocrine disturbances. Endocrine dysfunction can precede diagnosis from months to years, necessitating a comprehensive endocrinological evaluation. Hypothalamic lesions often manifest with endocrine disturbances, including diabetes insipidus (polyuria/polydipsia), growth hormone deficiency leading to poor growth, and precocious or delayed puberty.

Diencephalic syndrome, almost always associated with tumors of the hypothalamus or of the suprasellar region, is a distinct presentation of pLGG that is defined as failure to thrive with severe emaciation despite adequate caloric intake, hyperactivity, and euphoria. Diencephalic syndrome independently predicts worse prognosis in pLGG [37, 38].

15.4.2.4 Ataxia

Cerebellar and brainstem tumors frequently manifest with ataxia and dysmetria [17], presenting as clumsiness, gait instability, or coordination difficulties. For example, cerebellar pilocytic astrocytomas may present with ataxia of long duration given their relatively slow growth rate. A longer prediagnostic symptom interval may influence the long-term incidence of ataxia and dysmetria [17]. Differentiating between cerebellar hemispheric (appendicular dysmetria) and midline/vermis (truncal ataxia) involvement is useful clinically.

15.4.3 Impact on Neurodevelopment and Quality of Life

pLGGs significantly impact the neurodevelopmental trajectory and overall quality of life (QoL) of affected children and adolescents. Despite their typically slow growth and favorable prognosis compared to high-grade gliomas, anatomical location and subsequent treatments frequently result in long-term neurological, cognitive, and psychosocial sequelae [39]. Survival rates are excellent, with overall survival (OS) approaching 100% for completely resected tumors and above 90% at 5 years for tumors treated with chemotherapy. However, recurrence rates remain significant, with progression-free survival (PFS) after conventional chemotherapy typically around 40–50% at 5 years [40–42]. Both tumor-related symptoms and treatment modalities, especially radiotherapy, contribute substantially to chronic morbidity, underscoring the chronic nature of pLGGs [14].

- Motor and sensory deficits: Persistent weakness, coordination difficulties, sensory disturbances, and gait abnormalities linked to tumors in motor pathways, cerebellum, brainstem, or spinal cord.
- Endocrine dysfunction: Chronic endocrine disorders, including growth hormone deficiency, diabetes insipidus, and pubertal abnormalities, often arise from hypothalamic and pituitary tumors. Radiotherapy significantly increases endocrine complications, notably growth and thyroid hormone deficiencies [43].
- Visual impairment: Frequently permanent and severe, substantially affecting QoL. Approximately 60% of optic pathway glioma (OPG) patients have severely impaired visual acuity (<1/10) in at least one eye, with binocular blindness eventually developing in up to 20% [44].
- Cognitive deficits: Commonly include impairments in executive functions, attention, memory, processing speed, and academic performance, particularly with tumors involving cortical areas, thalamus, or hypothalamus. Additional challenges include behavioral and emotional difficulties, reduced adaptive skills, and lower intellectual functioning, observed even in cerebellar tumor survivors [45, 46].

Quality-of-life considerations:

- Psychosocial impact: Anxiety, depression, social withdrawal, reduced self-esteem, and altered body image.
- Academic and social integration: Cognitive and physical impairments hinder academic achievement, school attendance, and social interactions with peers.
- Family burden: Chronic illness significantly affects family dynamics, causing emotional, financial, and practical strain.
- Treatment-related morbidity: While essential, surgery, chemotherapy, and radiotherapy can induce additional complications, such as neurotoxicity, hearing loss, and secondary malignancies.

Early identification and multidisciplinary management (including neuropsychology, endocrinology, rehabilitation, education, and mental health support) are critical to optimize neurodevelopmental outcomes and QoL for patients with pLGGs. Newer targeted therapies show promising preliminary results in terms of efficacy and toxicity compared to standard chemotherapy, and ongoing trials will compare their long-term morbidity and QoL impacts.

15.5 Diagnosis

15.5.1 Imaging Modalities

Imaging is central to the diagnosis, characterization, and longitudinal assessment of pLGGs, which represent a biologically and radiologically heterogeneous group of CNS tumors. Although the Radiologic Assessment in Neuro-Oncology (RANO) group has established guidelines for evaluating adult low-grade gliomas (LGGs), pediatric LGGs (pLGGs) represent a distinct clinical and biological entity that warrants separate imaging assessment criteria. This distinction arises from fundamental differences in tumor biology between adult and pediatric LGGs. Notably, malignant transformation—a common feature in adult LGGs—is exceedingly rare in pediatric cases.

These needs prompted the formation of the Radiologic Assessment in Pediatric Neuro-Oncology (RAPNO) group to address challenges in standardizing imaging protocols and response evaluation [47]. This international consortium, composed of pediatric and adult neuro-oncologists, neuroradiologists, radiation oncologists, neurosurgeons, and other specialists, was established to develop specific imaging criteria tailored to the unique features of pLGG. The working group proposed detailed recommendations for radiologic response assessment, including supplementary guidelines for evaluating visual outcomes in patients with optic pathway gliomas. They offer a unified framework that facilitates consistent evaluation and improves comparability across clinical studies.

The RAPNO consortium recommends that baseline MRI of the brain—or spine, depending on tumor location—be performed both preoperatively and within 24–72 hours postoperatively. The early postoperative scan should serve as the new reference point for evaluating response to systemic therapies and radiotherapy. For patients enrolled in clinical trials, imaging should be conducted every 12 weeks during active treatment. In cases of optic pathway or hypothalamic tumors, dedicated orbital MRI sequences are advised in addition to standard brain imaging. Furthermore, RAPNO provides standardized protocols for assessing visual acuity and monitoring changes over time in patients with optic pathway gliomas.

Standard imaging practices, primarily based on magnetic resonance imaging (MRI), continue to evolve with the development of advanced imaging techniques and integration of computational tools such as machine learning. Conventional MRI remains the gold standard for initial evaluation and follow-up of pLGGs. Core sequences include T1-weighted (pre- and post-contrast), T2-weighted, and FLAIR, which together help define tumor extent, location, and enhancement patterns [48]. These features are particularly important for classifying tumors such as pilocytic astrocytomas, gangliogliomas, and optic pathway gliomas.

In recent years, advanced multiparametric MRI techniques have gained increasing relevance. These include diffusion-weighted imaging (DWI), diffusion tensor imaging (DTI) for the evaluation of microstructural integrity, MR perfusion for vascular characterization, and MR spectroscopy (MRS) for metabolic profiling of gliomas. These modalities enhance diagnostic specificity and may help distinguish between indolent tumor behavior and early progression.

15.5.2 Histopathological Evaluation

The histopathological diagnosis of pediatric low-grade gliomas (pLGGs) integrates clinical presentation, neuroimaging findings, and microscopic tissue analysis, which together inform tumor classification and WHO grading.

Following tissue sampling, standard hematoxylin and eosin (H&E) staining is employed to evaluate tumor architecture and cytology. Key microscopic features include

- Cellularity: Typically low to moderate, with relatively uniform cells and minimal mitotic activity.
- Growth pattern: Varies by histological subtype. Some tumors exhibit a diffuse infiltrative pattern (e.g., pediatric-type diffuse astrocytoma), while others are well-circumscribed and biphasic (e.g., pilocytic astrocytoma).
- Cytological features:
  - Pilocytic astrocytoma: Characterized by a biphasic architecture with compact and microcystic areas, Rosenthal fibers, and eosinophilic granular bodies.
  - Pediatric-type diffuse astrocytoma: Displays mild nuclear atypia, infiltrative margins, and lacks necrosis or microvascular proliferation.
  - Angiocentric glioma: Shows a distinctive perivascular arrangement of tumor cells, often with ependymoma-like morphology.
- Mitotic activity: Generally absent or rare; a higher mitotic index may suggest anaplastic transformation or an alternative diagnosis.

Immunohistochemistry (IHC) supports diagnosis and classification:

- GFAP (glial fibrillary acidic protein): Commonly positive, indicating astrocytic differentiation.
- Olig2: Expressed in most glial neoplasms, including astrocytic and oligodendroglial tumors.
- Ki-67/MIB-1 labeling index: Typically low in pLGG, helping differentiate low-grade from high-grade gliomas by assessing proliferative activity.

15.5.3 Molecular Diagnostic Techniques

15.5.3.1 Next-Generation Sequencing

Next-generation sequencing (NGS) is a high-throughput DNA sequencing technology that allows for the simultaneous analysis of multiple genes or even entire genomes. Unlike traditional Sanger sequencing, which sequences one gene at a time, NGS can examine hundreds to thousands of genes in parallel, making it especially valuable for complex diseases like pLGGs, molecularly heterogeneous. Specific genetic alterations often guide both diagnosis and treatment. NGS enables identification of driver mutations, molecular classification, targeted therapy decisions, and prognostic assessment.

NGS can detect a range of alterations, including single-nucleotide variants (SNVs), gene fusions, and copy number variations (CNVs). Key alterations frequently found in pLGGs include BRAF mutations and fusions, FGFR1 alterations, NTRK gene fusions, MYB and MYBL1 alterations. Types of NGS panels used are targeted gene panels (focus on known glioma-associated genes), whole-exome sequencing (WES, broader view, useful in atypical cases), and RNA sequencing that detects gene fusions and abnormal gene expression.

15.5.3.2 Fluorescence In Situ Hybridization (FISH)

Fluorescence in situ hybridization (FISH) is a cytogenetic technique widely employed in the diagnostic workup of pLGGs to detect specific genetic alterations with high sensitivity and spatial resolution. In particular, FISH is commonly used to identify gene fusions such as *KIAA1549-BRAF*, which is a hallmark of pilocytic astrocytomas, the most frequent subtype of pLGGs. FISH enables the detection of these rearrangements directly in formalin-fixed, paraffin-embedded (FFPE) tissue sections, aiding in tumor classification and guiding therapeutic decisions. As molecular characterization becomes increasingly critical in the diagnosis and risk stratification of pediatric brain tumors, FISH remains a valuable tool due to its accessibility, speed, and ability to complement more advanced sequencing-based assays [49].

15.5.3.3 Liquid Biopsy Approaches

Liquid biopsy is an emerging, minimally invasive technique that analyzes tumor-derived genetic material—such as circulating tumor DNA (ctDNA) or cell-free DNA (cfDNA)—from fluids like blood or cerebrospinal fluid (CSF) [50]. pLGG liquid biopsy offers a promising alternative or complement to surgical biopsy, especially in cases where tumor location poses a high surgical risk. Recent studies have shown that key genetic alterations, such as BRAF fusions or mutations (e.g., BRAF V600E), can be detected in CSF-derived ctDNA, facilitating molecular diagnosis and potentially enabling real-time monitoring of treatment response or disease progression. Although still under clinical investigation, liquid biopsy holds significant potential to improve diagnostic accuracy and patient safety in pediatric neuro-oncology.

15.5.4 Challenges in Diagnosis and the Importance of Multidisciplinary Collaboration

The diagnosis of pLGGs continues to evolve, driven by advances in molecular biology and imaging. However, the inherent diagnostic challenges—ranging from surgical inaccessibility to molecular complexity—underscore the indispensable value of a multidisciplinary, precision medicine approach. Integrating cutting-edge techniques such as liquid biopsy, within a collaborative framework, holds the potential to transform diagnostic pathways and improve outcomes for children with these tumors.

15.5.4.1 Diagnostic Challenges

15.5.4.1.1 Clinical and Radiologic Ambiguity

The clinical presentation of pLGGs is highly variable, ranging from subtle neurological symptoms to acute presentations depending on tumor location. Radiologically, these tumors often show overlapping features with other pediatric CNS neoplasms. MRI findings, while essential, are not always definitive for distinguishing between low-grade and high-grade lesions or for determining histological subtype.

15.5.4.1.2 Anatomic Constraints and Surgical Risk

Many pLGGs arise in deep or eloquent brain regions (e.g., brainstem, optic pathway), where surgical biopsy or resection carries significant risk. In such cases, neurosurgical access may be limited, and obtaining tissue for histopathological confirmation may not be feasible.

15.5.4.1.3 Histopathological and Molecular Complexity

Even when tissue is available, histopathological classification can be complicated by tumor heterogeneity and sampling limitations. Moreover, the 2021 WHO CNS tumor classification emphasizes the importance of molecular features—particularly genetic alterations such as BRAF mutations or fusions (e.g., *KIAA1549-BRAF*)—which guide both prognosis and treatment. However, identifying these molecular alterations typically requires specialized testing not universally available in all centers.

15.5.4.1.4 Limitations of Current Diagnostic Tools

Traditional diagnostics rely heavily on tissue-based analysis. These methods can be supplemented or potentially replaced by noninvasive approaches like liquid biopsy. Their study demonstrated the feasibility of detecting the *KIAA1549-BRAF* fusion in circulating tumor DNA (ctDNA) from plasma samples of children with pilocytic astrocytoma. This method could significantly reduce diagnostic risk, particularly for tumors in surgically inaccessible regions.

Given these complexities, a multidisciplinary approach (pediatric neuro-oncologists, neurosurgeons, neuropathologists, neuroradiologists, molecular geneticists) is essential for optimal diagnosis and management of pLGGs. Collaboration among specialists enhances diagnostic accuracy, allows for tailored treatment planning, and ensures comprehensive care.

15.6 Treatment Strategies

Treatment strategies are always individualized in pLGG because they are a very heterogeneous group of tumors with often erratic behavior. Main factors that influence therapeutic decisions include tumor location, surgical resectability, tumor biology and molecular diagnostics, clinical presentation, and patient age. Options include surgery, chemotherapy, and radiotherapy, with an increasing role for molecularly targeted therapies. An initial "watch-and-wait" approach may be appropriate for asymptomatic and stable lesions, particularly in eloquent or surgically inaccessible areas, provided that careful radiologic and clinical surveillance is ensured. However, most patients eventually require active treatment, particularly those with progressive disease or significant neurological, visual, or endocrine symptoms.

15.6.1 Surgical Management

Surgical removal remains the most effective treatment and offers the highest chance of cure; despite advances in diagnostic and therapeutic techniques, it continues to be the cornerstone of care.

The choice to operate the patient is usually based on clinical presentation, surgical risk, and tumor location and is usually the first treatment modality when treatment is indicated [51, 52].

15.6.1.1 Surgical Techniques and Considerations

Gross total resection (GTR) is the goal, when possible, as it offers the best chance of cure, particularly for tumors located in the cerebellum or cerebral hemispheres (e.g., pilocytic astrocytoma). Long-term PFS approaches 100% following complete resection in these settings.

Subtotal resection or biopsy is more appropriate for deep-seated lesions involving eloquent regions such as the optic pathway, hypothalamus, thalamus, and brainstem. In these cases with elevated surgical risk, the goal becomes obtaining tumor tissue for histological and molecular diagnosis, which can be inform subsequent treatment decisions [4, 53]. Tumors that usually do not require biopsy are NF1-associated OPGs, or SEGA in tuberous sclerosis, with classical imaging and clinical features.

Surgical planning should be performed in a multidisciplinary tumor board, particularly for complex or borderline cases. Techniques such as neuronavigation, electrophysiological monitoring, and intraoperative MRI can reduce morbidity and improve surgical outcomes.

15.6.2 Chemotherapy

Chemotherapy is the primary nonsurgical treatment modality for pLGGs that are not amenable to GTR or that have progressed after surgery. It is typically preferred over radiotherapy, especially in younger children, to avoid long-term toxicities.

15.6.2.1 Standard Regimens

Several regimens have demonstrated efficacy in both newly diagnosed and progressive pLGGs:

- Carboplatin and vincristine (CV) [54]: This regimen is widely used and has a well-documented safety and efficacy profile. However, hypersensitivity reactions to carboplatin may occur in up to 40% of cases, necessitating treatment modification. The 5-year EFS of 39% is reached with this regimen [41].
- Vinblastine monotherapy [42]: Increasingly adopted as a first-line alternative, particularly in NF1-associated tumors and older children. It is well tolerated, with 5-year PFS of 53.2% (85.1% in NF1 patients) according to phase II results. The most common adverse effect is hematological toxicity.
- TPCV (thioguanine, procarbazine, lomustine, vincristine): This combination demonstrates a 5-year EFS of 52%, though with increased hematological toxicity [41].
- Vincristine/cisplatin/cyclophosphamide regimen: Considered after carboplatin hypersensitivity. Alternating cycles of vincristine with cisplatin or cyclophosphamide are administered every 6 weeks, up to 10 cycles. However, this regimen should be avoided in patients with pre-existing visual or auditory deficits due to ototoxicity risk.
- Bevacizumab-based regimens have shown promising activity in pLGG, such as bevacizumab + irinotecan [40, 55] or bevacizumab + vinblastine (NCT02840409).

15.6.2.2 Considerations for Children with NF1

Children with NF1-associated pLGGs have distinct considerations. Observation first is often appropriate for typical OPG with no significant progression or symptoms. When treatment is needed, vinblastine monotherapy is favored due to its tolerability, avoiding platinum-associated long-term toxicities, and due to the good efficacy results in clinical trials [42].

15.6.3 Radiotherapy

Radiotherapy is now generally reserved for selected or refractory cases, owing to the substantial risk of long-term sequelae in the developing brain [56].

15.6.3.1 Indications and Timing

Radiotherapy should be delayed as long as possible, especially in children <5 years of age, due to higher vulnerability to neurocognitive decline, endocrinopathies, and vascular complications (e.g., Moyamoya disease) [43]. Modern techniques, including conformal radiotherapy and proton beam therapy, possess unique physical characteristics that allow for a considerable decrease in the total radiation dose delivered to the patient. As a result, healthy brain tissue can be better preserved, which may lower the likelihood of neurocognitive side effects following treatment [54]. Radiotherapy can be considered for tumors that progress or recur after multiple lines of chemotherapy in older children, especially in case there are no actionable molecular targets. It is also an important option for disseminated disease when chemotherapy fails. Radiation should be avoided in patients with NF1, unless no other effective options exist due to increased risk of vasculopathy (e.g., moyamoya), second malignancies, and global increase of radiation-induced toxicities.

15.6.4 Targeted Therapies

Recent advances in the molecular biology of pLGGs have led to new treatment strategies. Targeted therapy has provided new treatment options for patients with pLGGs with the hope of reducing long-term morbidity due to their disease. These effective agents have changed the treatment paradigm for patients with improved outcomes compared to historical treatments such as chemotherapy. Most pLGGs are driven by activation of the MAPK pathway, often through a single genetic alteration such as *KIAA1549::BRAF* fusion or *BRAF* V600E mutation. Other alterations include mutations in *FGFR1/2/3* and *NF1*. These discoveries have supported the development and clinical study of small-molecule inhibitors targeting the MAPK pathway. pLGGs have a distinct molecular profile compared to adult gliomas, which more commonly harbor *IDH1/2* mutations, and some pediatric cases involve genetic changes (e.g., *MYB/MYBL1*) that currently lack targeted therapies.

15.6.4.1 MEK and BRAF Inhibitors

MEK inhibition is a promising treatment approach for tumors with BRAF fusions or single-nucleotide variants (SNVs). Several MEK inhibitors (MEKis) are in clinical use or trials, including selumetinib, trametinib, binimetinib, cobimetinib, and mirdametinib, showing efficacy in pediatric low-grade gliomas. BRAF inhibitors, including dabrafenib and vemurafenib, have shown significant efficacy in treating pLGGs with the BRAF p.V600E mutation, particularly in ganglioglioma and pleomorphic xanthoastrocytoma [57–60]. Clinical trials demonstrated favorable response rates and safety profiles, especially with dabrafenib plus trametinib, which outperformed standard chemotherapy in upfront treatment [61]. Rapid tumor progression may occur upon discontinuation, though retreatment often remains effective. Ongoing research focuses on optimizing therapy duration and discontinuation strategies.

15.6.4.2 FGFR Inhibitors

Erdafitinib, a pan-FGFR inhibitor initially approved for adult urinary tract cancers with FGFR2/3 mutations, has been increasingly explored in pLGGs harboring FGFR1 alterations. Early data [62] demonstrated promising efficacy, with 54% of patients showing partial response or stable disease. Pemigatinib, a selective FGFR1-3 inhibitor with superior blood–brain barrier penetration compared to erdafitinib, remains under investigation. Although pediatric-specific data are limited, adult CNS tumor studies such as the FIGHT-207 phase II trial revealed partial or complete responses in 23% of patients and stable disease in an additional 23%. The ongoing FIGHT-209 trial is evaluating pemigatinib in recurrent FGFR1-3 rearranged solid and CNS tumors in adults, with potential implications for future pediatric use [63]. These findings highlight the therapeutic potential of FGFR-targeted agents in pLGGs but underscore the need for larger, pediatric-focused clinical trials to clarify efficacy and optimize treatment strategies.

15.6.4.3 BRAF Inhibitors

BRAF inhibitors such as dabrafenib, vemurafenib, and encorafenib target the BRAF p.V600E mutation. These agents have demonstrated significant clinical efficacy, with rapid and durable radiographic responses. Combination therapy with dabrafenib and the MEK inhibitor trametinib further improves outcomes, with phase II trials reporting higher response rates, longer progression PFS, and better safety compared to chemotherapy [59]. However, therapy discontinuation often leads to rapid tumor progression, although retreatment typically restores response. Consensus recommends gradual tapering of BRAFi to reduce the risk of rebound growth. Ongoing efforts by international coalitions aim to develop guidelines on therapy duration, resistance, and safe discontinuation strategies.

15.6.4.4 Next-Generation RAF Inhibitors

Tovorafenib (DAY101) and plixorafenib (FORE8394) are emerging next-generation RAF inhibitors targeting the RAS-MAPK pathway in pLGGs [64]. Tovorafenib is an oral, CNS-penetrant pan-RAF type II inhibitor that has shown notable efficacy in relapsed or refractory BRAF- and RAF-altered pLGGs. Importantly, it is effective even in patients previously treated with RAF or MEK inhibitors. Plixorafenib, a novel inhibitor targeting both BRAF V600E and non-V600 mutations without inducing paradoxical MAPK activation, is currently being evaluated in ongoing trials in pediatric and adult populations [65]. Ongoing clinical trials are assessing tovorafenib as upfront therapy versus standard chemotherapy and in combination with vinblastine for recurrent or progressive RAF-altered pLGGs, highlighting its potential as a key component of targeted treatment strategies in this setting [66].

15.6.4.5 NTRK Inhibitors

NTRK gene fusions, while rare in adults (<2%), occur in up to 3% of pLGGs. Pediatric patients, especially infants, show better outcomes with TRK fusion-driven tumors compared to adults, with LGGs faring better than HGGs [67]. Larotrectinib, a selective TRK inhibitor, has demonstrated strong antitumor activity across TRK fusion-driven malignancies. Entrectinib targets TRK-A/B/C, ROS1, and ALK, showing a 50% ORR in pediatric and young adult patients with TRK fusion-positive CNS tumors in the STARTRK-NG trial. It has been well tolerated with confirmed safety in this population [68]. Ongoing trials are evaluating its efficacy in pediatric and young adult patients with advanced tumors harboring ALK, ROS1, or NTRK alterations.

15.6.4.6 mTOR Inhibitors

The mTOR pathway is a key therapeutic target in pLGGs, often activated by mutations in receptor tyrosine kinases or BRAF alterations. Everolimus, an mTOR inhibitor, has shown promising disease control in pLGGs [69]. The POETIC phase I–II and PNOC001 phase II trials demonstrated its ability to stabilize or reduce tumors. Notably, a phase II study in NF1-associated pLGGs reported tumor control or shrinkage in 68% of patients. Currently, the PNOC021 trial is exploring combined everolimus and trametinib treatment in recurrent low-grade gliomas [70].

15.6.4.7 Clinical Trial Data and Future Directions

The clinical development of targeted therapies for pLGGs has advanced significantly, particularly with the introduction of BRAF and MEK inhibitors. These agents have transformed the therapeutic landscape by offering more precise, less toxic alternatives to conventional chemotherapy and radiation. Trials involving BRAF inhibitors such as dabrafenib and vemurafenib have demonstrated notable efficacy in pLGGs harboring the BRAF p.V600E mutation. These studies report rapid and durable radiographic responses, improved progression-free survival, and favorable safety profiles compared to traditional treatments. However, challenges remain regarding optimal treatment duration and management of tumor progression after drug discontinuation, which may require careful tapering or reinitiation of therapy.

15.6.4.7.1 Future Directions

Ongoing research aims to refine targeted therapy strategies. Key areas include defining the optimal duration of treatment to balance efficacy and toxicity, understanding mechanisms of resistance, and developing protocols for safely discontinuing therapy. Additionally, combination regimens—such as MEK inhibitors with mTOR inhibitors or chemotherapy—are under investigation to enhance therapeutic efficacy and overcome resistance.

Emerging molecular profiling, techniques will further enable personalized treatment approaches, tailoring therapies to individual tumor biology. Collaborative efforts like the International Pediatric Low-Grade Glioma Coalition are establishing consensus guidelines to address challenges related to resistance, rebound progression, and long-term management.

In summary, the integration of molecularly targeted agents into pLGG treatment represents a paradigm shift, improving outcomes and quality of life. Continued clinical trials and translational research will be critical to optimize these therapies and expand their benefits to all affected patients.

15.7 Prognosis

15.7.1 Factors Influencing Prognosis

15.7.1.1 Tumor and Patient Characteristics

Tumor location is a critical determinant of prognosis in pLGGs. Tumors located in accessible, noneloquent cortical regions (e.g., superficial cerebral hemispheres) generally allow for GTR, correlating with excellent outcomes [14, 51]. Conversely, tumors in deep-seated or eloquent areas (brainstem, optic pathway, hypothalamus, thalamus, and basal ganglia) are often not amenable to complete resection due to the risk of significant morbidity [71], leading to increased risk of recurrence and requiring adjuvant therapy. Tumor size at diagnosis may also impact prognosis [72, 73] by influencing surgical feasibility and symptom burden, with larger tumors potentially associated with increased perioperative complications and neurological sequelae.

Leptomeningeal dissemination is seen in 4–12% of children with pLGG either at diagnosis or progression and results in worse outcomes (15-year OS of 50.9%) [74].

Patient age is also a factor in survival rates for pLGG, with infants having a worse prognosis. Infantile gliomas more commonly involve the hypothalamus and optic pathway, limiting resectability and increasing the likelihood of progression or metastasis: a spine MRI is typically recommended in infants at diagnosis (otherwise only when there is concern for metastatic disease or for clinical trials) [74]. Diencephalic syndrome is also a negative prognostic factor.

15.7.1.2 Tumor Location and Size

Tumor location plays a critical role in both treatment options and prognosis. LGGs located in accessible regions like the cerebral hemispheres are often amenable to gross total resection (GTR), which is associated with excellent outcomes and a high likelihood of cure. In contrast, tumors in deep or critical areas—such as the brainstem, optic pathway, or thalamus—pose surgical challenges due to the risk of neurological damage. In these cases, subtotal resection or nonsurgical treatments (e.g., chemotherapy, radiation) may be necessary, and the risk of recurrence or progression is generally higher [75].

Tumor size also impacts prognosis. Larger tumors may be more difficult to remove completely and can cause significant mass effect or hydrocephalus, leading to earlier symptom onset and potential neurological deficits. While size alone is not always a direct predictor of malignancy or survival, it can influence the extent of surgical resection and the need for adjuvant therapy.

15.7.1.3 Extent of Surgical Resection

The extent of resection is one of the strongest predictors of progression-free survival (PFS), and overall survival (OS) in pLGG gross total or near-total resection, achievable in around 50–70% of patients, is associated with 5-year PFS >90% and OS approaching 100% [72, 73, 76]. On the other hand, subtotal resection or biopsy-only approaches, often required for deep-seated or eloquent-location tumors, are associated with higher recurrence rates, though these tumors can remain stable, indolent, or show good response to medical therapies over prolonged periods. Reoperation may be considered for tumor progression in selected cases, particularly when resection is achievable with a low risk of morbidity. However, given the expanding landscape of medical therapies, especially targeted therapies, for pLGG, the surgical option should be discussed in multidisciplinary tumor boards, with functional preservation in mind.

15.7.1.4 Molecular Profile

The molecular understanding of pLGG is constantly expanding, with the 2021 WHO classification integrating molecular data in the definition of specific tumor entities. Molecular profiling has important ramifications for risk stratification, therapeutic decision-making, and general prognosis of pLGG [4, 53].

Activation of the RAS/MAPK pathway (e.g., *KIAA1549: BRAF* fusions, BRAF V600E mutations) is nearly universal in pLGG, and the specific underlying mutation has prognostic and therapeutic significance. Tumors harboring BRAF V600E mutations have a higher recurrence risk compared to pLGG with BRAF fusions [4, 53], but are amenable to treatment with targeted agents such as the combination of dabrafenib + trametinib with dramatically better efficacy results compared to standard chemotherapy (median PFS of 20.1 months vs 7.4 months) and better safety profile [59].

Also in the case of FGFR1, which is the second most commonly altered gene in pLGG, point mutations are associated with worse outcomes compared to FGFR1 fusions [4].

NF1-associated pLGG shows distinct biological and treatment response, and many patients will develop a pLGG in the first two decades of life with a tendency to progress, especially in the optic pathway, but with good response to medical therapy (both chemotherapy and targeted agents such as selumetinib) [77–81]. NF1-associated OPGs are a challenging entity with a variable course and consequent visual impairment can greatly affect quality of life.

CDKN2A/B deletions are associated with more aggressive behavior and increased risk of malignant transformation, particularly if combined with BRAF V600E mutation [82].

H3.3 p.K27M mutations, which are common in childhood HGG, can sometimes be found in cases of pLGG: these patients have unfavorable outcomes, supporting the role of this mutation as a marker of high-risk, aggressive tumors regardless of morphology [4].

IDH1 mutations are rare in pLGG compared to adult-type gliomas. The clinical significance of this mutation in pediatric gliomas is not completely understood, but might reflect adult-type malignancies that are identified early and might have a more aggressive course compared to typical pLGGs [53].

MYB/MYBL1 alterations in diffuse astrocytomas typically predict indolent courses with favorable outcomes.

Some rarer molecular alterations are targetable and offer the possibility of better outcomes or chemo-free approaches through newer agents; among these, FGFR, NTRK, or ALK are the most promising.

Data suggests that routine molecular profiling should be performed in pediatric gliomas in order to identify molecular alterations that confer additional risk for poor outcome, as histology does not always provide a perfect correlation [16]. Methylation profiling of pLGG may provide additional diagnostic and prognostic information, especially in difficult tumor entities, even if it is still expensive and not widely available [83].

15.7.2 Long-Term Outcomes

15.7.2.1 Survival Rates

pLGGs generally have excellent long-term survival rates, with 10-year OS exceeding 90% in most series, particularly in cases with gross total resection. However, PFS varies, with reported 5-year PFS around 40–50% for patients requiring chemotherapy or with subtotal resections [40–42]. There is evidence supporting the concept that, for children with progressive pLGG, treatment efficacy declines with subsequent treatment lines, yet is still higher for patients with NF1-associated pLGG [84].

Moreover, anatomical location and subsequent treatments frequently result in long-term neurological, cognitive, and psychosocial sequelae [39]. Therefore, despite the high survival rates, pLGGs are chronic diseases, often requiring multiple interventions and prolonged surveillance over years. Malignant transformation, while a possibility, is a rare phenomenon in pLGG compared to the adult population [85].

15.7.2.2 Neurocognitive and Endocrine Sequelae

Survivors of pLGG frequently experience long-term sequelae impacting quality of life and neurodevelopment. These complications are more frequent for pLGG involving midline structures and in children receiving radiotherapy, and also the involvement of the hypothalamus and chronic hydrocephalus play an important role in long-term morbidity [86].

Neurocognitive deficits: Impairments in attention, processing speed, executive function, and memory, particularly in patients with cortical, thalamic, or hypothalamic involvement, or those who received radiotherapy [87].

Endocrine dysfunction: Growth hormone deficiency, hypothyroidism, pubertal disturbances, and diabetes insipidus, particularly in patients with hypothalamic/pituitary involvement and those treated with cranial irradiation [88].

Visual impairment: Optic pathway gliomas frequently result in permanent vision loss; up to 60% may have severe visual impairment, with binocular blindness in 10–20% of cases [44].

Motor and sensory deficits: Persistent weakness, gait abnormalities, and ataxia are common in tumors involving motor pathways or the cerebellum.

Psychosocial challenges: Anxiety, depression, reduced social integration, and academic difficulties are frequently reported, necessitating long-term psychosocial support.

15.7.3 Importance of Long-Term Follow-Up and Surveillance

Both tumor-related symptoms and treatment modalities, especially radiotherapy, contribute substantially to chronic morbidity, underscoring the chronic nature of pLGGs.

Tumor progression or recurrence can occur years after initial treatment, necessitating periodic MRI surveillance, particularly for subtotally resected or deep-seated tumors.

Neurocognitive and endocrine complications require routine neuropsychological assessments and lifelong endocrinological follow-up for early identification and management of deficits, especially during puberty and growth.

Ophthalmological follow-up in patients with optic pathway gliomas, even if asymptomatic, given the risk of insidious progression.

Treatment-related sequelae, including secondary malignancies in irradiated patients and late effects of chemotherapy.

A multidisciplinary approach involving neuro-oncology, endocrinology, neurology, ophthalmology, rehabilitation, psychology, and education specialists is critical to optimize outcomes and quality of life for children with pLGGs.

Emerging targeted therapies (e.g., MEK inhibitors) offer the potential to improve disease control while reducing long-term toxicity compared to conventional chemotherapy and radiotherapy, warranting close monitoring of their impact on long-term outcomes in ongoing trials.

15.8 Conclusions

15.8.1 The Evolving Landscape of pLGG Management: Advances in Molecular Diagnostics and Their Impact on Treatment

Pediatric low-grade gliomas represent a heterogeneous group of CNS tumors characterized by generally favorable prognosis but with significant variability in the outcome and quality of life, influenced by tumor location, histology, and molecular features. Advances in molecular diagnostics, particularly since the 2021 WHO CNS tumor classification update, have revolutionized the understanding, classification, and management of pLGGs. Integration of next-generation sequencing, methylation profile, and liquid biopsy techniques has enabled precise identification of key genetic alterations, including BRAF mutations and fusions, FGFR alterations, and NTRK gene rearrangements. This molecular stratification not only refines diagnostic accuracy but also guides personalized treatment strategies. Targeted therapies, especially MEK and BRAF inhibitors, have transformed the therapeutic landscape by offering effective and less toxic alternatives to conventional chemotherapy and radiotherapy, with ongoing trials continuously expanding their indications. Despite these advances, challenges remain in optimizing treatment duration, managing resistance and tumor progression upon therapy discontinuation, and mitigating long-term sequelae including neurocognitive and endocrine dysfunction. Multidisciplinary collaboration among neuro-oncologists, neurosurgeons, pathologists, and geneticists is essential to ensure accurate diagnosis and individualized care. Long-term surveillance remains crucial due to potential late effects and tumor recurrence. Future directions include expanding the role of immunotherapy, gene therapy, and combination regimens to improve outcomes further.

Bibliography

1. Ostrom QT, Price M, Neff C, Cioffi G, Waite KA, Kruchko C, Barnholtz-Sloan JS. CBTRUS statistical report: primary brain and other central nervous system tumors diagnosed in the United States in 2015-2019. Neuro-Oncol. 2022;24:v1–v95. https://doi.org/10.1093/neuonc/noac202.
2. Louis DN, Perry A, Wesseling P, Brat DJ, Cree IA, Figarella-Branger D, Hawkins C, Ng HK, Pfister SM, Reifenberger G, et al. The 2021 WHO classification of tumors of the central nervous system: a summary. Neuro-Oncol. 2021;23:1231–51. https://doi.org/10.1093/neuonc/noab106.
3. Bandopadhayay P, Bergthold G, London WB, Goumnerova LC, Morales La Madrid A, Marcus KJ, Guo D, Ullrich NJ, Robison NJ, Chi SN, et al. Long-term outcome of 4,040 children diagnosed with pediatric low-grade gliomas: an analysis of the surveillance epidemiology and end results (SEER) database. Pediatr Blood Cancer. 2014;61:1173–9. https://doi.org/10.1002/pbc.24958.
4. Ryall S, Zapotocky M, Fukuoka K, Nobre L, Guerreiro Stucklin A, Bennett J, Siddaway R, Li C, Pajovic S, Arnoldo A, et al. Integrated molecular and clinical analysis of 1,000 pediatric low-grade gliomas. Cancer Cell. 2020;37:569–583.e5. https://doi.org/10.1016/j.ccell.2020.03.011.
5. Northrup H, Aronow ME, Bebin EM, Bissler J, Darling TN, de Vries PJ, Frost MD, Fuchs Z, Gosnell ES, Gupta N, et al. Updated international tuberous sclerosis complex diagnostic criteria and surveillance and management recommendations. Pediatr Neurol. 2021;123:50–66. https://doi.org/10.1016/j.pediatrneurol.2021.07.011.
6. Cockerell I, Christensen J, Hoei-Hansen CE, Holst L, Grenaa Frederiksen M, Issa-Epe AI, Nedregaard B, Solhoff R, Heimdal K, Johannessen Landmark C, et al. Effectiveness and safety of everolimus treatment in patients with tuberous sclerosis complex in real-world clinical practice. Orphanet J Rare Dis. 2023;18:377. https://doi.org/10.1186/s13023-023-02982-1.
7. Ogórek B, Hamieh L, Hulshof HM, Lasseter K, Klonowska K, Kuijf H, Moavero R, Hertzberg C, Weschke B, Riney K, et al. TSC2 pathogenic variants are predictive of severe clinical manifestations in TSC infants: results of the EPISTOP study. Genet Med. 2020;22:1489–97. https://doi.org/10.1038/s41436-020-0823-4.
8. Moavero R, Carai A, Mastronuzzi A, Marciano S, Graziola F, Vigevano F, Curatolo P. Everolimus alleviates obstructive hydrocephalus due to subependymal giant cell astrocytomas. Pediatr Neurol. 2017;68:59–63. https://doi.org/10.1016/j.pediatrneurol.2016.11.003.
9. Becker L-L, Agricola K, Ritter DM, Caré MM, Krueger DA, Franz DN. Long-term efficacy and safety of mammalian target of rapamycin inhibitor treatment for subependymal giant cell astrocytoma in tuberous sclerosis. Pediatr Neurol. 2025;168:90–5. https://doi.org/10.1016/j.pediatrneurol.2025.04.007.
10. Sturm D, Pfister SM, Jones DTW. Pediatric gliomas: current concepts on diagnosis, biology, and clinical management. J Clin Oncol Off J Am Soc Clin Oncol. 2017;35:2370–7. https://doi.org/10.1200/JCO.2017.73.0242.
11. Greuter L, Guzman R, Soleman J. Pediatric and adult low-grade gliomas: where do the differences lie? Children. 2021;8:1075. https://doi.org/10.3390/children8111075.

12. Jett K, Friedman JM. Clinical and genetic aspects of neurofibromatosis 1. Genet Med. 2010;12:1–11. https://doi.org/10.1097/GIM.0b013e3181bf15e3.
13. Chen Y, Yu J, Ge S, Jia R, Song X, Wang Y, Fan X. An overview of optic pathway glioma with neurofibromatosis type 1: pathogenesis, risk factors, and therapeutic strategies. Invest Ophthalmol Vis Sci. 2024;65:8. https://doi.org/10.1167/iovs.65.6.8.
14. Fangusaro J, Jones DT, Packer RJ, Gutmann DH, Milde T, Witt O, Mueller S, Fisher MJ, Hansford JR, Tabori U, et al. Pediatric low-grade glioma: state-of-the-art and ongoing challenges. Neuro-Oncol. 2024;26:25–37. https://doi.org/10.1093/neuonc/noad195.
15. Czyzyk E, Jóźwiak S, Roszkowski M, Schwartz RA. Optic pathway gliomas in children with and without neurofibromatosis 1. J Child Neurol. 2003;18:471–8. https://doi.org/10.1177/08830738030180070401.
16. Renzi S, Bennett J, Thacker N, Cacciotti C. Precision medicine for pediatric glioma and NF1-associated tumors: the role of small molecule inhibitors. Curr Oncol Tor Ont. 2025;32:280. https://doi.org/10.3390/curroncol32050280.
17. Sadighi ZS, Curtis E, Zabrowksi J, Billups C, Gajjar A, Khan R, Qaddoumi I. Neurologic impairments from pediatric low-grade glioma by tumor location and timing of diagnosis. Pediatr Blood Cancer. 2018;65:e27063. https://doi.org/10.1002/pbc.27063.
18. Arnautovic A, Billups C, Broniscer A, Gajjar A, Boop F, Qaddoumi I. Delayed diagnosis of childhood low-grade glioma: causes, consequences, and potential solutions. Childs Nerv Syst. 2015;31:1067–77. https://doi.org/10.1007/s00381-015-2670-1.
19. Jones DTW, Gronych J, Lichter P, Witt O, Pfister SM. MAPK pathway activation in pilocytic astrocytoma. Cell Mol Life Sci CMLS. 2012;69:1799–811. https://doi.org/10.1007/s00018-011-0898-9.
20. Louis DN, Perry A, Burger P, Ellison DW, Reifenberger G, von Deimling A, Aldape K, Brat D, Collins VP, Eberhart C, et al. International Society Of Neuropathology--haarlem consensus guidelines for nervous system tumor classification and grading. Brain Pathol Zurich Switz. 2014;24:429–35. https://doi.org/10.1111/bpa.12171.
21. Aisner DL, Newell KL, Pollack AG, Kleinschmidt-Demasters BK, Steinberg GK, Smyth LT, Vogel H. Composite pleomorphic xanthoastrocytoma-epithelioid glioneuronal tumor with BRAF V600E mutation - report of three cases. Clin Neuropathol. 2014;33:112–21. https://doi.org/10.5414/NP300679.
22. Komori T, Arai N. Dysembryoplastic neuroepithelial tumor, a pure glial tumor? Immunohistochemical and morphometric studies. Neuropathol. 2013;33:459–68. https://doi.org/10.1111/neup.12033.
23. Ryall S, Arnoldo A, Krishnatry R, Mistry M, Khor K, Sheth J, Ling C, Leung S, Zapotocky M, Guerreiro Stucklin A, et al. Multiplex detection of pediatric low-grade glioma signature fusion transcripts and duplications using the NanoString nCounter system. J Neuropathol Exp Neurol. 2017;76:562–70. https://doi.org/10.1093/jnen/nlx042.
24. Schindler G, Capper D, Meyer J, Janzarik W, Omran H, Herold-Mende C, Schmieder K, Wesseling P, Mawrin C, Hasselblatt M, et al. Analysis of BRAF V600E mutation in 1,320 nervous system tumors reveals high mutation frequencies in pleomorphic xanthoastrocytoma, ganglioglioma and extra-cerebellar Pilocytic astrocytoma. Acta Neuropathol (Berl). 2011;121:397–405. https://doi.org/10.1007/s00401-011-0802-6.
25. Qaddoumi I, Orisme W, Wen J, Santiago T, Gupta K, Dalton JD, Tang B, Haupfear K, Punchihewa C, Easton J, et al. Genetic alterations in uncommon low-grade neuroepithelial tumors: BRAF, FGFR1, and MYB mutations occur at high frequency and align with morphology. Acta Neuropathol. (Berl.). 2016;131:833–45. https://doi.org/10.1007/s00401-016-1539-z.
26. D'Angelo F, Ceccarelli M, Tala n, Garofano L, Zhang J, Frattini V, Caruso FP, Lewis G, Alfaro KD, Bauchet L, et al. The molecular landscape of glioma in patients with Neurofibromatosis 1. Nat Med. 2019;25:176–87. https://doi.org/10.1038/s41591-018-0263-8.
27. Soleman J, Kozyrev DA, Ben-Sira L, Constantini S, Roth J. Management of incidental brain tumors in children: a systematic review. Childs Nerv Syst. 2020;36:1607–19. https://doi.org/10.1007/s00381-020-04658-8.
28. Soleman J, Constantini S, Roth J. Incidental brain tumor findings in children: prevalence, natural history, management, controversies, challenges, and dilemmas. Childs Nerv Syst. 2024;40:3179–87. https://doi.org/10.1007/s00381-024-06598-z.
29. Ramírez-Melo JL, Moreira DC, Orozco-Alvarado AL, Sánchez-Zubieta F, Navarro-Martín Del Campo RM. Challenges in treating children with optic pathway gliomas: an 18-year experience from a middle-income country. Front Oncol. 2024;14:1329729. https://doi.org/10.3389/fonc.2024.1329729.
30. Liu APY, Harreld JH, Jacola LM, Gero M, Acharya S, Ghazwani Y, Wu S, Li X, Klimo P, Gajjar A, et al. Tectal glioma as a distinct diagnostic entity: a comprehensive clinical, imaging, histologic and molecular analysis. Acta Neuropathol Commun. 2018;6:101. https://doi.org/10.1186/s40478-018-0602-5.
31. Rudà R, Bello L, Duffau H, Soffietti R. Seizures in low-grade gliomas: natural history, pathogenesis, and outcome after treatments. Neuro-Oncol. 2012;14(Suppl 4):iv55–64. https://doi.org/10.1093/neuonc/nos199.

32. Ettinger AB. Structural causes of epilepsy. Tumors, cysts, stroke, and vascular malformations. Neurol Clin. 1994;12:41–56.
33. Slegers RJ, Blumcke I. Low-grade developmental and epilepsy associated brain tumors: a critical update 2020. Acta Neuropathol Commun. 2020;8:27. https://doi.org/10.1186/s40478-020-00904-x.
34. Fabbri VP, Caporalini C, Asioli S, Buccoliero A. Paediatric-type diffuse low-grade gliomas: a clinically and biologically distinct group of tumours with a favourable outcome. Pathologica. 2022;114:410–21. https://doi.org/10.32074/1591-951X-828.
35. Binning MJ, Liu JK, Kestle JRW, Brockmeyer DL, Walker ML. Optic pathway gliomas: a review. Neurosurg Focus. 2007;23:E2. https://doi.org/10.3171/FOC-07/11/E2.
36. Robert-Boire V, Rosca L, Samson Y, Ospina LH, Perreault S. Clinical presentation and outcome of patients with optic pathway glioma. Pediatr Neurol. 2017;75:55–60. https://doi.org/10.1016/j.pediatrneurol.2017.06.019.
37. Trapani S, Bortone B, Bianconi M, Rubino C, Sardi I, Lionetti P, Indolfi G. Diencephalic syndrome in childhood, a challenging cause of failure to thrive: miniseries and literature review. Ital J Pediatr. 2022;48:147. https://doi.org/10.1186/s13052-022-01316-4.
38. Fleischman A, Brue C, Poussaint TY, Kieran M, Pomeroy SL, Goumnerova L, Scott RM, Cohen LE. Diencephalic syndrome: a cause of failure to thrive and a model of partial growth hormone resistance. Pediatrics. 2005;115:e742–8. https://doi.org/10.1542/peds.2004-2237.
39. Benesch M, Lackner H, Sovinz P, Suppan E, Schwinger W, Eder H-G, Dornbusch HJ, Moser A, Triebl-Roth K, Urban C. Late sequela after treatment of childhood low-grade gliomas: a retrospective analysis of 69 long-term survivors treated between 1983 and 2003. J Neuro-Oncol. 2006;78:199–205. https://doi.org/10.1007/s11060-005-9091-z.
40. Gururangan S, Fangusaro J, Poussaint TY, McLendon RE, Onar-Thomas A, Wu S, Packer RJ, Banerjee A, Gilbertson RJ, Fahey F, et al. Efficacy of bevacizumab plus irinotecan in children with recurrent low-grade gliomas—a pediatric brain tumor consortium study. Neuro-Oncol. 2014;16:310–7. https://doi.org/10.1093/neuonc/not154.
41. Ater JL, Zhou T, Holmes E, Mazewski CM, Booth TN, Freyer DR, Lazarus KH, Packer RJ, Prados M, Sposto R, et al. Randomized study of two chemotherapy regimens for treatment of low-grade glioma in young children: a report from the children's oncology group. J Clin Oncol. 2012;30:2641–7. https://doi.org/10.1200/JCO.2011.36.6054.
42. Lassaletta A, Scheinemann K, Zelcer SM, Hukin J, Wilson BA, Jabado N, Carret AS, Lafay-Cousin L, Larouche V, Hawkins CE, et al. Phase II weekly vinblastine for chemotherapy-naïve children with progressive low-grade glioma: a Canadian pediatric brain tumor consortium study. J Clin Oncol. 2016;34:3537–43. https://doi.org/10.1200/JCO.2016.68.1585.
43. Merchant TE, Conklin HM, Wu S, Lustig RH, Xiong X. Late effects of conformal radiation therapy for pediatric patients with low-grade glioma: prospective evaluation of cognitive, endocrine, and hearing deficits. J Clin Oncol Off J Am Soc Clin Oncol. 2009;27:3691–7. https://doi.org/10.1200/JCO.2008.21.2738.
44. Morin A, Allodji R, Kariyawasam D, Touraine P, Puget S, Beccaria K, De Carli E, Kieffer V, Rivollet S, Abbou S, et al. Very long-term outcomes of pediatric patients treated for optic pathway gliomas: a longitudinal cohort study. Neuro-Oncol. 2024;26:1310–24. https://doi.org/10.1093/neuonc/noae045.
45. Traunwieser T, Kandels D, Pauls F, Pietsch T, Warmuth-Metz M, Bison B, Krauss J, Kortmann R-D, Timmermann B, Thomale U-W, et al. Long-term cognitive deficits in pediatric low-grade glioma (LGG) survivors reflect pretreatment conditions-report from the German LGG studies. Neuro-Oncol Adv. 2020;2:vdaa094. https://doi.org/10.1093/noajnl/vdaa094.
46. Walker DA, Aquilina K, Spoudeas H, Pilotto C, Gan H-W, Meijer L. A new era for optic pathway glioma: a developmental brain tumor with life-long health consequences. Front Pediatr. 2023;11:1038937. https://doi.org/10.3389/fped.2023.1038937.
47. Fangusaro J, Witt O, Hernáiz Driever P, Bag AK, de Blank P, Kadom N, Kilburn L, Lober RM, Robison NJ, Fisher MJ, et al. Response assessment in paediatric low-grade glioma: recommendations from the Response Assessment in Pediatric Neuro-Oncology (RAPNO) working group. Lancet Oncol. 2020;21:e305–16. https://doi.org/10.1016/S1470-2045(20)30064-4.
48. Kim M, Jung SY, Park JE, Jo Y, Park SY, Nam SJ, Kim JH, Kim HS. Diffusion- and perfusion-weighted MRI radiomics model may predict Isocitrate Dehydrogenase (IDH) mutation and tumor aggressiveness in diffuse lower grade glioma. Eur Radiol. 2020;30:2142–51. https://doi.org/10.1007/s00330-019-06548-3.
49. Buckner J, Giannini C, Eckel-Passow J, Lachance D, Parney I, Laack N, Jenkins R. Management of diffuse low-grade gliomas in adults - use of molecular diagnostics. Nat Rev Neurol. 2017;13:340–51. https://doi.org/10.1038/nrneurol.2017.54.
50. Krynina O, de Ståhl TD, Jylhä C, Arthur C, Giraud G, Nyman P, Fritzberg A, Sandgren J, Tham E, Sandvik U. The potential of liquid biopsy for detection of the KIAA1549-BRAF fusion in circulating tumor DNA from children with pilocytic astrocytoma. Neuro-Oncol Adv. 2024;6:vdae008. https://doi.org/10.1093/noajnl/vdae008.

51. Wisoff JH, Sanford RA, Heier LA, Sposto R, Burger PC, Yates AJ, Holmes EJ, Kun LE. Primary neurosurgery for pediatric low-grade gliomas: a prospective multi-institutional study from the children's oncology group. Neurosurgery. 2011;68:1548–54; discussion 1554-1555. https://doi.org/10.1227/NEU.0b013e318214a66e.
52. Boop S, Shimony N, Boop F. How modern treatments have modified the role of surgery in pediatric low-grade glioma. Childs Nerv Syst. 2024;40:3357–65. https://doi.org/10.1007/s00381-024-06412-w.
53. Ryall S, Tabori U, Hawkins C. Pediatric low-grade glioma in the era of molecular diagnostics. Acta Neuropathol Commun. 2020;8:30. https://doi.org/10.1186/s40478-020-00902-z.
54. Gnekow AK, Walker DA, Kandels D, Picton S, Giorgio Perilongo, Grill J, Stokland T, Sandstrom PE, Warmuth-Metz M, Pietsch T, et al. A European randomised controlled trial of the addition of etoposide to standard vincristine and carboplatin induction as part of an 18-month treatment programme for childhood (≤16 years) low grade glioma—a final report. Eur J Cancer. 2017;81:206–25. https://doi.org/10.1016/j.ejca.2017.04.019.
55. Zhukova N, Rajagopal R, Lam A, Coleman L, Shipman P, Walwyn T, Williams M, Sullivan M, Campbell M, Bhatia K, et al. Use of bevacizumab as a single agent or in adjunct with traditional chemotherapy regimens in children with unresectable or progressive low-grade glioma. Cancer Med. 2019;8:40–50. https://doi.org/10.1002/cam4.1799.
56. Krishnatry R, Zhukova N, Guerreiro Stucklin AS, Pole JD, Mistry M, Fried I, Ramaswamy V, Bartels U, Huang A, Laperriere N, et al. Clinical and treatment factors determining long-term outcomes for adult survivors of childhood low-grade glioma: a population-based study. Cancer. 2016;122:1261–9. https://doi.org/10.1002/cncr.29907.
57. Fangusaro J, Onar-Thomas A, Poussaint TY, Wu S, Ligon AH, Lindeman N, Campagne O, Banerjee A, Gururangan S, Kilburn LB, et al. A phase II trial of Selumetinib in children with recurrent optic pathway and hypothalamic low-grade glioma without NF1: a pediatric brain tumor consortium study. Neuro-Oncol. 2021;23:1777–88. https://doi.org/10.1093/neuonc/noab047.
58. Bouffet E, Geoerger B, Moertel C, Whitlock JA, Aerts I, Hargrave D, Osterloh L, Tan E, Choi J, Russo M, et al. Efficacy and safety of Trametinib monotherapy or in combination with Dabrafenib in pediatric BRAF V600-mutant low-grade glioma. J Clin Oncol Off J Am Soc Clin Oncol. 2023;41:664–74. https://doi.org/10.1200/JCO.22.01000.
59. Bouffet E, Hansford JR, Garrè ML, Hara J, Plant-Fox A, Aerts I, Locatelli F, van der Lugt J, Papusha L, Sahm F, et al. Dabrafenib plus trametinib in pediatric glioma with BRAF V600 mutations. N Engl J Med. 2023;389:1108–20. https://doi.org/10.1056/NEJMoa2303815.
60. Kieran MW, Geoerger B, Dunkel IJ, Broniscer A, Hargrave D, Hingorani P, Aerts I, Bertozzi A-I, Cohen KJ, Hummel TR, et al. A phase I and pharmacokinetic study of oral dabrafenib in children and adolescent patients with recurrent or refractory BRAF V600 mutation-positive solid tumors. Clin Cancer Res. 2019;25:7294–302. https://doi.org/10.1158/1078-0432.CCR-17-3572.
61. Erker C, Vanan MI, Larouche V, Nobre L, Cacciotti C, Vairy S, Zelcer S, Fleming A, Bouffet E, Jabado N, et al. Canadian consensus for treatment of BRAF V600E mutated pediatric and AYA gliomas. Curr Oncol. 2024;31:4022–9. https://doi.org/10.3390/curroncol31070299.
62. Eckstein OS, Allen CE, Williams PM, Roy-Chowdhuri S, Patton DR, Coffey B, Reid JM, Piao J, Saguilig L, Alonzo TA, et al. Phase II study of selumetinib in children and young adults with tumors harboring activating mitogen-activated protein kinase pathway genetic alterations: arm E of the NCI-COG pediatric MATCH trial. J Clin Oncol Off J Am Soc Clin Oncol. 2022;40:2235–45. https://doi.org/10.1200/JCO.21.02840.
63. Rodón J, Damian S, Furqan M, García-Donas J, Imai H, Italiano A, Spanggaard I, Ueno M, Yokota T, Veronese ML, et al. Pemigatinib in previously treated solid tumors with activating FGFR1-FGFR3 alterations: phase 2 FIGHT-207 basket trial. Nat Med. 2024;30:1645–54. https://doi.org/10.1038/s41591-024-02934-7.
64. Kilburn LB, Khuong-Quang D-A, Hansford JR, Landi D, van der Lugt J, Leary SES, Driever PH, Bailey S, Perreault S, McCowage G, et al. The type II RAF inhibitor tovorafenib in relapsed/refractory pediatric low-grade glioma: the phase 2 FIREFLY-1 trial. Nat Med. 2024;30:207–17. https://doi.org/10.1038/s41591-023-02668-y.
65. De La Fuente M, Butowski NA, Taylor J, Yaeger R, Tsai FY-C, Janku F, Allen CE, Ammakkanavar N, Michelson G, Jiang P, et al. TRLS-02. Safety and efficacy of BRAF inhibitor PLIXORAFENIB (FORE8394; PLX8394) in children and adults with recurrent, BRAF-altered primary central nervous system tumors (PCNST). Neuro-Oncol. 2024;26 https://doi.org/10.1093/neuonc/noae064.155.
66. van Tilburg CM, Kilburn LB, Perreault S, Schmidt R, Azizi AA, Cruz-Martínez O, Zápotocký M, Scheinemann K, Meeteren AYNS, Sehested A, et al. LOGGIC/FIREFLY-2: a phase 3, randomized trial of Tovorafenib vs chemotherapy in pediatric and young adult patients with newly diagnosed low-grade glioma harboring an activating RAF alteration. BMC Cancer. 2024;24:147. https://doi.org/10.1186/s12885-024-11820-x.
67. Lamoureux A-A, Fisher MJ, Lemelle L, Pfaff E, Amir-Yazdani P, Kramm C, De Wilde B, Kazanowska B, Hutter C, Pfister SM, et al. Clinical characteristics and outcomes of central nervous system tumors harboring NTRK gene fusions. Clin Cancer Res.

2025;31:561–72. https://doi.org/10.1158/1078-0432.CCR-24-0581.

68. Desai AV, Robinson GW, Gauvain K, Basu EM, Macy ME, Maese L, Whipple NS, Sabnis AJ, Foster JH, Shusterman S, et al. Entrectinib in children and Young adults with solid or primary CNS tumors harboring NTRK, ROS1, or ALK aberrations (STARTRK-NG). Neuro-Oncol. 2022;24:1776–89. https://doi.org/10.1093/neuonc/noac087.
69. Cacchione A, Lodi M, Carai A, Miele E, Tartaglia M, Megaro G, Del Baldo G, Alessi I, Colafati GS, Carboni A, et al. Upfront treatment with mTOR inhibitor Everolimus in pediatric low-grade gliomas: a single-center experience. Int J Cancer. 2021;148:2522–34. https://doi.org/10.1002/ijc.33438.
70. Wright KD, Yao X, London WB, Kao P-C, Gore L, Hunger S, Geyer R, Cohen KJ, Allen JC, Katzenstein HM, et al. A POETIC phase II study of continuous oral everolimus in recurrent, radiographically progressive pediatric low-grade glioma. Pediatr Blood Cancer. 2021;68:e28787. https://doi.org/10.1002/pbc.28787.
71. Weiß S, Thomale U-W, Schulz M, Kandels D, Schuhmann MU, El Damaty A, Krauss J, Driever PH, Witt O, Bison B, et al. Neurosurgical morbidity in pediatric supratentorial midline low-grade glioma: results from the German LGG studies. Int J Cancer. 2023;153:1487–500. https://doi.org/10.1002/ijc.34615.
72. Chen Z, Guo Z, Wang J, Cao D, Xu Y, Dong F, Wan F. Clinical features and outcomes of pediatric intracranial gliomas: results from single center's 226 cases and corroborated with SEER database. Childs Nerv Syst. 2023;39:593–601. https://doi.org/10.1007/s00381-023-05841-3.
73. Garzón M, García-Fructuoso G, Suñol M, Mora J, Cruz O. Low-grade gliomas in children: single institutional experience in 198 cases. Childs Nerv Syst. 2015;31:1447–59. https://doi.org/10.1007/s00381-015-2800-9.
74. Roka K, Scheinemann K, Avula S, Maduro JH, Thomale UW, Sehested A, Schouten-Van Meeteren AYN. European standard clinical practice recommendations for primary pediatric low-grade gliomas. EJC Paediatr Oncol. 2024;4:100169. https://doi.org/10.1016/j.ejcped.2024.100169.
75. Albalkhi I, Shafqat A, Bin-Alamer O, Mallela AN, Gersey ZC, Fernandes Cabral D, Sabbagh AJ, Hadjipanayis CG, González-Martínez JA, Friedlander RM, et al. Complications and visual outcomes following surgical resection of pediatric optic pathway/hypothalamic gliomas: a systematic review and meta-analysis. Childs Nerv Syst. 2024;40:2033–42. https://doi.org/10.1007/s00381-024-06407-7.
76. Dodgshun AJ, Maixner WJ, Hansford JR, Sullivan MJ. Low rates of recurrence and slow progression of pediatric pilocytic astrocytoma after gross-total resection: justification for reducing surveillance imaging. J Neurosurg Pediatr. 2016;17:569–72. https://doi.org/10.3171/2015.9.PEDS15449.
77. Ruggiero A, Attinà G, Campanelli A, Maurizi P, Triarico S, Romano A, Massimi L, Tamburrini G, Verdolotti T, Mastrangelo S. Pediatric low-grade glioma and neurofibromatosis type 1: a single-institution experience. J Cancer Res Ther. 2023;19:228–34. https://doi.org/10.4103/jcrt.jcrt_1677_21.
78. Hernáiz Driever P, von Hornstein S, Pietsch T, Kortmann R, Warmuth-Metz M, Emser A, Gnekow AK. Natural history and management of low-grade glioma in NF-1 children. J Neuro-Oncol. 2010;100:199–207. https://doi.org/10.1007/s11060-010-0159-z.
79. Packer RJ, Iavarone A, Jones DTW, Blakeley JO, Bouffet E, Fisher MJ, Hwang E, Hawkins C, Kilburn L, MacDonald T, et al. Implications of new understandings of gliomas in children and adults with NF1: report of a consensus conference. Neuro-Oncol. 2020;22:773–84. https://doi.org/10.1093/neuonc/noaa036.
80. Kotch C, de Blank P, Gutmann DH, Fisher MJ. Low-grade glioma in children with neurofibromatosis type 1: surveillance, treatment indications, management, and future directions. Childs Nerv Syst. 2024;40:3241–50. https://doi.org/10.1007/s00381-024-06430-8.
81. Fangusaro J, Onar-Thomas A, Young Poussaint T, Wu S, Ligon AH, Lindeman N, Banerjee A, Packer RJ, Kilburn LB, Goldman S, et al. Selumetinib in paediatric patients with *BRAF*-Aberrant or neurofibromatosis type 1-associated recurrent, refractory, or progressive low-grade glioma: a multicentre, phase 2 trial. Lancet Oncol. 2019;20:1011–22. https://doi.org/10.1016/S1470-2045(19)30277-3.
82. Ahrendsen JT, Sinai C, Meredith DM, Malinowski SW, Cooney TM, Bandopadhayay P, Ligon KL, Alexandrescu S. Molecular alterations in pediatric low-grade gliomas that led to death. J Neuropathol Exp Neurol. 2021;80:1052–9. https://doi.org/10.1093/jnen/nlab097.
83. Sexton-Oates A, Dodgshun A, Hovestadt V, Jones DTW, Ashley DM, Sullivan M, MacGregor D, Saffery R. Methylation profiling of paediatric pilocytic astrocytoma reveals variants specifically associated with tumour location and predictive of recurrence. Mol Oncol. 2018;12:1219–32. https://doi.org/10.1002/1878-0261.12062.
84. Kandels D, Pietsch T, Bison B, Warmuth-Metz M, Thomale U-W, Kortmann R-D, Timmermann B, Hernáiz Driever P, Witt O, Schmidt R, et al. Loss of efficacy of subsequent nonsurgical therapy after primary treatment failure in pediatric low-grade glioma patients-report from the German SIOP-LGG 2004 cohort. Int J Cancer. 2020;147:3471–89. https://doi.org/10.1002/ijc.33170.
85. Broniscer A, Baker SJ, West AN, Fraser MM, Proko E, Kocak M, Dalton J, Zambetti GP, Ellison DW, Kun LE, et al. Clinical and molecular characteristics of malignant transformation of low-grade glioma in children. J Clin Oncol. 2007;25:682–9. https://doi.org/10.1200/JCO.2006.06.8213.

86. Jujui-Eam A, Sirachainan N, Hongeng S, Hansasuta A, Boongird A, Tritanon O, Dhanachai M, Swangsilpa T, Ruangkanchanasetr R, Worawongsakul R, et al. Long-term treatment outcomes of pediatric low-grade gliomas treated at a university-based hospital. Childs Nerv Syst. 2023;39:1173–82. https://doi.org/10.1007/s00381-022-05809-9.
87. Plant-Fox AS, O'Halloran K, Goldman S. Pediatric brain tumors: the era of molecular diagnostics, targeted and immune-based therapeutics, and a focus on long term neurologic sequelae. Curr Probl Cancer. 2021;45:100777. https://doi.org/10.1016/j.currproblcancer.2021.100777.
88. Gan H-W, Phipps K, Aquilina K, Gaze MN, Hayward R, Spoudeas HA. Neuroendocrine morbidity after pediatric optic gliomas: a longitudinal analysis of 166 children over 30 years. J Clin Endocrinol Metab. 2015;100:3787–99. https://doi.org/10.1210/jc.2015-2028.

16 Pediatric-Type Diffuse High-Grade Gliomas

Maria Vinci and Veronica Biassoni

16.1 Introduction

Pediatric high-grade gliomas (pHGGs) are highly invasive brain tumors accounting for approximately 15% of all central nervous system (CNS) tumors in children and adolescents, with a dismal prognosis [1].

The 2021 World Health Organization (WHO) Classification of CNS tumors introduced significant updates and changes to the categorization of pHGG by grouping them within the family of pediatric-type diffuse high-grade glioma (pDHGG). In recent years, advancements in DNA and RNA sequencing and methylation profiling have largely contributed to expanding the classical pathology knowledge of pHGG, providing an integrated approach for the definition of new tumor entities characterized by distinct genetic and epigenetic alterations. Here, we outline the different pDHGG tumor entities as defined by the 2021 WHO classification: (1) diffuse midline gliomas, H3 K27-altered; (2) diffuse hemispheric glioma, H3 G34-mutant; (3) diffuse pediatric-type high-grade glioma, H3-wildtype, and IDH-wildtype; and (4) infant-type hemispheric glioma [2]. We report on the epidemiology, clinical presentation, imaging characteristics, molecular biology, and histology and include an extended section on standard and advanced therapies. For this review, we will not focus on other high-grade glial tumors outside the family of pDHGG, such as high-grade astrocytoma with piloid features, grade 3 pleomorphic xantoastrocytoma, and astroblastoma MN1-altered.

In addition to the newly recognized pDHGG entities by the 2021 WHO classification, we provide an overview of *gliomatosis cerebri,* a tumor type no longer considered a distinct entity by the WHO but characterized by a unique growth pattern [3]. We report on the history of GC, the differences between adult and pediatric GC, and the recent advances in the field.

Understanding the distinct characteristics of the different pHGG tumor type is crucial for accurate diagnosis, prognostication, and development of targeted therapies.

16.2 Definition

*Diffuse midline glioma, H3 K27-altered (*DMG-H3K27*)* is the term adopted to identify a pDHGG tumor entity that encompasses a broad range of tumor subtypes beyond the DMG H3 K27M mutant previously acknowledged in the 2016 WHO classification [1]. DMG-H3K27 is charac-

M. Vinci (✉)
Research Unit of Genetics and Epigenetics of Pediatric Tumors, Bambino Gesù Children's Hospital-IRCCS, Rome, Italy
e-mail: maria.vinci@opbg.net

V. Biassoni
Pediatric Oncology Unit, Fondazione IRCCS Istituto Nazionale dei Tumori, Milan, Italy

A. Mastronuzzi, A. Carai (eds.), *Navigating Pediatric Brain Tumors*,
https://doi.org/10.1007/978-3-032-18992-9_16

terized by the loss of the H3K27me3 histone modification, which can result from either a K27M mutation in one of the H3 histone isoforms, aberrant overexpression of the EZHIP gene, or EGFR alterations [2]. These highly aggressive tumors predominantly affect children and young adults, infiltrating midline brain and spinal cord structures. In children, they arise more often in the pons and are also known as diffuse intrinsic pontine glioma (DIPG), while in adolescents and young adults, they are more likely to arise in the thalamus or spinal cord [1]. *Diffuse hemispheric glioma, H3 G34-mutant (*DHG-H3G34*)*, identifies a new pDHGG tumor subtype characterized by a missense mutation in the H3.3 histone variant, specifically a glycine-to-arginine or glycine-to-valine substitution at codon 34. This aggressive tumor predominantly affects adolescents and young adults, comprising approximately 16% of pediatric hemispheric high-grade gliomas [2]. *Diffuse pediatric-type high-grade glioma, H3-wildtype and IDH-wildtype* (DHGG-WT) is the term used to identify the highly infiltrative hemispheric pDHGG that do not carry mutations in histone H3 genes and lack mutations in isocitrate dehydrogenase (IDH1/IDH2), distinguishing them from adult HGG. DHGG-WT typically occurs in the cerebral hemispheres of children, adolescents, or young adults. A combination of histological, molecular, and clinical features has to be considered to make a diagnosis of DHGG-WT [2]. *Infant-type hemispheric glioma (*IHG*)* is the term used to identify the primary aggressive brain tumor arising within the cerebral hemispheres in young children, typically under the age of 1 and associated with gene fusions involving receptor tyrosine kinase (RTK) pathways, most notably ALK, ROS1, MET, NTRK1/2/3, or with the specific methylation profile [2].

16.3 Epidemiology and Prognosis

The majority of cases of *DMG-H3K27* occur in children, with a peak incidence between 5 and 10 years of age with a smaller subset of cases seen in adolescents and young adults and occasional rare cases reported in older adults. DMG-H3K27 represents approximately 20–40% of pHGG. Within the DMG-H3K27, the pontine tumors defined as diffuse intrinsic pontine glioma (DIPG) represent 10–15% of all pediatric brain tumors, while the thalamic DMG are rarer, representing 1–5% of pediatric brain tumors. The prognosis for DMG-H3K27 remains extremely poor, with a median survival of approximately 10–12 months for H3- and EGFR-mutant tumors and slightly longer survival for EZHIP-overexpressing tumors [4, 5]. Interestingly for DIPG, patients with H3.1 K27M mutation have a better prognosis with a median overall survival (OS) of 15 months compared to 9.2 months for the H3.3K27M patients. Several factors contribute to this dismal prognosis in DMG-H3K27 such as the critical location that makes surgical resection extremely challenging, with the pontine region inoperable and the diffuse infiltration in adjacent structures.

DHG-H3G34 most frequently occurs in adolescents and young adult patients (median age 15–19 years), with most cases reported in individuals between 10 and 30 years of age, and rarely seen in younger children and older adults. DHG-H3G34 accounts for approximately 7% of pHGG and 16% of hemispheric pHGG [6]. A slight male predominance is described, although the difference is not statistically significant. The prognosis is poor, with a median OS of 18–22 months. MGMT methylation is associated with longer OS while the amplification of genes such *EGFR* confers a worse outcome [7]. *DHGG-WT* accounts for approximately 40% of pDHGG. This tumor subgroup occurs primarily in children and young adults with a poor prognosis and a median OS of 17 months. Of the three main methylation classes identified, pedHGG-RTK1, pedHGG-RTK2 and pedHGG_MYCN, the latter is associated with the lowest survival rates while the pedHGG-RTK2 is the less aggressive; pedHGG-RTK1 is generally related to radiation-induced HGG or HGG arising within cancer predisposition syndromes [8, 9]. *IHG* is rare compared to other pHGG with a frequency of 5% of pHGG, occurs in infants under the age of 1, and often presents as congenital tumors [6].

The prognosis of IHG is better compared to other pDHGG and interestingly the presence of gene fusions seems to confer a longer OS compared to IHG without fusions [10]. In addition, also surgery (e.g., the extent of resection) also has an impact on prognosis with a better outcome when gross total resection is achievable [11].

16.4 CNS Location and Clinical Features

Disease presentation varies largely depending on the specific tumor location and patient age. *DMG-H3K27* can arise in any of the midline structures, including the brainstem, the thalamus, and the spinal cord (Fig. 16.1) [6]. Patients with tumor lesions affecting the brainstem and pontine region present multiple cranial nerve palsy, motor deficits (long trait signs), and cerebellar dysfunction. Headache and vomiting may also be present as signs of increased intracranial pressure (ICP). Patients with lesions in the thalamic region present motor deficits, sensory disturbances, as well as cognitive impairment and increased ICP, while tumor lesions in the spinal cord are associated with bowel and bladder dysfunction, sensitive and motori signs according to the level of the lesion, and back pain in addition to other symptoms more common in the other midline structures. Symptoms typically develop gradually over weeks to months, but then disease progression can be rapid, leading to significant neurological deterioration (Table 16.1) [12, 13]. In *DHG-H3G34*, tumor arise in the cerebral hemispheres (Fig. 16.1), with the frontal lobe and left hemisphere being the most frequently affected, even if multiple lobes can be involved. Its clinical presentation is dictated by its location in the cerebral hemispheres, rapid growth, and infiltrative behavior. Seizures are a common and often the first symptom for patients with DHG-H3G34 tumors. They can be focal or progress to generalized seizures depending on the specific tumor's location. Neurological deficits as motor weakness may be present if the tumor lesion involves the motor pathways. Other symptoms include numbness or tingling when the parietal lobe is involved and speech difficulties if the tumor affects the dominant hemisphere's language areas. Cognitive and behavioral changes may be

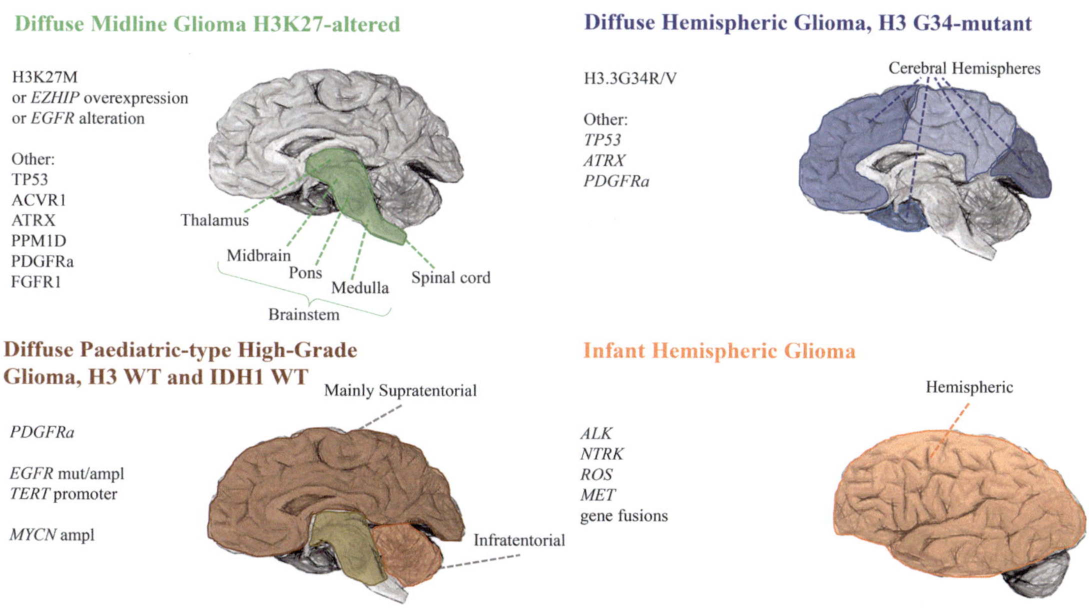

Fig. 16.1 Schematic representation of the different pDHGG tumor types showing their specific CNS locations and the main molecular alterations

Table 16.1 Summary of the clinical, imaging, histological, and immunophenotypic features of pDHGG

Type	Clinical presentation	Imaging	Histology	Phenotype
Diffuse midline glioma, H3 K27-altered (DMG-H3K27)	Cranial nerve palsies Motor deficits Cerebellar dysfunction Headache, vomiting Cognitive impairment Bowel and bladder dysfunction Back pain	Large, infiltrative masses Hypointense T1-weighted Hyperintense T2-weighted Variable contrast enhancement Infiltration of surrounding tissue Focal hemorrhage and necrosis	Diffusely infiltrative growth pattern, monomorphic or polymorphic cells, variable mitotic activity, necrosis, and microvascular proliferation	Positive for OLIG2 and S100 variable GFAP expression H3K27M or EZHIP overexpression loss of H3K27me3
Diffuse hemispheric glioma, H3 G34-mutant (DHG-G34)	Seizures Focal neurological deficits Headache, nausea, vomiting Cognitive and behavioral changes	Large, contrast-enhancing masses Hyperintense T2-weighted images Multifocal lesions, necrosis, cystic changes, calcifications	Diffusely infiltrative growth pattern dual phenotype: Astrocytic and PNET-like High mitotic activity, necrosis, and microvascular proliferation	Negative for OLIG2 and ATRX Positive for p53 Variable GFAP expression
Diffuse pediatric-type high-grade glioma, H3-wildtype and IDH-wildtype (DHGG-WT)	Headache, nausea, vomiting Seizures Focal neurological deficits Cognitive and behavioral changes	Large, contrast-enhancing masses Hyperintense T2-weighted Diffuse parenchymal infiltration, softening, discoloration, hemorrhage, necrosis	Diffuse astrocytic morphology Variable mitotic activity, necrosis, and microvascular proliferation	Positive for p53 Expression of GFAP and OLIG2
Infant-type hemispheric glioma (IHG)	Polyhydramnios Macrocephaly Increased head circumference Lethargy, irritability Seizures, vomiting Abnormal eye movements	Large, intra-axial mass Solid and cystic components Mass effect, compression of surrounding tissue hemorrhage	Hypercellular with clear boundaries Astrocytic cytomorphology with gemistocytic-like cells and spindle cell differentiation High-grade features: Mitoses, microvascular proliferation, necrosis	Positive for OLIG2 and GFAP negative for synaptophysin; H3K27me3, INI-1 and BRG1 nuclear expression is retained

present as well as headache, nausea, and vomiting associated with raised ICP (Table 16.1) ([6, 14, 15, 16]. The vast majority of *DHGG-WT* arise in the supratentorial compartment, a minority of cases of specific type can also occur in the brainstem (pHGG MYCN) and more generally in the infratentorial structures (pHGG RTK1) (Fig. 16.1) [8]. General symptoms include ICP, headaches, nausea, vomiting, and focal or generalized seizures, but the clinical presentation varies depending on the specific location (Table 16.1). *IHG* are hemispheric tumors (Fig. 16.1) that present mainly in the supratentorial compartments as large masses and may include both cystic and solid components. Although "*hemispheric*" is the term used for defining this pDHGG subtype, the term may be too restrictive since brainstem and spinal locations have also been reported for IHG. In very young children, interpreting symptoms can be difficult. Common clinical presentation signs include agitation, lethargy, and increased head circumference, typically appearing acutely within the first year of life. Congenital cases may show noticeable signs such as bulging fontanelles. During the antenatal period, polyhydramnios—caused by depressed swallowing due to hypothalamic dysfunction—occurs in about one-third of patients. Additionally, macrocephaly may arise from tumor expansion or hydrocephalus (Table 16.1) [8, 17].

16.5 Imaging and Diagnostics

DMG-H3K27 typically presents as large, infiltrative masses on neuroimaging. Magnetic resonance imaging (MRI) characteristics include hypointense T1-weighted images and hyperintense T2-weighted images, with rare and variable contrast enhancement, when present with a ring enhancement. DMG infiltrate the surrounding tissue, distorting normal brain anatomy. Focal areas of hemorrhage and necrosis may be evident. In the brainstem, tumors typically appear as large, expansive lesions often involving the pons, encasing the basilar artery, with infiltration of cerebellar peduncles, midbrain, or medulla. Cranial nerve involvement, especially cranial nerves V, VII, and VIII, may occur. Thalamic DMG may be unilateral or bilateral, with infiltration into adjacent structures like the internal capsule or basal ganglia (Table 16.1) [18, 19]. The clinic–radiological diagnosis of DIPG remains relevant. Many children suspected of a brainstem tumor centered in the pons, in the absence of a biopsy, are still diagnosed with a DIPG based on typical brainstem symptoms (cranial nerve deficits, long tract signs, or ataxia) and the onset of symptoms should be short, preferably less than 3 months and at maximum 6 months. If MR imaging alone, diagnosis is based on the appearance of an intrinsic, pontine-based infiltrative lesion hypointense on T1- and hyperintense on T2-weighted sequences, involving at least 2/3 of the pons [20]. *DHG-H3G34* and *DHGG-WT* tumors share several common neuroimaging and gross pathological characteristics. They appear as large, sometimes contrast-enhancing masses and are typically hyperintense on T2-weighted images. The DHG-H3G34 may exhibit multifocal lesions, necrosis, cystic changes, and calcifications while the DHGG-WT often demonstrate diffuse parenchymal infiltration, softening, discoloration, and hemorrhagic/necrotic zones. Hemorrhage and necrosis may be present, especially in more aggressive tumors (Table 16.1) [21]. Within the DHGG-WT, it is worth noting the recent description of distinct radiological (and histo-molecular) features in two different subclasses: pedHGG-RTK2A, which tend to be hemispheric, with a *gliomatosis cerebri* growth pattern, and the pedHGG-RTK2B, which frequently showed a bithalamic involvement at diagnosis [22].

For *IHG*, unlike in children of older age, different signs or symptoms need to be considered in the clinical and diagnostic evaluation. In the antenatal period, polyhydramnios and macrocephaly are common presentations of a congenital brain tumor, usually detected by ultrasound, but fetal MRI can also be employed. Later in infancy, the following symptoms may appear: apneic episodes, irritability, delay in developmental milestones, drowsiness, irritability, but also seizures, vomiting, and abnormal eye movements [17]. On neuroimaging, IHG generally presents as a huge intra-axial mass with both solid and cystic components. Some features include the evident mass effect with compression of the surrounding tissue and in some cases intratumoral hemorrhage. Although cranial ultrasound is useful for initial screening, MRI is the gold standard for diagnosis, providing detailed information on tumor size, location, and relationship with the surrounding anatomical structures and internal characteristics.

Alongside imaging, *liquid biopsy* (LB) is another noninvasive technique that offers a promising alternative by detecting tumor-derived biomarkers in blood or cerebrospinal fluid (CSF). In particular, LB is an emerging approach for DMG-H3K27M tumors, for which surgery is less amenable than other pDHGG. Digital droplet PCR and next-generation sequencing (NGS) represent sensitive techniques with diagnostic value for detecting circulating tumor DNA (ctDNA) with histone mutations. Recently, extracellular histone profiles have also been detected in DMG-H3K27M in plasma and CSF. Besides the future diagnostic application, LB is also useful for disease monitoring by tracking changes in ctDNA levels to assess tumor dynamics and response to therapy and for prognostication by correlating ctDNA levels with tumor burden and prognosis [23–25]. Due to their potential utility, LB is increasingly being incorporated into several clinical protocols of different CNS tumors, though still at an investigational level.

16.6 Molecular Biology

DMG-H3K27 is mainly characterized by the oncogenic driver mutation in H3 histone genes (*H3F3A*, *HIST1H3B*, *HIST1H3C*, or *HIST2H3C*) that leads to the amino acid substitution of the lysine (K) to methionine (M) [26, 27] or isoleucine (I) [5] in the position 27. These mutations cause a global methylation loss on the H3K27me3 mark through the inhibition of the Polycomb Repressive Complex2 (PRC2), resulting in the upregulation of gene expression [28]. Following recent molecular profiling studies and based on the 2021 WHO classification, four distinct tumor subtypes have been grouped in the DMG-H3K27-altered tumor entity: H3.3 K27M-mutant, H3.1/H3.2 K27M-mutant; H3-WT with *EZHIP* overexpression [4] and DMG-H3K27 with EGFR mutation or amplification [29], all associated with the loss of H3K27m3. Recently, a new DMG-H3K27 subtype has been described as characterized by a co-occurring mutation in H3K27M and BRAFV600E or FGFR1 [30], also presenting loss of trimethylation, though it differs from the other DMG-H3K27 tumors for a unique methylation profile, longer survival, and histopathological features. DMG-H3K27 often presents other co-occurring gene alterations such as TP53, ACVR1, PPM1D, and *ATRX* mutations, *PDGFRA*, *CDK4/6*, *CCND1–3*, and *MYC/PVT1* amplifications, and *CDKN2A/B* homozygous deletion, with varying frequencies (Fig. 16.1).

DHG-H3G34 is characterized by the driver mutation in the histone H3 gene H3F3A, which substitutes the glycin (G) with the arginine (R) or less frequently the valine (V) on position 34 [26, 27]. This mutation is associated with altered gene expression as a result of the SETD2 methyltransferase inhibition [31] and downregulation of DNA damage repair pathways [32]. DHG-H3G34 presents concurrent mutations with H3.3G34R/V with the most frequent being mutations in *TP53*, *ATRX*, and *PDGFRA* (Fig. 16.1). Other co-occurring alterations are *CCND2*, *PDGFRA*, and *MYC* amplifications; and chromosomal abnormalities, such as deletions of the long arm of chromosomes 3 and 4. MGMT promotor is frequently methylated in these tumors [9, 33].

DHGG-WT comprises a mixture of different molecular subtypes all characterized by histone H3 WT and IDH WT. Genetic investigations and the analysis of methylation profiles have contributed to identifying three different subgroups defined as pedHGG-RTK1, pedHGG-RTK2, and pedHGG-MYCN [34, 35]. Tumors of the pedHGG-RTK1 are associated with *PDGFRA* alterations and are frequently found in patients with *Lynch syndrome* and in the context of *germline mismatch repair deficiency* (CMMRD), as well as in the radiation-induced HGG [9]. The pHGG-MYCN subclass is characterized by *MYCN* activation, mostly amplification. The co-amplification of *MYCN* with *ID2* on the short arm of chromosome 2 seems to define the pedHGG-MYCN class better than the *MYCN* amplification alone [36]. The pedHGG-RTK2 subclass is frequently characterized by *EGFR* amplification and mutations in the promoter of *TERT*. A recent study has warranted a refinement of the pedHGG-RTK2 methylation subclass, distinguishing the 2A and 2B subtypes, based on radiological and histomolecular features. From the molecular point of view, besides the most common *EGFR* alteration in both classes, the pedHGG-RTK2A is characterized by mutations in *BCOR*, *SETD2*, and *TERT* promoter while the pedHGG-RTK2B is enriched in alterations in *TP53* [22] (Fig. 16.1). Finally, several tumors fall into the DHGG-WT tumor entity as they are H3 WT and IDH1 WT, but do not classify as pHGG RTK1, pHGG RTK2 or pHGG MYCN, are negative for receptor RTK fusions, and are designated as "NEC" by the WHO 2021 classification [2]. This highlights that further molecular, clinical, histological, and radiological characterization is needed for this heterogeneous group of pDHGG.

IHG is characterized by gene fusions involving receptor tyrosine kinase (RTK) genes. The most common alterations are fusions in *ALK*, *NTRK1/2/3, ROS1,* and *MET* genes [10, 37] (Fig. 16.1). *NTRK* encode for the tropomyosin receptor kinase (Trk) A, B, and C proteins. These fusions typically combine the C-terminal kinase domain of NTRK genes with N-terminal sequences from diverse partner genes, producing chimeric proteins with constitutively active kinase functions that drive oncogenesis.

These alterations arise through structural genomic variants and form a distinct molecular subgroup based on DNA methylation profiling. This subgrouping is consistent regardless of the specific RTK fusion present. The diagnosis of IHG relies on either the detection of RTK fusions, such as those involving NTRK, or the characteristic DNA methylation profile of the tumor. However, identifying RTK fusions alone is not sufficient to confirm a diagnosis of IHG, as similar rearrangements can occasionally occur in adult-type glioblastoma (IDH-wildtype), where they likely result from clonal evolution rather than serving as primary oncogenic drivers [38].

An element worth mentioning is the elevated *intratumor heterogeneity* that characterizes pDHGG. These tumors hold a complex subclonal architecture given by the coexistence of multiple codominant subclonal populations, regardless of tumor location or mutational subgroup. Tumors with H3.3 G34R mutations show a higher number of subclones compared with other pDHGG while the infant cases have the least [39]. Moreover, driver somatic mutations such as histone mutations and *ACVR1* are clonal event, conserved across time and space, while other mutations such as *PDGFRA* are often found to be later events in clonal expansion and spatially heterogeneous [39, 40].

16.7 Histology and Immunophenotype

DMG-H3K27 microscopic analysis reveals a diffusely invasive growth pattern, with tumor cells extensively interspersed among neurons and infiltrating adjacent structures. The majority of DMG cells appear typically small and monomorphic, although they can also exhibit polymorphism with cells presenting astrocytic, piloid, oligodendroglial, giant cell, or undifferentiated features. While some cases do not display mitotic activity, necrosis, and microvascular proliferation, and have a histological appearance of grade 2, DMG-H3K27 are now classified as grade 4, independently of the histology (WHO Classification of Tumours, 5th edn.) The immunophenotype of DMG-H3K27, regardless of the molecular subtypes, shows positive staining for OLIG2 and S100 and variable positivity for GFAP. It is diagnostic practice to use antibodies for H3K27M, H3K27me3, and EZHIP. Immunostaining for these markers can identify the different DMG subtypes and immunohistochemistry can be diagnostic. Positive and negative IHC nuclear staining to H3K27M and H3K27me3 is useful in identifying DMG-H3K27 mutant subtype while negative IHC staining for both H3K27M and H3K27me3 but positive staining for EZHIP can identify DMG-H3K27 H3 wild-type with EZHIP overexpression. Some cases show p53 expression and/or nuclear loss of *ATRX*, which can be indicative of the presence of somatic mutations in these genes [8]. The recently described DMG-H3K27M/BRAFV600E or FGFR1 co-altered subtype presents features of heterogeneous histopathological profiles with calcifications and solid tumor components, unique to this subtype and not present in the classical DMG-H3K27M [30].

DHG-H3G34 are hypercellular tumors displaying a diffusely infiltrating pattern. Tumor cells appear heterogeneous exhibiting often a dual phenotype, with astrocytic morphology, high mitotic activity microvascular proliferation and necrosis (glioblastoma-like phenotype), and small monomorphic cells with hyperchromatic nuclei and scant cytoplasms (PNET-like phenotype) [8]. These phenotypes can coexist within the same tumor, but even when the glioblastoma-like features are absent, the presence of the H3.3G34R/V mutation is enough to confer grade 4. Differently from the DMG-H3K27, although there are antibodies suitable for the immunostaining of H3.3G34R [41] and V variants [42], these are not sensitive or specific enough to be used with a diagnostic value [43]. The immunophenotype of DHG-H3G34 is characterized by negative expression of OLIG2 and ATRX, and expression of p53. The immunoreactivity of ATRX and p53 is often correlated to the presence of mutations in the corresponding genes. GFAP is strongly expressed in the glioblastoma-like phenotype while it appears focal in the PNET-like phenotype, which also displays a diffuse positive staining for synaptophysin [8].

DHGG-WT typically exhibits a classic diffuse astrocytic morphology characterized by brisk mitotic activity, necrosis, and microvascular proliferation. Some cases, particularly those belonging to the pedHGG-MYCN methylation class, or, less commonly, the pedHGG-RTK1 class, may present with a primitive or embryonal morphology and well-defined borders, showing only minimal infiltration of the surrounding brain tissue. Notably, DHGG-WT tumors arising in syndromic contexts, such as Li–Fraumeni syndrome, may display remarkable nuclear pleomorphism. The pedHGG-RTK MYCN subclass is characterized by well-circumscribed nodules and isolated tumoral cells infiltrating the brain. In all DHGG-WT subtypes, immunohistochemical analyses typically reveal negative nuclear staining for H3 K27M, H3K27me3, and IDH1. Neoplastic cells generally exhibit extensive and intense immunostaining for p53, while focal positivity for glial fibrillary acidic protein (GFAP) and OLIG2 is also observed. The pedHGG-MYCN subclass is marked by the expression of certain glial markers, such as GFAP and OLIG2, although undifferentiated cases may lose both markers. Additionally, neuronal markers such as NeuN, neurofilaments, and CD56 may be expressed. Other notable features include strong nuclear positivity for p53, loss of PTEN, and preserved ATRX expression. Within the pedHGG-RTK2 class, there are interesting distinctions between subclass 2A and 2B. Subclass 2A may exhibit pleomorphic xanthoastrocytoma-like features, which are absent in subclass 2B. Conversely, subclass 2B can contain giant, multinucleated cells, a feature absent in subclass 2A. Tumors in subclass 2A are generally negative for OLIG2, whereas this marker is found in at least a subset of tumor cells in subclass 2B. Both subclasses express EGFR but with differing patterns. ATRX expression is preserved in subclass 2A and may be lost in subclass 2B [8, 9, 22].

IHG are hypercellular tumors characterized by a clear boundary with minimal neoplastic infiltration of surrounding cerebral tissue. IHG typically presents uniform astrocytic cytomorphology, featuring sheets of gemistocytic-like cells and spindle cell differentiation. Ependymal differentiation has been observed in the context of ALK fusion cases. Most cases demonstrate high-grade features, such as brisk mitoses, microvascular proliferation, and palisading necrosis, although low-grade components may occasionally coexist with high-grade. The NTRK-fusion-positive tumors show a significantly higher proliferation index (Ki67) than fusion-negative tumors. The immunophenotype shows the expression of glial markers OLIG2 and GFAP, with dot-like EMA patterns; synaptophysin, IDH1 R132H, and H3K27M are negative. H3K27me3, INI-1, and BRG1 nuclear expressions are retained [8, 10].

16.8 Standard and Advanced Therapy

In spite of biological insight into pHGGs and the promise for more effective therapies, little progress has been made in the treatment and outcome of these tumors in the last four decades. Although most children receive adjuvant chemotherapy, the "standard" regimen to offer to newly diagnosed pHGG patients has not been established, also due to the heterogeneity of these tumors [44]. Given the rarity of the disease, it is fundamental that children with HGG are treated within clinical trials, for the same reason registries that can collect such rare diseases are advocated to better understand the real impact of this disease and the specific treatments in the pediatric population.

For *DMG-H3K27*, standard therapy includes radiation therapy (RT), which provides only a transient benefit. In general, focal RT (up to 54 Gy) is considered the standard of care for all patients with DMG older than 3 years at diagnosis. Perioperative corticosteroids may be used to manage peritumoral edema and raised intracranial pressure. There is no standard systemic treatment in addition to RT that has been acknowledged in the scientific community. For this group of patients, an international consensus on the role of adjuvant chemotherapy [e.g., temozolomide (TMZ)] or any other drug regimen (e.g., mTOR inhibitors) is still lacking. However, previous findings suggest that any chemotherapy or drug treatment in addition to radiotherapy (RT) may be beneficial for DIPG/DMG patients compared to RT alone [45]. Pontine DMG-H3K27 are surgically unresectable. Given their clear radiological features and considering the delicate pontine location, stereotactic biopsy is not routinely performed but it is becoming more frequently practiced in several centers providing precious samples for refined diagnostic assessment of patient tumors, guiding toward a more personalized treatment approach. Recent clinical studies have demonstrated the possibility of targeted therapies in DIPG patients, underscoring the value of safety biopsy procedures, which also offer the opportunity to advance research in the DIPG field when tissue is available [46, 47].

Based on the experience of the adult glioblastoma EORTC trial with oral TMZ and RT, a phase II trial with TMZ in parallel to RT and as subsequent consolidation treatment for pediatric patients ($\geq$3 years $\leq$18 years of age) with primary high-grade glioma, DIPG, or gliomatosis cerebri, has been performed in Germany (HIT-HGG-2007 trial, ISRCTN19852453). The preliminary results reported so far within a subgroup analysis showed a 3-month event-free survival (EFS) and OS benefit for patients with nonpontine pHGG treated with TMZ compared with a more intensive cisplatinum-based chemotherapy regimen (median EFS 10.7 versus 7.4 months and 19.3 versus 16.2 months, respectively) [48]. The definitive results and the analysis within the DMG group patients will help elucidate the role of TMZ in this subset of patients.

There are several collaborative trials ongoing in Europe and all around the world to ensure uniform patient accrual and treatment for newly diagnosed pHGG, including children with DMG-H3K27-altered. For example, CONNECT (Collaborative Network for Neuro-oncology Clinical Trials, a network of 18 institutions across the globe covering different pediatric malignancies: HGG/DIPG, medulloblastoma, craniopharyngioma, and recurrent CNS tumors) and PNOC (Pediatric Neuro-Oncology consortium, dedicated to precision therapies for pediatric CNS tumors with sites opened all around the world) have ongoing trials for children with DMG. In addition, the BIOMEDE 2.0 trial is currently recruiting patients with DMG-H3K27 who are randomized to receive either ONC201 or everolimus. ONC201 (dordaviprone) is a molecule acting in DMG-H3K27 with two different pathways: it acts as DRD2 antagonist and as mitochondrial ClpP agonist. The result of these interactions is the suppression of the producing-metabolism pathways with subsequent apoptosis and the restoring of the histone trimethylation. Several publications have reported the clinical activity of this compound in DMG patients [49, 50], but a recent paper expressed some concerns about them, mainly related to the selection of the patients, the lack of uniform enrolment criteria, the fact that some patients were treated before a progression of the disease, and the unclear role of reirradiation [51]. What is known by now about its mechanism of action is that high EGFR expression and ClpP mutations are predictive of a poor response to ONC201 while DMG with RAS/MAPK activation have a better response. Preclinically, ONC201 has given promising results when used in combination with an oncolytic virus [52] or with the PI3K inhibitor paxalisib [53], with the latter that led to an ongoing clinical trial (NCT05009992).

Some light will be shed by the ongoing prospective trials, including this molecule upfront (PNOC022—phase II trial with ONC201 combined with different drugs, panobinostat or paxalisib, for DMG; BIOMEDE 2.0 phase III multicenter, randomized, open-label, controlled trial evaluating the efficacy of ONC201 compared with everolimus in children and adults with pontine and nonpontine DMG; ACTION phase III, ONC201 for the treatment of newly diagnosed H3 K27M-mutant diffuse glioma following completion of RT: a randomized double-blind, placebo-controlled, multicenter study).

Other national efforts are ongoing focused on different compounds or alternative RT schedules (e.g., the use of a reduced-dose RT schedule approach followed by further cycles of irradiation at definitive timepoints in the absence of progression has been evaluated within the recently closed Italian phase II open-label randomized study of RT, concomitant nimotuzumab and vinorelbine and reirradiation at relapse versus RT and multiple elective RT courses with concomitant vinorelbine and nimotuzumab for newly diagnosed childhood and adolescence diffuse intrinsic pontine glioma/DIPG and an observational study for DMG with K27 mutation).

Other promising treatment strategies at the moment investigated either at diagnosis or in the relapse setting include

- Chimeric antigen receptor T (CAR-T) cell therapy, with several ongoing clinical trials focusing on two main targets being GD2 ([54, 55]; NCT04196413, NCT05544526, NCT05298995, NCT05438368) and B7-H3 ([56]; NCT05835687, NCT05768880, NCT04185038). Despite many hopes for this immunotherapy approach, there are open issues that will need to be addressed that include the antigen escape, the optimal route of administration (intravenous, intrathecal, combined) to obtain adequate tumor access with durable engraftment and minimum toxicity [55, 57–59].
- Oncolytic viruses: Their use is sustained by high tumor selectivity, low probability of resistance, high oncolytic capacity, and the possibility of genetic manipulation. The result of a phase 1 study (NCT03178032) with DNX-2401 in relapsing DIPG patients has been published [60] showing promising results with a single intratumoral infusion of the oncolytic virus.
- Alternative methods of drug delivery such as convention enhanced delivery (CED) [61] and focused ultrasound (FUS) [62, 63] are under investigation (NCT04264143, NCT05762419, NCT04804709) with a potential need to combine them with systemic treatment to avoid dissemination.

Cancer neuroscience is another evolving field in the treatment of pHGG. Neuronal activity increases tumor growth in pediatric HGG through paracrine factors such as neuroligin 3, GABAergic synapsis, and AMPAR signaling, so they represent potential targets [64–66].

Since it is well recognized that TME plays a key role in pHGG maintenance, targeting the main hallmarks of TME through anticancer therapies, repurposed drugs and multimodal immunotherapy are also issues that need to be further investigated [67, 68].

For *DHG-H3G34* and *DHGG-WT*, the standard of care involves a multimodal approach combining surgery, RT, and chemotherapy. The extent of surgical resection should be maximized while minimizing neurological deficits (maximal safe resection). Perioperative focal RT is crucial for local control of residual disease. While adjuvant chemotherapy is standard practice, the optimal regimen remains uncertain, with Stupp regimen or TMZ-containing regimens being the most commonly and widely used. *DHG-H3G34* has generally high levels of MGMT promoter methylation and might have better responses to TMZ than those with low MGMT promoter methylation, even if the role of MGMT status in pHGG has to be determined yet.

Interestingly, while DHG-H3G34 tumors are classified as gliomas, two recent studies have revealed that interneuron-like progenitors are the actual cells of origin for these tumors [69, 70]. This particular cellular lineage may facilitate the co-option of PDGFRA, which helps explain the high percentage of activating PDGFRA mutations found in DHG-H3G34 tumors [69]. These findings point toward new, clinically relevant actionable targets for treating patients with DHG-H3G34, particularly by directly targeting PDGFRA signaling [69] or exploring emerging specific vulnerabilities such as CDK6 [70]. The H3.3-G34R mutation causes significant DNA damage and contributes to genomic instability. This instability activates the cGAS/STING signaling pathway, leading to a pro-inflammatory immune response. In this context, research suggests that combining DNA damage response inhibitors with radiotherapy (RT) is a promising approach. In preclinical studies using DHG-H3G34 mouse models, this combination has been shown to extend survival [32]. Currently, two phase I trials are underway focusing on peptide-pulsed dendritic cell vaccination for DHG-H3G34. The first trial, NCT06342908, aims to evaluate the safety and feasibility of the vaccine and is limited to patients with DHG-H3G34 who are older than 18 years. The second trial, NCT05457959, seeks to assess the safety, tolerability, and immunogenicity of the vaccine in combination with the immunotherapy drugs nivolumab and ipilimumab. This trial is open to DHG-H3G34 patients aged 13 years and older.

DHGG-WT hypermutant tumors that occur in the context of CMMRD may respond more favorably to immune checkpoint inhibitors. In particular, gliomas with primary replication repair deficiencies are inherently resistant to TMZ (temozolomide) due to the lack of a functional mismatch repair system that is essential for the drug's cytotoxic effects. As a result, these tumors often experience rapid recurrence after chemoradiation.

The first prospective randomized clinical trial (CCG-943) for pHGG was published in 1989 by the American Children's Cancer Study Group (CCG) reporting a significant improvement in the outcome of RT followed by PCV (procarbazine/chloroethyl-cyclohexyl nitrosourea [CCNU]/vincristine), over RT alone, after maximal safe surgical resection [71]. Five-year OS rates of 43% (±9%) and 17% (±7%) were reported for RT + PCV vs. RT alone, respectively. The following CCG-945 study compared the RT + PCV regimen 8-in-1 chemotherapy with no significant difference between the arms (5-year OS 36% ±6%) [72]. Later, a pathology central review of the CCG-945 study (but not of the CCG-943) was performed and 30% of patients were low-grade gliomas misclassified as HGG, with an adjusted OS rate of 22% (±3%) for HGG in CCG-945 [73].

In a randomized-controlled phase III trial conducted between 2000 and 2002 by Stupp and colleagues, the role of the alkylating agent TMZ was investigated in adult glioblastoma patients. They compared RT combined with concomitant and adjuvant TMZ therapy to RT alone in patients with newly diagnosed HGG. The results, published in 2005 [74], documented a median OS of 14.6 months in the TMZ plus RT arm vs. 12.1 months in the RT alone arm. This survival advantage was maintained also in the follow-up cohort where the 5-year OS of the experimental group was 9.8% vs. 1.9% in the control group [75].

After these results in adult patients with TMZ, the Children's Oncology Group (COG) phase II ACNS0126 pediatric trial failed to demonstrate significant improvement of the outcome with radiochemotherapy with TMZ compared with previous radiochemotherapy regimens in pediatric patients with HGG.

In contrast, the German HIT-HGG-2007 trial was launched by the German Society for Paediatric Oncology and Haematology (GPOH) to investigate the noninferiority of a less toxic TMZ radiochemotherapy for pHGG (including DIPG) compared to the previous protocols HIT-GBM-C and D with different chemotherapy compounds. Results did not only confirm noninferiority and less toxicity for the analyzed 438 HIT-HGG-2007 patients but demonstrated increased OS in nonpontine HGG (median OS: 19.3 months) and improved EFS rates for patients with both nonpontine and pontine HGG (median EFS +3.3/+2 months) compared with the historical cohort. The significance of MGMT overexpression in predicting response to alkylating agents remains a matter of debate in pediatric HGG. With its comparatively favorable toxicity profile and the possibility of an oral outpatient treatment, TMZ radiochemotherapy is nowadays widely considered as the treatment of choice in pediatric patients with (non-DIPG/non-DMG) hemispheric HGG. The role of CCNU added to TMZ was investigated in the subsequent ACNS-0423 study that resulted in better 3-year EFS and OS rates of 22 ± 8% and 28 ± 8%, respectively, most pronounced for selected patients (methylation of the MGMT promoter and non-GTR) and at the expense of increased toxicity [76].

The addition of bevacizumab to a backbone of TMZ/RT (Herby trial) failed to improve EFS and OS in non-brainstem pedHGGs [77].

The German cooperative group is currently conducting the HIT-HGG-2013 trial (DRKS-ID:DRKS00012806), comparing the combination of TMZ and valproate with historical data from their previous studies, HIT-HGG-2007 (NCT03243461), using single-agent TMZ.

Other phase II studies are exploring the combination of TMZ with nivolumab and immunotherapy (NCT02960230, NCT04267146).

IHG show unique biological traits and generally respond better to treatments than older children [37]. They have higher survival rates and improved outcomes with chemotherapy and delayed radiation therapy, which is usually avoided due to potential neurocognitive side effects. Surgical resection should be tailored to each patient, weighing tumor removal against neurological risks. For large hemispheric tumors, a different surgical approach may be necessary. If aggressive resection poses significant risks or will not achieve complete tumor removal, debulking surgery or biopsy might be appropriate.

In the past years, different treatment schedules have been developed to delay or avoid irradiation for infants with HGG.

The CCG-945 study evaluated the 8-in-1 regimen (that includes vincristine 1.5 mg/m^2 i.v., methylprednisolone 300 mg/m^2 × 3 doses q6h iv, lomustine 100 mg/m^2 by mouth, procarbazine 75 mg/m^2 by mouth, hydroxyurea 3000 mg/m^2 by mouth, cisplatin 90 mg/m^2 over 6 h iv, cytosine arabinoside 300 mg/m^2 iv and imidazole carboximide 150 mg/m^2 iv, all within a 12 h period) with reported 3-year PFS and OS of 36% and 51%, respectively, better than older children treated with this regimen combined with RT [78].

From 1986 to 1996, the Baby POG I study reported cases cured with 24 months of chemotherapy alone using prolonged alternating chemotherapy consisting of two cycles of cyclophosphamide and vincristine followed by a third cycle of cisplatin and etoposide. The study reported 5-year PFS and OS of 43% and 50% for the 18 pHGG patients [79].

The French chemotherapy-only BBSFOP protocol is a 16-month schedule of seven cycles of three drug pairs of carboplatin–procarbazine, cisplatin–etoposide, and vincristine–cyclophosphamide used in pHGG patients under the age of 5 years with the aim of developing a mild chemotherapy that could be given for a long period to delay/avoid RT and with reported 5-year PFS and OS of 35.3% and 58.8%, respectively [80].

The German HIT-SKK chemotherapy is a similar chemo-only strategy to delay and avoid RT in patients with brain tumors. It consists of three 2-month cycles of chemotherapy as follows: intravenous methotrexate, cyclophosphamide, vincristine, carboplatin, and etoposide. The HIT-SKK chemotherapy—in combination with intraventricular methotrexate for young children with medulloblastoma patients—is feasible and well tolerated. In IHG, the modified HIT-SKK chemotherapy (without intraventricular methotrexate) is frequently used [81].

In the UKCCSG/SIOP CNS 9204 trial, infants with non-brainstem HGG were treated without intraventricular chemotherapy and with courses of carboplatin/vincristine, high-dose methotrexate/vincristine, cyclophosphamide monotherapy, and cisplatin monotherapy, resulting in PFS and OS rates of 13.0% and 30.9%. The aim was to enhance treatment intensity with chemotherapy given every 2 weeks [82].

The emerging evidence of the different biology between the infant and older pHGG may be a major contributing factor to the survival differences between these groups of patients. Interestingly, there have also been reports of spontaneous regression in rare instances [83].

Early clinical trials show that IHG may respond to targeted therapy directed at their respective RTK fusion (ALK, ROS1, NTRK1/2/3, and MET). Personalized therapy for IHG may be shaped by the identification of fusions and fusion gene partners for choosing the most appropriate molecular targeted agent, although the presence or type of fusions does not seem to correlate with better outcomes compared to IHG cases without fusions [11].

16.8.1 Targeting BRAFV600E in pHGG

Up to 5–10% of pHGG harbor the BRAFV600E mutation that is associated with favorable histological subtypes. Dabrafenib is a BRAF inhibitor that demonstrated clinical activity as monotherapy in phase I/II trial in relapsed/refractory BRAF V600 mutant pHGG [84, 85]. After the publication of the results of the phase I/II trial [85], a subsequent phase II trial with dabrafenib and trametinib in relapsing/refractory HGG was performed. From December 2017 to August 2020, 41 pediatric patients (median age 13 years) from 28 sites of 13 countries were enrolled at a median time since diagnosis of 17.4 months and with a median follow-up of 25.1 months. Overall response rate (complete + partial remission) was observed in 56% of patients with a median duration of response of 22.2 months and most responses occurring within 4 months of treatment. For the whole cohort, median PFS and OS were 9 months and 32.8 months, respectively. Treatment-related adverse events of grade ≥ 3 were observed in 26.8% of patients with a manageable safety profile. These findings suggest that the combination of dabrafenib plus trametinib is a promising targeted therapy option for children and adolescents with relapsed/refractory BRAF V600E–mutant HGG [86].

Based on this, the European Medical Agency (EMA) has recently approved the combination of MEK inhibitors, such as trametinib, to address the acquired resistance to the MAPK pathway. This approval is for children older than 1 year with BRAFV600 mutant low-grade gliomas (LGG) requiring treatment and for BRAFV600 mutant high-grade gliomas (HGG) that have relapsed after first-line therapy.

16.8.2 Treatment at Relapse

Median survival following the recurrence of pediatric high-grade glioma (pHGG) is typically just a few months, and there is no established standard of care. Different medical centers often pursue various strategies, with most patients receiving multimodal treatments that show very limited success. Before considering management strategies for relapsing patients, it is essential to conduct a complete restaging to determine the most appropriate approach. The evidence for selecting specific treatments for recurrent or progressive pHGG is limited, largely based on retrospective cohort studies involving patients who have received a variety of treatments. Due to the lack of international collaborative trials for recurrent or progressive pHGG, it is reasonable to integrate standard multimodal treatment approaches—including reirradiation—with targeted therapies informed by molecular and genetic findings. A meta-analysis of therapeutic approaches over the past two decades in recurrent nonpontine pHGG reports a cumulative overall survival (OS) of 5.6 months. Reirradiation (re-RT) has been associated with the longest survival, while chemotherapy approaches have shown an OS of only 4 months in pediatric patients with recurrent high-grade glioma [87]. Focusing on reirradiation, there are only a few reported studies on its role in relapsing or progressive pHGG. Some of these studies primarily discuss patterns of failure but all document a clinical benefit from reirradiation [88, 89]. The two most extensive studies are from Canada and Italy. The Canadian study is a retrospective cohort analysis of 40 children with recurrent pHGG. In this study, 14 out of 40 patients received reirradiation at relapse, leading to an improved median survival time from the first disease progression (9.4 months for those who received reirradiation compared to 3.8 months for the 26 patients who did not; $P = 0.005$) [90]. The Italian study is the largest retrospective series, reporting data on 21 relapsed pHGG patients, all of whom were reirradiated (three received a third course of radiation therapy). The median time to progression and survival after re-RT was 3.7 months and 6.9 months, respectively, with improved outcomes for patients who had a longer interval between the first and reirradiation ($P = 0.017$) and for those who did not progress after re-RT ($P < 0.001$). The first marginal relapse suggested a potential association with dissemination after re-RT ($P = 0.081$). Considering that 9 out of 21 patients exhibited dissemination at relapse, the results may warrant investigation into different first-line radiation therapy fields in a randomized trial [91].

16.9 Cancer Predisposition Syndrome

At least 10% of children with cancer are primarily affected by a cancer predisposition syndrome (CPS). The more prominent syndrome associated with pHGG are Li–Fraumeni syndrome (LFS), constitutional mismatch repair deficiency (CMMRD), and in a small percentage neurofibromatosis 1. Specific consensus recommendations have been published by international expert groups concerning surveillance of patients with CPS [51].

LFS: The median age of onset of brain tumors in LFS is 16 years, the tumors most frequently observed are choroid plexus carcinoma, medulloblastoma SHH/TP53 mutant, and at a lower extent HGG. Currently, there are no TP53-specific therapies and the prognosis for LFS-associated HGG remains poor [92].

NF1: The most common CNS neoplasia in NF1 is optic pathway glioma while the rate of higher grade brain malignancies in NF1 is low. It is still unclear whether NF1-pHGG are secondary gliomas arising from low-grade lesions or can be primary pHGG. Also in this case, there are no specific treatment suggestions for a patient harboring a pHGG in NF1 [93].

CMMRD: It arises from alterations within one of the two recognized mechanisms of DNA replication during cell division, the mismatch repair (MMR) system (involving PMS2, MLH1, MSH2, MSH6) and the internal proofreading capability of the DNA polymerase (POLE, POLD1). For pHGG driven by germline or somatic DNA replication repair deficiency, including both mismatch repair and/or polymerase-proofreading deficiency, focal irradiation is recommended. TMZ should be avoided in those circumstances, but CCNU can be considered as an adjuvant therapy [94]. Moreover, immune checkpoint inhibition is well established to improve survival at progression for these hypermutant gliomas and may be considered as a frontline treatment for some patients with favorable genomic and immune biomarkers [95, 96].

16.10 Gliomatosis Cerebri

Even though gliomatosis cerebri (GC) is not recognized as a tumor entity in the latest WHO classification of CNS tumors [2], we believe it is important to report here about GC given its highly aggressive and infiltrative nature. GC is a rare form of diffuse glioma with a unique diffuse growth pattern characterized by extensive infiltration of tumor cells across multiple brain regions (Fig. 16.2). GC was initially described in 1938 by Samuel Nevin [97], an English pathologist who analyzed three autopsy cases and reported on tumor-like gliomas affecting an extensive area of the brain. He described these conditions in which the brain swells extensively without forming grossly visible tumor nodules while maintaining normal gross architecture as *gliomatosis cerebri* [97]. In 1979, GC was described in the first edition of the WHO classification as "poorly differentiated and embryonal tumors" [98]. Later on, from the second to the third edition of the WHO classification, GC was defined as a glial tumor infiltrating multiple lobes, two lobes in the third edition (2000) [99, 100], revised to three lobes in the four edition (2007) [101], with detailed criteria emphasizing bilateral involvement and wide tissue spread. In the revised fourth edition (2016) [1], GC was removed as a distinct entity due to molecular studies showing GC as molecularly equivalent to

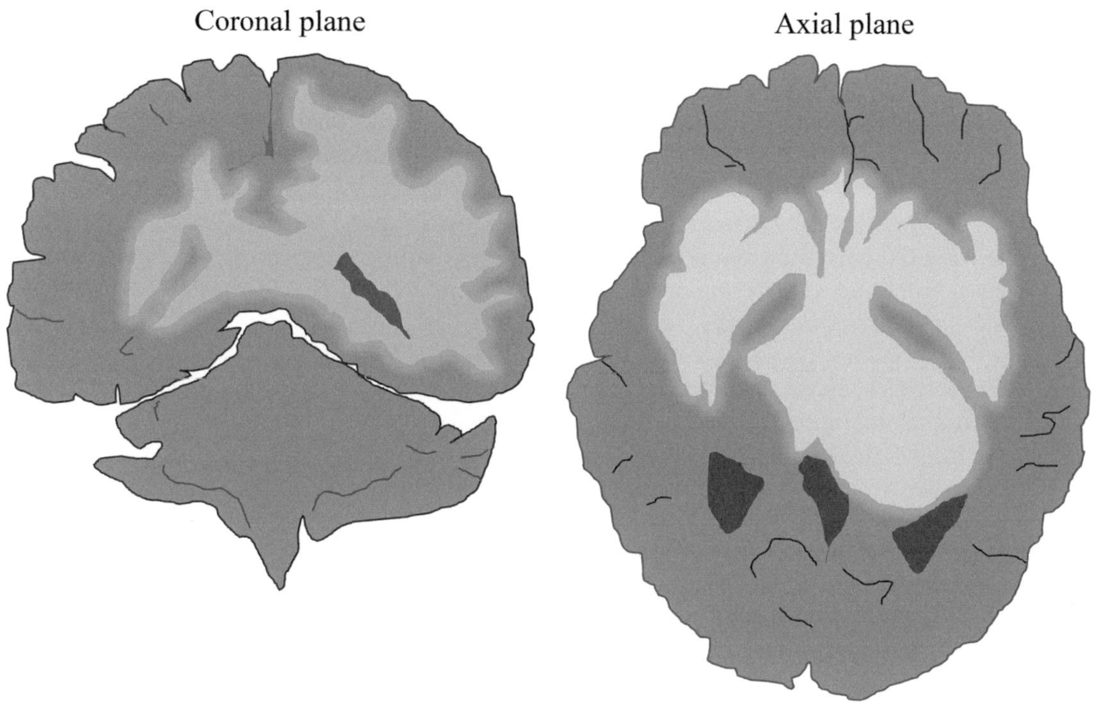

Fig. 16.2 Schematic representation of the typical radiological appearance of *Gliomatosis Cerebri* in sagittal and coronal planes

diffuse gliomas. It was reclassified as a "gliomatosis cerebri pattern of invasion" [102]. Finally, in the fifth edition (2021), the classification included even more molecular data compared to previous editions, and GC was only briefly described as a spreading pattern of diffuse glioma [103]. Thus, GC transitioned from being a recognized entity (2007) to being excluded from CNS tumor classifications (2016 onward).

The origin of GC is still debated, though it is mainly reported as a tumor of astrocytic origin but can present also oligodendroglioma features.

Unlike other gliomas, GC involves at least three cerebral lobes, with frequent infiltration into the deep gray matter, brainstem, and spinal cord (Fig. 16.2). This diffuse nature complicates early detection and treatment, resulting in a poor prognosis. We do not know the precise incidence of GC since several cases, especially in the United States, have been diagnosed at autopsy [104]. GC affects individuals across all age groups but is more commonly diagnosed in adult patients [105]. In the pediatric age, affects children and adolescents with a median age of 11.8 years and a gender predominance for male to female as 2:1 [3]. The etiology of GC remains poorly understood, with no clear links to environmental or genetic risk factors.

Patients with GC typically present varied *symptoms* depending on the regions of the brain affected. Common symptoms include focal neurological deficits, headaches, sensory loss, or manifestations of increased intracranial pressure, and behavioral and personality changes, with seizures reported as most frequent in the pediatric age [3, 104]. These symptoms often lead to misdiagnosis or delayed recognition, further complicating patient outcomes. Moreover, various conditions can mimic GC's clinical and radiological features, leading to misdiagnosis and inappropriate treatments. Among these, it is worth mentioning viral encephalitis and acute disseminated encephalomyelitis (ADEM), multiple sclerosis, leukodystrophies, and vasculitis [104]. The diagnosis of GC relies on a combination of clinical, radiological, and histopathological findings.

On MRI, T2-weighted and FLAIR sequences typically show diffuse hyperintensity across multiple brain regions with minimal mass effect or contrast enhancement. Lesions are typically non-enhancing, but small enhancing areas may occur. Two patterns of GC have been described: *type 1*, with diffuse neoplastic growth without a solid tumor, and *type 2*, showing a mass component alongside diffuse infiltration. Compared to multifocal gliomas, GC is uniquely characterized by continuous tumor infiltration and lack of clear boundaries from normal brain tissue [104].

Histologically, the main characteristic of these tumors is a diffuse pattern of neoplastic glial cells that infiltrate brain tissue without forming a distinct mass. Despite the high infiltration in the white matter, GC cells preserve the axonal structures, but it is often associated with myelin damage. The mitotic index varies, with no evidence of vascular proliferation or necrosis. GFAP expression suggests an astrocytic origin, though it may be minimal or absent. These tumors typically correspond to WHO grade III astrocytoma but can also be grade II or IV. Oligodendroglial gliomatosis may occur, showing a uniform population of rounded cells with perinuclear clearing in biopsies [104, 106, 107].

Since the majority of the available molecular data come from adults or small pediatric series, the biology of GC in children has not been well elucidated yet. A recently published large multinational retrospective study on 104 children and adolescents with GC sheds light on this tumor type. Nussbaumer and colleagues conducted a comprehensive analysis of pediatric GC revealing that it is associated with a particularly poor prognosis and exhibits a unique molecular profile and specific genetic alterations distinct from other diffuse gliomas as well as from adult GC [3]. In particular, the study shows that GC has a worse prognosis compared to hemispheric pediatric high-grade gliomas (pedHGG), that low-grade GC does not clinically behave like pediatric low-grade gliomas (pedLGG), and that WHO grading remains a key prognostic marker. Interestingly, pediatric GC is primarily associated with pedHGG_RTK2A/B and pedHGG_A/B methylation classes and the presence of high frequencies of EGFR mutations, BCOR alterations, and structural aberrations in chromosome 6. Moreover, differently from other hemispheric pedHGG, pediatric GC show a low frequency of common alterations such as CDKN2A/B deletion, ATRX mutation/deletion, or PDGFRA activating mutation/amplification [3]. The management of GC is challenging due to its diffuse infiltration and resistance to conventional therapies. Almost 76% of the patients received upfront irradiation while TMZ-containing regimens were the most frequently used. Target-therapies (anti-EGFR or anti-VEGF) were mostly used in combination with other agents. Reirradiation was an option at relapse [3].

There is a continuous debate on GC and the need for more in-depth studies that would allow a reevaluation of GC as a distinct tumor entity (ref). For this, neuro-oncologists and scientists have established the "International Gliomatosis Cerebri Working Group," initially established by NIH, that already held four conferences (Paris, 2015; Bethesda, 2017; Barcelona, 2019, New York 2022). Major initiatives include creating an international GC tissue registry, investigating immunotherapeutics, and advancing GC-specific clinical and preclinical research focusing on tumor invasiveness, biomarkers, single-cell analysis, and imaging techniques. The Dana-Farber Cancer Institute has established an international GC platform supporting collaborative research on pediatric GC (ref).

Despite its exclusion from the WHO classification, continued efforts are essential to improve treatment and understanding of this disease.

References

1. Louis DN, et al. The 2016 World Health Organization classification of tumors of the central nervous system: a summary. Acta Neuropathol. 2016;131(6):803–20. https://doi.org/10.1007/s00401-016-1545-1. Epub 2016 May 9. PMID: 27157931.
2. Louis DN, et al. The 2021 WHO classification of tumors of the central nervous system: a summary. Neuro-Oncology. 2021;23(8):1231–51. https://doi.org/10.1093/neuonc/noab106. PMID: 34185076; PMCID: PMC8328013.
3. Nussbaumer G, et al. Gliomatosis cerebri in children: a poor prognostic phenotype of diffuse gliomas with a distinct molecular profile. Neuro-Oncology. 2024;26(9):1723–37. https://doi.org/10.1093/neuonc/noae080.
4. Castel D, et al. Histone H3 wild-type DIPG/DMG overexpressing EZHIP extend the spectrum diffuse midline gliomas with PRC2 inhibition beyond H3-K27M mutation. Acta Neuropathol. 2020;139:1109–13.https://doi.org/10.1007/S00401--020-02142-W. Epub 2020 Mar 19. PMID: 32193787.
5. Castel D, et al. Histone H3F3A and HIST1H3B K27M mutations define two subgroups of diffuse intrinsic pontine gliomas with different prognosis and phenotypes. Acta Neuropathol. 2015;130(6):815–27. https://doi.org/10.1007/s00401-015-1478-0. Epub 2015 Sep 23. PMID: 26399631; PMCID: PMC4654747.
6. Mackay A, et al. Integrated molecular meta-analysis of 1,000 pediatric high-grade and diffuse intrinsic pontine glioma. Cancer Cell. 2017;32(4):520–537.e5. https://doi.org/10.1016/j.ccell.2017.08.017. Epub 2017 Sep 28. PMID: 28966033; PMCID: PMC5637314.
7. Korshunov A, et al. Histologically distinct neuroepithelial tumors with histone 3 G34 mutation are molecularly similar and comprise a single nosologic entity. Acta Neuropathol. 2016;131(1):137–46. https://doi.org/10.1007/s00401-015-1493-1. PMID: 26482474.
8. Gianno F, et al. Paediatric-type diffuse high-grade gliomas in the 5th CNS WHO classification. Pathologica. 2022;114:422–35. https://doi.org/10.32074/1591-951X-830.
9. Blasco-Santana L, Colmenero I. Molecular and pathological features of paediatric high-grade gliomas. Int J Mol Sci. 2024;25:8498. https://doi.org/10.3390/ijms25158498.
10. Clarke M, et al. Infant high-grade gliomas comprise multiple subgroups characterized by novel targetable gene fusions and favorable outcomes. Cancer Discov. 2020;10(7):942–63. https://doi.org/10.1158/2159-8290.CD-19-1030. Epub 2020 Apr 1. PMID: 32238360; PMCID: PMC8313225.
11. Chavaz L, Bagchi A, Dhanda SK, Toutain F, Pfister SM, Sturm D, Pietsch T, Gielen GH, Waha A, Clarke M, Lu C, Karremann M, Benesch M, Perwein T, Nussbaumer G, Kramm C, Massimino M, Biassoni V, Vinci M, Mastronuzzi A, van Vuurden D, Sophie EM, van Zanten V, Mackay A, Jones DTW, Ana S, Stucklin G, Tabori U, Hawkins C, Ryall S, La Madrid AM, Lassaletta A, Bailey S, Hargrave D, Chiang J, El-Ayadi M, Mançano BM, Reis RM, Hagel C, Gorsi H, Silvestrini N, Gilani A, Papusha L, Klimo Jr P, Zhou X, Gajjar A, Robinson GW, von Bueren AO. A systematic study of molecular diagnosis, treatment, and prognosis in infant-type hemispheric glioma: An individual patient data meta-analysis of 164 patients, Neuro-Oncology. 2025;264. https://doi.org/10.1093/neuonc/noaf264.
12. Manjunath N, et al. Clinico-pathological and molecular characterization of diffuse midline gliomas: is there a prognostic significance? Neurol Sci. 2021;42:925–34. https://doi.org/10.1007/s10072-020-04489-0.
13. Wang Y, et al. Clinical features and molecular markers on diffuse midline gliomas with H3K27M mutations: a 43 cases retrospective cohort study. Front Oncol. 2021;10:602553. https://doi.org/10.3389/fonc.2020.602553. PMID: 33659209; PMCID: PMC7917281.
14. Crowell C, et al. Systematic review of diffuse hemispheric glioma, H3 G34-mutant: outcomes and associated clinical factors. Neuro-Oncol Adv. 2022;4(1):vdac133. https://doi.org/10.1093/noajnl/vdac133.
15. Lavrador JP, et al. H3 G34-mutant high-grade gliomas: integrated clinical, imaging and pathological characterisation of a single-centre case series. Acta Neurochir. 2023;165:1615–33. https://doi.org/10.1007/s00701-023-05545-2.
16. Nguyen AV, Soto JM, Gonzalez SM, Murillo J, Trumble ER, Shan FY, Huang JH. H3G34-Mutant Gliomas-A Review of Molecular Pathogenesis and Therapeutic Options. Biomedicines. 2023 15;11(7):2002. https://doi.org/10.3390/biomedicines11072002. PMID: 37509641; PMCID: PMC10377039..
17. Ceglie G, et al. Infantile/congenital high-grade gliomas: molecular features and therapeutic perspectives. Diagnostics (Basel). 2020;10(9):648. https://doi.org/10.3390/diagnostics10090648. PMID: 32872331; PMCID: PMC7555400.
18. Colafati GS, et al. Direct involvement of cranial nerve V at diagnosis in patients with diffuse intrinsic pontine glioma: a potential magnetic resonance predictor of short-term survival. Front Oncol. 2019;9:204. https://doi.org/10.3389/fonc.2019.00204. PMID: 31019890; PMCID: PMC6458256.
19. Lacruz CR, et al. Pediatric-type diffuse gliomas. In: Lacruz CR, editor. Central nervous system tumors. Cham: Springer; 2023. https://doi.org/10.1007/978-3-031-51078-6_4.
20. Fischbein NJ, et al. Radiologic classification of brain stem tumors: correlation of magnetic resonance imaging appearance with clinical outcome.

Pediatr Neurosurg. 1996;24(1):9–23. https://doi.org/10.1159/000121010. PMID: 8817611.
21. Kurokawa R, et al. Neuroimaging features of diffuse hemispheric glioma, H3 G34-mutant: a case series and systematic review. J Neuroimaging. 2022;32(1):17–27. https://doi.org/10.1111/join.12939.
22. Tauziède-Espariat A, et al. Diffuse pediatric high-grade glioma of methylation-based RTK2A and RTK2B subclasses present distinct radiological and histomolecular features including Gliomatosis cerebri phenotype. Acta Neuropathol Commun. 2024;12(1):176. https://doi.org/10.1186/s40478-024-01881-1. PMID: 39558399; PMCID: PMC11575044.
23. Izquierdo E, et al. Droplet digital PCR-based detection of circulating tumor DNA from pediatric high grade and diffuse midline glioma patients. Neuro-Oncol Adv. 2021;3(1):vdab013. https://doi.org/10.1093/noajnl/vdab013.
24. Cantor E, et al. Serial H3K27M cell-free tumor DNA (cf-tDNA) tracking predicts ONC201 treatment response and progression in diffuse midline glioma. Neuro Oncol. 2022;24(8):1366–74. https://doi.org/10.1093/neuonc/noac030. PMID: 35137228; PMCID: PMC9340643.
25. Buzova D, et al. Extracellular histones profiles of pediatric H3K27-altered diffuse midline glioma. Mol Diagn Ther. 2024;29(1):129–41. https://doi.org/10.1007/s40291-024-00754-6.
26. Wu G, et al. Somatic histone H3 alterations in pediatric diffuse intrinsic pontine gliomas and non-brainstem glioblastomas. Nat Genet. 2012;44:251–3. https://doi.org/10.1038/ng.1102.
27. Schwartzentruber J, et al. Driver mutations in histone H3.3 and chromatin remodelling genes in paediatric glioblastoma. Nature. 2012;482:226–31. https://doi.org/10.1038/nature10833.
28. Bender S, et al. Reduced H3K27me3 and DNA hypomethylation are major drivers of gene expression in K27M mutant pediatric high-grade gliomas. Cancer Cell. 2013;24(5):660–72. https://doi.org/10.1016/j.ccr.2013.10.006. Epub 2013 Oct 31. PMID: 24183680.
29. Sievers P, et al. A subset of pediatric-type thalamic gliomas share a distinct DNA methylation profile, H3K27me3 loss and frequent alteration of *EGFR*. Neuro-Oncology. 2021;23(1):34–43. https://doi.org/10.1093/neuonc/noaa251.
30. Auffret L, et al. A new subtype of diffuse midline glioma, H3 K27 and BRAF/FGFR1 co-altered: a clinico-radiological and histomolecular characterisation. Acta Neuropathol. 2023;147(1):2. https://doi.org/10.1007/s00401-023-02651-4. PMID: 38066305; PMCID: PMC10709479.
31. Jain SU, Khazaei S, Marchione DM, et al. Histone H3.3 G34 mutations promote aberrant PRC2 activity and drive tumor progression. Proc Natl Acad Sci USA. 2020;117:27354–64. https://doi.org/10.1073/PNAS.2006076117/.
32. Haase S, et al. H3.3-G34 mutations impair DNA repair and promote cGAS/STING-mediated immune responses in pediatric high-grade glioma models. J Clin Invest. 2022;132(22):e154229. https://doi.org/10.1172/JCI154229. PMID: 36125896; PMCID: PMC9663161.
33. Lim KY, et al. H3 G34-mutant high-grade glioma. Brain Tumor Pathol. 2021;38:4–13. https://doi.org/10.1007/s10014-020-00378-8.
34. Korshunov A, et al. H3-/IDH-wild type pediatric glioblastoma is comprised of molecularly and prognostically distinct subtypes with associated oncogenic drivers. Acta Neuropathol. 2017;134:507–16. https://doi.org/10.1007/s00401-017-1710-1.
35. Das S, et al. Pediatric high grade gliomas: a comprehensive histopathological, immunohistochemical and molecular integrated approach in routine practice. Pathol Res Pract. 2024;258:155347. https://doi.org/10.1016/j.prp.2024.155347. ISSN 0344-0338.
36. Tauziède-Espariat A, et al. Refinement of diagnostic criteria for pediatric-type diffuse high-grade glioma, *IDH*- and H3-wildtype, *MYCN*-subtype including histopathology, *TP53*, *MYCN* and *ID2* status. Acta Neuropathol Commun. 2023;11:170. https://doi.org/10.1186/s40478-023-01667-x.
37. Guerreiro Stucklin AS, et al. Alterations in ALK/ROS1/NTRK/MET drive a group of infantile hemispheric gliomas. Nat Commun. 2019;10(1):4343. https://doi.org/10.1038/s41467-019-12187-5. PMID: 31554817; PMCID: PMC6761184.
38. Woo HY, Na K, Yoo J, et al. Glioblastomas harboring gene fusions detected by next-generation sequencing. Brain Tumor Pathol. 2020;37(4):136–44. https://doi.org/10.1007/S10014-020-00377-9.
39. Vinci M, et al. Functional diversity and cooperativity between subclonal populations of pediatric glioblastoma and diffuse intrinsic pontine glioma cells. Nat Med. 2018;24(8):1204–15. https://doi.org/10.1038/s41591-018-0086-7. Epub 2018 Jul 2. PMID: 29967352; PMCID: PMC6086334.
40. Hoffman LM, et al. Spatial genomic heterogeneity in diffuse intrinsic pontine and midline high-grade glioma: implications for diagnostic biopsy and targeted therapeutics. Acta Neuropathol Commun. 2016;4:1. https://doi.org/10.1186/s40478-015-0269-0.
41. Haque F, Varlet P, Puntonet J, Storer L, Bountali A, Rahman R, Grill J, Carcaboso AM, Jones C, Layfield R, Grundy RG. Evaluation of a novel antibody to define histone 3.3 G34R mutant brain tumours. Acta Neuropathol Commun. 2017;5(1):45. https://doi.org/10.1186/s40478-017-0449-1. PMID: 28587626; PMCID: PMC5461722.
42. Yamamoto H, Iwasaki T, Yamada Y, Matsumoto Y, Otsuka H, Yoshimoto M, Kohashi K, Taguchi K, Yokoyama R, Nakashima Y, Oda Y. Diagnostic utility of histone H3.3 G34W, G34R, and G34V mutant-specific antibodies for giant cell tumors of bone. Hum Pathol. 2018;73:41–50. https://doi.org/10.1016/j.humpath.2017.11.020. Epub 2017 Dec 12. PMID: 29241742

43. Gianno F, et al. Correlation between immunohistochemistry and sequencing in H3G34-mutant gliomas. Am J Surg Pathol. 2021;45(2):200–4. https://doi.org/10.1097/PAS.0000000000001571. PMID: 33428336.
44. Szychit E, et al. European standard clinical practice recommendations for paediatric high-grade gliomas. EJC Paediatr Oncol. 2024;5:100210. https://doi.org/10.1016/j.ejcped.2024.100210.
45. Janssens GO, et al. Survival benefit for patients with diffuse intrinsic pontine glioma (DIPG) undergoing re-irradiation at first progression: a matched-cohort analysis on behalf of the SIOP-E-HGG/DIPG working group. Eur J Cancer. 2017;73:38–47. https://doi.org/10.1016/j.ejca.2016.12.007. Epub 2017 Feb 3. PMID: 28161497.
46. Carai A, et al. Robot-assisted stereotactic biopsy of diffuse intrinsic pontine glioma: a single-center experience. World Neurosurg. 2017;101:584–8. https://doi.org/10.1016/j.wneu.2017.02.088. Epub 2017 Feb 27. PMID: 28254596.
47. Del Baldo G, et al. Targeted therapy for pediatric diffuse intrinsic pontine glioma: a single-center experience. Ther Adv Med Oncol. 2022;14:17588359221113693. https://doi.org/10.1177/17588359221113693. PMID: 36090803; PMCID: PMC9459464.
48. von Bueren AO, et al. HGG-16. Final analysis of the HIT-HGG-2007 trial (ISRCTN19852453): significant survival benefit for pontine and non-pontine pediatric high-grade gliomas in comparison to previous HIT-GBM-C/-D trials. Neuro-oncol. 2022;24(Suppl 1):i63–4. https://doi.org/10.1093/neuonc/noac079.231. PMCID: PMC9164809.
49. Venneti S, et al. Clinical efficacy of ONC201 in H3K27M-mutant diffuse midline gliomas is driven by disruption of integrated metabolic and epigenetic pathways. Cancer Discov. 2023;13(11):2370–93. https://doi.org/10.1158/2159-8290.CD-23-0131. PMID: 37584601; PMCID: PMC10618742.
50. Di Carlo D, et al. Real life data of ONC201 (dordaviprone) in pediatric and adult H3K27-altered recurrent diffuse midline glioma: results of an international academia-driven compassionate use program. Eur J Cancer. 2024;216:115165. https://doi.org/10.1016/j.ejca.2024.115165. Epub ahead of print. PMID: 39700833.
51. Hansford JR, et al. Update on cancer predisposition syndromes and surveillance guidelines for childhood brain tumors. Clin Cancer Res. 2024;30(11):2342–50. https://doi.org/10.1158/1078-0432.CCR-23-4033. PMID: 38573059; PMCID: PMC11147702.
52. de la Nava D, et al. The oncolytic adenovirus Delta-24-RGD in combination with ONC201 induces a potent antitumor response in pediatric high-grade and diffuse midline glioma models. Neuro-Oncol. 2024;26(8):1509–25. https://doi.org/10.1093/neuonc/noae066. PMID: 38554031; PMCID: PMC11300018.
53. Jackson ER, et al. ONC201 in combination with paxalisib for the treatment of H3K27-altered diffuse midline glioma. Cancer Res. 2023;83(14):2421–37. https://doi.org/10.1158/0008-5472.CAN-23-0186. Epub ahead of print. PMID: 37145169; PMCID: PMC10345962.
54. Majzner RG, et al. GD2-CAR T cell therapy for H3K27M-mutated diffuse midline gliomas. Nature. 2022;603:934–41. https://doi.org/10.1038/s41586-022-04489-4.
55. Monje M, et al. Intravenous and intracranial GD2-CAR T cells for H3K27M+ diffuse midline gliomas. Nature. 2024;637(8046):708–15. https://doi.org/10.1038/s41586-024-08171-9.
56. Vitanza NA, et al. Intraventricular B7-H3 CAR T cells for diffuse intrinsic pontine glioma: preliminary first-in-human bioactivity and safety. Cancer Discov. 2023;13(1):114–31. https://doi.org/10.1158/2159-8290.CD-22-0750. PMID: 36259971; PMCID: PMC9827115.
57. Mahdi J, et al. Tumor inflammation-associated neurotoxicity. Nat Med. 2023;29(4):803–10. https://doi.org/10.1038/s41591-023-02276-w. Epub 2023 Apr 6. PMID: 37024595; PMCID: PMC10166099.
58. Zarychta J, et al. Strategies to overcome tumor microenvironment immunosuppressive effect on the functioning of CAR-T cells in high-grade glioma. Ther Adv Med Oncol. 2024;16:17588359241266140. https://doi.org/10.1177/17588359241266140.
59. Rankin AW, Duncan BB, Allen C, et al. Evolving strategies for addressing CAR T-cell toxicities. Cancer Metastasis Rev. 2024;44:17. https://doi.org/10.1007/s10555-024-10227-1.
60. Gállego Pérez-Larraya J, et al. Oncolytic DNX-2401 virus for pediatric diffuse intrinsic pontine glioma. N Engl J Med. 2022;386(26):2471–81. https://doi.org/10.1056/NEJMoa2202028. PMID: 35767439.
61. Singleton WGB, et al. The distribution, clearance, and brainstem toxicity of panobinostat administered by convection-enhanced delivery. J Neurosurg Pediatr. 2018;22(3):288–96. https://doi.org/10.3171/2018.2.PEDS17663.
62. Haumann R, et al. Imaged-guided focused ultrasound in combination with various formulations of doxorubicin for the treatment of diffuse intrinsic pontine glioma. Transl Med Commun. 2022;7:8. https://doi.org/10.1186/s41231-022-00115-7.
63. 't Hart E, et al. Radiosensitisation by olaparib through focused ultrasound delivery in a diffuse midline glioma model. J Control Release. 2023;357:287–98. https://doi.org/10.1016/j.jconrel.2023.03.058. Epub 2023 Apr 5. PMID: 37019285.
64. Venkatesh HS, et al. Neuronal activity promotes glioma growth through neuroligin-3 secretion. Cell. 2015;161(4):803–16. https://doi.org/10.1016/j.cell.2015.04.012. Epub 2015 Apr 23. PMID: 25913192; PMCID: PMC4447122.
65. Venkatesh HS, et al. Electrical and synaptic integration of glioma into neural circuits. Nature. 2019;573:539–45. https://doi.org/10.1038/s41586-019-1563-y.

66. Taylor KR, et al. Glioma synapses recruit mechanisms of adaptive plasticity. Nature. 2023;623:366–74. https://doi.org/10.1038/s41586-023-06678-1.
67. Bilotta MT, et al. Managing the TME to improve the efficacy of cancer therapy. Front Immunol. 2022;13:954992. https://doi.org/10.3389/fimmu.2022.954992. PMID: 36341428; PMCID: PMC9630343.
68. Messiaen J, et al. The tumor micro-environment in pediatric glioma: friend or foe? Front Immunol. 2023;14:1227126. https://doi.org/10.3389/fimmu.2023.1227126. PMID: 37901250; PMCID: PMC10611473.
69. Chen CCL, et al. Histone H3.3G34-mutant interneuron progenitors co-opt PDGFRA for gliomagenesis. Cell. 2020;183(6):1617–33. https://doi.org/10.1016/j.cell.2020.11.012.
70. Liu I, et al. GABAergic neuronal lineage development determines clinically actionable targets in diffuse hemispheric glioma, H3G34-mutant. Cancer Cell. 2024;42(9):1528–48. https://doi.org/10.1016/j.ccell.2024.08.006.
71. Sposto R, et al. The effectiveness of chemotherapy for treatment of high-grade astrocytoma in children: results of a randomized trial. A report from the Childrens cancer study group. J Neuro-Oncol. 1989;7(2):165–77. https://doi.org/10.1007/BF00165101. PMID: 2550594.
72. Finlay JL, Boyett JM, Yates AJ, Wisoff JH, Milstein JM, Geyer JR, Bertolone SJ, McGuire P, Cherlow JM, Tefft M, et al. Randomized phase III trial in childhood high-grade astrocytoma comparing vincristine, lomustine, and prednisone with the eight-drugs-in-1-day regimen. Childrens Cancer Group. J Clin Oncol. 1995;13(1):112–23. https://doi.org/10.1200/JCO.1995.13.1.112. PMID: 7799011.
73. Fouladi M, Hunt DL, Pollack IF, Dueckers G, Burger PC, Becker LE, Yates AJ, Gilles FH, Davis RL, Boyett JM, Finlay JL. Outcome of children with centrally reviewed low-grade gliomas treated with chemotherapy with or without RT on Children's Cancer Group high-grade glioma study CCG-945. Cancer. 2003;98(6):1243–52. https://doi.org/10.1002/cncr.11637. PMID: 12973849.
74. Stupp R, et al. RT plus concomitant and adjuvant TMZ for glioblastoma. N Engl J Med. 2005;352(10):987–96.
75. Stupp R, et al. Effects of RT with concomitant and adjuvant TMZ versus RT alone on survival in glioblastoma in a randomised phase III study: 5-year analysis of the EORTC-NCIC trial. Lancet Oncol. 2009;10(5):459–66.
76. Jakacki RI, et al. Phase 2 study of concurrent RT and TMZ followed by TMZ and lomustine in the treatment of children with high-grade glioma: a report of the Children's Oncology Group ACNS0423 study. Neuro-Oncology. 2016;18(10):1442–50. https://doi.org/10.1093/neuonc/now038. Epub 2016 Mar 22. PMID: 27006176; PMCID: PMC5035517.
77. Grill J, et al. Phase II, open-label, randomized, multicenter trial (HERBY) of bevacizumab in pediatric patients with newly diagnosed high-grade glioma. J Clin Oncol. 2018;36(10):951–8. https://doi.org/10.1200/JCO.2017.76.0611. Epub 2018 Feb 7. PMID: 29412784.
78. Geyer JR, et al. Survival of infants with malignant astrocytomas. A report of the Children's Cancer Group. Cancer. 1995;75:1045–50.
79. Duffner PK, et al. The treatment of malignant brain tumors in infants and very young children: an update of the Pediatric Oncology Group experience. Neuro-Oncology. 1999;1(2):152–61. https://doi.org/10.1093/neuonc/1.2.152. PMID: 11554387; PMCID: PMC1920752.
80. Dufour C, et al. High-grade glioma in children under 5 years of age: a chemotherapy only approach with the BBSFOP protocol. Eur J Cancer. 2006;42(17):2939–45. https://doi.org/10.1016/j.ejca.2006.06.021. Epub 2006 Sep 7. PMID: 16962317.
81. Kuehl J, et al. Delayed radiation therapy after postoperative chemotherapy in children less than 3 years of age with medulloblastoma: results of the trial HIT-SKK'87 and preliminary results of the pilot trial HIT-SKK'92. Med Pediatr Oncol. 1995;25(Suppl):250. abstract.
82. Grundy RG, et al. Primary postoperative chemotherapy without RT for treatment of brain tumours other than ependymoma in children under 3 years: results of the first UKCCSG/SIOP CNS 9204 trial. Eur J Cancer. 2010;46(1):120–33. https://doi.org/10.1016/j.ejca.2009.09.013. PMID: 19818598.
83. Riedmeier M, et al. Spontaneous regression of a congenital high-grade glioma-a case report. Neuro-Oncol Adv. 2021;3(1):vdab120. https://doi.org/10.1093/noajnl/vdab120. PMID: 34704035; PMCID: PMC8541705.
84. Hargrave DR, et al. Dabrafenib in pediatric patients with BRAF V600–positive high-grade glioma (HGG). J Clin Oncol. 2018;36:10505. https://doi.org/10.1200/JCO.2018.36.15_suppl.10505.
85. Kieran MW, et al. A phase I and pharmacokinetic study of oral dabrafenib in children and adolescent patients with recurrent or refractory BRAF V600 mutation-positive solid tumors. Clin Cancer Res. 2019;25(24):7294–302. https://doi.org/10.1158/1078-0432.CCR-17-3572. Epub 2019 Sep 10. PMID: 31506385.
86. Hargrave DR, et al. Phase II trial of dabrafenib plus trametinib in relapsed/refractory BRAF V600–mutant pediatric high-grade glioma. J Clin Oncol. 2023;41:5174–83. https://doi.org/10.1200/JCO23.00558.
87. Kline C, et al. Survival outcomes in pediatric recurrent high-grade glioma: results of a 20-year systematic review and meta-analysis. J Neurooncol. 2018;137(1):103–10. https://doi.org/10.1007/

s11060-017-2701-8. Epub 2017 Dec 4. PMID: 29204840; PMCID: PMC5823744.
88. Müller K, et al. Reirradiation as part of a salvage treatment approach for progressive nonpontine pediatric high-grade gliomas: preliminary experiences from the German HIT-HGG study group. Radiat Oncol. 2014;9:177. https://doi.org/10.1186/1748-717X-9-177.
89. Lucas JT Jr, Cooper DA, Hwang S, Tinkle C, Li X, Li Y, Orr B, Merchant TE, Broniscer A. Prognostic relevance of treatment failure patterns in pediatric high-grade glioma: is there a role for a revised failure classification system? Int J Radiat Oncol Biol Phys. 2017;99:450–8. https://doi.org/10.1016/j.ijrobp.2017.04.039.
90. Tsang DS, et al. Repeat irradiation for children with supratentorial high-grade glioma. Pediatr Blood Cancer. 2019;66(9):e27881. https://doi.org/10.1002/pbc.27881. Epub 2019 Jun 17. PMID: 31207154.
91. Massimino M, et al. How ten-years of reirradiation for paediatric high-grade glioma may shed light on first line treatment. J Neuro-Oncol. 2022;159(2):437–45. https://doi.org/10.1007/s11060-022-04079-4. Epub 2022 Jul 9. PMID: 35809148.
92. Mai PL, Best AF, Peters JA, et al. Risks of first and subsequent cancers among TP53 mutation carriers in the National Cancer Institute Li-Fraumeni syndrome cohort. Cancer. 2016;122(23):3673–81. [PubMed: 27496084].
93. Perrino MR, et al. Update on pediatric cancer surveillance recommendations for patients with neurofibromatosis type 1, Noonan syndrome, CBL syndrome, Costello syndrome, and related RASopathies. Clin Cancer Res. 2024;30(21):4834–43. https://doi.org/10.1158/1078-0432.CCR-24-1611. PMID: 39196581; PMCID: PMC11530332.
94. Touat M, et al. Mechanisms and therapeutic implications of hypermutation in gliomas. Nature. 2020;580(7804):517–23. https://doi.org/10.1038/s41586-020-2209-9. Epub 2020 Apr 15. PMID: 32322066; PMCID: PMC8235024.
95. Larkin T, et al. Upfront adjuvant immunotherapy of replication repair-deficient pediatric glioblastoma with chemoradiation-sparing approach. JCO Precis Oncol. 2021;5:1426–31. https://doi.org/10.1200/PO.21.00153. PMID: 34994637.
96. Tabori U, et al. Clinical management and tumor surveillance recommendations of inherited mismatch repair deficiency in childhood. Clin Cancer Res. 2017;23(11):e32–7. https://doi.org/10.1158/1078-0432.CCR-17-0574. PMID: 28572265.
97. Nevin S. Gliomatosis cerebri. Brain. 1938;61(2):170–91. https://doi.org/10.1093/brain/61.2.170.
98. Zülch KJ. Histological typing of tumours of the central nervous system. Geneva: World Health Organization; 1979.
99. Kleihues P, et al. Histological typing of tumours of the central nervous system. World Health Organization international histological classification of tumours. Heidelberg: Springer; 1993.
100. Kleihues P, Cavenee WK, Health Organization Classification of Tumours. Pathology and genetics of tumours of the nervous system. Lyon: IARC Press; 2000.
101. Louis DN, Ohgaki H, Wiestler OD, Cavenee WK, editors. WHO classification of tumours of the central nervous system, vol. 1. 4th ed. Lyon: International Agency for Research on Cancer; 2007.
102. Herrlinger U, et al. Gliomatosis cerebri: no evidence for a separate brain tumor entity. Acta Neuropathol. 2016;131(2):309–19. https://doi.org/10.1007/s00401-015-1495-z. Epub 2015 Oct 22.
103. WHO Classification of Tumours Editorial Board. WHO classification of Tumours. 5th ed. Lyon: IARC; 2021.
104. Greenfield JP, et al. Gliomatosis cerebri: a consensus summary report from the First International Gliomatosis cerebri Group Meeting, March 26–27, 2015, Paris, France. Pediatr Blood Cancer. 2016;63(12):2072–7. https://doi.org/10.1002/pbc.26169. Epub 2016 Jul 28. PMID: 27466787.
105. Broniscer A, et al. Gliomatosis cerebri in children shares molecular characteristics with other pediatric gliomas. Acta Neuropathol. 2016;131(2):299–307. https://doi.org/10.1007/s00401-015-1532-y. Epub 2016 Jan 7. PMID: 26744350; PMCID: PMC4886851.
106. Pal L, et al. Gliomatosis cerebri: an uncommon neuroepithelial tumor in children with oligodendroglial phenotype. Pediatr Neurosurg. 2008;44:212–5. https://doi.org/10.1159/000120153.
107. Chen S, et al. Gliomatosis cerebri: clinical characteristics, management, and outcomes. J Neurooncol. 2013;112(2):267–75. https://doi.org/10.1007/s11060-013-1058-x. Epub 2013 Jan 23. PMID: 23341100; PMCID: PMC3907195.

17 Central Nervous System Germ Cell Tumors

Giacomina Megaro, Giada Del Baldo, Rossana Pavone, Assunta Tornesello, Andrea Carai, and Angela Mastronuzzi

17.1 Introduction

Intracranial germ cell tumors (iGCTs) are heterogeneous rare tumors of childhood and adolescence. They represent a subset of brain tumors classified based on histological and immunohistochemical characteristics and are further supported by the detection of tumor-secreted biomarkers in serum and/or cerebrospinal fluid (CSF) [1].

The prognosis of iGCTs depends on histological subtype. They are broadly divided into germinomas and non-germinomatous germ cell tumors (NGGCTs) [2, 3].

Standard treatment includes surgery, chemotherapy, and radiotherapy.

Germinomas are the most common subtype of iGCTs and are highly sensitive to both chemotherapy and radiotherapy, resulting in a more favorable prognosis compared with NGGCTs [4].

Overall, intracranial germ cell tumors have an excellent long-term outcome, with a 10-year overall survival rate exceeding 90% [5].

17.2 Epidemiology

iGCTs are rare tumors, accounting for approximately 2–3% of pediatric brain tumors [1].

Germinomas represent about two-thirds of iGCTs, with an incidence of 60–77% [6, 7].

Between 80% and 90% of iGCTs arise in patients younger than 25 years, with a peak incidence between 10 and 14 years of age. Teratomas tend to be diagnosed earlier in life, especially during infancy [8, 9].

There is a clear geographic variation in the incidence of iGCTs: they are more prevalent in East Asia compared to the USA. In the USA, they account for 2–3% of all primary intracranial neoplasms, whereas in Japan, China, and South Korea, they represent 8–15%. The reasons for this disparity remain unclear [10–13].

Germ cell tumors develop more frequently in males than in females with a 2:1 ratio, but this male predominance is observed only in tumors

G. Megaro · G. Del Baldo
Area of Hematology-Oncology, Cell Therapy, Gene Therapies, and Hematopoietic Transplantation, Bambino Gesù Children's Hospital, IRCCS, Rome, Italy

A. Mastronuzzi (✉)
Area of Hematology-Oncology, Cell Therapy, Gene Therapies, and Hematopoietic Transplantation, Bambino Gesù Children's Hospital, IRCCS, Rome, Italy

Department of Life Sciences and Public Health, Università Cattolica del Sacro Cuore, Rome, Italy
e-mail: angela.mastronuzzi@opbg.net

R. Pavone · A. Tornesello
Pediatric Hematology-Oncology Unit, Ospedale Vito Fazzi, Lecce, Italy

A. Carai
Neurosurgery Unit, Bambino Gesù Children's Hospital, IRCCS, Rome, Italy

A. Mastronuzzi, A. Carai (eds.), *Navigating Pediatric Brain Tumors*,
https://doi.org/10.1007/978-3-032-18992-9_17

arising in the pineal region. This is more evident in Japanese tumor registries. By contrast, females have a higher risk of developing suprasellar germinomas and choriocarcinoma [14].

17.3 Classification and Histopathology

According to the WHO classification, iGCTs include different types from mature teratomas to highly aggressive NGGCTs [15].

2021 WHO classification of intracranial germ cell tumors (iGCTs)
Mature teratoma
Immature teratoma
Teratoma with somatic-type malignancy
Germinoma
Embryonal carcinoma
Yolk sac tumor
Choriocarcinoma
Mixed germ cell tumor

These tumors are typically classified into three main categories: teratomas, pure germinomas, or NGGCTs. The production of beta-human chorionic gonadotrophin (β-HCG) and alpha-fetoprotein (AFP) supports the diagnosis.

Teilum proposed that all germ cell tumors originate from a primordial germ cell differentiated into a germinoma or totipotent cells, giving rise to the other tumor subtypes [9, 16].

An alternative theory (from Takei and Pearl) proposed that the primordial germ cell tumor arise from the fetal yolk sac developing into multiple different pathways [17].

Sano et al., in turn, suggested that germinomas derive directly from germ cells, whereas other germ cell tumors are dysembryogenic in origin and arise through involvement of the lateral mesoderm and developing brain regions [18].

Germinomas are the malignant counterparts of a normal embryonic stage of development, which explains their close resemblance to normal tissue at both the macroscopic and microscopic levels, similar to other extracranial germ cell tumors. Macroscopically, a germinoma appears as a solid, circumscribed and soft mass. The surface is pink-gray and may occasionally contain small cysts. There are no areas of hemorrhage or necrosis. Germinomas are composed of large, undifferentiated cells embedded within fibrous connective tissue. These tumor cells exhibit high mitotic activity and are arranged in sheets, lobules, or nests. Germinomas are highly immunogenic, leading to recruitment of inflammatory cells into the tumor microenvironment. This results in a prominent lymphocytic infiltrate and the characteristic histological appearance commonly referred to as a "two-cell pattern" [19–22].

NGGCTs exhibit a heterogeneous histological pattern characterized by different components (Fig. 17.1).

Typical immunohistochemical markers supporting the diagnosis of germinoma include D2–40, c-kit, OCT 3/4, SALL-4, LIN28A, CD30, and PLAP (normally expressed by primordial germ cells) [23–28].

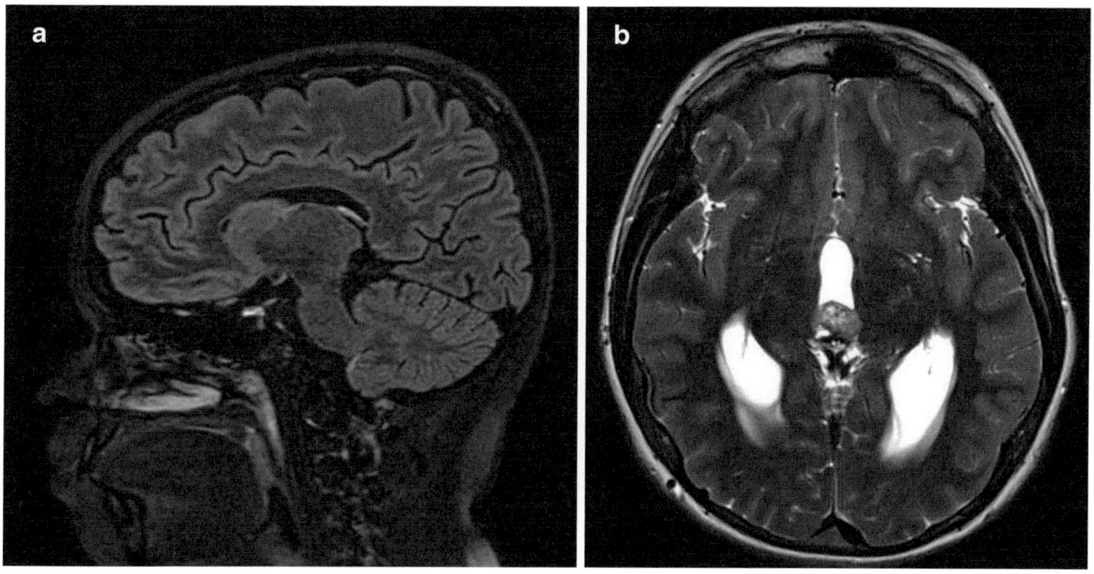

Fig. 17.1 (**a**) Suprasellar germinoma: Pathological tissue located in the suprasellar/hypothalamic region involving the optic chiasm, the prechiasmatic tracts of the optic nerves and optic tracts, the (thickened) pituitary stalk, and the pituitary gland. It is characterized by the presence of cyst-like components and likely intralesional hemorrhagic/calcified areas and shows inhomogeneous enhancement after contrast medium. (**b**) Pineal germinoma: Pathological tissue with inhomogeneously hyperintense signal on T2, due to the presence of some intralesional calcifications that takes up contrast medium

17.4 Molecular Biology of iGCTs

Recent transcriptomic and integrated genomic analyses have demonstrated that iGCTs are characterized by substantial biological heterogeneity that extends beyond conventional histopathological classification. While germinomas have traditionally been regarded as a relatively homogeneous entity based on their morphology, molecular profiling studies have revealed the existence of biologically distinct tumor populations with different patterns of immune activation, proliferative activity, and developmental signaling pathways [29].

Using transcriptomic clustering approaches, three major molecular subtypes of iGCTs have been identified—Immune-hot, MYC/E2F, and SHH—each displaying unique genomic, immunological, and clinical characteristics [30]. This molecular classification provides important insights into tumor pathogenesis and may facilitate the development of more personalized therapeutic strategies.

The Immune-hot subtype, composed predominantly of germinomas, is characterized by marked activation of immune-related pathways and a highly inflamed tumor microenvironment. These tumors show extensive infiltration by CD8+ and CD4+ T lymphocytes, regulatory T cells, and macrophages, together with elevated expression of immune checkpoint molecules including PD-1, PD-L1, PD-L2, CTLA-4, LAG3, and IDO1. Such findings are consistent with previous studies demonstrating abundant immune cell infiltration and frequent PD-L1 expression in germinomas [31]. Patients belonging to this subgroup tend to present at an older age and more frequently harbor tumors located in the pineal or sellar regions. The pronounced immune activation observed in this subtype provides a strong biological rationale for the use of immune checkpoint inhibitors, and preliminary clinical evidence suggests that anti-PD-1 therapies may achieve meaningful responses in relapsed germinoma patients [30].

The MYC/E2F subtype is also composed mainly of germinomas but differs substantially from the Immune-hot group by exhibiting enrichment of cell cycle-related pathways and increased expression of MYC and E2F target genes. Tumors within this subgroup demonstrate the highest levels of cell-cycle activity among all iGCT categories, reflecting enhanced proliferative potential and dysregulated cell-cycle control. In addition, these tumors are characterized by increased chromosomal instability, frequent whole-genome doubling events, and a greater burden of copy-number alterations, suggesting that genomic instability is a major driver of tumorigenesis [30]. Clinically, patients tend to present at a younger age and have a lower incidence of disseminated disease at diagnosis.

The SHH subtype is characterized by activation of the Sonic Hedgehog (SHH) and epithelial-mesenchymal transition (EMT) signaling pathways. In contrast to the previous subgroups, it includes both germinomas and NGGCTs, with the majority of NGGCTs clustering within this category. The molecular similarities observed between germinomatous and NGGCTs in this subgroup suggest a possible developmental continuum and support the hypothesis that SHH and EMT signaling may contribute to tumor differentiation, progression, and malignant transformation [30]. These observations provide novel insights into the biological mechanisms underlying NGGCTs' development and may help explain the marked clinical and pathological diversity observed among iGCTs.

Beyond transcriptomic classification, comprehensive genomic analyses have further expanded the molecular landscape of iGCTs. Recurrent alterations involving the KIT/RAS/MAPK and PI3K/AKT/mTOR pathways have been consistently reported and appear to represent early oncogenic events in tumor development [29]. More recently, novel genomic abnormalities have been identified, including truncating mutations of USP28 and high-level amplifications of KRAS and CRKL mediated by extrachromosomal DNA [30]. Functional studies demonstrated that loss-of-function USP28 mutations can activate MAPK signaling and increase sensitivity to MEK inhibition, thereby identifying a potentially actionable therapeutic target. Similarly, the discovery of distinct immune signatures and molecular subtypes provides a framework for the development of subtype-specific therapeutic approaches, including immunotherapy, targeted inhibition of MAPK signaling, and potentially therapies directed against SHH pathway activation [30].

Overall, the identification of molecularly defined iGCT subgroups represents a major advance in the understanding of germ cell tumor biology. Molecular classification is likely to complement conventional histopathological diagnosis, improve risk stratification, and facilitate the implementation of precision medicine approaches aimed at reducing treatment-related toxicity while maintaining excellent survival outcomes [29–32].

17.5 Clinical Presentation and Diagnosis

iGCTs are characterized by a wide range of clinical manifestations, largely determined by tumor location. The most common presenting symptoms include fatigue, irritability, headache, diplopia, endocrine dysfunction, vomiting, and behavioral changes [33–36]. Symptom onset is often insidious, progressive, and nonspecific, leading to delays in diagnosis and treatment.

We mainly distinguish three areas of occurrence for iGCTs: sellar-suprasellar region, pineal region, thalamic and basal ganglia region.

Tumors arising in the sellar and suprasellar regions typically present with symptoms resulting from mass effect and/or infiltration of adjacent structures, most notably the pituitary gland and hypothalamus. Consequently, endocrine dysfunction is a prominent feature of these lesions. These symptoms are primarily related to pituitary or hypothalamic involvement. The most common are diabetes insipidus, delayed pubertal development, growth retardation, precocious puberty, and panhypopituitarism [37]. Diabetes insipidus is present in approximately 90% of sellar region tumors, with a long history of polyuria and polydipsia.

Visual disturbances resulting from compression of the optic pathways occur in 40% to 90% of cases.

Tumors arising in the pineal region typically present with symptoms secondary to obstructive hydrocephalus (vomiting and headache leading to drowsiness) and Parinaud syndrome (upward vertical conjugate gaze palsy) caused by compression of the midbrain [38]. In most cases, symptoms of pineal tumors develop more rapidly than those arising in the sellar region, largely due to the early onset of obstructive hydrocephalus. Approximately, 75% of patients with pineal region tumors present with Parinaud syndrome [39].

By contrast, germ cell tumors involving the thalamus and basal ganglia typically have an insidious onset and a slowly progressive clinical course. The main clinical manifestations include cognitive impairment and alterations in mental status. Involvement of the extrapyramidal system results in movement disorders such as hemiparesis, rigidity, dystonia, and bradykinesia [39, 40].

Germinomas can be located synchronously in the pineal and pituitary regions, a presentation referred to as a "bifocal germinoma". This diagnosis (exclusively pituitary and pineal iGCT localization) may obviate the need for histological confirmation by biopsy.

The radiological diagnosis of iGCTs relies on magnetic resonance imaging (MRI), which provides detailed information regarding tumor characteristics, location, extent, and relationships with adjacent anatomical structures. On MRI images, germinomas appear as well-defined round or oval masses. Larger lesions often contain cystic portions and calcifications. Germ cell tumors are isointense on T1-weighted sequences and iso- or hyperintense on T2-weighted sequences (Fig. 17.1a, b). Contrast enhancement may be homogeneous or inhomogeneous; in some cases, perilesional edema may be observed [41, 42]. Germinomas of the sellar region may initially manifest as isolated thickening of the pituitary stalk on MRI, a finding that can precede the development of a more evident mass lesion.

Because the location of iGCTs may limit safe access for biopsy or result in insufficient tissue sampling, histological confirmation is not always feasible. Therefore, accurate radiological evaluation combined with the assessment of tumor markers characteristic is essential for establishing the diagnosis. Germ cell tumors can secrete proteins into the blood and CSF, which play a key role in their diagnosis, staging, and risk stratification. The two principal biomarkers used in the iGCTs diagnosis are AFP and β-HCG [43]. Assessment of these markers in both serum and CSF is essential for diagnostic workup. The detection of values above a certain threshold can support a definitive diagnosis without the need for biopsy.

iGCTs represent a heterogeneous group of neoplasms with their biological and clinical diversity partly reflected by the production of tumor markers: yolk sac tumors secrete AFP, and choriocarcinomas secrete β-HCG; pure embryonal carcinomas and teratomas generally do not secrete specific markers; germinomas may secrete β-HCG, suggesting the presence of syncytiotrophoblastic cells.

In summary, in staging iGCTs and guiding appropriate treatment selection, comprehensive evaluation is essential and includes brain and spine MRI, CSF cytology, and AFP and β-HCG assessment in both serum and CSF.

The disease is classified as metastatic in the presence of multiple intracranial and/or spinal cord lesions (excluding pineal-pituitary bifocality) and/or positive CSF cytology. CSF must be collected before any neurosurgical intervention (biopsy, ventriculostomy, or shunt placement) (Fig. 17.2).

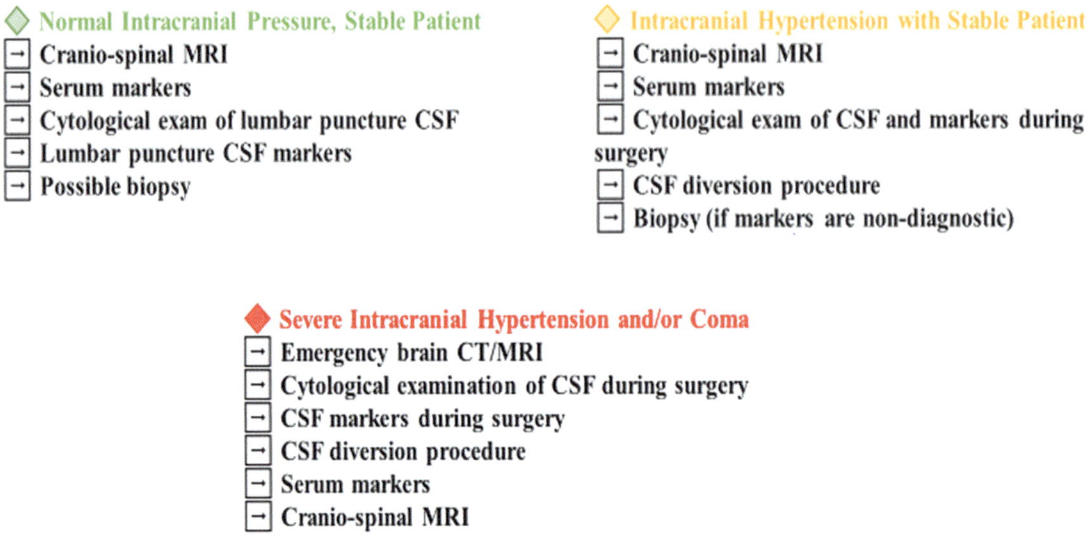

Fig. 17.2 Diagnostic algorithm in intracranial germ cell tumors

17.6 Treatment

17.6.1 Surgery

The key neurosurgical considerations for pediatric iGCTs span several domains: management of hydrocephalus, tissue diagnosis, surgical approach selection, the role of resection by histologic subtype, second-look surgery for residual disease, and postoperative management.

17.6.1.1 Management of Obstructive Hydrocephalus

Over 50% of iGCTs present with symptomatic obstructive hydrocephalus, making CSF diversion a frequent first neurosurgical intervention [44, 45].

In pineal region tumors with obstruction of the Silvian aqueduct, endoscopic third ventriculostomy (ETV) is the favored procedure, as it avoids the long-term complications of a permanent shunt. Given the significant risk of bleeding in the first week of adjuvant treatment, positioning of a ventricula access device at the time of third ventriculostomy could be considered and is a standard practice at our institution.

If ETV is not possible as in presence of tumor tissue in the anterior part or at the floor of the third ventricle, an external ventricular drain (EVD) is preferred over a permanent ventriculoperitoneal (VP) shunt, because chemotherapy-induced tumor shrinkage (especially in germinomas) often restores CSF pathways within days.

In the context of hydrocephalus, CSF collection for tumor markers (AFP, β-HCG) should be performed at the time of any CSF diversion procedure before tumor manipulation occurs.

17.6.1.2 Tissue Diagnosis: Biopsy Versus Marker-Based Diagnosis

The need for surgical biopsy depends on serum/CSF tumor marker levels [45].

In marker-negative tumors (AFP and β-HCG below protocol thresholds), surgical biopsy is required regardless of imaging findings. Endoscopic biopsy is the preferred method, as it can be combined with ETV and minimizes neurological sequelae compared to open surgery [46–48].

In marker-positive tumors with consistent imaging, treatment may be initiated without surgical biopsy, based on the diagnosis suggested by the markers [45]. Biopsy methods include endoscopic, stereotactic, open, or transsphenoidal approaches. Endoscopic biopsy is by far the preferred method, allowing administration of chemotherapy within days and having a diagnostic accuracy of approximately 90% [47, 48].

17.6.1.3 Role of Resection

The need for surgical resection in the context of first-line treatment varies significantly by tumor type [46, 47, 49]. In germinomas, an aggressive upfront resection is not recommended. These tumors are highly chemo- and radiosensitive and can be managed without surgery (>90% 5-year EFS with chemotherapy + whole ventricular irradiation) [47, 49]. Surgical resection, whenever feasible, can be considered after adjuvant treatment to obtain absence of measurable disease.

NGGCTs benefit from neoadjuvant chemotherapy followed by delayed (second-look) surgery for residual disease. Residual disease is associated with worse outcomes and may represent growing teratoma syndrome [45, 46, 49]. Current treatment protocols provide specific guidance about the timing of surgical resection, allowing elective programming of such complex procedures.

On the other hand, mature teratomas benefit from complete surgical resection, as it is curative for the majority without malignant components representing the recommended treatment [45].

For localized brain recurrence, maximal safe resection should be considered, followed by adjuvant systemic therapy and/or radiation. Resection may also be considered in specific cases for palliation of symptoms in disseminated recurrent disease [50]. An early post-operative MRI should always be obtained to assess the extent of resection and post-operative complications.

17.6.1.4 Surgical Approaches

Germ cell tumors typically present in the third ventricle. Most frequent locations include the infundibular and the pineal regions.

For anteriorly located lesions, surgical approaches include the anterior transcallosal and trans-lamina terminalis approach. Extreme care should be taken not to violate the ventricular walls for the risk of subsequent pituitary and hypothalamic syndromes. Additional risks include visual and vascular damage [49, 51].

For posteriorly located tumors, approaches to the pineal region include considerations include the supracerebellar infratentorial, which is most commonly used and preferred for midline tumors with extension into the third ventricle, and the occipital transtentorial, which is preferred for lesions extending toward the quadrigeminal cystern and the fourth ventricle. Less commonly used additional options include the occipital interhemispheric transtentorial and transcallosal routes [48, 50]. Transient postoperative morbidity occurs in 15–25% of cases, with Parinaud syndrome and ataxia being the most frequent complications. Permanent neurological deficits occur in less than 10% of patients [50].

Gross total resection rates range from 40% to 100%, depending on histology and tumor extension, with the highest GTR rates (~77%) achieved in GCTs and smaller lesions.

Endoscopic or endoscope-assisted techniques are increasingly complementing traditional microsurgical routes, aiming to reduce morbidity and improve CSF management. However, a significant experience and a refined technical armamentarium are necessary to obtain the radicality of resection offered by the microsurgical techniques.

In any case, referral to a pediatric brain tumor center with multidisciplinary expertise is strongly recommended [52].

17.6.2 Radiotherapy and Chemotherapy

Germ cell tumors are a group of highly radiosensitive and chemosensitive neoplasms.

Radiotherapy has long been considered the cornerstone of treatment for intracranial germ cell tumors, particularly craniospinal irradiation (CSI) [53–56].

Over the past two decades, the high rate of endocrine and neurocognitive sequelae has prompted experts to conduct studies focused on reducing the radiation field and dose [57, 58].

Modern radiotherapy (RT) techniques include volumetric-modulated arc therapy (VMAT), intensity-modulated radiotherapy (IMRT), and proton beam radiotherapy (PBRT), which may reduce the risk of long-term treatment-related sequelae [59, 60].

Because of the long-term adverse effects associated with radiotherapy, chemotherapy has been incorporated into the treatment of localized germinomas and all cases of NGGCTs. The role of chemotherapy in iGCTs has been extensively investigated. In particular, chemotherapy has been evaluated as a possible alternative to radiotherapy. Several studies have investigated the possibility of increasing chemotherapy doses or replacing certain cytotoxic agents; available evidence has consistently demonstrated that chemotherapy alone is less effective than combined chemoradiotherapy or radiotherapy alone [61–63].

The addition of chemotherapy has enabled reductions in both radiation dose and treatment volume without compromising clinical outcomes [64, 65].

The most commonly used chemotherapeutics currently in the first-line treatment of germ cell tumors are platinum salts, nitrogen mustards, and etoposide. These are combined in neoadjuvant multichemotherapy regimens that vary according to histology and risk category [66–68].

Current European treatment recommendations for iGCTs are based on the SIOP CNS GCT (International Society of Paediatric Oncology Central Nervous System Germ Cell Tumour) II protocol (2012–2018), which remains the reference framework for risk stratification and therapeutic management across European centers. The SIOP CNS GCT III trial will represent the next European multinational framework for the diagnosis, staging, and treatment of primary iGCTs. Scheduled to be implemented in 2027, it builds upon the experience and outcomes of the previous SIOP CNS GCT II study, with the aim of further refining risk-adapted treatment strategies while reducing long-term treatment-related toxicity. The GCT III study is expected to harmonize European and North American therapeutic approaches, promoting a unified international framework that emphasizes de-escalation of radiotherapy and chemotherapy, and refinement of diagnostic biomarker cutoffs. In addition, it introduces the clinical integration of circulating microRNAs in serum and CSF for noninvasive diagnosis, tumor monitoring, and early detection of relapse [69].

The use and combination of radiotherapy and chemotherapy in germ cell tumors is based on histology and staging.

17.6.2.1 Germinoma

Historically, the standard treatment for germinoma was CSI, which, however, was associated with long-term endocrine and neurocognitive impairment. For this reason, the use of chemotherapy was introduced in the late 1990s by various European, North American, and Japanese working groups.

Chemotherapy alone has failed to achieve acceptable cure rates when compared with radiotherapy [70].

Non-metastatic Germinoma

During the 1990s, the North American group investigated neoadjuvant chemotherapy followed by focal radiotherapy, achieving a 3-year event-free survival (EFS) of approximately 92%, but several working groups observed an increased risk of ventricular recurrence in cases treated with neoadjuvant chemotherapy and focal RT. These results led global experts, in subsequent years, to recommend whole ventricular irradiation over focal irradiation alone [71–74].

The European group currently recommends whole ventricular irradiation (WVI) (24 Gy, performed after chemotherapy) and possible boosting of residual disease (16 or 30 Gy). This approach avoids CSI while maintaining comparable disease control.

In the SIOP CNS GCT II trial, the primary objective was to maintain high EFS rates using a risk-adapted approach; specifically, focal radiotherapy of 16 Gy could be omitted in patients in complete remission. In the forthcoming SIOP CNS GCT III, trial patients with localized germinoma will receive a WVI reduced to 12 Gy, while the boost dose to the primary tumor site will range from 12 to 18 Gy according to the radiological response to induction chemotherapy [69].

Bifocal germinomas (involving both the sellar and pineal regions) are treated as localized disease; when treated with chemo-radiotherapy combination, they reach a 3-year PFS and OS of 100% [75].

For both unifocal and bifocal germinomas, in the future European trial, the boost volume will encompass the post-chemotherapy tumor bed with a 5-mm margin.

Basal ganglia and thalamus germinomas are rare and no clear consensus currently exists regarding their optimal treatment: CSI, WVI, and focal RT have all been utilized [76].

For atypical location diseases, dose and field reduction strategies are less widely accepted in this setting. Accordingly, in the forthcoming SIOP CNS GCT III protocol, a more conservative boost volume is planned for these tumors, encompassing the post-chemotherapy tumor bed with a 10-mm margin [69].

The chemotherapy regimens currently recommended in Europe for patients with localized germinomas consist of four alternating cycles of carboplatin/etoposide (carboplatin 600 mg/m^2 on day 1 and etoposide 100 mg/m^2/day on days 1–3) and ifosfamide/etoposide (ifosfamide 1800 mg/m^2/day on days 1–5 and etoposide 100 mg/m^2/day on days 1–3), administered before radiotherapy. Under the forthcoming SIOP CNS GCT III protocol, this regimen will be simplified to four cycles of carboplatin/etoposide only, with carboplatin administered at 600 mg/m^2 on day 1 and etoposide at 150 mg/m^2/day on days 1–3. An additional major modification in the SIOP CNS GCT III protocol concerns the diagnostic classification of germinomas and NGGCTs. In the current European protocol, patients are classified as having germinoma when serum and/or CSF AFP levels are <25 ng/mL and serum and/or CSF β-HCG levels are <50 IU/L. In the upcoming SIOP CNS GCT III protocol, these thresholds will be revised to AFP <10 ng/mL and β-HCG <100 IU/L. These revised biomarker thresholds are intended to improve biological stratification and diagnostic classification within future European treatment protocols [69].

Metastatic Germinoma

Approximately 20% of patients present with metastatic disease at diagnosis.

Craniospinal irradiation (24 Gy) remains the only treatment shown to improve survival. Currently, it is the sole available option. An additional boost is administered to the disease site (16 Gy).

By contrast, in the forthcoming SIOP CNS GCT III protocol, chemotherapy will be added before craniospinal irradiation-based treatment for metastatic germinoma, reinforcing a combined modality approach [69].

Relapsed Germinoma

Relapses in germinomas are rare. Treatment options include chemotherapy and re-irradiation or high-dose chemotherapy (HDCT) followed by autologous stem-cell transplantation (with or without irradiation) [77, 78]. Regimens used for standard care chemotherapy are platinum and ifosfamide based followed by Melphalan based HDCT.

17.6.2.2 Non-germinomatous Germ Cell Tumors (NGGCTs)

NGGCTs are more aggressive than germinomas and are associated with a less favorable prognosis. Their higher risk of recurrence requires a more intensive multimodal approach combining chemotherapy and radiotherapy (fields and doses are yet unclear).

According to the European treatment strategy, patients with NGGCTs receive four cycles of dose-intense cisplatin-based chemotherapy (PEI: cisplatin 20 mg/m^2 D1-5, etoposide 100 mg/m^2 D1-3, ifosfamide 1.5 g/m^2 D1-5), followed by RT 54 Gy to tumor bed (involving ventricular irradiation) in localized disease, and CSI in metastatic disease (30 Gy CSI and boost 24 Gy) [79].

The GCT III trial will recommend a WVI for all localized NGGCTs, with a proposed dose range of 24–30 Gy, currently under evaluation [69].

Patients considered at high risk of recurrence—based on elevated CSF AFP levels, suboptimal response to induction therapy, and/or age younger than 6 years—may receive intensified PEI chemotherapy followed by autologous stem-cell rescue.

In cases of recurrence, treatment with HDCT and reinfusion of stem cells is highly recommended for curative purposes. Regarding re-irradiation, the fields, doses, and timing are still being debated.

17.7 Conclusions

iGCTs have an excellent prognosis, largely due to chemotherapy and radiosensitivity.

Long-term survival rates have improved substantially over recent decades, with 10-year overall survival exceeding 90% in several contemporary series.

Treatment strategies have progressively evolved toward reducing radiation dose and treatment volume while preserving disease control, thereby minimizing long-term neurocognitive, endocrine, and other treatment-related sequelae.

Given the high cure rate, proper follow-up with careful monitoring of long-term toxicities is essential.

Molecular biology studies are expected to provide deeper insights into the cellular microenvironment and alterations in signal transduction pathways. These findings may support the development of novel targeted and immunotherapeutic strategies, with the potential to improve clinical outcomes while minimizing treatment-related morbidity.

References

1. Brain Tumor Registry of Japan. Brain tumor registry of Japan (2005-2008). Neurol Med Chir (Tokyo). 2017;57(suppl 1):9–102.
2. Matsutani M, Sano K, Takakura K, et al. Primary intracranial germ cell tumors: a clinical analysis of 153 histologically verified cases. J Neurosurg. 1997;86:446–55.
3. Kamoshima Y, Sawamura Y. Update on current standard treatments in central nervous system germ cell tumors. Curr Opin Neurol. 2010;23:571–5.
4. Kellie SJ, Boyce H, Dunkel I, et al. Primary chemiotherapy for intracranial non germinomatous germ cell tumors: results of the second international CNS germ cell study group protocol. J Clin Oncol. 2004;22:846–53.
5. Acharya S, DeWees T, Shinoharam ET, et al. Long-term outcomes and late affects for childhood and young adulthood intracranial germinomas. Neuro-Oncology. 2015;17:741–6.
6. McCarthy BJ, Shibui S, Kayakama T, et al. Primary CNS germ cell tumors in Japan and the United States: an analysis of 4 tumor registries. Neuro-Oncology. 2012;14(9):1194–200.
7. Gittleman H, Cioffi G, Vecchione-Koval T, et al. Descriptive epidemiology of germ cell tumors of the central nervous system diagnosed in the United States from 2006 to 2015. J Neuro-Oncol. 2019;143(2):251–60.
8. Laughton SJI, Merchant TE, al Sklar CA e. Endocrine outcomes for children with embryonal brain tumors after risk adapted craniospinal and conformal primary-site irradiation and high-dose chemotherapy with stem cell rescue on the SJMB-96 trial. J Clin Oncol. 2008;26(7):1112–8.
9. Packer RJ, Cohen BH, Cooney K. Intracranial germ cell tumors. Oncologist. 2000;5:312.
10. Poynter JN, Fonstad R, Tolar J, et al. Incidence of intracranial germ cell tumors by race in the United States,1992–2010. J Neuro-Oncol. 2014;120(2):381–8.
11. Ostrom QT, Cioffi G, Waite K, et al. CBTRUS statistical report: primary brain and the other central nervous system tumors diagnosed in the United States in 2014–2018. Neuro Oncol. 2012;23(12 Suppl 2):iii1.
12. Lee SH, Jung KW, Ha J, et al. Nation-wide population-based incidence and survival rates of malignant central nervous system germ cell tumors in Korea. 2005-2012. Cancer Res Treat. 2017;49(2):494–501.
13. Kremenevski N, Buchfelder M, Hore N. Intracranial germinomas: diagnosis, pathogenesis, clinical presentation and management. Curr Oncol Rep. 2023;25:765–75.
14. Pizzo PA, Poplack DG. Principles and practice of pediatric oncology, 6th edn. 2016.
15. Louis DN, Perry A, Wesseling P, et al. The 2021 WHO classification of Tumors of the central nervous system: a summary. Neuro-Oncology. 2021;23(8):1231–51.
16. Teilum G. Special tumors of the ovary and testis and related extragonadal lesions. Philadelphia, PA: JB. Lippincott; 1976.
17. Takey Y, Pearl GS. Ultrastructure study of intracranial yolk sac tumor: with special reference to the oncologic phylogeny of germ-cell tumors. Cancer. 1981;48:2038–46.
18. Sano K, Matsutani M. Pinealoma (germinoma) treated by direct surgery and post-operative irradiation. Childs Brain. 1981;8:81–97.
19. Bentley AJ, Parkinson MCHBN, et al. A comparative morphological and immunoistochimical study of testicular seminomas and intracranial germinomas. Histopathology. 1990;17(5):443–9.
20. Bjornsson J, Scheithauer BW, al Okazaki H e. Intracranial germ cell tumors: pathobiological and immunoistochimical aspects of 70 cases. J Neuropathol Exp Neurol. 1985;44(1):32–46.
21. Utsuki S, Oka H, Tanizaki Y, et al. Pathological features of intracranial germinomas with references to fibrous tissue and granulomatous change. Brain Tuor Pathol. 2005;22(1):9–13.
22. Utsuki S, Oka HTY, et al. Histological features of intracranial germinomas not disappearing immediately after radiotherapy. Neurol Med Chir (Tokyo). 2006;46(9):429–33.
23. Mishima K, Kato Y, Kaneko MK, et al. Podoplanin expression in primary central nervous system

germ cell tumors: a useful histological marker for the diagnosis of germinoma. Acta Neuropathol. 2006;111(6):563–8.
24. Hattab EM, Tu PH, al Wilson JD e. OCT4 immunoistochemistry is superior to placental alkaline phosphatase (PLAP) in the diagnosis of central nervous system germinoma. Am J Surg Pathol. 2005;29(3):368–71.
25. Nakamura H, Takeshima H, Makino K, et al. C-kit expression in germinoma: an immunohistochemistry-based study. J Neuro-Oncol. 2005;75(2):163–217.
26. Mei K, Liu A, Allan RW, et al. Diagnostic utility of SALL4 in primary germ cell tumors of the central nervous system: a study of 77 cases. Mod Pathol. 2009;22(12):1628–36.
27. Pantazis G, Harter PN, al Capper D e. The embry9onic stem cell factor UTF1 serves as a reliable diagnostic marker for germinmas. Pathology. 2014;46(3):225–9.
28. Shinoda J, Miwa Y, al Sakai N e. Immunoistochemical study of placental alkaline phosphatase in primary intracranial germ-cell tumors. J Neurosurg. 1985;63(5):733–9.
29. Wang L, Yamaguchi S, Burstein MD, et al. Integrated genomic characterization of intracranial germ cell tumors. Nat Commun. 2018;9:4964.
30. Li B, Zhao S, Li S, et al. Novel molecular subtypes of intracranial germ cell tumors expand therapeutic opportunities. Neuro-Oncology. 2024;26(7):1335–51.
31. Takami H, Fukuoka K, Fukushima S, et al. Integrated clinical, histopathological, and molecular data analysis of intracranial germ cell tumors. Acta Neuropathol Commun. 2020;8:190.
32. Liu X, Wang Y, Zhang J, et al. Novel molecular subtypes of intracranial germ cell tumors expand therapeutic opportunities. Neuro-Oncology. 2024;26(8):1454–68.
33. Jorsal T, Rorth M. Intracranial germ cell tumors. A review with special reference to endocrine manifestations. Acta Oncol. 2012;51(1):3–9.
34. Wataya T, Ishizaki R, Kitagawa M, et al. Germinoma in the bilateral basal ganglia presented with cognitive deterioration. Childs Nerv Syst. 2015;31(6):953–8.
35. Sethi RV, Marino R, Niemerko A, et al. Delayed diagnosis in children with intracranial germ cell tumors. J Pediatr. 2013;163(5):1448–53.
36. Esfahani DR, Alden T, al DiPatri A e. Pediatric suprasellar germ cell tumors: a clinical and radiographic review of solitary vs bifocal tumors and its therapeutic implications. Cancers (Basel). 2020;12(9):2621.
37. Partenope C, Pozzobon G, al Weber G e. Endocrine manifestations of pediatric intracranial germ cell tumors: from diagnosis to longe term follow-up. Endocrine. 2022;77(3):546–55.
38. Crawford J, Vezina LG, Packer RJ. Central nervous system germ cell tumors of childhood, presentation and delay in diagnosis. Neurology. 2007;68:1668–73.
39. Matsutani M, Sano K, al Takakura K e. Primary intracranial germ cell tumors: a clinical analysis of 153 histologically verified cases. Neurosurgery. 1997;86(3):446–55.
40. Sonoda Y, Kumabe T, al Sugiyama S e. Germ cell tumors in the basal ganglia: problems of early diagnosis and treatment. J Neurosurg Pediatr. 2008;2(2):118–24.
41. Liang L, Korogi Y, Sugiyama S, et al. MRI of intracranial germ-cell tumors. Neuroradiology. 2002;44(5):382–8.
42. Wang Y, Zou L, Gao B. Intracranial germinoma: clinical and MRI findings in 56 patients. Childs Nerv Syst. 2010;26(12):1773–7.
43. Seregni E, Massimino M, al Nerini Molteni S e. Serum cerebrospinal fluid human chorionic gonadotropin (HCG) and alpha-fetoprotein (AFP) in intracranial germ cell tumors. Int J Biol Markers. 2002;17(2):112–8.
44. Wong TT, Tsai ML, Chang H, et al. Brain and spinal tumors originating from the germ line cells. Adv Exp Med Biol. 2023;1405:421–55. https://doi.org/10.1007/978-3-031-23705-8_16.
45. Murray MJ, Bartels U, Nishikawa R, et al. Consensus on the management of intracranial germ-cell tumours. Lancet Oncol. 2015;16(9):e470–7. https://doi.org/10.1016/S1470-2045(15)00244-2.
46. Frappaz D, Dhall G, Murray MJ, et al. EANO, SNO and Euracan Consensus Review on the current management and future development of intracranial germ cell tumors in adolescents and young adults. Neuro-Oncology. 2022;24(4):516–27. https://doi.org/10.1093/neuonc/noab252.
47. Carlos Chung KH, Owler BK, Dexter M, Chaseling R. Paediatric germ cell TUMOURS of the central nervous system: results and experience from a tertiary-referral Paediatric institution in Australia. J Clin Neurosci. 2013;20(4):514–9. https://doi.org/10.1016/j.jocn.2012.04.017.
48. Cavalheiro S, Valsechi LC, Dastoli PA, et al. Outcomes and surgical approaches for pineal region tumors in children: 30 years' experience. J Neurosurg Pediatr. 2023;32(2):184–93. https://doi.org/10.3171/2023.3.PEDS22468.
49. McCrea HJ, George E, Settler A, Schwartz TH, Greenfield JP. Pediatric suprasellar tumors. J Child Neurol. 2016. Review.
50. Yeoh TDYY, Nga V, Kimpo M, Lo SS, Vellayappan B. Intracranial germ cell tumors. Semin Neurol. 2023;43(6):897–908. https://doi.org/10.1055/s-0043-1776763.
51. Weiner HL, Finlay JL. Surgery in the management of primary intracranial germ cell tumors. Child's Nerv Syst. 1999.
52. Vitulli F, Berardinelli J, Bove I, et al. Surgical management of pediatric pineal region tumors: an overview of current strategies. Child's Nerv Syst. 2026;42(1):117. https://doi.org/10.1007/s00381-026-07209-9.
53. Rich TA, Cassady JR, Strand RD, et al. Radiation therapy for pineal and suprasellar germ cell tumors. Cancer. 1985;55(5):932–40.
54. Wolden SL, Wara WM, al Larson DA e. Radiation therapy for primary intracranial germ cell tumors. Int H Radiat Oncol Biol Phys. 1995;32(4):943–9.

55. Lafay-Cousin L, Millar BA, Mabbott D, et al. Limited filed radiation for bifocal germinoma. Int J Radiat Oncol Biol Phys. 2006;65(2):486–92.
56. Maity A, Shu HK, al Janss A e. Craniospinal radiation in the treatment of biopsy proven intracranial germinomas: twenty-five years' experience in a single center. Int J Radiat Oncol Biol Phys. 2004;58(4):1165–70.
57. Acharya S, DeWees T, Shinohara ET, et al. Long-term outcomes and late effects for childhood and young adulthood intracranial germinomas. Neuro-Oncology. 2015;17(5):741–6.
58. Hale GA, Marina NM, Jones-Wallace D, et al. Late effects of treatment form germ cell tumors during childhood and adolescence. J Pediatr Hematol Oncol. 1999;21(2):115–22.
59. Park J, Park Y, Lee SU, et al. Differential dosimetric benefit of proton beam therapy over intensity modulated radiotherapy for a variety of targets in patients with intracranial germ cell tumors. Radiat Oncol. 2015;10(1):135.
60. Nota 36:Correia D, Terribilini D, Zepter S, et al. Whole ventricular irradiation for intracranial germ cell tumors: dosimetric comparison of pencil beam scanned protons, intensity-modulated radiotherapy and volumetric-modulated arc therapy. Clin Transl Radiat Oncol. 2019;15:53–61.
61. Calaminus G, Kortmann R, al Worch J e. SIOP CNS GCT 96: final report of outcome of a prospective, multinational nonrandomized trial for children and adults with intracranial germinoma, comparing cranispinal alone with chemotherapy followed by focal primary site irradiation for patients with localized disease. Neuro-Oncology. 2013;15(6):788–96.
62. Rogers SJ, Mosleh-Shizari MA, Saran FH. Radiotherapy of localized intracranial germinoma: time to sever historical ties? Lancet Oncol. 2005;6(7):509–19.
63. Shikama N, Ogawa K, al Tanaka S e. Lack of benefit of spinal irradiation in the primary treatment of intracranial germinoma: a multi-institutional, retrospective review of 180 patients. Cancer. 2005;104(1):126–34.
64. Balmaceda C, Heller G, al Rosenblum M e. Chemotherapy without irradiation- a novel approach for newly diagnosed CNS germ cell tumors: results of an international cooperative trial. The first international central nervous system germ cell tumor study. J Clinic Oncol. 1996;14(11):2908–15.
65. Kellie SJ, Boyce H, al Dunkel IJ e. Primary chemiotherapy for intracranial nongerminomatous germ cell tumors: results of the second international CNS germ cell study group protocol. J Clin Oncol. 2004;22(5):846–53.
66. Da Silva NS, Cappellano AM, al Diez B e. Primary chemiotherapy for intracranial germ cell tumors: results of the third international CNS germ cell tumor study. Pediatr Blood Cancer. 2010;54(3):377–83.
67. Bouffet E, Baranzelli MC, al Patte C e. Combined treatment modality for intracranial germinomas: results of a multicentre SFOP experience. Societé Francaise d'Oncologie Pediatrique. Br J Cancer. 1999;79(7–8):1199–204.
68. Bartels U, Onar-Thomas A, al Patel SK e. Phase II trial of response-based radioation therapy for patients with localized germinoma: a Children's oncology group study. Neuro-Oncology. 2022;24(6):974–83.
69. International symposium on intracranial germ cell tumors; Essen, Germany; 2025. Congress proceedings. SIOPE Annual Congress; Glasgow, United Kingdom; 2026. Congress proceedings.
70. Kellie SJ, et al. Intensive cisplatin and cyclophosphamide-based chemotherapy without radiotherapy for intracranial germinomas: failure of a primary chemotherapy approach. Pediatr Blood Cancer. 2004;43(2):126–33.
71. Kretschmar C, et al. Pre-radiation chemotherapy with response-based radiation therapy in children with central nervous system germ cell tumors: a report from the Children's oncology group. Pediatr Blood Cancer. 2007;48(3):285–91.
72. Matsutani, M. and G. Japanese Pediatric Brain Tumor Study. Combined chemotherapy and radiation therapy for CNS germ cell tumors--the Japanese experience. J Neuro-Oncol. 2001;54(3):311–6.
73. Alapetite C, et al. Pattern of relapse and outcome of non-metastatic germinoma patients treated with chemotherapy and limited field radiation: the SFOP experience. Neuro-Oncology. 2010;12(12):1318–25.
74. Calaminus G, et al. SIOP CNS GCT 96: final report of outcome of a prospective, multinational nonrandomized trial for children and adults with intracranial germinoma, comparing craniospinal irradiation alone with chemotherapy followed by focal primary site irradiation for patients with localized disease. Neuro-Oncology. 2013;15(6):788–96.
75. Al-Mahfoudh R, Zakaria R, Irvine E, Pizer B, Mallucci CL. The management of bifocal intracranial germinoma in children. Childs Nerv Syst. 2014;30:625–30.
76. Schuetze SM, Wathen JK, Lucas DR, Choy E, Samuels BL, Staddon AP, Ganjoo KN, von Mehren M, Chow WA, Loeb DM, et al. SARC009: phase 2 study of dasatinib in patients with previously treated, high-grade, advanced sarcoma. Cancer. 2016;122:868–74.
77. Murray MJ, et al. Treatment and outcomes of UK and German patients with relapsed intracranial germ cell tumors following uniform first-line therapy. Int J Cancer. 2017;141(3):621–35.
78. Kubota H, et al. High-dose chemotherapy with autologous stem cell transplantation spares re irradiation for recurrent intracranial germinoma. Pediatr Blood Cancer. 2018;65(8):e27104.
79. Calaminus G, et al. Outcome of patients with intracranial non-germinomatous germ cell tumors lessons from the SIOP-CNS-GCT-96 trial. Neuro-Oncology. 2017;19(12):1661–72.

Craniopharyngiomas

18

B. J. Hall, M. A. Cinalli, C. Mallucci,
and B. L. Pettorini

18.1 Embryology and Development

The buccopharyngeal membrane represents a junction between ecto- and endoderm, forming a septum between the pharynx and oral cavity [1]. Arising anterior to the membrane, Rathke's pouch is an evagination of ectoderm through the buccopharyngeal membrane that, when ultimately disconnected from the pharynx, gives rise to the anterior pituitary [2]. For this to occur, the anterior wall of Rathke's pouch proliferates and, in normal embryogenesis, results in the development of pars distalis and pars tuberalis. In up to a third of individuals, the eventual involution of the pouch does not occur completely, and Rathke's cleft cyst may persist: a residual space often measuring only a few millimetres and rarely symptomatic [2, 3]. The epithelial lining of this persistent duct provides the cellular origin of craniopharyngiomas and explains their typical suprasellar location. Craniopharyngiomas have also been described arising from sites remote to the suprasellar region, ranging from the clivus to as distant as the pineal gland and Sylvian fissure. Causation for such tumors is not easily explained through any embryological route, with dissemination via cerebrospinal fluid (CSF) one proposed mechanism, or in the rare case of distant recurrence after a previous surgical resection, 'seeding' along the surgical tract [4].

B. J. Hall
Department of Neurosurgery, Alder Hey Children's Hospital NHS Foundation Trust, Liverpool, UK

Institute of Infection, Veterinary and Ecological Sciences, University of Liverpool, Liverpool, UK
e-mail: benjaminhall@doctors.org.uk

M. A. Cinalli
Department of Medicine and Surgery, University of Milan Bicocca, Milan, Italy

Neurosurgery Department, Fondazione IRCCS San Gerardo dei Tintori, Monza, Italy

C. Mallucci · B. L. Pettorini (✉)
Department of Neurosurgery, Alder Hey Children's Hospital NHS Foundation Trust, Liverpool, UK
e-mail: conor.mallucci@alderhey.nhs.uk;
benedetta.pettorini@alderhey.nhs.uk

18.2 Clinical Presentation

Childhood craniopharyngioma (CP) diagnosis tends to happen years after the symptoms' onset [5, 6]. The initial presentation most often includes symptoms of raised intracranial pressure, such as headaches—in 60–75% of cases—and nausea [5, 7].

Visual impairment is seen in 62–84% of patients [5, 8] and is usually caused by compression and/or direct infiltration of the visual pathway. The classical visual field abnormality observed is bitemporal hemianopia (seen in 50% of patients), although abnormal pupillary

A. Mastronuzzi, A. Carai (eds.), *Navigating Pediatric Brain Tumors*,
https://doi.org/10.1007/978-3-032-18992-9_18

responses and visual acuity deficits can be observed as well. Obstructive hydrocephalus caused by the tumor can lead to a rise in intracranial pressure, with consequent papilledema (present in 20% of patients), optic atrophy, and loss of vision [9, 10]. Visual disturbances at diagnosis (in particular if <6 years old), along with papilledema or optic atrophy, correlate with poorer visual outcomes [11].

Endocrine deficiencies are the first manifestation of CP in 40–87% of patients [5, 12, 13]. Craniopharyngiomas arise from embryonic epithelial remnants of the Rathke's pouch. Due to their location, the hypothalamic–pituitary axis is often affected. Growth hormone deficiencies are seen in up to 75% of patients, followed by gonadotropins (40% of patients), adrenocorticotropic hormone (ACTH; 25% of patients), and thyroid-stimulating hormone (TSH; 25% of patients) deficiency. Central diabetes insipidus (DI) is seen in 17–27% of patients before treatment [5]. These hormonal disturbances need to be investigated and addressed thoroughly when a suspicious suprasellar lesion is found, as they can lead to serious complications in a peri-operative setting [10]. Around 15–30% of patients experience weight gain as a late manifestation before the diagnosis. It is a sign of hypothalamic dysfunction, and it is predictive of hypothalamic obesity [14–16].

Diencephalic syndrome (DS) is characterised by profound emaciation with normal caloric intake, euphoria, locomotor hyperactivity, and absence of cutaneous adipose tissue. Mostly associated with optic chiasm glioma, it can rarely (4.3%) be a manifestation of CP with hypothalamic involvement. Its presence at the time of diagnosis does not preclude weight gain afterwards [17].

18.3 Diagnosis: Radiological and Histological

Adamantinomatous craniopharyngiomas have characteristic radiologic features. 90% are cystic, 90% have prominent calcifications, and 90% have contrast-enhancing cystic walls [5, 18]. On magnetic resonance imaging (MRI), both on T1 and T2 sequences, the signal can be highly heterogeneous, depending on the distribution of calcifications and/or on the presence of one or more cysts.

MRI is not always sufficient to differentiate calcifications from other entities, due to the peculiar position of CPs, which lie in proximity of central skull base sinuses. The air content of the sinuses can interfere with susceptibility-weighted and T2*-weighted sequences. Therefore, for the identification of calcifications in CPs, CT scan remains the gold standard [5]. Also, a CT scan can be useful when planning the surgical approach to study the skull base anatomy, as well as to assess the presence of secondary changes such as erosion of the dorsum sellae provoked by the tumor [19]. The solid portion of the tumor and the cyst wall are typically contrast enhancing [10].

Identification of the relation between the tumor and the delicate structures around it is one of the main purposes of MRI imaging. The optic chiasm, hypothalamus, pituitary gland, the third ventricle, circle of Willis, frontal and temporal lobes, and brainstem need to be evaluated thoroughly to plan the appropriate surgical corridor and estimate the extent of resection [10]. The posterior hypothalamic nuclei are located in the lateral walls of the third ventricle, with the mammillary bodies (MB) representing the anterior limit. Therefore, since MB are easily identifiable on MRI, they have been used as a radiologic landmark to estimate the relation between CPs and the hypothalamus [5].

Puget et al. [20] have described a radiologic grading system for craniopharyngiomas, mainly focusing on hypothalamus involvement on MRI. In the pre-operative imaging, grade 0 means the hypothalamus is not involved, grade 1 describes displacement of the hypothalamus, and grade 2 represents infiltration of the hypothalamus by the tumor. The post-operative assessment includes 3 grades as well, with 0 meaning no damage to the hypothalamus, and 2 denoting severe hypothalamus damage. This classification is not just descriptive, as it also provides a practical approach for the surgical management of

CPs. In tumors with hypothalamic involvement, gross total resection (GTR) is not a suitable option, due to the unacceptable morbidity associated with surgical damage to the hypothalamus [21].

Craniopharyngiomas are Grade I tumors according to the World Health Organization (WHO) classification. Two subtypes have been identified: adamantinomatous (aCP) and papillary (pCP). The most common subtype of CP in the paediatric population is the adamantinomatous, although sporadic cases of papillary CP have been described in children [22, 23]. The two craniopharyngioma subtypes are driven by distinct somatic mutations. While pCPs frequently (57% to 100%) harbour somatic BRAF-V600E mutation [24], mutations of the CTNNB1 gene are found in 63–100% of aCPs [10, 25, 26]. The CTNNB1 gene codes for the β-catenin. A mutation in CTNNB1 improves β-catenin stability, resulting in its accumulation in the cellular nuclei, and determining the constitutive activation of the WNT-β-catenin pathway and cell proliferation [27–29].

Adamantinomatous CPs express inflammatory mediators in the solid and cystic portions. The cholesterol crystals characteristic of aCPs are considered responsible for inflammasome activation, with elevated expression of numerous cytokines (IL1β, IL6, IL8, IL10, IL18, TNF). Programmed death ligand (PD-L1) and its receptor PD-1 have been reported, as well as other immunosuppressive factors, which might lead to tumor's escape to immune surveillance [30–32]. Pathological features of adamantinomatous CPs show both cystic and solid components, with three layers surrounding the cyst lumen. A keratinised epithelium faces the cyst lumen, with sporadic formation of keratin nodules that can become calcified over time; the middle layer is composed of a loose stellate reticulum, while the basal layer is composed of palisaded small cells abutting a chronically inflamed fibrous stroma [33, 34]. On the other hand, pCPs are characterised by a papillary structure, they are preferentially solid, and they rarely develop calcifications [35].

18.4 Principles of Care

Heterogeneity in the management approaches between centres has resulted in recent efforts by the UK Children's Cancer and Leukaemia Group and the British Society for Paediatric Endocrinology and Diabetes to develop a standardised framework by which to approach craniopharyngiomas [11]. Primarily, given the overall scarcity of the tumors, it is crucial that newly diagnosed CPs are referred to and managed in a centre capable of delivering specialist paediatric neuro-endocrine care. This necessitates the regular cooperation of a broad multidisciplinary team (MDT), composed of representatives from paediatric endocrinology, ophthalmology, neuro-oncology, neuroradiology, neuropathology, and neurosurgery. Neurosurgical representation should furthermore be able to provide a multimodal approach to any surgical intervention by having experience in both transcranial and transsphenoidal approaches to CPs [11]. Most importantly, communication should not be limited to single centres, regardless of how experienced a particular MDT may be. As such, discussion at regional and national MDTs should be available for particularly complex cases to ensure all possible avenues are explored prior to intervention [11].

The benign nature of CPs against the backdrop of their usual complex anatomical origin results in an excellent survival rate, but with the potential for severe and chronic morbidity. Crucial then, to establishing a high standard of care, is ensuring that all paediatric patients diagnosed with CPs are safely and effectively transitioned to appropriate adult services upon reaching adulthood. Transition of care between paediatric and adult services is reputedly challenging across healthcare, though individuals with the rarest diagnoses such as CP are set to suffer the most without adequate support. Thus, it is important that active cooperation is maintained between the initial treating paediatric unit and the respective adult unit that the patient is ultimately transitioned to [11].

As discussed, the low mortality associated with craniopharyngiomas is often accompanied by multifaceted morbidity, often due to ophthalmological or neuro-endocrine deficits. In order to establish the effectiveness of the ongoing care provided, there must be regular review of the service and its constituent parts. Paediatric neuro-oncology is limited by a paucity of core outcome sets; therefore, establishing these in the coming years to facilitate objective outcome assessment is a priority for the neurosurgical community.

18.5 Therapeutic Dilemmas and Surgical Considerations

The management of craniopharyngiomas poses a number of formidable challenges to neurosurgeons and oncologists alike. As in any WHO Grade 1 tumor, gross total resection invariably remains the ideal outcome to halt disease progression and limit the functional impact on adjacent structures. Unlike histologically benign lesions located elsewhere, however, the complex anatomical relationships of suprasellar craniopharyngiomas make the decision to operate—and indeed how to operate—more nuanced.

The slow growth pattern of craniopharyngiomas and the subsequently insidious onset of symptoms can permit extraordinarily large tumors to develop with little clinical indication. In such cases, superior extension from above the sellar and into the floor of the third ventricle can eventually result in obstruction of either or both foramina of Monro. In these circumstances, the resultant hydrocephalus can become imminently life threatening and may ultimately be the point at which the patient is first diagnosed with an intracranial tumor. In such scenarios, urgent CSF diversion is the mainstay of treatment, usually in the form of a temporary external ventricular drain (EVD). Except in certain emergency circumstances, or when there is clear evidence supporting the likely diagnosis, it is generally considered optimal to obtain histological confirmation of craniopharyngioma prior to embarking on definitive management.

Obtaining tissue diagnosis can be achieved through two main routes: tissue biopsy or cyst aspiration [36]. By definition, the feasibility of either of these diagnostic routes is dependent on the morphology of the tumor itself, with most CPs demonstrating a combination of both cystic and solid components [5]. In the case of large, cystic CPs, the size of the cyst itself may be responsible for symptomatic deterioration. As such, aspiration of the main cystic component provides a minimally invasive option through which to obtain tissue diagnosis, while also decompressing adjacent structures such as the optic nerves and chiasm [36, 37]. Depending on the clinical status of the patient, cyst decompression alone may be less suitable in the setting of acute hydrocephalus, given the propensity for such patients to rapidly deteriorate, unless an additional route of CSF diversion is also implemented. Implantation of an Ommaya reservoir into any residual cyst may also serve as a simple temporising measure to permit serial fluid aspiration whilst formulating a definitive management plan [37].

Ensconced amidst the critical neurovascular structures surrounding the sella, the operative aspect of craniopharyngioma management exemplifies what it means to achieve ‘maximal safe resection’. As in all neuro-oncological surgery, an increasing number of surgical adjuncts may be considered to assist in this goal. These include primarily stereotactic image guidance, ultrasound probes, and, in some circumstances, intraoperative MRI scanning. While gross total resection, defined as >95% resection [38], is well recognised as achieving the lowest recurrence rates, improved risk stratification has led to a shift away from this radical approach in many patients. Variables including the presence of hydrocephalus, large tumor size with multiple compartments, clinical evidence of hypothalamic dysfunction, and younger age (≤5 years) are often applied to discern patients at higher risk of morbidity with more radical surgery [37], while others such as the Liverpool group also incorporate the Paris radiological grading criteria [39].

By grading risk of morbidity preoperatively, the treating team are able to tailor their intended surgical approach. In those with multiple high-risk features, particularly the inclusion of hypothalamic syndrome at the time of diagnosis, subtotal resection (STR) was deemed the maximum achievable surgical outcome to preserve function and avoid excess morbidity [39]. In those with hypothalamic syndrome, resecting hypothalamic tissue invariably leads to neuroendocrine dysfunction [40]. Thus, the goal should be to leave any hypothalamic tumor in situ whilst debulking the remainder of the lesion to decompress surrounding neurovascular structures, ameliorate any hydrocephalus, and slow disease progression. In patients presenting with no high-risk features, the operative goal should be to obtain gross total resection, guided by case-specific, intraoperative findings. For those patients with 1–2 high-risk features, excluding hypothalamic syndrome, then variability in initial surgical intent remains. As such, gross total or near-total resection should be the goal, while also allowing intraoperative findings (e.g. tumor adherent to the hypothalamus) to guide the surgeon in their decision-making [39].

18.6 Surgical Approaches

While multiple surgical approaches may be employed in the management of craniopharyngiomas, a common goal among them is to ensure adequate exposure of the critical surrounding structures. While historically transcranial approaches were favoured, improving endoscopic techniques have led to an increased adoption of endonasal approaches. Ultimately, the decision for either route depends on the experience of the surgeon in question, with some opting for a combination of the two.

18.6.1 Transcranial

In the setting of transcranial surgery, subfrontal or frontotemporal approaches are frequently employed by beginning from the non-dominant side and extending towards the midline, facilitating access to tumors between the superior aspect of the pituitary and the chiasm. The frontobasal burr hole is situated lateral to the superior sagittal sinus, at the level of the anterior cranial fossa floor. After durotomy and exposure of the chiasmatic region, the prechiasmatic and carotid cisterns are opened to allow continued arachnoid dissection in the direction of the Sylvian fissure. By releasing the frontal lobe from any arachnoid adhesions with the temporal lobe, minimal pressure is then required to enable retraction and adequate exposure of the chiasm. For those with components lateral to the anterior clinoid, a pterional or orbitozygomatic craniotomy may be favoured, permitting better access to the supraclinoid component of the internal carotid. To access tumors with intraventricular extension, the surgeon can approach directly through the lamina terminalis, with the tumor often pressed against it [41, 42].

18.6.2 Endoscopic Endonasal

Given their anatomical origin, an endonasal approach is an oft-employed route by which to manage craniopharyngiomas. As such, a comprehensive understanding of nasal anatomy is a necessary tool in the armamentarium of neurosurgeons.

A well-vascularised, nasoseptal mucoperiosteal flap is the appropriate means by which to repair the surgical defect after an endonasal approach to CPs, which should be harvested prior to exploration and debulking of the tumor itself. After flap harvesting, the first step in an endonasal approach involves identifying and opening the ostium of the sphenoid sinus, usually at the medial aspect of the superior turbinate. After opening the sphenoid rostrum, the sphenoidotomy is widened, and accessing the anterior skull base is most often performed with a drill. The degree of bony work can be titrated according to the extent of exposure required, with large tumors necessitating removal of the sella, tuberculum sella, and entire planum sphenoidale in some instances. Following durotomy, meticulous inspection of the surrounding neurovascular structures is necessary, as even vessels that appear to be superfluous at first glance may constitute the vascular supply of either the chiasm or pituitary. The heterogeneity of craniopharyngioma consistency makes each operation unique, with solid component debulking and cyst decompression both usually required along the way. To facilitate collapse of the tumor onto itself, an ultrasonic aspirator is often employed to 'core out' the central tumor, before dissecting the capsule away from surrounding structures. It is during this planar dissection that particular attention must be paid to the hypothalamic–tumor interface, ensuring that any disease firmly adherent to or involving the hypothalamus is left in situ to avoid significant neuro-endocrine injury. The advent of angled endoscopes has enabled previously inaccessible endoscopic views, supporting surgeons in ensuring that all tumor tissue that can be safely resected is ultimately removed [41, 43–45].

18.7 Endoscopic Transventricular

Sixty percent of paediatric craniopharyngiomas have a pure or predominant cystic component. CP cysts, due to their location, tend to impinge or grow into the third ventricle [46].

In these cases, the main purpose of the surgical management of CPs is to treat the mass effect caused by the cystic portion of the tumor. Neuroendoscopy has been proposed as a less invasive approach for cyst drainage and fenestration. Hence, it allows a direct visualisation of the cyst wall, as well as wider fenestration if compared with blind techniques, while being less invasive than the microsurgical approach [47, 48].

Historically, CPs have not been considered the most suitable tumors for an endoscopic resection since they often have calcified portions. More recently, the availability of the endoscopic ultrasonic aspirator has opened a new possible path for resection of the solid portions of CPs in selected cases [49, 50].

18.8 Oncologists' Role

The effectiveness of radiotherapy (RT) in reducing craniopharyngioma recurrence has long been recognised, though much like surgery it is not without risk. Traditionally, adjuvant external beam radiation therapy (EBRT) has been employed following surgery for CPs, particularly for those in whom gross total resection was unobtainable [51, 52]. While EBRT is targeted at tumor residuum in order to minimise damage to adjacent tissues, such an impact cannot be entirely mitigated. Both stereotactic radiosurgery (SRS) and proton beam therapy (PBT) [53, 54] aim to further limit the dose of radiation delivered to adjacent structures, focusing instead on maximal dose delivery to target tissues. Whilst these modalities may present potentially effective alternatives to EBRT in the future [55], the current evidence base is yet to definitively identify either as superior [11].

The effects of radiation therapy on the developing brain are numerous and can be devastating in the long term [56]. In a patient cohort with an intrinsically high risk of postoperative morbidity, this may represent an unacceptable additional risk. Accordingly, UK guidance on the use of radiotherapy specifies that, when GTR is achieved, there is no benefit to upfront radiotherapy and its use may be deferred. While adjuvant RT following STR can achieve outcomes comparable to those of GTR, the timing of RT should be considered on a case-by-case basis to minimise radiotherapy-related risks, particularly in younger patients.

18.9 Long-Term Surveillance and Quality of Life

Despite their benign classification and overall excellent survival rates, craniopharyngioma recurrence is well recognised, with rates highly dependent on the extent of resection. Recurrence rates in those undergoing radical resection with adjuvant radiotherapy are reported between 11% and 17.6% [57–59] compared to between 28.5% and 42.8% [58] in subtotal resection. As a result, long-term neurosurgical and neuro-oncological follow-up is an absolute necessity for patients diagnosed with CP, with interval imaging usually performed at 3–6 months postoperatively, while further surveillance may be guided by MDT discussion and patient symptomatology. The need for protracted care for a benign tumor also extends to the rest of the MDT, including both ophthalmology and endocrinology. Visual deficits are historically reported to occur in as many as 75% of patients [60, 61], which, particularly during childhood development and schooling, are of the utmost importance to monitor to ensure adequate support is provided. From a developmental perspective, preserving hypothalamic–pituitary function is also critical. Any evidence of preoperative hypopituitarism is rarely corrected following resection of the tumor, and while surgery provides the theoretical benefit of preventing further deterioration, in real terms this is not without risk of causing deterioration in and of itself. Across the literature, postoperative panhypopituitarism ranged from 12.8% [62] to 67% [58], with over 94% of patients requiring at least one hormone replacement therapy in one series [63].

Ultimately, CPs necessitate an active approach towards long-term surveillance and holistic care. Regular clinical assessments, radiological surveillance, and endocrine monitoring are imperative to detect tumor recurrence, assess hormonal status, and address late treatment sequelae. Collectively, the MDT remains indispensable throughout the patient's journey, optimising quality of life and mitigating long-term disability.

18.10 The Future

In spite of advancements in both diagnostic and therapeutic modalities, craniopharyngiomas remain a challenging clinical entity, inherently associated with substantial morbidity. Ongoing research endeavours seek to elucidate the molecular underpinnings of tumor pathogenesis, unravel the intricate neuroendocrine interactions disrupted by tumor growth, and explore novel therapeutic avenues aimed at improving outcomes and minimising treatment-related morbidity. A recent systematic review summarised the landscape of novel therapies in craniopharyngioma, with a number of clinical trials evaluating novel agents targeting key signalling pathways, ranging from MEK and BRAF inhibitors through to pegylated IFN-α-2b and IL-6 inhibitors such as tocilizumab. While adverse events were identified in a number of cases, positive responses were seen in both adamantinomatous and papillary CPs, suggesting that the outlook for novel targeted therapies in CP is an optimistic one [64].

18.11 Summary

In summary, craniopharyngiomas epitomise the intricacies of neuro-oncology, requiring clinicians and researchers to continue striving for advances in care. With the advent of increasingly standardised and centralised care pathways, increased exposure to such complex cases will support future generations of neurosurgeons in their efforts to redefine therapeutic paradigms towards craniopharyngiomas and advance towards personalised, patient-centred care.

References

1. Momin AA, Recinos MA, Cioffi G, Patil N, Soni P, Almeida JP, et al. Descriptive epidemiology of craniopharyngiomas in the United States. Pituitary. 2021;24(4):517–22.
2. Yachnis AT. Craniopharyngioma. In: Craniopharyngiomas [internet]. Elsevier; 2015 [cited 2024 May 31]. p. 95–105. Available from: https://linkinghub.elsevier.com/retrieve/pii/B9780124167063000040.
3. Bunin GR, Surawicz TS, Witman PA, Preston-Martin S, Davis F, Bruner JM. The descriptive epidemiology of craniopharyngioma. J Neurosurg. 1998;89(4):547–51.
4. Clark SW, Kenning TJ, Evans JJ. Recurrent ectopic craniopharyngioma in the sylvian fissure thirty years after resection through a pterional approach: a case report and review of the literature. Nagoya J Med Sci. 2015;77(1–2):297–306.
5. Müller HL, Merchant TE, Warmuth-Metz M, Martinez-Barbera JP, Puget S. Craniopharyngioma. Nat Rev Dis Primers. 2019;5(1):75.

6. Hoffmann A, Boekhoff S, Gebhardt U, Sterkenburg AS, Daubenbüchel AMM, Eveslage M, et al. History before diagnosis in childhood craniopharyngioma: associations with initial presentation and long-term prognosis. Eur J Endocrinol. 2015;173(6):853–62.
7. Ohmori K, Collins J, Fukushima T. Craniopharyngiomas in children. Pediatr Neurosurg. 2007;43(4):265–78.
8. Prieto R, Pascual JM, Barrios L. Optic chiasm distortions caused by craniopharyngiomas: clinical and magnetic resonance imaging correlation and influence on visual outcome. World Neurosurg. 2015;83(4):500–29.
9. Nuijts MA, Veldhuis N, Stegeman I, Van Santen HM, Porro GL, Imhof SM, et al. Visual functions in children with craniopharyngioma at diagnosis: a systematic review. Awadein A, editor. PLoS One. 2020;15(10):e0240016.
10. Drapeau A, Walz PC, Eide JG, Rugino AJ, Shaikhouni A, Mohyeldin A, et al. Pediatric craniopharyngioma. Childs Nerv Syst. 2019;35(11):2133–45.
11. Gan HW, Morillon P, Albanese A, Aquilina K, Chandler C, Chang YC, et al. National UK guidelines for the management of paediatric craniopharyngioma. Lancet Diabetes Endocrinol. 2023;11(9):694–706.
12. Hoffman HJ, Silva MD, Humphreys RP, Drake JM, Smith ML, Blaser SI. Aggressive surgical management of craniopharyngiomas in children. J Neurosurg. 1992;76(1):47–52.
13. Elliott RE, Jane JA, Wisoff JH. Surgical management of craniopharyngiomas in children: meta-analysis and comparison of transcranial and transsphenoidal approaches. Neurosurgery. 2011;69(3):630–43.
14. Müller HL, Gebhardt U, Etavard-Gorris N, Korenke E, Warmuth-Metz M, Kolb R, et al. Prognosis and sequela in patients with childhood craniopharyngioma - results of HIT-ENDO and update on KRANIOPHARYNGEOM 2000. Klin Padiatr. 2004;216(6):343–8.
15. Roth CL. Hypothalamic obesity in patients with craniopharyngioma: profound changes of several weight regulatory circuits. Front Endocrin [Internet]. 2011 [cited 2024 May 31];2. Available from: http://journal.frontiersin.org/article/10.3389/fendo.2011.00049/abstract.
16. Vinchon M, Weill J, Delestret I, Dhellemmes P. Craniopharyngioma and hypothalamic obesity in children. Childs Nerv Syst. 2009;25(3):347–52.
17. Hoffmann A, Gebhardt U, Sterkenburg AS, Warmuth-Metz M, Müller HL. Diencephalic syndrome in childhood craniopharyngioma—results of German multicenter studies on 485 long-term survivors of childhood craniopharyngioma. J Clin Endocrinol Metabol. 2014;99(11):3972–7.
18. Johnson LN, Hepler RS, Yee RD, Frazee JG, Simons KB. Magnetic resonance imaging of craniopharyngioma. Am J Ophthalmol. 1986;102(2):242–4.
19. Harwood-Nash DC. Neuroimaging of childhood craniopharyngioma. Pediatr Neurosurg. 1994;21(1):2–10.
20. Puget S, Garnett M, Wray A, Grill J, Habrand JL, Bodaert N, et al. Pediatric craniopharyngiomas: classification and treatment according to the degree of hypothalamic involvement. J Neurosurg Pediatr. 2007;106(1):3–12.
21. Whelan R, Prince E, Mirsky DM, Naftel R, Bhatia A, Pettorini B, et al. Interrater reliability of a method to assess hypothalamic involvement in pediatric adamantinomatous craniopharyngioma. J Neurosurg Pediatr. 2020;25(1):37–42.
22. Zhang YQ, Wang CC, Ma ZY. Pediatric craniopharyngiomas: clinicomorphological study of 189 cases. Pediatr Neurosurg. 2002;36(2):80–4.
23. Borrill R, Cheesman E, Stivaros S, Kamaly-Asl ID, Gnanalingham K, Kilday JP. Papillary craniopharyngioma in a 4-year-old girl with BRAF V600E mutation: a case report and review of the literature. Childs Nerv Syst. 2019;35(1):169–73.
24. Brastianos PK, Taylor-Weiner A, Manley PE, Jones RT, Dias-Santagata D, Thorner AR, et al. Exome sequencing identifies BRAF mutations in papillary craniopharyngiomas. Nat Genet. 2014;46(2):161–5.
25. Yoshimoto K, Hatae R, Suzuki SO, Hata N, Kuga D, Akagi Y, et al. High-resolution melting and immunohistochemical analysis efficiently detects mutually exclusive genetic alterations of adamantinomatous and papillary craniopharyngiomas. Neuropathology. 2018;38(1):3–10.
26. Martinez-Gutierrez JC, D'Andrea MR, Cahill DP, Santagata S, Barker FG, Brastianos PK. Diagnosis and management of craniopharyngiomas in the era of genomics and targeted therapy. FOC. 2016;41(6):E2.
27. Buslei R, Nolde M, Hofmann B, Meissner S, Eyupoglu IY, Siebzehnrübl F, et al. Common mutations of β-catenin in adamantinomatous craniopharyngiomas but not in other tumours originating from the sellar region. Acta Neuropathol. 2005;109(6):589–97.
28. Hölsken A, Buchfelder M, Fahlbusch R, Blümcke I, Buslei R. Tumour cell migration in adamantinomatous craniopharyngiomas is promoted by activated Wnt-signalling. Acta Neuropathol. 2010;119(5):631–9.
29. Gaston-Massuet C, Andoniadou CL, Signore M, Jayakody SA, Charolidi N, Kyeyune R, et al. Increased Wingless (*Wnt*) signaling in pituitary progenitor/stem cells gives rise to pituitary tumors in mice and humans. Proc Natl Acad Sci USA. 2011;108(28):11482–7.
30. Hölsken A, Sill M, Merkle J, Schweizer L, Buchfelder M, Flitsch J, et al. Adamantinomatous and papillary craniopharyngiomas are characterized by distinct epigenomic as well as mutational and transcriptomic profiles. Acta Neuropathol Commun. 2016;4(1):20.
31. Gump JM, Donson AM, Birks DK, Amani VM, Rao KK, Griesinger AM, et al. Identification of targets for rational pharmacological therapy in childhood craniopharyngioma. Acta Neuropathol Commun. 2015;3(1):30.
32. Donson AM, Apps J, Griesinger AM, Amani V, Witt DA, Anderson RCE, et al. Molecular analyses reveal inflammatory mediators in the solid component and cyst fluid of human adamantinomatous

craniopharyngioma. J Neuropathol Exp Neurol. 2017;76(9):779–88.

33. Miller DC. Pathology of craniopharyngiomas: clinical import of pathological findings. Pediatr Neurosurg. 1994;21(1):11–7.
34. Zada G, Lin N, Ojerholm E, Ramkissoon S, Laws ER. Craniopharyngioma and other cystic epithelial lesions of the sellar region: a review of clinical, imaging, and histopathological relationships. Neurosurg Focus. 2010;28(4):E4.
35. Crotty TB, Scheithauer BW, Young WF, Davis DH, Shaw EG, Miller GM, et al. Papillary craniopharyngioma: a clinicopathological study of 48 cases. J Neurosurg. 1995;83(2):206–14.
36. Rahmathulla G, Barnett G. Minimally invasive management of adult craniopharyngiomas: an analysis of our series and review of literature. Surg Neurol Int. 2013;4(7):411.
37. Thompson D, Aquilina K. Surgical approaches. In: Craniopharyngiomas [internet]. Elsevier; 2015 [cited 2024 May 31]. p. 259–70. Available from: https://linkinghub.elsevier.com/retrieve/pii/B9780124167063000167.
38. Flitsch J, Müller HL, Burkhardt T. Surgical strategies in childhood craniopharyngioma. Front Endocrin [Internet] 2011 [cited 2024 May 31];2. Available from: http://journal.frontiersin.org/article/10.3389/fendo.2011.00096/abstract.
39. Mallucci C, Pizer B, Blair J, Didi M, Doss A, Upadrasta S, et al. Management of craniopharyngioma: the Liverpool experience following the introduction of the CCLG guidelines. Introducing a new risk assessment grading system. Childs Nerv Syst. 2012;28(8):1181–92.
40. Yang L, Xie S, Tang B, Wu X, Tong Z, Fang C, et al. Hypothalamic injury patterns after resection of craniopharyngiomas and correlation to tumor origin: a study based on endoscopic observation. Cancer Med. 2020;9(23):8950–61.
41. Cappabianca P, Maria Cavallo L, Solari D, Di Somma A, Del Basso De Caro ML. Surgical approaches. In: Craniopharyngiomas [internet]. Elsevier; 2015 [cited 2024 May 31]. p. 137–53. Available from: https://linkinghub.elsevier.com/retrieve/pii/B9780124167063000076.
42. Mortini P, Gagliardi F, Bailo M, Losa M. Surgical approach to craniopharyngiomas: transcranial routes. In: Lania A, Spada A, Lasio G, editors. Diagnosis and management of craniopharyngiomas [internet]. Cham: Springer International Publishing; 2016 [cited 2024 May 31]. p. 85–99. Available from: https://link.springer.com/10.1007/978-3-319-22297-4_5.
43. Hong CS, Omay SB. The role of surgical approaches in the multi-modal management of adult craniopharyngiomas. Curr Oncol. 2022;29(3):1408–21.
44. Cavallo LM, Solari D, Esposito F, Villa A, Minniti G, Cappabianca P. The role of the endoscopic endonasal route in the management of craniopharyngiomas. World Neurosurg. 2014;82(6):S32–40.
45. Baldauf J, Hosemann W, Schroeder HWS. Endoscopic endonasal approach for craniopharyngiomas. Neurosurg Clin N Am. 2015;26(3):363–75.
46. Delitala A, Brunori A, Chiappetta F. Purely neuroendoscopic transventricular management of cystic craniopharyngiomas. Childs Nerv Syst. 2004;20(11–12):858–62.
47. Nakahara Y, Koga H, Maeda K, Takagi M, Tabuchi K. Neuroendoscopic transventricular surgery for suprasellar cystic mass lesions such as cystic craniopharyngioma and Rathke cleft cyst. Neurol Med Chir(Tokyo). 2004;44(8):408–15.
48. Abdullah J, Caemaert J. Endoscopic management of craniopharyngiomas: a review of 3 cases. Minim Invasive Neurosurg. 1995;38(02):79–84.
49. Cinalli G, Spennato P, Cianciulli E, Fiorillo A, Di Maio S, Maggi G. The role of transventricular neuroendoscopy in the management of craniopharyngiomas: three patient reports and review of the literature. J Pediatr Endocrinol Metab. 2006;19(Suppl 1):341–54.
50. Cinalli G, Imperato A, Mirone G, Di Martino G, Nicosia G, Ruggiero C, et al. Initial experience with endoscopic ultrasonic aspirator in purely neuroendoscopic removal of intraventricular tumors. J Neurosurg Pediatr. 2017;19(3):325–32.
51. Iannalfi A, Fragkandrea I, Brock J, Saran F. Radiotherapy in craniopharyngiomas. Clin Oncol. 2013;25(11):654–67.
52. Clark AJ, Cage TA, Aranda D, Parsa AT, Sun PP, Auguste KI, et al. A systematic review of the results of surgery and radiotherapy on tumor control for pediatric craniopharyngioma. Childs Nerv Syst. 2013;29(2):231–8.
53. Beltran C, Roca M, Merchant TE. On the benefits and risks of proton therapy in pediatric craniopharyngioma. Int J Radiat Oncol Biol Phys. 2012;82(2):e281–7.
54. Boehling NS, Grosshans DR, Bluett JB, Palmer MT, Song X, Amos RA, et al. Dosimetric comparison of three-dimensional conformal proton radiotherapy, intensity-modulated proton therapy, and intensity-modulated radiotherapy for treatment of pediatric craniopharyngiomas. Int J Radiat Oncol Biol Phys. 2012;82(2):643–52.
55. Kamogawa M, Shuto T, Matsunaga S. Effects of two different radiotherapies for craniopharyngiomas using stereotactic radiosurgery/ stereotactic radiotherapy or fractionated stereotactic radiotherapy. Surg Neurol Int. 2022;13:563.
56. Duffner PK. Long-term effects of radiation therapy on cognitive and endocrine function in children with leukemia and brain tumors. Neurologist. 2004;10(6):293–310.
57. Tomei G, Bello L, Sganzerla E, Ambrosi B, Re T, Barilari MG, et al. Long-term results of treatment for craniopharyngioma in children. Childs Nerv Syst. 1997;13(7):397–405.
58. Jane JA, Kiehna E, Payne SC, Early SV, Laws ER. Early outcomes of endoscopic transsphenoidal surgery for adult craniopharyngiomas. Neurosurg Focus. 2010;28(4):E9.

59. Fahlbusch R, Honegger J, Paulus W, Huk W, Buchfelder M. Surgical treatment of craniopharyngiomas: experience with 168 patients. J Neurosurg. 1999;90(2):237–50.
60. Laws ER. Transsphenoidal microsurgery in the management of craniopharyngioma. J Neurosurg. 1980;52(5):661–6.
61. Yaşargil MG, Curcic M, Kis M, Siegenthaler G, Teddy PJ, Roth P. Total removal of craniopharyngiomas: approaches and long-term results in 144 patients. J Neurosurg. 1990;73(1):3–11.
62. Dusick JR, Esposito F, Kelly DF, Cohan P, DeSalles A, Becker DP, et al. The extended direct endonasal transsphenoidal approach for non-adenomatous suprasellar tumors. J Neurosurg. 2005;102(5):832–41.
63. Miao Y, Fan K, Peng X, Li S, Chen J, Bai RN, et al. Postoperative hypothalamic-pituitary dysfunction and long-term hormone replacement in patients with childhood-onset craniopharyngioma. Front Endocrinol. 2023;14:1241145.
64. Agosti E, Zeppieri M, Antonietti S, Piazza A, Ius T, Fontanella MM, et al. Advancing craniopharyngioma management: a systematic review of current targeted therapies and future perspectives. IJMS. 2024;25(2):723.

Choroid Plexus Tumors

19

Carla De Luca Picione, Maria Elena Errico, Carmela Russo, Pietro Spennato, Serena De' Santi, Lucia De Martino, Stefania Picariello, Eugenio Covelli, Vittoria Donofrio, Giuseppe Cinalli, and Lucia Quaglietta

19.1 Background and Epidemiology

Choroid plexus tumors (CPTs) are rare, highly vascularized neoplasms that originate from the choroid plexus. The choroid plexus is located inside the ventricular system, attached to its walls. Its typical structure is lobulated and "cauliflower-like," with a central highly vascularized stroma surrounded by neuroectoderm-derived cells [102]. The choroid plexus has multiple functions: producing cerebrospinal fluid (CSF), maintaining the blood–CSF barrier, and secreting growth factors. Unlike the adjacent choroid plexus epithelial cells that have tight junctions, the fenestrated endothelial cells of the choroid plexus capillaries allow free movement of small molecules through fenestration [60].

The choroid plexus is present in all the ventricular cavities. There is a tight attachment between the ventricular wall and the choroid plexus, and through this attachment, vascular loops enter the epithelium of the choroid plexus. The attachment of the choroid plexus to the ventricle wall forms the taenia choroidea, which is a linear structure on the ventricular wall. Other parts of the choroid plexus move freely within the CSF [58].

CPTs include low-grade choroid plexus papilloma (CPPCNS WHO grade 1), intermediate-grade atypical choroid plexus papilloma, characterized by increased mitotic activity (APPCNS WHO grade 2), and high-grade choroid plexus carcinoma, which display clear signs of malignancy (CPCCNS WHO grade 3) [49]. The age-standardized incidence rate is 1.0 per million, with an incidence peak in the first year of life at 6.1 per million [40]. They represent only 0.2% of all CNS tumors, but are relatively more frequent in pediatric age (in which they represent up to 2% of CNS tumors) and even more so in children younger than 5 years of age (5% of all CNS tumors) and in the first year of life (12–20% of all tumors) [7, 65]. CPTs comprise 7.9% of prenatally diagnosed fetal brain tumors [58]. The median age of onset is 3.5 years, with 20% of patients presenting in the first year of life and

C. De Luca Picione · L. De Martino · S. Picariello · L. Quaglietta (✉)
Neuro-Oncology Unit, Department of Pediatric Hematology, Oncology and Cell Therapy, Santobono-Pausilipon Children's Hospital, Naples, Italy
e-mail: l.quaglietta@santobonopausilipon.it

M. E. Errico · V. Donofrio
Pathology Unit, Department of Health Services, Santobono-Pausilipon Children's Hospital, Naples, Italy

C. Russo · E. Covelli
Neuroradiology Unit, Department of Pediatric Neuroscience and Rehabilitation, Santobono-Pausilipon Children's Hospital, Naples, Italy

P. Spennato · S. D. Santi · G. Cinalli
Neurosurgery Unit, Department of Pediatric Neuroscience and Rehabilitation, Santobono-Pausilipon Children's Hospital, Naples, Italy

A. Mastronuzzi, A. Carai (eds.), *Navigating Pediatric Brain Tumors*,
https://doi.org/10.1007/978-3-032-18992-9_19

almost 50% in the first decade [18]. While CPPs are more evenly distributed throughout all pediatric age groups, the great majority of CPCs occur in very young children (usually in children less than 3 years of age). When relating malignancy to location, CPCs are more frequent in the lateral ventricles [103]. More than 10% of patients present with metastatic disease. The metastases occur predominantly along the cerebrospinal fluid pathways, even if other sites, including abdomen, bone, and lung, have been reported [103]. Choroid plexus tumors, in particular carcinomas, are more frequent in patients affected by a cancer-predisposing syndrome, such as Li–Fraumeni syndrome [64].

19.2 Genetics, Immunology, and Molecular Biology

19.2.1 Genetics of Choroid Plexus Tumors

The majority of CPTs occur sporadically; however, CPCs are strongly correlated with Li–Fraumeni syndrome (LFS), a classic cancer predisposition disorder caused by germline mutations of the TP53 tumor suppressor gene [44, 51]. The frequency of TP53 germline mutations in patients affected by CPC ranges from 26% [56] to 44% [89]. Rare cases of constitutional mosaicism are also on record [97].

Thomas et al. performed DNA methylation profiling, RNA-sequencing, whole exome sequencing, and linked-read whole genome sequencing in a large cohort of choroid plexus tumors. They showed that pediatric choroid plexus tumors lack recurrent driver alterations except for TP53, whereas choroid plexus tumors in adults show TERT promoter mutations and gain of chromosome 5 or, in one patient, a novel CCDC47-PRKCA gene fusion with underlying inversion on chromosome 17 [95]. While the majority of TP53-mutant choroid plexus tumors were encountered in the molecular subgroup "pediatric B," TERT promoter mutations resulting in new binding sites for members of the E-twenty-six (ETS) transcription factor family [38] were exclusively detected in choroid plexus papillomas (CPP and aCPP) from adult patients [95].

Patients with CPC and somatic TP53 mutations show more severe outcomes in terms of decreased overall survival (OS) and event-free survival (EFS) [89]. Thus, in a clinical setting, TP53 mutation status may be supportive of risk stratification of CPCs, and an accurate family history to rule out Li–Fraumeni syndrome (LFS) should be obtained.

Although likely pathogenic variants of SF3B1, ERBB4, ERCC2, MSH6, TSC2, and SMARCA4 were found in CPP and aCPP samples, variant enhancers associated with atrial fibrillation (VAFs) of the missense mutations (except for TSC2) were around 50%, and their potential role in the pathogenesis of CPTs needs to be determined by functional assays in the context of germ line testing, which was not available for the cases of the retrospective series [95].

Additional rare genetic diseases associated with CPTs include Aicardi syndrome, an X-linked genetic disorder characterized by agenesis of the corpus callosum, chorioretinal lacunae, infantile spasms, and high risk of developing (sometimes multifocal) CPPs. Cases of CPP have also been found in the context of Hypomelanosis of Ito with translocation (X;17) [88] and of CPC in a family with Lynch syndrome (hereditary nonpolyposis colorectal cancer) with MSH6 mutation [110]. Additional reports of familial clustering of CPPs also exist [112]. Cloning of the chromosome 22q11.2 breakpoint region revealed deletions of the SNF5 (INI/SMARCB1) gene, a member of the SWI/SNF (switch/sucrose nonfermentable) ATP-dependent chromatin-remodeling complex [98]. These patients are predisposed to malignant rhabdoid tumors when occurring in the CNS, but mutations in hSNF5/INI1 have also been associated with CPCs [41]. Recently, whole exome sequencing (WES) identified homologous recombination deficiency (HRD), amplification of mesenchymal-epithelial transition (MET), and loss of retinoblastoma susceptibility gene in two CPC patients [66]. Taher et al. performed Next Generation Sequencing (NGS) analysis of an aCPP, identifying 12 novel missense mutations in the following genes: NOTCH1, ATM, STK36, MAGI1, DST, RECQL4, NUMA1, THBS1, MYH11, MALT1, SMARCA4, and CDH20 [90]. Oliveira et al. investigated the occurrence of H3F3A K27M and G34R/V mutations in a cohort of pediatric tumors that included CPTs, and no H3F3A/K27M mutations were detected [63].

On a structural level, CPTs are characterized by an elevated degree of chromosomal imbalances. Early cytogenetic analyses have shown hyperdiploid chromosome sets in CPPs [17, 76] and mainly hypodiploid genomes in CPCs [61]. By using array comparative genomic hybridization (CGH), Rickert et al. have associated chromosomal imbalances of 34 CPPs and 15 CPCs with clinical follow-up [75], observing longer survival in the case of gains of chromosome 9p and losses of chromosome 10q. In a recent study including 26 CPCs, loss of chromosome 12q was significantly related to shorter survival on multivariate analysis, taking into consideration neurosurgery and radiotherapy [77]. Additional studies involving larger cohorts confirmed that CPPs and aCPPs are mainly characterized by whole chromosomal gains, whereas CPCs mainly display chromosomal losses [39, 96]. Recently, an institutional review of all congenital CNS tumors (surgical and autopsy specimens from 1990 to 2019), including 8 CPTs, identified, in 1 patient with CPP, loss of partial chromosome 1p, and gains of whole chromosomes 2, 7, 12, and 13, detected by NGS [99].

Interestingly, Merino et al. separated CPCs into two different groups of hypo- and hyperdiploid CPCs. Allele-specific analyses pinpoint that most hyperdiploid CPCs are characterized by acquired uniparental disomy (aUPD) of several chromosomes, with chromosome 17 (containing TP53 on 17p13.1) being most affected by this modification [56]. In summary, chromosomal imbalances occur frequently in CPTs, but it remains to be determined whether all these alterations are tumor-driving events or rather represent a passenger effect during tumor growth and progression. At the gene expression level, unsupervised clustering certainly segregates CPC from CPP and aCPP [39, 56]. In infants, CPP and aCPP have molecular similarities based on copy-number profiling, DNA methylation, and gene expression signatures, but aCPP shows higher frequency in newborns and in proliferation activity, suggesting that at this age aCPP may represent the immature variant of CPP but not a separate entity. Given that aCPP is related to recurrence only in older children (≥ 3y) and adults [92], underlying biological factors explaining these age-dependent prognostic variations in aCPP remain to be determined.

19.2.2 Epigenetic Profile of Choroid Plexus Tumors

Epigenetic dysregulation, including alterations of DNA methylation, has long been recognized as an important factor contributing to tumorigenesis and tumor maintenance. Moreover, specific changes in DNA methylation in small genomic regions can be considered powerful prognostic and predictive biomarkers [21]. In contrast, global DNA methylation alterations occur due to wide somatically acquired changes [21], while retaining features that reflect the cell of origin [23]. In this context, DNA methylation-based tumor classification has a substantial impact on diagnostic accuracy and allows the identification of clinically relevant subgroups [8, 36, 92]. Merino et al. demonstrated that CPPs and aCPPs in children differ from most CPCs on DNA methylation profiling [56]. In another series of 92 choroid plexus tumors comprising 29 CPPs, 32 aCPPs, and 31 CPCs of pediatric and adult patients, DNA methylation profiling revealed three epigenetically distinct and clinically relevant subgroups [93].

Tumors of methylation cluster 1 comprised CPPs and aCPPs characterized by young age and mainly supratentorial location, while methylation cluster 2 comprised mainly infratentorial CPP and aCPPs of adult patients. In contrast, all 31 CPCs were in methylation cluster 3 and were characterized by young age and mainly supratentorial location. Importantly, 14 of 32 aCPPs (44%) and 5 of 29 CPPs (17%) shared epigenetic similarities with CPCs and were also in methylation cluster 3. The majority of CPPs and aCPPs were encountered within methylation cluster 1 and methylation cluster 2. However, clusters 1 and 2 differed significantly by age and tumor location. Both methylation clusters also differed on the genetic level, with gains of chromosome 5 and losses of chromosome 21q being more frequently encountered in methylation cluster 2. While outcomes in methylation cluster 1 and methylation cluster 2 were favorable, the prognosis for patients in methylation cluster 3 was worse. In this cluster, which contained all CPCs and all p53-positive tumors examined, a total of eight tumor-related deaths occurred, whereas none of the patients in methylation cluster 1 and methylation cluster 2 succumbed to their disease. On multivariate analysis considering WHO grade, age, location, copy-number alterations, and p53 status as cofactors, WHO grade (but not methylation clustering) was the only independent predictor of OS, while WHO grade and p53 status remained the only predictors of PFS. Analyzing the prognostic role of methylation clustering according to WHO grade revealed that all recurrences observed in aCPPs occurred in methylation cluster 3, whereas none of the aCPPs of the low-risk clusters (cluster 1 and cluster 2) recurred. Taken together, these data suggest that DNA methylation profiling might be especially useful (and superior to histopathology) for identifying aCPPs at increased risk of recurrence [94].

DNA methylation profiling is becoming part of routine neuro-oncologic diagnostics [8] and is available as a web-based platform (www.molecularneuropathology.org).

In CNS tumor methylation classifiers of choroid plexus tumor, subclasses pediatric A and B represent methylation clusters 1 and 3, respectively, whereas the plexus tumor, subclass adult, is considered methylation cluster 2. Moreover, CPP and aCPP can be detected in all three methylation groups, while CPC cases are associated with methylation subclass pediatric B [92, 93], indicating that this classification is lacking additional molecular layers for CPCs. Pienkowska et al. generated a genome-wide DNA profile for CPTs to identify a correlation between epigenetic alterations and specific phenotypes [70]. They found significant genome-wide hypermethylation in CPCs in comparison with CPPs or aCPPs, but no difference was found between CPPs and aCPPs. They concluded that DNA profiling can distinguish severe and aggressive forms of CPTs from benign forms. However, further investigation in a larger cohort study is required before this result can be employed in the clinical setting.

Numerous studies demonstrated that microRNAs (miRNAs) may play important roles in regulating cancer initiation and progression [16, 63]. Redshaw et al. identified miR-449, an important regulator of choroid plexus development and function, suggesting that its dysregulation could be associated with tumorigenesis [73], but its contribution to tumor development needs to be better explored. Recently, Li–Fraumeni patients with CPT underwent a genome-wide DNA methylation analysis in CPT, showing that the hypermethylation of miR34a was associated with cancer susceptibility [78].

Recently, Granberg et al. detected moderate expression of fibroblast growth factor receptor (FGFR)1 or FGFR3 in one-third of the studied CPTs [31]. Targeted sequencing of a CPC and an aCPP, both with moderate-to-strong FGFR3 expression, revealed a lack of protein-altering mutations or fusions in FGFR1 or FGFR3, but TP53 was altered in both tumors. Deregulation of FGFR signaling is highly related to several human benign and malignant tumors. Further studies on larger cohorts of patients are essential to identify the clinical significance of FGFR1 and FGFR3 expression in CPTs.

19.3 Histopathology and Morphology

CPTs encompass a morphologic spectrum of neoplasms ranging from well-differentiated tumors to highly aggressive carcinomas. According to the current WHO CNS fifth edition, they are classified and graded as papilloma (Grade 1), atypical papilloma (Grade 2), and carcinoma (Grade 3); the classification, largely unchanged compared to the fourth edition, is based on architecture (preservation or blurring of papillary pattern), cellular density, degree of nuclear pleomorphism, necrosis, and mitoses (WHO Classification of Tumors of the Central Nervous System. Revised 4th ed 2016).

19.3.1 Macroscopic Features

CPP and aCPP are discrete, cauliflower-like masses, usually well demarcated from the surrounding brain tissue; the tumors are pinkish-gray, friable, soft, with a tufted surface, and granular texture; calcifications, cysts [68], and old or recent hemorrhages may be seen.

Carcinomas are fleshy, reddish-gray masses with variable necrosis and hemorrhage; adherence to ventricular walls, along with invasion into adjacent brain parenchyma, may be present in some cases.

19.3.2 Histology

Most CPPs show a basic architecture similar to that of normal choroid plexus, but with more cellular crowding (Fig. 19.1); they are constituted by papillary fibrovascular projections, covered by a variably pseudostratified layer of flat, cuboidal to columnar cells (Fig. 19.2); the cells have monotonous, bland nuclei, and abundant, eosinophilic, vacuolated or clear cytoplasm. Necrosis or loss of the papillary pattern is rarely found. Mitotic activity is absent or < 2 mitoses/10 HPF. Calcospherites and confluent calcifications may be present (Fig. 19.3).

On occasion, papillomas may show oncocytic change, cytoplasmic vacuolization reminiscent of signet ring cells, tubular-glandular architecture, focal ependymal differentiation, or neuropil-like islands [34]. Degenerative features may be quite prominent, including xanthomatous or mucinous change, angioma–like increase of blood vessels, formation of metaplastic bone, cartilage, or adipose tissue [13].

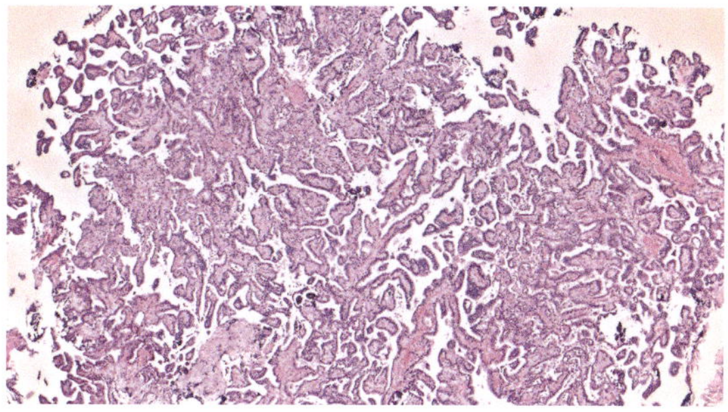

Fig. 19.1 CPP: distinctive papillary architecture; papillae are more irregular and complex than those of normal choroid plexus

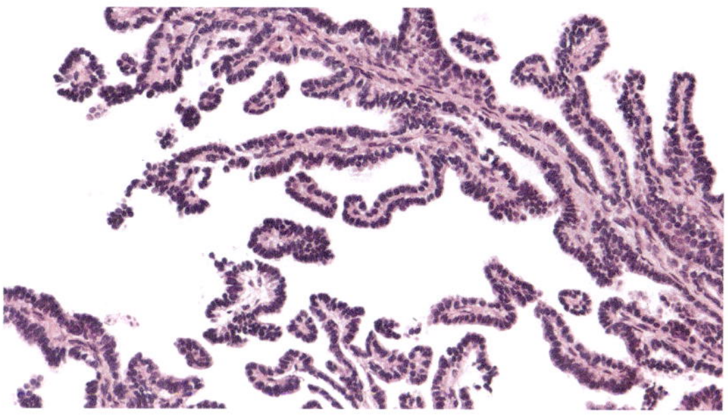

Fig. 19.2 CPP: finger-like papillary structures are lined by a single layer of cuboidal or columnar epithelium

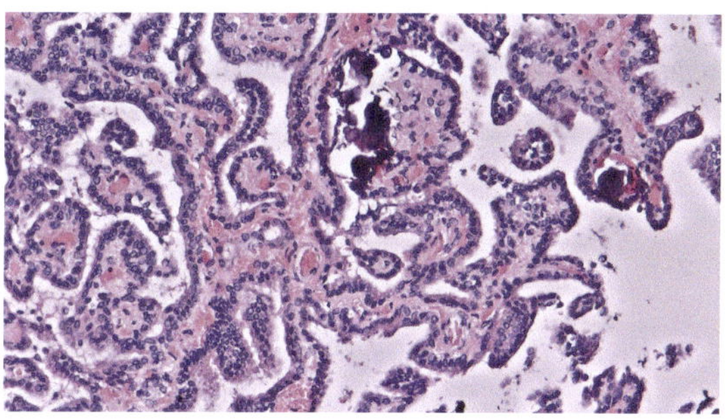

Fig. 19.3 CPP: the cells retain their polarity with basal, round nuclei and apical eosinophilic cytoplasm. Calcific concretions are not uncommon

19.3.3 Atypical Papilloma

These tumors show same features as papillomas (Fig. 19.4), but compared to CPP, demonstrate increased mitotic activity (2–5 mitoses/10 HPF) (Fig. 19.5); moreover, some of the following features may also be observed: increased cell den-

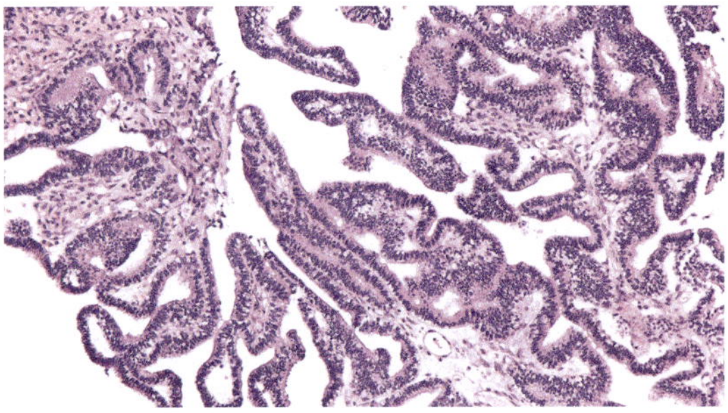

Fig. 19.4 ACPP: papillary architecture

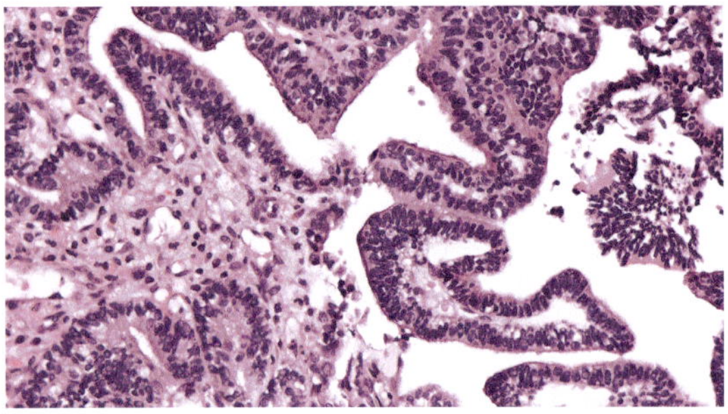

Fig. 19.5 APPC: cellular crowding, pseudostratification, and mitosis (arrow)

sity, moderate nuclear pleomorphism, blurring of papillary pattern, and areas of necrosis (Fig. 19.6). Complex architectural change, with cribriform and anastomosing papillary structures, may sometimes be found.

19.3.4 Choroid Plexus Carcinoma

CPCs are malignant epithelial neoplasms; according to WHO criteria, they must harbor at least four of the five following features: frequent mitoses (usually >5 per 10 high power fields), increased cellular density, nuclear pleomorphism, blurring of the papillary pattern and solid growth with sheets of tumor cells, and necrosis (Fig. 19.7). There is nearly always invasion of the adjacent brain tissue (Fig. 19.8).

These tumors show architectural disarray with sheets, complex glands, cribriform arrangement and only poorly formed papillae, and they display significant morphologic heterogeneity with

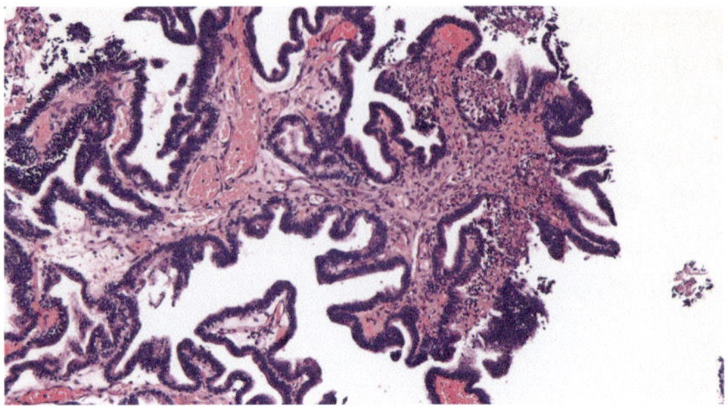

Fig. 19.6 ACPP: small foci of necrosis are present

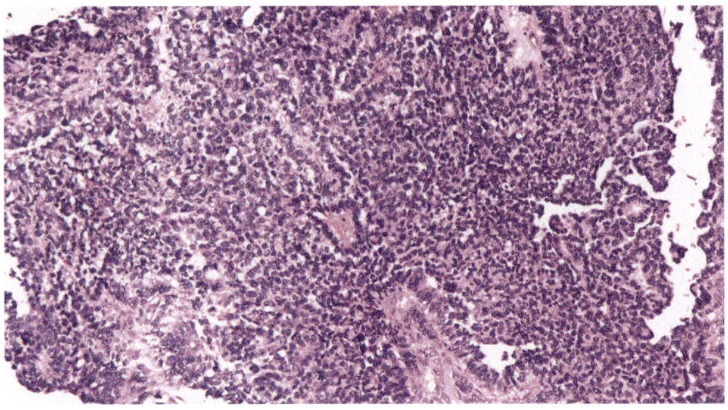

Fig. 19.7 CPC: blurring of papillary pattern, increased cellularity, and mitoses

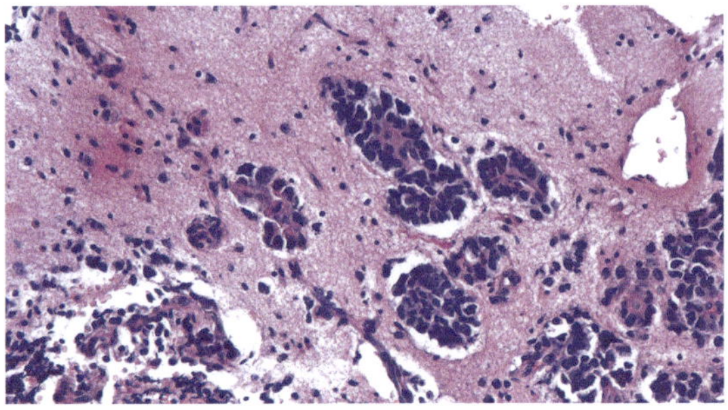

Fig. 19.8 CPC: area of invasion into the adjacent parenchyma

considerable variation in cellular size, form and degree of anaplasia (Fig. 19.9); both small cell with high nuclear to cytoplasmic ratio, and large pleomorphic elements with occasional features such as eccentric, vesicular, and nucleated nuclei, and abundant eosinophilic cytoplasm can be present (Fig. 19.10). Eosinophilic globules may be found in markedly pleomorphic areas (Fig. 19.11).

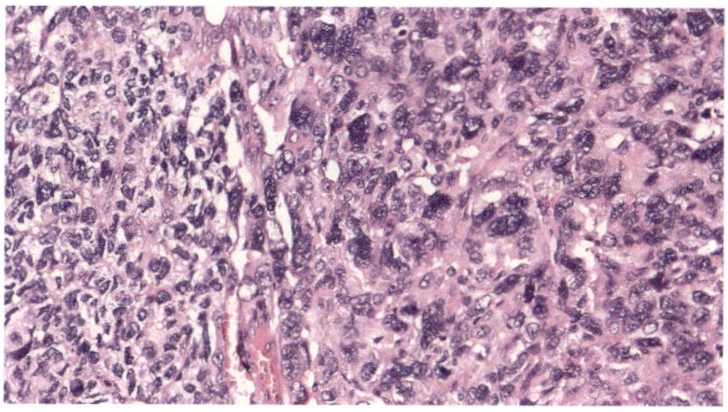

Fig. 19.9 CPC: high cellular and nuclear pleomorphism

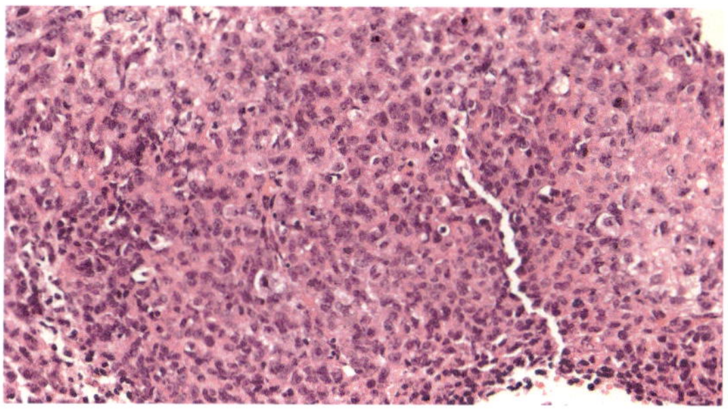

Fig. 19.10 CPC: solid, compact sheets of cell with rhabdoid morphology

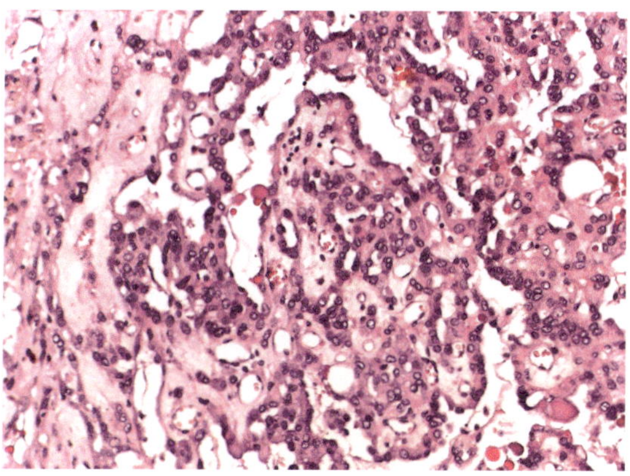

Fig. 19.11 CPC: hyaline globule may be present in cytoplasm-rich areas

19.3.5 Immunohistochemistry

Almost all choroid plexus tumors are immunoreactive for cytokeratins (CKs), usually panCK and CK7 (Fig. 19.12) and vimentin, whereas

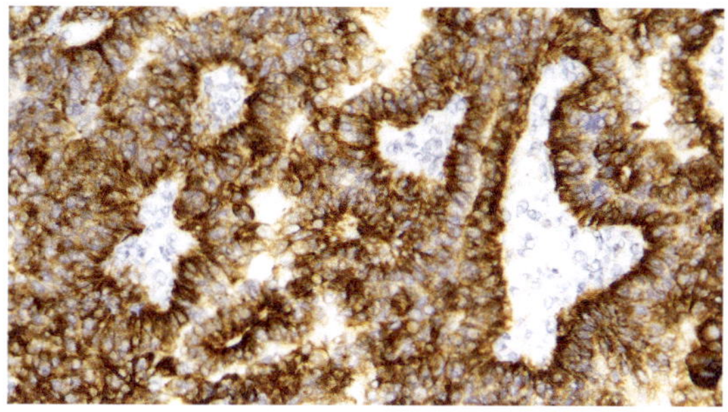

Fig. 19.12 Immunohistochemical stain for CKAE1/AE3 in CPC

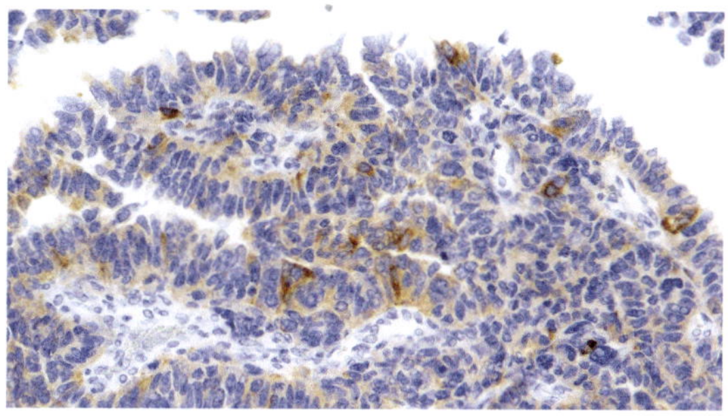

Fig. 19.13 Focal transthyretin reactivity in CPC

S100 protein and glial fibrillary acidic protein (GFAP) may show variable and weak staining, mostly in CPP; transthyretin, which is positive in normal choroid plexus cells, may be only focally expressed in papillomas and carcinomas (Fig. 19.13), as is also the case for synaptophysin. EMA and CEA are usually negative.

The MIB-1 (Ki67) proliferative index is typically brisk in choroid plexus carcinomas (>10–15%) (Fig. 19.14), while it is approximately 1–2% in CPP and 5–10% in aCPP [74]; the majority of carcinomas show nuclear accumulation of P53.

19.3.6 Differential Diagnosis

CPTs need to be distinguished from a wide spectrum of lesions, both neoplastic and non-neoplastic.

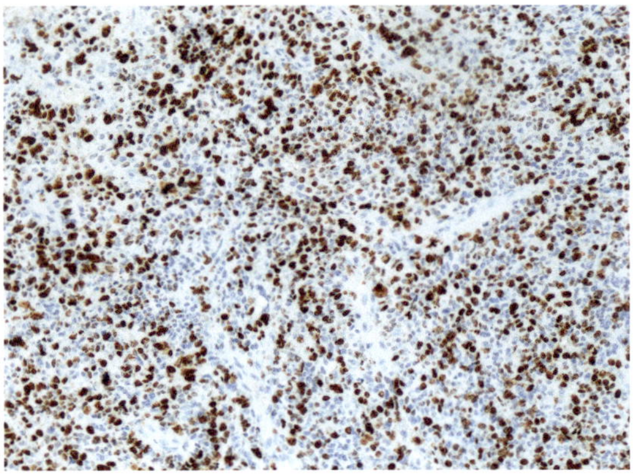

Fig. 19.14 CPC: brisk proliferative index Ki67

19.3.7 Choroid Plexus with Villous Hypertrophy

The papillomas must be distinguished from normal choroid plexus and villous hypertrophy of the choroid plexus; regular, uncrowded cells with cobblestone appearance, together with very low Ki67 labeling, should identify non-neoplastic lesions.

19.3.8 Intraventricular Meningioma

Whorl formation, vesicular nuclei, and syncytial cytoplasm, together with EMA positivity, help to differentiate intraventricular meningioma from CPP.

19.3.9 Ependymoma

CPP shares architectural features with papillary ependymoma, but the latter has perivascular anucleate processes and pseudorosettes, and immunohistochemically it shows characteristic dot-like positivity for EMA and in most cases for GFAP.

19.3.10 Anaplastic Ependymoma and Astroblastoma

Both these tumors may mimic CP carcinoma; lack of ependymal rosettes and perivascular pseudorosettes, absence of microvascular proliferation, lack of prominent hyalinization (typical of astroblastoma), and strong CK staining favor the diagnosis of choroid plexus tumor.

19.3.11 Germ Cell Tumors

Tumors like embryonal carcinoma and yolk sac tumor can be differentiated from CPC (especially tumors with hyaline globules); they are distinguished by characteristic immunohistochemical positivity for placental alkaline phosphatase (PLAP) and SALL4.

19.3.12 AT/TR

Atypical teratoid/rhabdoid tumor can be somewhat challenging to distinguish from poorly differentiated carcinomas of choroid plexus with rhabdoid morphology; the loss of nuclear staining with INI1 or BRG1, typical of AT/TR, reliably differentiates these tumors (Fig. 19.15).

19.3.13 Cribriform Neuroepithelial Tumor

Cribriform/trabecular growth pattern and distinct tyrosinase immunostaining, along with EMA positivity and loss of nuclear staining of INI1, distinguish these rare neoplasms from CPC [35].

19.3.14 Metastases

Especially in young adults, CPC must be differentiated from papillary or solid metastatic carcinoma; though CKs are not helpful in this setting, immunoreactivity with transthyretin, S100, GFAP, and/or synaptophysin positivity can be useful in recognizing choroid plexus tumors. Additional immunohistochemical stains may be needed in some cases, i.e., TTF1+ (lung adenocarcinoma), PAX8 and CAIX+ (clear cell renal cell carcinoma), etc.

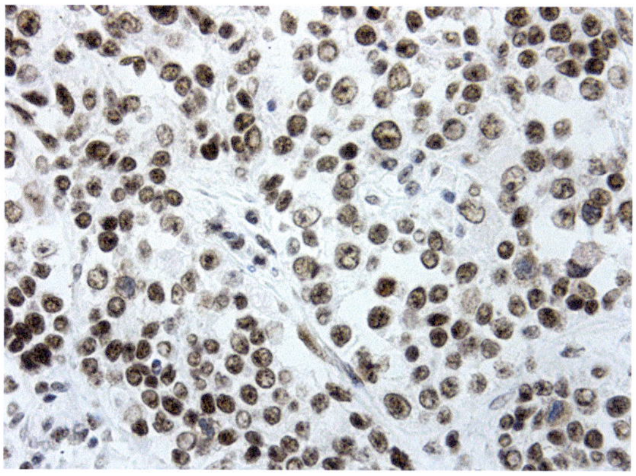

Fig. 19.15 Nuclear expression of INI1 is helpful in discriminating CPC from ATTR

19.4 Imaging and Radiologic Features

19.4.1 Overview of Imaging Features

A distinct radiological presentation characterizes CPT with a lobulated intraventricular mass displaying a frondlike pattern and intense enhancement, resembling a cauliflower [6]. However, imaging features of all three primary choroid plexus tumors may overlap, and so differentiating CPCs from ACPPs and CPP is frequently not possible on the basis of conventional radiological appearances.

Generally, CPPs are often well-delineated masses while CPCs frequently infiltrate adjacent brain tissue through the ventricular ependyma [5] and show necrosis, heterogeneous enhancement, and cystic components. Extensive edema in the brain parenchyma is suggestive of CPCs. CSF seeding is also more common in carcinomas [6].

19.4.2 CT Role and Findings

In the pediatric population, clinical symptoms of CPTs typically correlate with increased intracranial pressure. Despite concerns about radiation exposure, nonenhanced CT (NECT) plays a crucial role in rapidly assessing these tumors, identifying mass lesions, hydrocephalus, and potential complications necessitating urgent neurosurgery [47]. On NECT, CPTs typically exhibit heterogeneous features, with calcifications observed in approximately 25% of cases [47] (Fig. 19.16). CPPs are typically iso-hyperdense lesions with regular margins, while CPCs often display irregular margins, surrounding edema, and pronounced heterogeneity [5].

19.4.3 MRI Role

Contrast-enhanced MRI is the gold standard imaging modality for diagnosing and monitoring CPTs, providing superior soft tissue contrast without ionizing radiation [33]. Multiplanar imaging enables precise localization and assessment of tumor extent, while advanced techniques such as dynamic susceptibility contrast-enhanced perfusion-weighted imaging (DSC-PWI) and magnetic resonance spectroscopy (MRS) offer valuable insights into tumor biology [108]. Additionally, arterial spin-labeling (ASL) presents a promising noninvasive method for assessing cerebral blood flow in pediatric patients [108]. In conclusion, a comprehensive approach, integrating various imaging modalities, is essential for accurate diagnosis, treatment planning, and monitoring of CPTs in pediatric patients.

19.4.4 MRI Findings and Differential Diagnosis

Regardless of pathological grade, the choroid plexus tumors exhibit distinctive radiological features on MRI, often appearing as lobulated or cauliflower-like lesions, predominantly located in the atrium of the lateral ventricle. They appear slightly hypo- or isointense on T1WI (T1-weighted images), slightly hyper- or isointense on T2WI (T2-weighted images), and show moderately or strongly enhanced in post-contrast imaging [7]. Axial images often demonstrate a fan-shaped enlargement of the lateral ventricle, with some tumors connected to the choroid plexus by a vascular pedicle, which can lead to parenchymal ischemia. Diffusion-weighted imaging (DWI) and magnetic resonance spectroscopy (MRS) offer valuable insights into tumor biology, with lower apparent diffusion coefficient (ADC) values

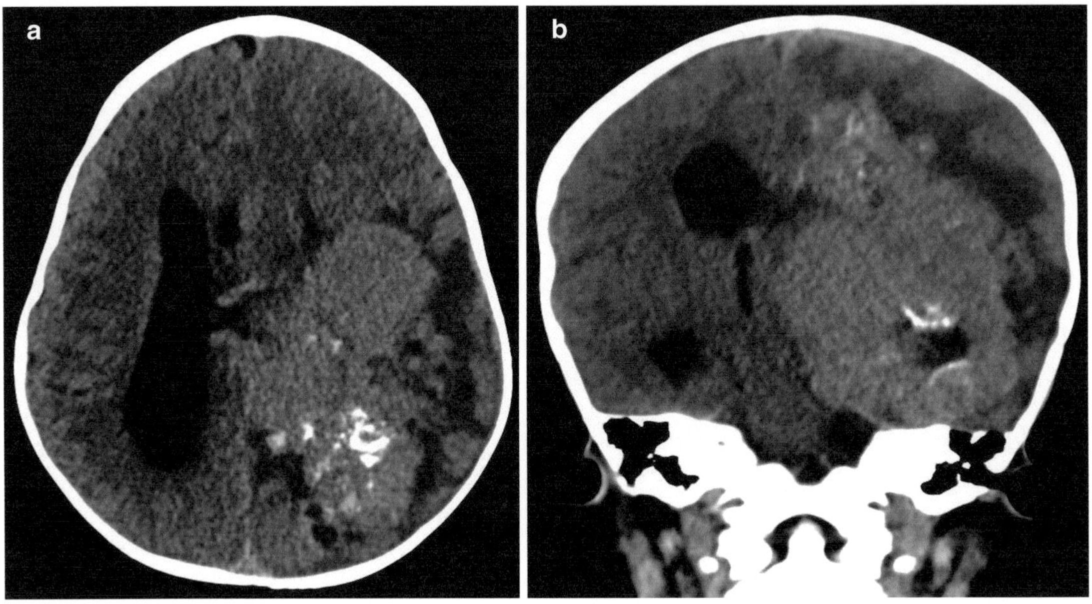

Fig. 19.16 Giant choroid plexus carcinoma in a 2-year-old baby girl. Axial nonenhanced CT images (**a**, **b**) show a heterogeneous mass from the atrium of the left lateral ventricle with some foci of hyperattenuation consistent with calcifications and some hypoattenuation due to cystic areas. Hydrocephalus is also present

(Fig. 19.17) and elevated choline (Cho) peaks associated with higher tumor grades and poorer prognoses [80]. Additionally, dynamic susceptibility contrast-enhanced MRI (DSC-MRI) and arterial spin-labeling (ASL) provide information about tumor vascularity, aiding in differential diagnosis and prognostic assessment [14]. Finally, diffusion tensor imaging (DTI) assists in surgical planning by delineating the relationship between the tumor and adjacent white matter tracts [111].

CPPs may be presented as intraventricular lobulated masses, homogeneously hypo- or isointense on T1WI. The central parts of the papilloma are hypointense in comparison with the gray matter on T2WI, even if CPP may be heterogeneous on T2WI when calcifications, hemorrhage, and flow voids corresponding to intratumoral vessels are present (Fig. 19.17).

Atypical choroid plexus papilloma can be difficult to differentiate from carcinoma on imaging. Generally, aCPPs tend to show smaller size, more regular margins, higher ADC values, and perilesional vasogenic edema, which are uncommon in CPPs (Fig. 19.17).

CPCs present as markedly heterogeneous lesions on both T1WI and T2WI, with areas of hyperintensity on T1WI possibly indicating hemorrhage and hypointense areas on T2WI suggestive of hypercellularity [106]. Marked enhancement and substantial nonenhancing components, often due to central necrosis, cysts, or hemorrhage, are typical features of CPCs (Tien, 1991) (Fig. 19.18). Other MRI techniques, such as susceptibility-weighted imaging (SWI) and T2*, are essential for detecting features like calcification or hemorrhage within the tumors [106] or associated superficial hemosiderosis (Fig. 19.19).

Peritumoral vasogenic edema, indicative of ventricular wall penetration and parenchymal infiltration, is characteristic of CPCs, but can also occur in CPPs and aCPPs [29, 91].

The differential diagnosis of CPTs can be narrowed down based on certain features observed on MRI. Ventricular dilatation, tumor conformity to the ventricular shape, and the presence of CSF outlining part of the tumor within a ventricle are suggestive of choroid plexus tumors. Choroid plexus carcinomas often present as large lesions with invasion of adjacent parenchyma and edema, which can make them challenging to distinguish from other aggressive parenchymal tumors like anaplastic ependymoma, atypical teratoid rhab-

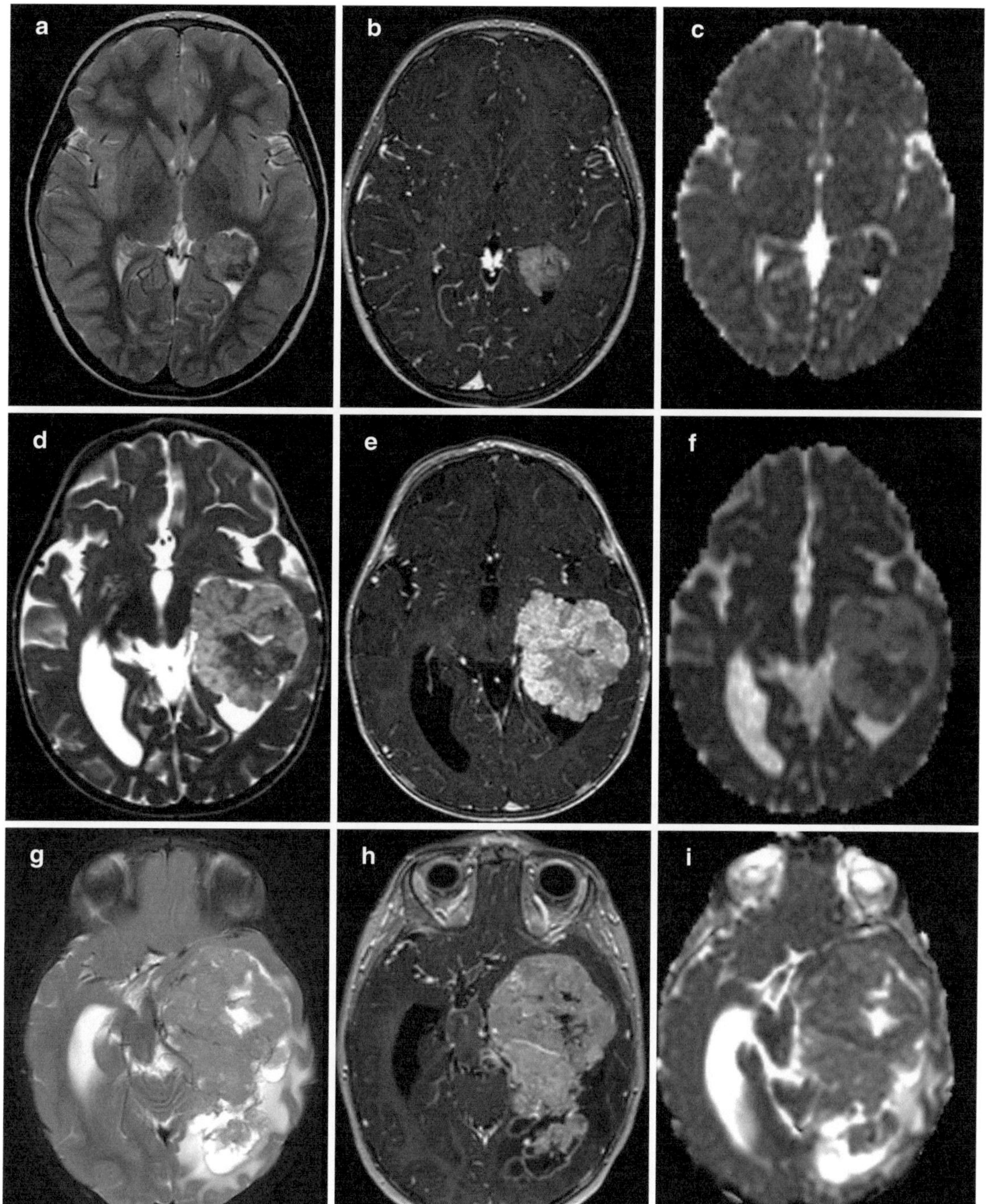

Fig. 19.17 Axial T2-weighted, contrast-enhanced T1-weighted sequences and ADC maps of three choroid plexus tumors: CPP (**a**–**c**), aCPP (**d**–**f**) and CPC (**g**–**i**). CPP and aCPP show smaller size, less illdefined margins and no perilesional edema compared to CPC. Note the differences in ADC values between the lesions with lower diffusivity of CPC (**c**, **f**, **i**), reflecting hypercellularity

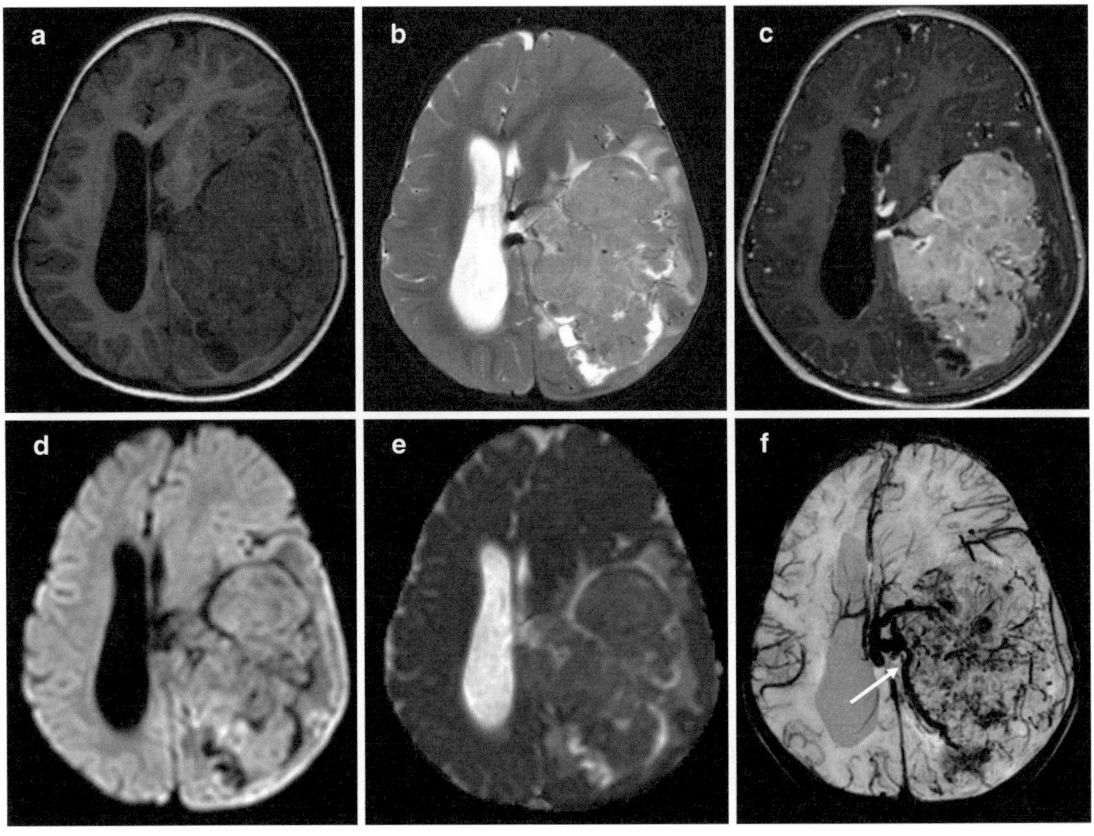

Fig. 19.18 Brain MRI study of the same patient of Fig. 19.16. Axial T1-weighted (**a**) and T2-weighted images (**b**) confirm a large heterogeneous mass with cystic and solid components arising from the atrium of the left lateral ventricle. Solid components show strong and inhomogeneous enhancement on contrast-enhanced T1-weighted sequence (**c**) and low diffusivity on DWI (**d**) and ADC map (**e**). Note multiple intratumoral microbleeds on SWI sequence (minimum intensity projection reconstructions, MinIP), as well as hypertrophy of left deep venous system (**f**). There are also perilesional vasogenic edema and obstructive hydrocephalus

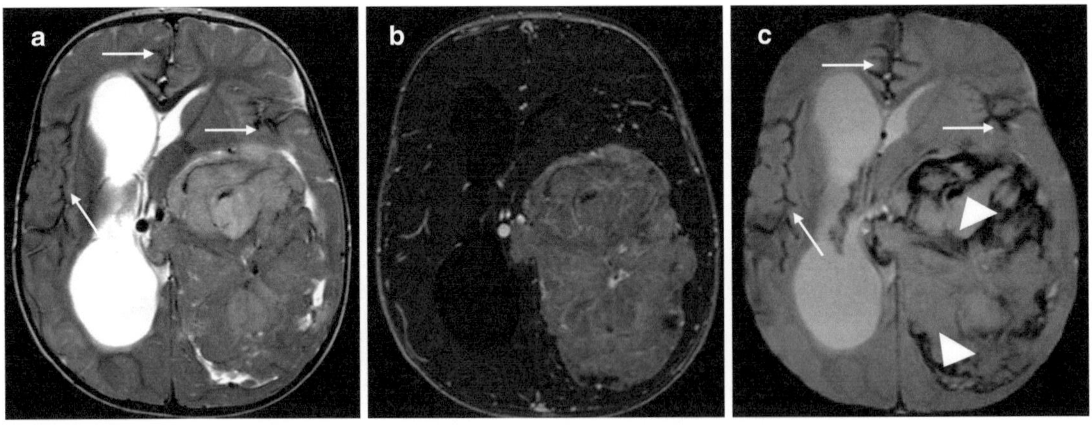

Fig. 19.19 Axial T2-weighted, contrast-enhanced T1-weighted and T2*-weighted MRI images (**a–c**) of a 1-year-old baby-boy with CPC. There are multiple foci of blooming on T2* (white arrowheads, **c**), reflecting tumoral hemorrhages and diffuse linear T2 and T2* hypointensities along the pial surfaces of frontal and insular regions (white arrows, **a** and **c**)

doid tumor (ATRT), or glioblastoma. Careful assessment of ventricular morphology, including the classic fan-shaped lateral ventricle dilatation, can aid in differentiation.

19.4.5 MRI Staging and Follow-Up

Cranial and spinal MRI plays a crucial role in the staging, monitoring of residual disease, and assessing treatment response in CPTs. Metastases can manifest as intraparenchymal or intraventricular nodules, particularly subarachnoid nodules, or less commonly as diffuse leptomeningeal seeding. MRI provides detailed anatomical localization of metastases, with post-contrast images and CISS sequences being essential for detecting small metastases, including ependymal dissemination and leptomeningeal seeding (Fig. 19.20). In some cases, complete resolution of leptomeningeal enhancement has been

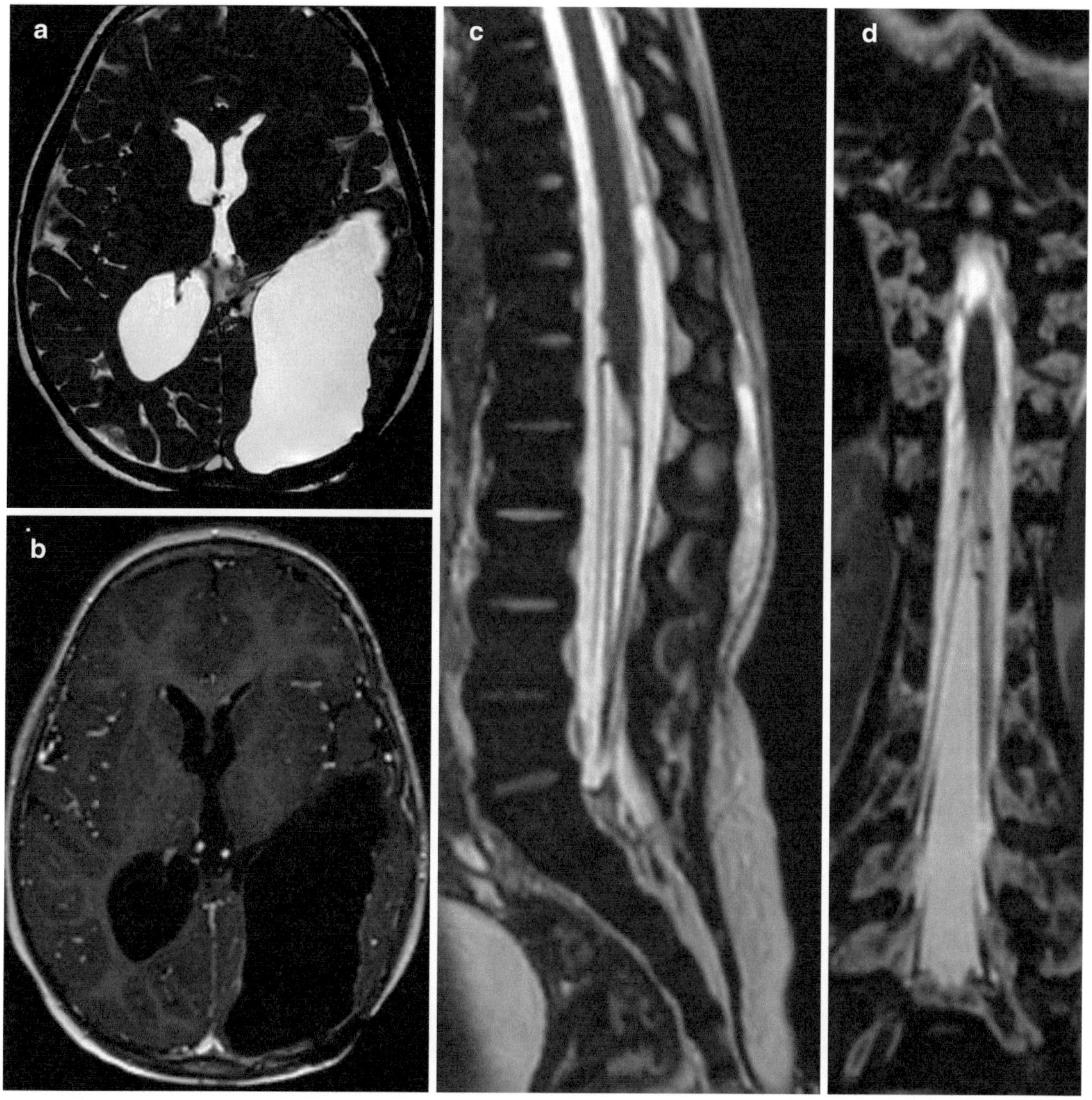

Fig. 19.20 Two-year follow-up MRI in a 4-year-old girl with CPC. Axial BFFE and contrast-enhanced T1-weighted images (**a**, **b**) show ependymal metastases. Sagittal and coronal MPR recostrunction of DRIVE sequence (**c**, **d**) demonstrate multiple micronodular lesions along cauda equina roots, consisting with leptomenigeal tumoral dissemination

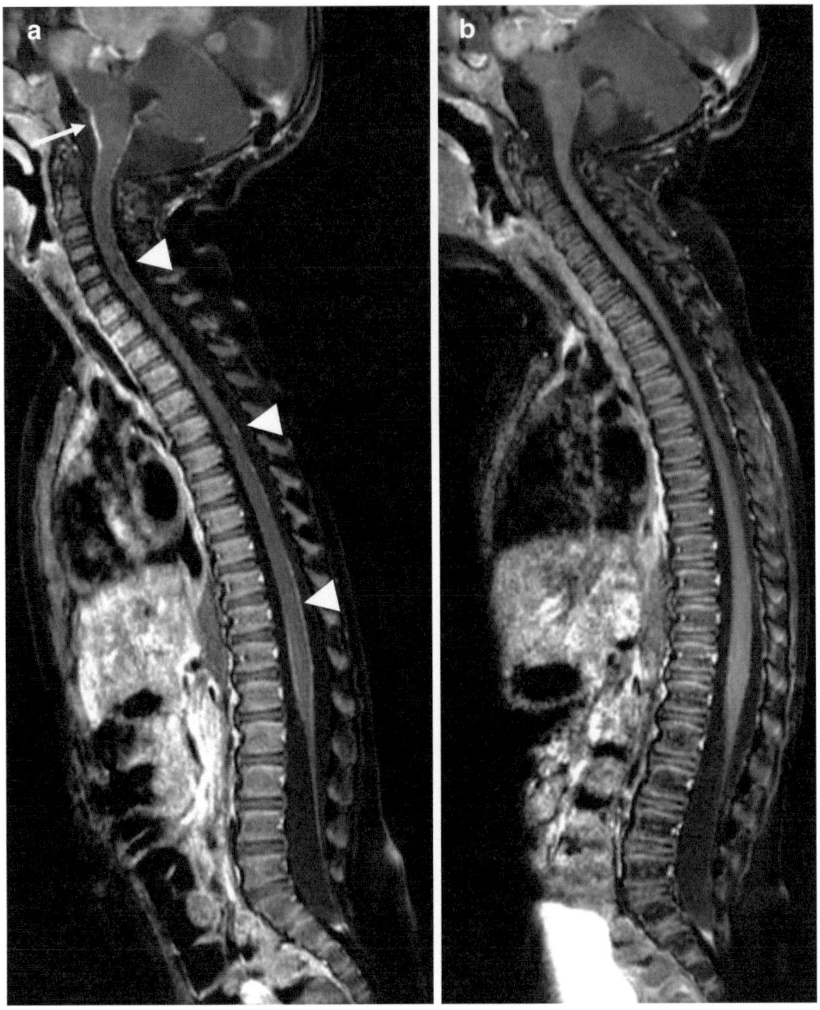

Fig. 19.21 Pathological enhancement along the pial surfaces of the brainstem (white arrows, a) and spinal cord (white arrowheads, a). One-week postoperative (partial removal) spinal contrast-enhanced T1-weighted images with fat-saturation show disappearence of leptomeningeal enhancement (**b**)

observed after surgical removal of the primary tumor, indicating a tumor-related effect rather than true tumor dissemination [81] (Fig. 19.21). In 2018, the Response Assessment in Pediatric NeuroOncology (RAPNO) working group proposed guidelines for the assessment of pediatric brain tumors with leptomeningeal seeding, including CPCs [101]. Objective response criteria include ≥50% volumetric decrease of all measurable lesions lasting at least 4 weeks, no progression of nonenhanced disease, negative CSF cytology, and absence of extra central nervous system (CNS) metastases. Disease progression is defined as ≥25% volumetric increase of all measurable lesions, significant progression of nonmeasurable disease not attributed to prior therapy, or any new tumor, with biopsy confirmation of suspected treatment-related lesions. These criteria can be useful in the follow-up of CPCs to evaluate their response to treatment.

19.5 Clinical Manifestations

Hydrocephalus is responsible for the presenting symptoms in most cases. Hydrocephalus was present in 78% of cases in the series of Ellenbogen [22], and in 95% in the series of Humphreys [37]. It can be caused by overproduction of CSF or, especially in the case of IV ventricle tumors, by obstruction of CSF [33, 110]. In the series of Zhou et al. [110], headache with nausea or vomiting was the most common primary presenting symptom (57.3%), followed by lower extremity weakness (46.9%) and ataxia (21.9%). Other common manifestations include visual impairment and papilledema. In children younger than 2 years, macrocrania, fontanelle bulging, irritability, seizures, and decreased level of consciousness are the most common complaints that lead to diagnosis [58]. A few patients present with hemiparesis or other lateralizing signs, usually as a consequence of asymmetric ventricular dilatation. In a significant percentage of cases (20% in the series of Zhou et al.), CPTs were incidentally detected [110]. The duration of symptoms before diagnosis usually varies from 2 to 6 months. However, the presence of stupor or coma as presenting symptoms was reported to be as high as 25%, suggesting acute decompensation. This can be secondary to massive hydrocephalus or intratumoral hemorrhage. Patients with tumors in the fourth ventricle tend to experience a higher incidence of acute hydrocephalus compared with patients with supratentorial tumors.

Zhou et al. [110] also noticed that patients with tumors in the fourth ventricle suffered from headaches at the early stage of hydrocephalus, whereas more patients with tumors in the lateral ventricle suffered from headaches at the late stage.

19.6 Surgery of Choroid Plexus Tumors

19.6.1 Preoperative Considerations

Complete surgical resection is curative for CPPs and significantly improves outcome for both CPCs and aCPPs [67]. However, CPTs are usually large, highly vascularized, and generally affect young children: the risk of intraoperative death secondary to hemorrhage is not negligible [33, 69]; therefore, patients with large intraventricular tumors, especially if they are young children, should be managed by an experienced neurosurgical and neuroanesthesiological team.

To reduce blood supply and intraoperative hemorrhage, preoperative angiography with embolization of the feeding vessels has been proposed, especially in cases in which the feeder arteries cannot be controlled at an initial stage of surgery. However, in clinical practice, unsuccessful embolization in CPTs is not uncommon: failure to cannulate the feeding vessels is the main reason [69].

Because most patients present with symptoms of intracranial hypertension secondary to hydrocephalus, the initial step is to decide whether CSF drainage is required [33]. In cases with a large cystic component, surgical drainage of the cyst may be an option. In patients with supratentorial tumors, the presence of ventricular dilatation may help microsurgical excision (especially papillomas): the tumors, in fact, are floating inside the dilated ventricles. On the contrary, in patients with infratentorial tumors, the presence of intracranial hypertension is detrimental for the surgeon. Therefore, if the patient, with a supratentorial tumor, is in a stable condition, it is better to schedule direct microsurgical tumor removal as soon as possible. However, if rapid neurologic deterioration is occurring or the patient is affected by a fourth ventricle tumor with significant hydrocephalus, treatment of hydrocephalus is required on an emergency basis.

Positioning of an external ventricular drainage (EVD) allows immediate resolution of intracranial hypertension. Usually, hydrocephalus resolves after tumor removal; thereafter, EVD can be removed. If it is necessary to delay definitive surgical treatment beyond a few days, a Ventricular Peritoneal (VP) shunt may allow time for the procedure to be performed electively [33, 69]. However, VP shunt should be used judiciously because metastatic seeding in the abdomen has been observed [54].

ETV should be reserved for patients with a fourth ventricle tumor and acute hydrocephalus, in which obstruction of the aqueduct or of the outlets of the fourth ventricle is evident. Resolution of intracranial hypertension facilitates subsequent posterior fossa surgery, decreasing cerebellar swelling and venous pressure.

Hydrocephalus can persist even after successful excision of the CPTs. In the series of Pancalet et al., 9 patients (24%) required ventriculoperitoneal shunt placement after surgery for persistent hydrocephalus (6/25 children with papillomas and 3/13 with carcinomas) [69]. In the series of Ellenbogen et al. [22], 37% of surviving patients required shunting.

Gross-total resection (GTR) is the goal of surgical treatment; it may be obtained by means of open microsurgical techniques or, in selected cases, by a minimally invasive endoscopic approach (via a single burr hole).

19.6.2 Microsurgery

Surgical approach is determined by the tumor site and its relationship with eloquent tissue (e.g., primary motor or sensory cortex, speech centers, visual cortex). Avoiding of eloquent areas and early control of vascular feeders are the most important factors in selecting the surgical approach [3].

Three main surgical positions can be used to approach intraventricular CPTs: supine position for most anterior lateral ventricles and third ventricle tumors; lateral position for trigone and temporal horn tumors; and prone position for occipital horn and fourth ventricle tumors.

Tumors located in the fontal horn, at the level of the foramen of Monro, in the anterior part of the body, and in the anterior third ventricle, can be removed via transcortical (crossing the cerebral mantle) or transcallosal (opening the interhemispheric fissure and cutting the corpus callosum, which is the roof of the lateral ventricles) approaches. Due to violation of the cortex, the incidence of postoperative epilepsy after the transcortical approach is higher than after the transcallosal approach. Another disadvantage is that it is more difficult to expose the contralateral ventricle. On the contrary, the advantage of the frontal transcortical approach is that with large tumors, the transcortical exposure provides better access to the tumor than the transcallosal approach. The frontal transcortical approach is facilitated in the presence of dilatation of the involved ventricle. The transcallosal approach may also be used in cases of small ventricles.

Neuro-navigation is of great help in this surgery (especially electromagnetic neuronavigation that avoids rigid skull fixation in young children). For both approaches, with the patient in supine position, a bicoronal or unilateral curvilinear skin incision is made. For the transcortical approach, a fronto-parietal flap is elevated and the dura overlying the middle frontal gyrus exposed, mostly anteriorly to the coronal suture. Corticectomy is planned along the long axis of the middle frontal gyrus anterior to the coronal suture and anterior to the premotor gyrus. White matter is dissected until the ventricle is reached. In many cases, the cortical mantle is thinned by chronic hydrocephalus. The length of the cortical exposure is extended as needed, and self-retaining retractors are placed to provide adequate exposure of the tumor. For the transcallosal approach, a bone flap that crosses the midline and the coronal suture (2 cm behind, 5 cm in front of the coronal suture) is drilled. The dura is opened in a U-shaped fashion with its base toward the sinus, making sure not to injure bridging veins in the subdural space. The falx–cortical interface is identified, and the hemisphere is gently retracted, dissecting the interhemispheric fissure. The corpus callosum is identified by its very white color and is incised on the midline for a length of 2 to 3 cm between the two pericallosal arteries, sparing the genu. Once inside the ventricle, the surgeon should check anatomical landmarks to recognize the anatomy of the ventricular system (foramen of Monro, choroid plexus, thalamostriate and septal veins). Regardless of the side of initial ventricular entry, it is generally possible to achieve adequate biventricular exposure by extending the callosotomy and fenestrating the septum pellucidum.

These two approaches may also offer a route to tumors of the third ventricle. There are three options for accessing the third ventricle: transforaminal, transchoroidal, and interforniceal. The anterior part of the third ventricle may be approached through the foramen of Monro, which is usually expanded by the tumor itself or by the concomitant obstructive hydrocephalus. Tumors of the middle and posterior third ventricle may be approached through the choroidal fissure. The third ventricle is exposed by opening the choroidal fissure along the tenia fornicis, beginning at the level of the foramen of Monro. The interforniceal approach is rarely used because of the risk of bilateral injury to the columns of the fornix and is reserved for cases in which a cavum septum pellucidum is present or the tumor has separated the columns of the fornix [43]. The septum pellucidum is incised (important landmark for midline union of the forniceal columns), and the raphe is identified at the site of septum attachment on the dorsal fornix. Incision is commenced at the level of Monro foramen and carried posteriorly not more than 2 cm: the third ventricle is reached from the roof, displacing the internal cerebral veins laterally.

For tumors located in the temporal horn and in the trigone, a transtemporal or transparietal approach can be used [3, 10, 107].

Once inside the ventricle, the tumor is exposed. The first goal is to identify and obliterate the vascular peduncle in order to minimize blood loss during the resection (the main blood source to such lesions is from the anterior and posterior choroidal arteries). If this is not possible, because of the large volume of the tumor, the capsule should be progressively devascularized with the help of bipolar coagulation, and the tumor should shrink. The use of intraoperative ultrasound may be helpful in order to inspect the surgical and ventricular cavity and verify the extent of tumor resection, together with neuro-navigation system surveillance. Also, endoscopy may be useful to control the entire surgical field. After tumor removal and accurate hemostasis, cortical or corpus callosum defects are closed with the aid of a fibrin adhesive and subsequent Ringer inflation of the ventricular system [57]. This should avoid cortical mantle collapse, preventing the development of subdural fluid collection.

CPTs of the fourth ventricle originate from the inferior half of the roof of the ventricle (where the choroid plexus is located). They tend to extend caudally through the foramen of Magendie and, more rarely, through the foramina of Luschka. Vascular supply comes from the posterior inferior cerebellar arteries (PICAs) [84]. Malignant tumors can invade the brain stem.

After adequate treatment of the hydrocephalus, the patient is positioned prone. Following midline skin incision, suboccipital craniotomy, and C1 laminectomy, the dura is opened in a Y-shaped fashion; the arachnoid of the cisterna magna is opened, and CSF is drained. Cerebellar tonsils are elevated and retracted laterally so that the cerebellomedullary fissure is exposed. The tumor (with its typical granular surface) usually appears at the level of the foramen of Magendie. The tela choroidea is incised to enlarge the foramen. Any vascular supply to the tumor from the PICAs is coagulated and cut, while the branches to the brain stem are preserved. The tumor is then detached from the inferior medullary velum, where it attaches. To avoid damage to the floor of the fourth ventricle, initial debulking is directed toward the aqueduct to identify the rostral part of the tumor. The tumor is resected using an ultrasonic surgical aspirator. To avoid postoperative sequelae, tumors attaching or infiltrating the floor of the fourth ventricle should be left untouched.

The first postoperative night and first postoperative day are spent in the Intensive Care Unit (ICU), with continued orotracheal intubation. Awakening is decided after post-gadolinium brain MRI, generally performed on the first postoperative day. Cortisone and antibiotic therapy are maintained for the immediate postoperative period. In cases of large clots in the surgical field or hemorrhagic infarction of the tumor residue, re-do surgery should not be deferred, in order to remove compression on the brain. In some cases, a decompressive craniotomy may be necessary to control intracranial hypertension.

19.6.3 Endoscopic Surgery

In selected cases, small intraventricular tumors may be totally resected through a minimally invasive transventricular endoscopic approach. Prerequisites for this kind of surgery are small size tumor (>3 cm in diameter), not hard consistency, and poor vascularization [11]. Some attempts at endoscopic removal of CPTs with vascularized lesions and a high potential for intraoperative hemorrhage have been reported in the literature. Meng et al. reported the first successful endoscopic removal of cystic CPP of the third ventricle in an 18-year-old patient [55]. Reddy et al. described a combined (endoscopic and microsurgical) approach to third ventricle CPP in a 6-month-old patient with secondary hydrocephalus [72]. Santos and Souweidane [79] and Sufianov et al. [86] reported a purely endoscopic surgical approach for the successful removal of solid third ventricle CPPs in two infants. These authors used conventional endoscopic instruments to dissect, coagulate, cut, and remove tumors. Early detection and control of the vascular tributary at the choroidal interface during endoscopic surgery should be the key to success. Our group recently reported endoscopic removal of two cases of tumors of the third ventricular choroid plexus [84]. The first case was a large aCPP associated with hydrocephalus; the second case was a smaller CPP without hydrocephalus. In both cases, an endoscopic ultrasonic aspirator was used. This tool made endoscopic surgery easier and faster. In fact, alternating surface coagulation with fragmentation and aspiration with the ultrasonic aspirator, the tumors were removed without difficult dissection maneuvers. Hemorrhage, which can obstruct endoscopic vision, can be reduced by continuous irrigation and keeping the tip of the ultrasound aspirator very close to the tumor. In cases of excessive bleeding, all CSF can be aspirated, and resection can be continued in a "dry field technique" as described by Oertel et al. [62].

Endoscopic techniques may also be used in cases of small residues of large tumors. A pure endoscopic transventricular approach may allow GTR, avoiding another major surgical procedure.

19.7 Chemotherapy and Radiotherapy

Given the rarity of CPTs, prospective randomized clinical trials are difficult to do, and treatments are based only on expert opinions and small case series. Therapeutic approaches are heterogeneous, including surgery, irradiation, and chemotherapy, such as myelo-suppressive high-dose chemotherapy (HDCTx) and autologous hematopoietic cell rescue (AuHCR) [105]. GTR is commonly reported as the most important predictor of survival, especially in CPC [25]. Based on the current cumulative literature and case studies, maximal safe resection and adjuvant treatment should be attempted. If GTR is not feasible, neoadjuvant chemotherapy may render delayed surgical resection more feasible. Management of incompletely resected aCPPs is questionable, considering that infants with aCPPs generally have higher event-free survival than older children with aCPPs, independent of adjuvant therapy, and hence, therapy de-escalation may be warranted in low-risk subgroups. Craniospinal irradiation as initial therapy for young children (<3 years of age) with CPC should be discouraged because of long-term effects in terms of neurocognitive outcomes and risk of second neoplasms. Radiotherapy (focal or craniospinal) should be avoided in children with germline TP53 mutations in the setting of LFS [109]. For the LFS cohort of CPC, further studies are needed to assess the role of intensive induction chemotherapy followed by myelosuppressive HDCTx and AuHCR versus conventional irradiation-free and alkylator-sparing therapy.

19.7.1 Chemotherapy

Due to the small number of enrolled patients in infant protocols with CPC, the advantage of using chemotherapy still needs to be studied and standardized; however, it has been suggested that chemotherapy may be beneficial for patients with partially resected CPC [9, 15, 25–27, 52, 71, 85, 104, 105, 109]. Different chemotherapy regimens were administered, including vincristine, etoposide, carboplatin, cyclophosphamide, doxorubicin, and high-dose methotrexate [24, 25, 48, 109].

In a literature review of 104 patients with CPC, the group who did not receive chemotherapy experienced significantly worse survival than the group with chemotherapy, even in non-irradiated tumors [105]. Fitzpatrick et al. showed a similar significant benefit of adjuvant treatment (irradiation with or without chemotherapy) for patients with CPC treated with less than GTR [25].

Children's Cancer Group study, CCG9921, randomized children <3 years of age affected by malignant brain tumors between two chemotherapy regimens following surgery with an attempt to delay irradiation [27]. Nine CPC patients were enrolled, of which 7 had progressive disease (PD); 5 within the first year with a 3-year PFS of 33% ± 16% and 3-year OS rate of 63 ± 17%. The UKCCSG/SIOP CNS 9204 trial utilized an intensive conventional-dose chemotherapy schedule and included 15 patients with CPC [32]. The health situation of 11 out of 15 patients following chemotherapy was improved, and their survival rate was increased. Only 2 patients had a GTR. The 5-year OS rate was reported as 26.7% (CI 8.3–49.6). The Canadian Pediatric Brain Tumor 2010 Consortium [48] also studied 16 children diagnosed with CPC who were younger than 3 years old. Fourteen of them had adjuvant conventional-dose chemotherapy. They reported that 10 of 14 patients developed PD at a median of 10 months with a 5-year OS rate of 31% ± 13.2%. The same group examined 17 children with CPC, and 12 of them received adjuvant chemotherapy with ifosfamide, carboplatin, and etoposide (ICE) and then underwent second-look surgery. The number of patients with GTR was increased from 2 to 9. Passariello et al. performed a retrospective study on 7 patients affected by CPC or aCPP [67]. In this series, surgery associated with sequential chemotherapy, including methotrexate and doxorubicin [24], led to long-term survival in 4/4 patients affected by aCPP and 2/3 of patients affected by CPC, suggesting that their therapeutic regimen was feasible and efficient as a possible adjuvant treatment for both CPC and aCPP.

The CPT-SIOP-2000 study (NCT00500890), the first intercontinental prospective clinical trial and the only randomized trial for CPT to date, included maximal surgical resection followed by observation for patients with CPP or completely resected aCPP and adjuvant chemotherapy for patients with CPC, metastases, or incompletely resected aCPP (six cycles of etoposide and vincristine, combined with either carboplatin or cyclophosphamide) [105]. Children >3 years old underwent irradiation after the second cycle of chemotherapy. Main outcomes (OS and EFS) of CPT patients were significantly impacted: 5-year OS and EFS were 100% and 96% in CPP ($n = 84$), 97% and 79% in aCPP (n = 88), and 58% and 35% in CPC (n = 76). Of note, infants (n = 22) with aCPP showed a better prognosis (5-year OS 100% and EFS 92%). Dissemination without local progression was observed in CPT patients on postoperative follow-up. The study group treated with carboplatin-based chemotherapy showed better results, while radiotherapy for CPC without LFS was associated with longer 5-year survival. Craniospinal treatment for localized CPC was not related to advantages. CPC infants ($n = 8$) irradiated after progression during chemotherapy demonstrated meaningful responses [46]. Using neoadjuvant chemotherapy to treat CPCs may contribute to decreasing the size and vascularity of the tumor and may be helpful in delayed GTR if incomplete resection or tumor dissemination has occurred [71, 85]. Schneider et al. investigated the role of neoadjuvant chemotherapy on the result of surgery, such as the extent of resection and intraoperative blood loss in pediatric patients with CPC [82]. A higher survival (38 vs. 6 months, $P = 0.01$), an increase in the rate of GTR (83% vs. 30%, $P = 0.03$), and decreased perioperative blood loss (22% vs. 96%, $P < 0.001$) were reported in those who received the neoadjuvant chemotherapy. It was concluded that the use of neoadjuvant chemotherapy in patients with CPC resulted in the reduction of intraoperative blood loss and an increase in the extent of resection, with a potentially positive impact on OS.

Final results of CPT-SIOP-2000 [104], an international registry for all CPT nesting a chemotherapy randomization for high-risk CPT with carboplatin/etoposide/vincristine (CarbEV) versus cyclophosphamide/etoposide/vincristine (CycEV), and the only randomized trial to date, were reported in 2022.

Patients older than three years received irradiation: focal fields for nonmetastatic CPC, incompletely resected aCPP, or metastatic CPP; craniospinal fields for metastatic CPC/aCPP and nonresponsive CPC. High risk was defined as CPC, incompletely resected aCPP, and all metastatic CPT. The registry enrolled 158 CPT patients from 23 countries from 2000 to 2010.

For randomized CPC, the 5/10-year PFSs of patients treated by CarbEV (n = 20) were 62%/47%, respectively, compared to 27%/18%, for children on CycEV (n = 15) (intention-to-treat, HR 2.6, p = 0.032). Histological grading seemed to be the most influential prognostic factor: for CPP (n = 55), the 5/10-year OS and the EFS probabilities were 100%/97% and 92%/92%, respectively; for aCPP (n = 49), 96%/96% and 76%/76%, respectively; and for CPC (n = 54), 65%/51% and 41%/39%, respectively. Twelve out of 33 patients with CPC younger than three years were alive for a median of 8.52 years without irradiation. The extent of surgery and metastases were not independent prognosticators. The study demonstrated that chemotherapy for CPC is feasible and effective. Standard chemotherapy for CPC is not yet established, although the results of CPT-SIOP-2000 showed that CarbEV is superior (for PFS but not OS) to CycEV; however, the number of patients randomized was low. In addition, a subset of CPC can be cured without irradiation.

19.8 Marrow-Ablative High-Dose Chemotherapy with Autologous Hematopoietic Cell Rescue

Intensive regimens utilizing chemotherapy and marrow ablative HDCTx with AuHCR have become the standard approach for the treatment of CNS tumors in infants and very young children in order to delay and possibly avoid irradiation, with its known profound adverse late effects [19, 20, 28, 59, 100, 109]. Zaky et al. assessed the effect of marrow ablation with chemotherapy in patients with CPCs, who received 5 cycles of chemotherapy and a single course of marrow ablative HDCTx and AuHCR. They found that 42% of the patients had no disease progression [109]. A retrospective study of 36 patients with CPC suggested that half of the CPC patients with TP53 mutation had a worse OS in comparison with not irradiated patients. This result confirmed the idea that tumor biology might influence long-term survival rather than the intensity of treatment [89]. Gozali et al. showed the outcome for CPC patients with and without LFS [30]. Three patients had TP53 germline mutations and underwent marrow ablative HDCTx followed by AuHCR, and all remained free of progression at the last follow-up between 12 and 84 months from diagnosis [30].

19.8.1 Radiation Therapy

Radiation therapy was reported to be beneficial in a variety of retrospective analyses, but its major limitation is the young age of patients with CPTs [25, 53, 103, 104]. Wolff et al. showed a significantly better 5-year survival of 68% for patients treated with irradiation versus 16% for those who were not [103]. Overall, the benefits of irradiation are more evident in subtotal resected tumors. A major deficiency of this analysis is not considering intent to treat, as some of the children in the nonirradiated group underwent palliative chemotherapy. Additionally, Dudley et al. did not show a statistically significant correlation between the use of irradiation and survival [18].

Of note, clinical studies on pediatric patients with CPC indicating advantages in terms of OS and EFS from radiotherapy may be biased by enrolling a higher proportion of relatively older children. Furthermore, Mazloom et al. observed better survival in patients who received craniospinal irradiation as opposed to limited-field irradiation [53].

This approach was adopted for patients with disseminated tumors or poor response to chemotherapy, while focal irradiation was proposed for those with nonmetastatic tumors with good chemotherapy response. Multiple issues remain uncertain concerning the respective advantages and disadvantages of adjuvant irradiation in this population, particularly in patients with germline TP53 mutation and a high risk of the second neoplasm. Survival for patients with CPC is also negatively impacted by TP53 mutations due to increased resistance to chemotherapy and irradiation [50, 89]. Bahar et al. investigated the impact of irradiation in 28 patients with CPC and LFS [4]. The survival of patients who did not receive irradiation was more favorable than that of those who received irradiation (2-year OS of 58% vs. 18%), suggesting a possible survival disadvantage with the use of irradiation for patients with CPC and LFS. This study had major limitations, which include the small number of patients, heterogeneity of treatment, and no statistical significance when the analysis was focused on upfront irradiation. Given the late toxicities in this population, including an increased cumulative risk for the second neoplasm, irradiation in LFS should not be pursued. Results of the CPT-SIOP-2000 study showed that patients with CPC without LFS had a benefit in terms of survival in the first 5 years of follow-up, while craniospinal irradiation did not improve survival for localized CPC [104]. In infants, delayed radiotherapy after the first progression during chemotherapy may have meaningful responses [46].

19.8.2 New Therapeutic Modalities

Revealing the molecular landscape of CPTs with the identification of multiple potential targets, including Shh, Notch, PDGFR, phosphatidylinositol-4, 5-bisphosphate 3-kinase (PI3K)-mTOR, and ATR inhibitors, may lead to better risk stratification and concrete opportunities for future therapeutic intervention. Tong et al. proposed that inhibitors of PI3K signaling (suppressed by PTEN) might also be used as new CPC therapies, as well as PI3K and mTOR inhibitors [96]. Furthermore, Tong et al. found three oncogenes controlling the epigenome and DNA repair in CPC. Using ATR inhibitors as DNA repair pathway inhibitors in vitro, CPC cells were observed to be remarkably sensitive to these drugs, indicating therapeutic potential in CPC. Additionally, PDGFR-b is functionally involved in the tumorigenesis of CPC and may represent a molecular target for therapy using tyrosine kinase inhibitors such as imatinib or dasatinib [45]. Recently, it was reported that the administration of bevacizumab, a humanized anti-angiogenic monoclonal antibody, in a small case series for progressive disseminated aCPP who had not responded to standard treatment, led to improvement of the disease [1, 2, 12, 42]. In the near future, epigenetic profiling may serve in detecting high-risk patients for recurrence and therefore could be the topic of future clinical trials in treatment stratification and clinical management of these patients.

19.8.3 Follow-Up and Prognosis

Maximal safe resection remains the mainstay for the treatment of these tumors, even though it is challenging due to their location, surrounding anatomy, size, and presence of hydrocephalus [83]. GTR has been recommended for CPCs with a five-year survival rate reported as 58% and 20% in cases of, respectively, total and partial resection. Intraoperative detection of brain invasion is, however, a predictor of recurrences. Indeed, the infiltrative growth pattern found in aCPPs, similar to that in CPCs, results in poor OS and PFS [87].

The extent of resection is important, also in cases of WHO grade I CPTs, for both pathologic confirmation and symptom relief with increased OS with respect to subtotal resection or biopsy alone. However, management of subtotally resected and recurrent CPPs and aCPPs remains controversial [109].

Since tumor recurrence has been observed up to 8 years after surgery, neuroradiological follow-up is highly recommended together with an MRI of the whole neuroaxis. Metastatic dissemination should be kept in mind in cases of CPCs; conversely, this is very rare for CPP and aCPPs [7, 103].

References

1. Abdulkader MM, Mansour NH, Van Gompel JJ, Bosh GA, Dropcho EJ, Bonnin JM, Cohen-Gadol AA. Disseminated choroid plexus papillomas in adults: a case series and review of the literature. J Clin Neurosci. 2016;32:148–54. https://doi.org/10.1016/j.jocn.2016.04.002.

2. Anderson MD, Theeler BJ, Penas-Prado M, Groves MD, Yung WKA. Bevacizumab use in disseminated choroid plexus papilloma. J Neuro-Oncol. 2013;114:251–3. https://doi.org/10.1007/s11060-013-1180-9.
3. Anderson RCE, Ghatan S, Feldstein NA. Surgical approaches to tumors of the lateral ventricle. Neurosurg Clin N Am. 2003;14:509–25. https://doi.org/10.1016/S1042-3680(03)00054-8.
4. Bahar M, Kordes U, Tekautz T, Wolff J. Radiation therapy for choroid plexus carcinoma patients with Li-Fraumeni syndrome: advantageous or detrimental? Anticancer Res. 2015;35:3013–7.
5. Barkovich AJ. Neuroimaging of pediatric brain tumors. Neurosurg Clin N Am. 1992;3:739–69. https://doi.org/10.1016/S1042-3680(18)30624-7.
6. Bisdas S, D'Arco F. Pediatric tumor neuroradiology. In: Barkhof F, Jager R, Thurnher M, Rovira Cañellas A, editors. Clinical neuroradiology. Cham: Springer International Publishing; 2019. p. 1–80.
7. Cannon DM, Mohindra P, Gondi V, Kruser TJ, Kozak KR. Choroid plexus tumor epidemiology and outcomes: implications for surgical and radiotherapeutic management. J Neuro-Oncol. 2015;121:151–7. https://doi.org/10.1007/s11060-014-1616-x.
8. Capper D, Stichel D, Sahm F, Jones DTW, Schrimpf D, Sill M, Schmid S, Hovestadt V, Reuss DE, Koelsche C, Reinhardt A, Wefers AK, Huang K, Sievers P, Ebrahimi A, Schöler A, Teichmann D, Koch A, Hänggi D, Unterberg A, Platten M, Wick W, Witt O, Milde T, Korshunov A, Pfister SM, von Deimling A. Practical implementation of DNA methylation and copy-number-based CNS tumor diagnostics: the Heidelberg experience. Acta Neuropathol (Berl). 2018;136:181–210. https://doi.org/10.1007/s00401-018-1879-y.
9. Chow E, Reardon DA, Shah AB, Jenkins JJ, Langston J, Heideman RL, Sanford RA, Kun LE, Merchant TE. Pediatric choroid plexus neoplasms. Int J Radiat Oncol. 1999;44:249–54. https://doi.org/10.1016/S0360-3016(98)00560-4.
10. Cikla U, Swanson KI, Tumturk A, Keser N, Uluc K, Cohen-Gadol A, Baskaya MK. Microsurgical resection of tumors of the lateral and third ventricles: operative corridors for difficult-to-reach lesions. J Neuro-Oncol. 2016;130:331–40. https://doi.org/10.1007/s11060-016-2126-9.
11. Cinalli G, Imperato A, Mirone G, Di Martino G, Nicosia G, Ruggiero C, Aliberti F, Spennato P. Initial experience with endoscopic ultrasonic aspirator in purely neuroendoscopic removal of intraventricular tumors. J Neurosurg Pediatr. 2017;19:325–32. https://doi.org/10.3171/2016.10.PEDS16352.
12. Colò F, Larrouquere L, Rivoirard R, Loiseau H, Mervoyer A, Lortholary A, Catry-Thomas I, Frappaz D. Bevacizumab in progressive disseminated atypical choroid plexus papilloma in adults. Neuro-Oncol. 2020;22:1046–7. https://doi.org/10.1093/neuonc/noaa073.
13. Corcoran GM, Frazier SR, Prayson RA. Choroid plexus papilloma with osseous and adipose metaplasia. Ann Diagn Pathol. 2001;5:43–7. https://doi.org/10.1053/adpa.2001.21478.
14. Dangouloff-Ros V, Grevent D, Pagès M, Blauwblomme T, Calmon R, Elie C, Puget S, Sainte-Rose C, Brunelle F, Varlet P, Boddaert N. Choroid plexus neoplasms: toward a distinction between carcinoma and papilloma using arterial spin-labeling. AJNR Am J Neuroradiol. 2015;36:1786–90. https://doi.org/10.3174/ajnr.A4332.
15. Dash C, Moorthy S, Garg K, Singh PK, Kumar A, Gurjar H, Chandra PS, Kale SS. Management of choroid plexus tumors in infants and young children up to 4 years of age: an institutional experience. World Neurosurg. 2019;121:e237–45. https://doi.org/10.1016/j.wneu.2018.09.089.
16. Delsin LEA, Salomao KB, Pezuk JA, Brassesco MS. Expression profiles and prognostic value of miRNAs in retinoblastoma. J Cancer Res Clin Oncol. 2019;145:1–10. https://doi.org/10.1007/s00432-018-2773-7.
17. Donovan MJ, Yunis EJ, Degirolami U, Fletcher JA, Schofield DE. Chromosome aberrations in choroid plexus papillomas. Genes Chromosomes Cancer. 1994;11:267–70. https://doi.org/10.1002/gcc.2870110410.
18. Dudley RWR, Torok MR, Gallegos D, Liu AK, Handler MH, Hankinson TC. Pediatric choroid plexus tumors: epidemiology, treatments, and outcome analysis on 202 children from the SEER database. J Neuro-Oncol. 2015;121:201–7. https://doi.org/10.1007/s11060-014-1628-6.
19. Duffner PK, Horowitz ME, Krischer JP, Friedman HS, Burger PC, Cohen ME, Sanford RA, Mulhern RK, James HE, Freeman CR, Seidel FG, Kun LE. Postoperative chemotherapy and delayed radiation in children less than three years of age with malignant brain tumors. N Engl J Med. 1993;328:1725–31. https://doi.org/10.1056/NEJM199306173282401.
20. Duffner PK, Kun LE, Burger PC, Horowitz ME, Cohen ME, Sanford RA, Krischer JP, Mulhern RK, James HE, Rekate HL, Friedman HS. Postoperative chemotherapy and delayed radiation in infants and very young children with choroid plexus carcinomas. Pediatr Neurosurg. 1995;22:189–96. https://doi.org/10.1159/000120900.
21. Dunn J, Baborie A, Alam F, Joyce K, Moxham M, Sibson R, Crooks D, Husband D, Shenoy A, Brodbelt A, Wong H, Liloglou T, Haylock B, Walker C. Extent of MGMT promoter methylation correlates with outcome in glioblastomas given temozolomide and radiotherapy. Br J Cancer. 2009;101:124–31. https://doi.org/10.1038/sj.bjc.6605127.
22. Ellenbogen RG, Winston KR, Kupsky WJ. Tumors of the choroid plexus in children. Neurosurgery. 1989:327. https://doi.org/10.1097/00006123-198909000-00001.
23. Fernandez AF, Assenov Y, Martin-Subero JI, Balint B, Siebert R, Taniguchi H, Yamamoto H, Hidalgo M, Tan A-C, Galm O, Ferrer I, Sanchez-Cespedes M, Villanueva A, Carmona J, Sanchez-Mut JV, Berdasco M, Moreno V, Capella G, Monk D,

Ballestar E, Ropero S, Martinez R, Sanchez-Carbayo M, Prosper F, Agirre X, Fraga MF, Grana O, Perez-Jurado L, Mora J, Puig S, Prat J, Badimon L, Puca AA, Meltzer SJ, Lengauer T, Bridgewater J, Bock C, Esteller M. A DNA methylation fingerprint of 1628 human samples. Genome Res. 2012;22:407–19. https://doi.org/10.1101/gr.119867.110.

24. Fiorillo A, Maggi G, Cirillo S, Migliorati R, Buffardi F, Alfieri E, Sabbatino MS, D'Amico A, DelBasso DeCaro ML. Efficacy of sequential chemotherapy including methotrexate and doxorubicin in an infant with partially resected choroid plexus carcinoma. Pediatr Neurosurg. 2003;38:21–6. https://doi.org/10.1159/000067559.
25. Fitzpatrick LK, Aronson LJ, Cohen KJ. Is there a requirement for adjuvant therapy for choroid plexus carcinoma that has been completely resected? J Neuro-Oncol. 2002;57:123–6. https://doi.org/10.1023/A:1015773624733.
26. Fouladi M, Gururangan S, Moghrabi A, Phillips P, Gronewold L, Wallace D, Sanford RA, Gajjar A, Kun LE, Heideman R. Carboplatin-based primary chemotherapy for infants and young children with CNS tumors. Cancer. 2009;115:3243–53. https://doi.org/10.1002/cncr.24362.
27. Geyer JR, Sposto R, Jennings M, Boyett JM, Axtell RA, Breiger D, Broxson E, Donahue B, Finlay JL, Goldwein JW, Heier LA, Johnson D, Mazewski C, Miller DC, Packer R, Puccetti D, Radcliffe J, Tao ML, Shiminski-Maher T. Multiagent chemotherapy and deferred radiotherapy in infants with malignant brain tumors: a report from the children's cancer group. J Clin Oncol. 2005;23:7621–31. https://doi.org/10.1200/JCO.2005.09.095.
28. Glauser TA, Packer RJ. Cognitive deficits in long-term survivors of childhood brain tumors. Childs Nerv Syst. 1991;7:2–12. https://doi.org/10.1007/BF00263824.
29. Gopal P, Parker JR, Debski R, Parker JC. Choroid plexus carcinoma. Arch Pathol Lab Med. 2008;132:1350–4. https://doi.org/10.1043/1543-2165(2008)132[1350:CPC]2.0.CO;2.
30. Gozali AE, Britt B, Shane L, Gonzalez I, Gilles F, McComb JG, Krieger MD, Lavey RS, Shlien A, Villablanca JG, Erdreich-Epstein A, Dhall G, Jubran R, Tabori U, Malkin D, Finlay JL. Choroid plexus tumors; management, outcome, and association with the Li-Fraumeni syndrome: the Children's Hospital Los Angeles (CHLA) experience, 1991–2010. Pediatr Blood Cancer. 2012;58:905–9. https://doi.org/10.1002/pbc.23349.
31. Granberg KJ, Raita A, Lehtinen B, Tihonen AM, Kesseli J, Annala M, Rodriguez-Martinez A, Nordfors K, Zhang W, Visakorpi T, Nykter M, Haapasalo H. Moderate-to-strong expression of FGFR3 and TP53 alterations in a subpopulation of choroid plexus tumors. Histol Histopathol. 2020;35:673–80. https://doi.org/10.14670/HH-18-180.
32. Grundy RG, Wilne SH, Robinson KJ, Ironside JW, Cox T, Chong WK, Michalski A, Campbell RHA, Bailey CC, Thorp N, Pizer B, Punt J, Walker DA, Ellison DW, Machin D. Primary postoperative chemotherapy without radiotherapy for treatment of brain tumours other than ependymoma in children under 3 years: results of the first UKCCSG/SIOP CNS 9204 trial. Eur J Cancer. 2010;46:120–33. https://doi.org/10.1016/j.ejca.2009.09.013.
33. Gupta N. Choroid plexus tumors in children. Neurosurg Clin N Am. 2003;14:621–31. https://doi.org/10.1016/S1042-3680(03)00058-5.
34. Hasselblatt M, Jeibmann A, Guerry M, Senner V, Paulus W, McLendon RE. Choroid plexus papilloma with neuropil-like islands. Am J Surg Pathol. 2008;32:162–6. https://doi.org/10.1097/PAS.0b013e3180cc2015.
35. Hasselblatt M, Mertsch S, Koos B, Riesmeier B, Stegemann H, Jeibmann A, Tomm M, Schmitz N, Wrede B, Wolff JE, Zheng W, Paulus W. TWIST-1 is overexpressed in neoplastic choroid plexus epithelial cells and promotes proliferation and invasion. Cancer Res. 2009;69:2219–23. https://doi.org/10.1158/0008-5472.CAN-08-3176.
36. Hovestadt V, Remke M, Kool M, Pietsch T, Northcott PA, Fischer R, Cavalli FMG, Ramaswamy V, Zapatka M, Reifenberger G, Rutkowski S, Schick M, Bewerunge-Hudler M, Korshunov A, Lichter P, Taylor MD, Pfister SM, Jones DTW. Robust molecular subgrouping and copy-number profiling of medulloblastoma from small amounts of archival tumour material using high-density DNA methylation arrays. Acta Neuropathol (Berl). 2013;125:913–6. https://doi.org/10.1007/s00401-013-1126-5.
37. Humphreys RP, Nemoto S, Hendrick EB, Hoffman NS, Hendrick EB, Hoffman HJ. Childhood choroid plexus tumors. Concepts Pediatr Neurosurg. 1987;7:1–18.
38. Huang FW, Hodis E, Xu MJ, Kryukov GV, Chin L, Garraway LA. Highly recurrent TERT promoter mutations in human melanoma. Science. 2013;339(6122):957–9.
39. Japp AS, Gessi M, Messing-Jünger M, Denkhaus D, zur Mühlen A, Wolff JE, Hartung S, Kordes U, Klein-Hitpass L, Pietsch T. High-resolution genomic analysis does not qualify atypical plexus papilloma as a separate entity among choroid plexus tumors. J Neuropathol Exp Neurol. 2015;74:110–20. https://doi.org/10.1097/NEN.0000000000000154.
40. Kaatsch PGD, Spix C (2019) German childhood cancer registry—annual report 2018 (1980–2017). https://www.kinderkrebsregister.de/dkkr-gb/latest-publications/annual-reports.html?L=1.
41. Kalimuthu SN, Chetty R. Gene of the month: SMARCB1. J Clin Pathol. 2016;69:484–9. https://doi.org/10.1136/jclinpath-2016-203650.
42. Kamar FG, Kairouz VF, Nasser SM, Faddoul SG, Saikali IC. Atypical choroid plexus papilloma treated with single agent bevacizumab. Rare Tumors. 2014;6:33–5. https://doi.org/10.4081/rt.2014.4687.

43. Kasowski H, Piepmeier JM. Transcallosal approach for tumors of the lateral and third ventricles. Neurosurg Focus. 2001;10:1–5. https://doi.org/10.3171/foc.2001.10.6.4.
44. Kim B, Tabori U, Hawkins C. An update on the CNS manifestations of brain tumor polyposis syndromes. Acta Neuropathol (Berl). 2020;139:703–15. https://doi.org/10.1007/s00401-020-02124-y.
45. Koos B, Paulsson J, Jarvius M, Sanchez BC, Wrede B, Mertsch S, Jeibmann A, Kruse A, Peters O, Wolff JEA, Galla H-J, Söderberg O, Paulus W, Östman A, Hasselblatt M. Platelet-derived growth factor receptor expression and activation in choroid plexus tumors. Am J Pathol. 2009;175:1631–7. https://doi.org/10.2353/ajpath.2009.081022.
46. Kordes UR, Hartung S, Löbel U, Ozga A-K, Traunecker H, Adamski J, Filipek I, Garami M, Solanki G, Hasselblatt M, Pietsch T, Kortmann R-D, Christoph R, Timmermann B, Wolff J. EMBR-08. Choroid plexus tumors in 2018: the CPT-SIOP experience and long-term outcome. Neuro-Oncol. 2018;20:i70–9. https://doi.org/10.1093/neuonc/noy059.192.
47. Kornienko VN, Pronin IN. Diagnostic neuroradiology: with 22 tables. Berlin: Springer; 2009.
48. Lafay-Cousin L, Mabbott DJ, Halliday W, Taylor MD, Tabori U, Kamaly-Asl ID, Kulkarni AV, Bartels U, Greenberg M, Bouffet E. Use of ifosfamide, carboplatin, and etoposide chemotherapy in choroid plexus carcinoma: clinical article. J Neurosurg Pediatr. 2010;5:615–21. https://doi.org/10.3171/2010.3.PEDS09354.
49. Louis DN, Perry A, Wesseling P, Brat DJ, Cree IA, FigarellaBranger D, Hawkins C, Ng HK, Pfster SM, Reifenberger G, Sofetti R, von Deimling A, Ellison DW. The 2021 WHO Classifcation of tumors of the central nervous system: a summary. Neuro-Oncol. 2021;23:1231–51. https://doi.org/10.1093/neuonc/noab1063.
50. Lu C, El-Deiry WS. Targeting p53 for enhanced radio- and chemo-sensitivity. Apoptosis. 2009;14:597–606. https://doi.org/10.1007/s10495-009-0330-1.
51. Malkin D. Li-Fraumeni Syndrome. Genes. Cancer. 2011;2:475–84. https://doi.org/10.1177/1947601911413466.
52. Mallick S, Benson R, Melgandi W, Rath GK. Effect of surgery, adjuvant therapy, and other prognostic factors on choroid plexus carcinoma: a systematic review and individual patient data analysis. Int J Radiat Oncol. 2017;99:1199–206. https://doi.org/10.1016/j.ijrobp.2017.08.012.
53. Mazloom A, Wolff JE, Paulino AC. The impact of radiotherapy fields in the treatment of patients with choroid plexus carcinoma. Int J Radiat Oncol. 2010;78:79–84. https://doi.org/10.1016/j.ijrobp.2009.07.1701.
54. McCallum S, Cooper K, Franks DN. Choroid plexus carcinoma. Cytologic identification of malignant cells in ascitic fluid. Acta Cytol. 1988;32:263–6.
55. Meng H, Feng H, Zhang L, Wang J. Endoscopic removal of a cystic choroid plexus papilloma of the third ventricle: a case report and review of the literature. Clin Neurol Neurosurg. 2011;113(7):582–5. https://doi.org/10.1016/j.clineuro.2011.02.010. Epub 2011 Mar 16. PMID: 21414714
56. Merino DM, Shlien A, Villani A, Pienkowska M, Mack S, Ramaswamy V, Shih D, Tatevossian R, Novokmet A, Choufani S, Dvir R, Ben-Arush M, Harris BT, Hwang EI, Lulla R, Pfister SM, Achatz MI, Jabado N, Finlay JL, Weksberg R, Bouffet E, Hawkins C, Taylor MD, Tabori U, Ellison DW, Gilbertson RJ, Malkin D. Molecular characterization of choroid plexus tumors reveals novel clinically relevant subgroups. Clin Cancer Res. 2015;21:184–92. https://doi.org/10.1158/1078-0432.CCR-14-1324.
57. Mirone G, Ruggiero C, Spennato P, Aliberti F, Trischitta V, Cinalli G. Cortical gluing and ringer lactate solution inflation to avoid cortical mantle collapse and subdural fluid collections in pediatric neurosurgery: safety and feasibility. Childs Nerv Syst. 2015;31:945–51. https://doi.org/10.1007/s00381-015-2660-3.
58. Morota N, Kumabe T, Kakita A. Posterior fossa choroid plexus tumor. In: Özek MM, Cinalli G, Maixner W, Sainte-Rose C, editors. Posterior fossa tumors in children. Cham: Springer International Publishing; 2015. p. 723–43.
59. Mosleh O, Tabori U, Bartels U, Huang A, Schechter T, Bouffet E. Successful treatment of a recurrent choroid plexus carcinoma with surgery followed by high-dose chemotherapy and stem cell rescue. Pediatr Hematol Oncol. 2013;30:386–91. https://doi.org/10.3109/08880018.2012.756089.
60. Naeini RM, Yoo JH, Hunter JV. Spectrum of choroid plexus lesions in children. Am J Roentgenol. 2009;192:32–40. https://doi.org/10.2214/AJR.08.1128.
61. Neumann E, Kalousek DK, Norman MG, Steinbok P, Cochrane DD, Goddard K. Cytogenetic analysis of 109 pediatric central nervous system tumors. Cancer Genet Cytogenet. 1993;71:40–9. https://doi.org/10.1016/0165-4608(93)90200-6.
62. Oertel J, Linsler S, Csokonay A, Schroeder HWS, Senger S. Management of severe intraoperative hemorrhage during intraventricular neuroendoscopic procedures: the dry field technique. J Neurosurg. 2018;131(3):931–5. https://doi.org/10.3171/2018.4.JNS172537. PMID: 30239311
63. Oliveira VF, De Sousa GR, dos Santos AC, Saggioro FP, Machado HR, de Oliveira RS, Tone LG, Valera ET. Evaluating H3F3A K27M and G34R/V somatic mutations in a cohort of pediatric brain tumors of different and rare histologies. Childs Nerv Syst. 2020; https://doi.org/10.1007/s00381-020-04852-8.
64. Orr BA, Clay MR, Pinto EM, Kesserwan C. An update on the central nervous system manifesta-

tions of Li–Fraumeni syndrome. Acta Neuropathol (Berl). 2020;139:669–87. https://doi.org/10.1007/s00401-019-02055-3.
65. Ostrom QT, Gittleman H, Farah P, Ondracek A, Chen Y, Wolinsky Y, Stroup NE, Kruchko C, Barnholtz-Sloan JS. CBTRUS statistical report: primary brain and central nervous system tumors diagnosed in the United States in 2006–2010. Neuro-Oncol. 2013;15:ii1–ii56. https://doi.org/10.1093/neuonc/not151.
66. Østrup O, Nysom K, Scheie D, Schmidt AY, Mathiasen R, Hjalgrim LL, Olsen TE, Skjøth-Rasmussen J, Henriksen BM, Nielsen FC, Wehner PS, Schrøder H, Sehested AM, Rechnitzer C, Rossing M. Importance of comprehensive molecular profiling for clinical outcome in children with recurrent cancer. Front Pediatr. 2018;6:114. https://doi.org/10.3389/fped.2018.00114.
67. Passariello A, Tufano M, Spennato P, Quaglietta L, Verrico A, Migliorati R, Cinalli G. The role of chemotherapy and surgical removal in the treatment of choroid plexus carcinomas and atypical papillomas. Childs Nerv Syst. 2015;31:1079–88. https://doi.org/10.1007/s00381-015-2697-3.
68. Patanakar T, Prasad S, Mukherji SK, Armao D. Cystic variant of choroid plexus papilloma. Clin Imaging. 2000;24:130–1. https://doi.org/10.1016/s0899-7071(00)00177-7.
69. Pencalet P, Sainte-Rose C, Lellouch-Tubiana A, Kalifa C, Brunelle F, Sgouros S, Meyer P, Cinalli G, Zerah M, Pierre-Kahn A, Renier D. Papillomas and carcinomas of the choroid plexus in children. J Neurosurg. 1998;88:521–8. https://doi.org/10.3171/jns.1998.88.3.0521.
70. Pienkowska M, Choufani S, Turinsky AL, Guha T, Merino DM, Novokmet A, Brudno M, Weksberg R, Shlien A, Hawkins C, Bouffet E, Tabori U, Gilbertson RJ, Finlay JL, Jabado N, Thomas C, Sill M, Capper D, Hasselblatt M, Malkin D. DNA methylation signature is prognostic of choroid plexus tumor aggressiveness. Clin Epigenetics. 2019;11:117. https://doi.org/10.1186/s13148-019-0708-z.
71. Razzaq AA, Cohen AR. Neoadjuvant chemotherapy for hypervascular malignant brain tumors of childhood. Pediatr Neurosurg. 1997;27:296–303. https://doi.org/10.1159/000121274.
72. Reddy D, Gunnarsson T, Scheinemann K, Provias JP, Singh SK. Combined staged endoscopic and microsurgical approach of a third ventricular choroid plexus papilloma in an infant. Minim Invasive Neurosurg. 2011;54(5–6):264–7. https://doi.org/10.1055/s-0031-1287775. Epub 2012 Jan 25
73. Redshaw N, Wheeler G, Hajihosseini MK, Dalmay T. microRNA-449 is a putative regulator of choroid plexus development and function. Brain Res. 2009;1250:20–6. https://doi.org/10.1016/j.brainres.2008.11.020.
74. Rickert CH, Paulus W. Tumors of the choroid plexus. Microsc Res Tech. 2001;52(1):104–11. https://doi.org/10.1002/1097-0029(20010101)52:1<104::AID-JEMT12>3.0.CO;2-3.
75. Rickert CH, Wiestler OD, Paulus W. Chromosomal imbalances in choroid plexus tumors. Am J Pathol. 2002;160:1105–13. https://doi.org/10.1016/S0002-9440(10)64931-0.
76. Roland B, Pinto A. Hyperdiploid karyotype in a choroid plexus papilloma. Cancer Genet Cytogenet. 1996;90:130–1. https://doi.org/10.1016/S0165-4608(96)00091-X.
77. Ruland V, Hartung S, Kordes U, Wolff JE, Paulus W, Hasselblatt M. Choroid plexus carcinomas are characterized by complex chromosomal alterations related to patient age and prognosis: genetic alterations in choroid plexus carcinoma. Genes Chromosomes Cancer. 2014;53:373–80. https://doi.org/10.1002/gcc.22148.
78. Samuel N, Wilson G, Lemire M, Id Said B, Lou Y, Li W, Merino D, Novokmet A, Tran J, Nichols KE, Finlay JL, Choufani S, Remke M, Ramaswamy V, Cavalli FMG, Elser C, Meister L, Taylor MD, Tabori U, Irwin M, Weksberg R, Wasserman JD, Paterson AD, Hansford JR, Achatz MIW, Hudson TJ, Malkin D. Genome-wide DNA methylation analysis reveals epigenetic dysregulation of microRNA-34A in TP53 -associated cancer susceptibility. J Clin Oncol. 2016;34:3697–704. https://doi.org/10.1200/JCO.2016.67.6940.
79. Santos MM, Souweidane MM. Purely endoscopic resection of a choroid plexus papilloma of the third ventricle: case report. J Neurosurg Pediatr. 2015;16(1):54–7. https://doi.org/10.3171/2014.12.PEDS14287. Epub 2015 Apr 10
80. Sasaki T, Kim J, Moritani T, Capizzano AA, Sato SP, Sato Y, Kirby P, Ishitoya S, Oya A, Toda M, Yuzawa S, Takahashi K. Roles of the apparent diffusion coefficient and tumor volume in predicting tumor grade in patients with choroid plexus tumors. Neuroradiology. 2018;60:479–86. https://doi.org/10.1007/s00234-018-2008-2.
81. Scala M, Morana G, Milanaccio C, Pavanello M, Nozza P, Garrè ML. Atypical choroid plexus papilloma: spontaneous resolution of diffuse leptomeningeal contrast enhancement after primary tumor removal in 2 pediatric cases. J Neurosurg Pediatr. 2017;20:284–8. https://doi.org/10.3171/2017.2.PEDS16526.
82. Schneider C, Kamaly-Asl I, Ramaswamy V, Lafay-Cousin L, Kulkarni AV, Rutka JT, Remke M, Coluccia D, Tabori U, Hawkins C, Bouffet E, Taylor MD. Neoadjuvant chemotherapy reduces blood loss during the resection of pediatric choroid plexus carcinomas. J Neurosurg Pediatr. 2015;16:126–33. https://doi.org/10.3171/2014.12.PEDS14372.
83. Siegfried A, Morin S, Munzer C, Delisle MB, Gambart M, Puget S, Maurage CA, Miquel C, Dufour C, Leblond P, André N, Branger DF, Kanold J, Kemeny J-L, Icher C, Vital A, Coste EU, Bertozzi AI. A French retrospective study on clinical outcome in 102 choroid plexus tumors in children. J Neuro-

Oncol. 2017;135:151–60. https://doi.org/10.1007/s11060-017-2561-2.
84. Spennato P, De Martino L, Russo C, Errico ME, Imperato A, Mazio F, Miccoli G, Quaglietta L, Abate M, Covelli E, Donofrio V, Cinalli G. Tumors of choroid plexus and other ventricular tumors. Adv Exp Med Biol. 2023;1405:175–223. https://doi.org/10.1007/978-3-031-23705-8_7. PMID: 37452939
85. St. Clair SK, Humphreys RP, Pillay PK, Hoffman HJ, Blaser SI, Becker LE. Current management of choroid plexus carcinoma in children. Pediatr Neurosurg. 1991;17:225–33. https://doi.org/10.1159/000120602.
86. Sufianov AA, Gaibov SS, Sufianov RA. Endoscopic monoportal removal of a choroid plexus papilloma in the posterior third ventricle in a child. J Neurosurg Pediatr. 2015;16(1):107–11. https://doi.org/10.3171/2014.12.PEDS14306. Epub 2015 Apr 24. PMID: 25910036
87. Sun MZ, Ivan ME, Oh MC, Delance AR, Clark AJ, Safaee M, Oh T, Kaur G, Molinaro A, Gupta N, Parsa AT. Effects of adjuvant chemotherapy and radiation on overall survival in children with choroid plexus carcinoma. J Neuro-Oncol. 2014;120:353–60. https://doi.org/10.1007/s11060-014-1559-2.
88. Sybert VP, Pagon RA. Hypomelanosis of Ito in a girl with plexus papilloma and translocation (X;17). Hum Genet. 1994;93 https://doi.org/10.1007/BF00210623.
89. Tabori U, Shlien A, Baskin B, Levitt S, Ray P, Alon N, Hawkins C, Bouffet E, Pienkowska M, Lafay-Cousin L, Gozali A, Zhukova N, Shane L, Gonzalez I, Finlay J, Malkin D. TP53 alterations determine clinical subgroups and survival of patients with choroid plexus tumors. J Clin Oncol. 2010;28:1995–2001. https://doi.org/10.1200/JCO.2009.26.8169.
90. Taher M, Hassan A, Saeed M, Jastania R, Nageeti T, Alkhalidi H, Dairi G, Abduljaleel Z, Athar M, Bouazzaoui A, ElBjeirami W, AlAllaf F. Next generation DNA sequencing of atypical choroid plexus papilloma of brain: identification of novel mutations in a female patient by Ion Proton. Oncol Lett. 2019; https://doi.org/10.3892/ol.2019.10882.
91. Taylor MB, Jackson RW, Hughes DG, Wright NB. Magnetic resonance imaging in the diagnosis and management of choroid plexus carcinoma in children. Pediatr Radiol. 2001;31:624–30. https://doi.org/10.1007/s002470100511.
92. Thomas C, Ruland V, Kordes U, Hartung S, Capper D, Pietsch T, Gerß J, Wolff JEA, Paulus W, Hasselblatt M. Pediatric atypical choroid plexus papilloma reconsidered: increased mitotic activity is prognostic only in older children. Acta Neuropathol (Berl). 2015;129:925–7. https://doi.org/10.1007/s00401-015-1434-z.
93. Thomas C, Sill M, Ruland V, Witten A, Hartung S, Kordes U, Jeibmann A, Beschorner R, Keyvani K, Bergmann M, Mittelbronn M, Pietsch T, Felsberg J, Monoranu CM, Varlet P, Hauser P, Olar A, Grundy RG, Wolff JE, Korshunov A, Jones DT, Bewerunge-Hudler M, Hovestadt V, von Deimling A, Pfister SM, Paulus W, Capper D, Hasselblatt M. Methylation profiling of choroid plexus tumors reveals 3 clinically distinct subgroups. Neuro-Oncol. 2016;18:790–6. https://doi.org/10.1093/neuonc/nov322.
94. Thomas C, Metrock K, Kordes U, Hasselblatt M, Dhall G. Epigenetics impacts upon prognosis and clinical management of choroid plexus tumors. J Neuro-Oncol. 2020;148(1):39–45. https://doi.org/10.1007/s11060-020-03509-5. Epub 2020 Apr 28. PMID: 32342334; PMCID: PMC7280353
95. Thomas C, Soschinski P, Zwaig M, Oikonomopoulos S, Okonechnikov K, Pajtler KW, Sill M, Schweizer L, Koch A, Neumann J, Schüller U, Sahm F, Rauschenbach L, Keyvani K, Proescholdt M, Riemenschneider MJ, Segewiß J, Ruckert C, Grauer O, Monoranu CM, Lamszus K, Patrizi A, Kordes U, Siebert R, Kool M, Ragoussis J, Foulkes WD, Paulus W, Rivera B, Hasselblatt M. The genetic landscape of choroid plexus tumors in children and adults. Neuro-Oncology. 2021;23(4):650–60. https://doi.org/10.1093/neuonc/noaa267. PMID: 33249490; PMCID: PMC8041331
96. Tong Y, Merino D, Nimmervoll B, Gupta K, Wang Y-D, Finkelstein D, Dalton J, Ellison DW, Ma X, Zhang J, Malkin D, Gilbertson RJ. Cross-species genomics identifies TAF12, NFYC, and RAD54L as choroid plexus carcinoma oncogenes. Cancer Cell. 2015;27:712–27. https://doi.org/10.1016/j.ccell.2015.04.005.
97. Trubicka J, Filipek I, Iwanowski P, Rydzanicz M, Grajkowska W, Piekutowska-Abramczuk D, Chrzanowska K, Karkucińska-Więckowska A, Iwanicka-Pronicka K, Pronicki M, Łastowska M, Płoski R, Dembowska-Bagińska B. Constitutional mosaicism of a de novo TP53 mutation in a patient with bilateral choroid plexus carcinoma. Cancer Genet. 2017;216–217:79–85. https://doi.org/10.1016/j.cancergen.2017.07.001.
98. Versteege I, Sévenet N, Lange J, Rousseau-Merck M-F, Ambros P, Handgretinger R, Aurias A, Delattre O. Truncating mutations of hSNF5/INI1 in aggressive paediatric cancer. Nature. 1998;394:203–6. https://doi.org/10.1038/28212.
99. Viaene AN, Pu C, Perry A, Li MM, Luo M, Santi M. Congenital tumors of the central nervous system: an institutional review of 64 cases with emphasis on tumors with unique histologic and molecular characteristics. Brain Pathol. 2020:bpa.12885. https://doi.org/10.1111/bpa.12885.
100. Walter AW, Mulhern RK, Gajjar A, Heideman RL, Reardon D, Sanford RA, Xiong X, Kun LE. Survival and neurodevelopmental outcome of young children with Medulloblastoma at St Jude children's research hospital. J Clin Oncol. 1999;17:3720–8. https://doi.org/10.1200/JCO.1999.17.12.3720.
101. Warren KE, Vezina G, Poussaint TY, Warmuth-Metz M, Chamberlain MC, Packer RJ, Brandes AA,

Reiss M, Goldman S, Fisher MJ, Pollack IF, Prados MD, Wen PY, Chang SM, Dufour C, Zurakowski D, Kortmann RD, Kieran MW. Response assessment in medulloblastoma and leptomeningeal seeding tumors: recommendations from the response assessment in pediatric neuro-oncology committee. Neuro-Oncol. 2018;20:13–23. https://doi.org/10.1093/neuonc/nox087.
102. Wolburg H, Paulus W. Choroid plexus: biology and pathology. Acta Neuropathol (Berl). 2010;119:75–88. https://doi.org/10.1007/s00401-009-0627-8.
103. Wolff JEA, Sajedi M, Brant R, Coppes MJ, Egeler RM. Choroid plexus tumours. Br J Cancer. 2002;87:1086–91. https://doi.org/10.1038/sj.bjc.6600609.
104. Wolff JE, Van Gool SW, Kutluk T, Diez B, Kebudi R, Timmermann B, Garami M, Sterba J, Fuller GN, Bison B, Kordes UR. Final results of the Choroid Plexus Tumor study CPT-SIOP-2000. J Neurooncol. 2022;156(3):599–613. https://doi.org/10.1007/s11060-021-03942-0. Epub 2022 Jan 8. PMID: 34997889; PMCID: PMC8860833
105. Wrede B, Hasselblatt M, Peters O, Thall PF, Kutluk T, Moghrabi A, Mahajan A, Rutkowski S, Diez B, Wang X, Pietsch T, Kortmann R-D, Paulus W, Jeibmann A, Wolff JEA. Atypical choroid plexus papilloma: clinical experience in the CPT-SIOP-2000 study. J Neuro-Oncol. 2009;95:383–92. https://doi.org/10.1007/s11060-009-9936-y.
106. Yan C, Xu Y, Feng J, Sun C, Zhang G, Shi J, Hao P, Wu Y, Lin B. Choroid plexus tumours: classification, MR imaging findings and pathological correlation: MRI of CPTs. J Med Imaging Radiat Oncol. 2013;57:176–83. https://doi.org/10.1111/1754-9485.12013.
107. Yasargil MG, Abdulrauf SI. Surgery of intraventricular tumors. Neurosurgery. 2008; https://doi.org/10.1227/01.NEU.0000316427.57165.01.
108. Yeom KW, Mitchell LA, Lober RM, Barnes PD, Vogel H, Fisher PG, Edwards MS. Arterial spin-labeled perfusion of pediatric brain tumors. Am J Neuroradiol. 2014;35:395–401. https://doi.org/10.3174/ajnr.A3670.
109. Zaky W, Dhall G, Khatua S, Brown RJ, Ginn KF, Gardner SL, Yildiz VO, Yankelevich M, Finlay JL. Choroid plexus carcinoma in children: the head start experience: choroid plexus carcinoma, therapy and outcome. Pediatr Blood Cancer. 2015;62:784–9. https://doi.org/10.1002/pbc.25436.
110. Zhou W-J-L, Wang X, Peng J-Y, Ma S-C, Zhang D-N, Guan X-D, Diao J-F, Niu J-X, Li C-D, Jia W. Clinical Features and Prognostic Risk Factors of Choroid Plexus Tumors in Children. Chin Med J (Engl). 2018;131:2938–46. https://doi.org/10.4103/0366-6999.247195.
111. Zimny A, Sasiadek M. Contribution of perfusion-weighted magnetic resonance imaging in the differentiation of meningiomas and other extra-axial tumors: case reports and literature review. J Neuro-Oncol. 2011;103:777–83. https://doi.org/10.1007/s11060-010-0445-9.
112. Zwetsloot CP, Kros JM, Paz y Gueze HD. Familial occurrence of tumours of the choroid plexus. J Med Genet. 1991;28:492–4. https://doi.org/10.1136/jmg.28.7.492.

Post-operative Cerebellar Mutism Syndrome

20

Maria Allegra Cinalli and Andrea Carai

20.1 Introduction

Pediatric central nervous system tumors are the second most common type of cancer in children with an overall incidence rate of 2.99 per 100.000 [1]. About 45–60% of pediatric brain lesions are in the posterior fossa [2, 3]. Medulloblastoma (MB) accounting for 30–40% of posterior fossa tumors in children, followed by pilocytic astrocytoma (25–35%), brainstem glioma (20–25%), ependymoma (10–15%), and atypical teratoid rhabdoid tumor (less than 2%) [4].

The prognosis of these different types of tumors has improved in the past few decades, due to advances in different technologies as well as surgical and oncological treatments, with a generalized improvement in survival in this patient population [5–7]. This has brought attention to a fundamental aspect of pediatric neurosurgery which is the quality of life of children with central nervous system tumors.

Despite the significant advances observed in the oncological field, surgical resection is still necessary to help achieve acceptable outcome and reduce treatment toxicity. Nevertheless, posterior fossa approaches are associated with a significant set of transient and/or permanent complications. Finding a balance between surgical and oncological treatment, aiming for the best possible prognosis not only in terms of overall survival but also in terms of quality of life, is therefore crucial for children with posterior fossa tumors [6, 8, 9].

Cerebellar mutism syndrome (CMS) is a well-known severe complication most seen in the pediatric population after posterior fossa surgery for tumor resection. It is a complex set of linguistic, cognitive, behavioral, and motor signs, which can be variably associated. The incidence of CMS after resection of posterior fossa tumors ranges between 8% and 50% [10, 11]. Medulloblastoma histology has the strongest association with CMS, with an incidence of 40% after tumor resection, followed by pilocytic astrocytoma (16%) and ependymoma (4%) [12, 13].

20.2 Historical Overview and Definition

In 1939, Bailey et al. first reported the case of a patient who developed delayed onset (3 days after surgery) dysarthria and dysphagia after excision of a fourth ventricle ependymoma, with complete recovery after 3 weeks [14].

M. A. Cinalli
Department of Paediatric Neurosurgery, Alder Hey Children's Hospital, NHS Foundation Trust, Liverpool, UK

A. Carai (✉)
Neurosurgery Unit, IRCCS Bambino Gesù Children's Hospital, Rome, Italy
e-mail: andrea.carai@opbg.net

A. Mastronuzzi, A. Carai (eds.), *Navigating Pediatric Brain Tumors*,
https://doi.org/10.1007/978-3-032-18992-9_20

The term akinetic mutism (AM) was first used by Cairns in 1941 to describe a patient who presented with a clinical syndrome characterized by mutism, whispering of monosyllables, absence of voluntary movements, and inability to chew caused by a Rathke's cyst invading the third ventricle; his symptoms regressed after surgical drainage of the cyst [15].

After that report, in 1958, Daly and Love used the same expression to refer to a case of mutism that occurred after posterior fossa tumor resection in a child. The patient was a 14-year-old boy with obstructive hydrocephalus caused by a pilocytic astrocytoma located in the upper portion of the fourth ventricle, which was resected through a transvermian approach. The post-operative course was characterized by slow lightening of an initial deep coma, with inconstant movement in all four limbs, dysphagia, inability to speak or make any sounds, decreased motor initiative, and indifference to his environment. The symptoms improved gradually; dysphagia was the first symptom that improved, with complete remission occurring within 2 weeks after tumor excision. By that time, the patient was able to communicate with his parents by sign language, although with no emotional response to them, and he still had low motor initiative, with a tendency to sleep excessively. After the administration of methylphenidate, hydrochloride alertness and responsiveness markedly improved. Approximately 1 month after the operation, the patient spoke, and in the subsequent days he rapidly improved his speech with increasing complexity of verbal production. Cerebellar dysarthria persisted, although with progressive improvement, until it almost disappeared by the time of discharge [16].

In 1979, Hirsch and colleagues reported a case series of 57 pediatric patients who underwent medulloblastoma resection and noted that these patients frequently experienced "post-operative mutism" and a complex of other neurological and behavioral disorders. Regarding surgical excision, they found correlation of these neuropsychogical sequelae with tumor adhesion to the brainstem, although patients with medulloblastoma usually face adverse effects from radiotherapy, which can lead to poor cognitive outcomes [17].

In the 1980s, Wisoff and Epstein used the term pseudobulbar palsy to refer to a syndrome characterized by "delayed onset, the presence of supranuclear lesions, the frequent association of emotional incontinence and lability, and complete recovery over several weeks or months." They postulated that the cause of this syndrome was cerebellar retraction and vermis splitting, causing edema along the middle and superior cerebellar peduncles [18].

In 1985, Rekate et al. reported six cases of "cerebellar muteness" after acute bilateral surgical injury (during posterior fossa tumor resection) to the cerebellar hemispheres, including the dentate nuclei. In this study, no associations were found between mutism and motor paralysis, cranial nerve dysfunction or loss of higher cognitive function [19].

In 1995, contrary to what was reported by Rekate, Pollack and colleagues reported 12 cases, the majority of which had mutism variably associated with other neurological symptoms, and in 1997, he renamed the combination of mutism and pseudobulbar signs "Posterior Fossa Syndrome" [20, 21].

A new entity introduced by Schmahmann and Sherman in 1997 after a series of studies investigating cerebellar involvement in higher functions was "cerebellar cognitive affective syndrome" (CCAS). This prospective study included 20 adult patients with purely cerebellar lesions associated with significant behavioral manifestations. Identification of this clinical entity helped understanding the deep connection between the cerebellum and higher functions [22]. In 2000, Levisohn et al. analyzed the cognitive outcomes of children who underwent surgery for posterior fossa tumors without receiving radiation therapy. The same CCAS affective component described in adults was found in the pediatric population [23].

"Mutism and subsequent dysarthria" (MSD) is the expression used by van Dogen and colleagues to refer more specifically to speech-related post-operative disorders after posterior fossa surgery [24].

The definition "cerebellar mutism syndrome" was first reported by the Children's Cancer Group in the USA, who performed a survey that examined the time of onset and duration of mutism, ataxia, hypotonia, and irritability severity [25].

As described above, there are many studies on this clinical syndrome in the literature, with a wide variety of terms used to describe it. The significant variability in clinical features and nomenclature of this syndrome was addressed by a group of researchers and clinicians in 2016, and an international consensus document was produced with the aim of finding a universal denomination and definition for this specific pediatric clinical issue.

The expression chosen among the many available was Cerebellar Mutism Syndrome and the international consensus document states: "post-operative pediatric CMS is characterized by delayed onset mutism/reduced speech and emotional lability after cerebellar or 4th ventricle tumor surgery in children. Additional common features include hypotonia and oropharyngeal dysfunction/dysphagia. It may frequently be accompanied by cerebellar motor syndrome, cerebellar cognitive affective syndrome, and brain stem dysfunction, including long tract signs and cranial neuropathies. Mutism is always transient, but recovery from CMS may be prolonged. Speech and language may not return to normal, and other deficits of cognitive, affective, and motor function often persist" [26].

Although consensus on the nomenclature of this clinical condition is far to be universal, with the recent resurgence of the posterior fossa syndrome (PFS) appellative by eminent research groups [27], precisely defining a problem is the first indispensable step in the path toward its solution. Despite many efforts are still ongoing to circumstantiate the semantic boundaries of CMS/PFS more precisely, we will refer to the definition proposed by the international consensus paper by the posterior fossa society throughout this chapter [26].

20.3 Clinical Features

Cerebellar mutism syndrome comprehends a spectrum of signs and symptoms that include delayed onset of linguistic, neuropsychological, and neurological signs and symptoms after posterior fossa surgery for tumor resection in children [26].

CMS typically occurs after a 1–15 days symptom-free interval after surgery, with a mean of 2 days. The hallmark of cerebellar mutism syndrome is mutism or severe speech impairment, which is limited to single words or brief sentences obtained through robust stimulation. This is the core symptom and is usually transient, ranging from 1 day to 2.5 years, with a mean of 43 days [13]. After the acute phase, patients experience a gradual improvement of mutism, with dysarthric speech characterized by slow speech rate and ataxic, monotonous speech that can persist for a variable amount of time [10]. Long-term language disabilities, such as slowed speech [10], word finding difficulties [23], agrammatism [28, 29], writing and reading problems [30, 31], and adynamic spontaneous speech production characterized by a lack of verbal initiative often persist [28, 31, 32]. An objective quantitative measure of speech impairment is not currently available; however, it is commonly accepted that both complete mutism and its duration are associated to more severe associated cerebellar injury manifestations in the acute phase and to lifelong persistence of disability [27]. In this regard, Ricci et al. [33] proposed a validated post-operative CMS severity scale that featured clinical signs and their duration to derive a three-tiered severity assessment. When assessed at least 4 weeks after surgery, the scale showed a good prognostic ability. However, scoring single items was not straightforward in all cases, posing the challenge of a multidisciplinary assessment in selected cases.

Discriminating the core symptoms of CMS from the general clinical picture might be difficult as associated cerebellar injury symptoms might include any of the features configuring a CCAS [22], extending from emotional changes such as emotional lability, depression [34], apathy [28], to cognitive impairment manifesting as inattention, long-term intelligence impairment, memory loss, and visual-spatial skills impairment [13].

A constellation of cerebellar motor symptoms can also be observed in combination to mutism and CCAS including manifestations such as

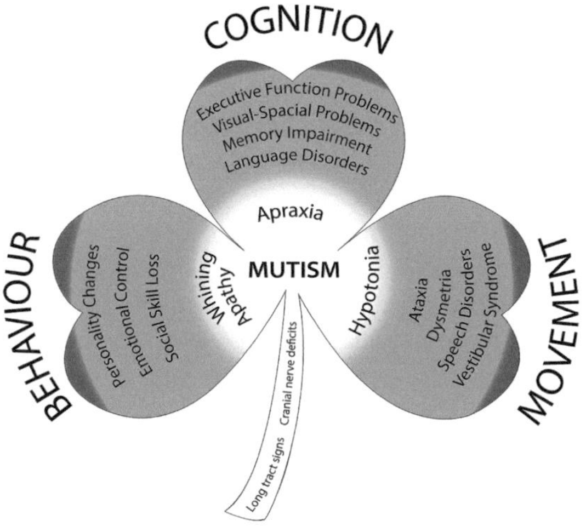

Fig. 20.1 The constellation of CMS clinical manifestations graphically visualized as a clover. The clover metaphor was historically used by St.Patrick to illustrate the concept of Trinity in Christianity, meaning the coexistence of three different people albeit in unity. Similarly, impairment of the three functional domains of the cerebellum: motor, cognitive, and behavioral (the latter two configuring the cognitive-affective cerebellar syndrome - CCAS) are represented in CMS. The core of the syndrome includes mutism and the most severe clinical manifestations from the three functional domains (inner white circle). Milder cerebellar damage and persistent symptoms after long-term recovery are represented with a constellation of symptoms at the periphery of the foils. Associated cranial nerve and long tract signs (the trunk of the trifoil) are not of direct cerebellar origin and represent brainstem damage due to anatomical contiguity to cerebellum and its white matter outflow tracts. Accurate clinical assessment would reveal coexistence of features from the three domains, due to damage of the cerebellar outflow system, where functional compartmentalization is virtually absent. (*Graphics by Matteo Barba*)

hypotonia, ataxia, dysmetria, and apraxia often resulting in a marked reduction in spontaneous initiation of movements such as eye opening and chewing.

Finally, anatomical proximity of brainstem explains the possibility of additional long tract injury and cranial nerve impairment, manifesting as alternating brainstem syndromes of variable entity and including hemiparesis, hemihypoesthesia, urinary retention or incontinence, and cranial nerve palsies (VI-XII) determining strabism, peripheral facial palsy, hypoacusia, nystagmus, dysphonia, and dysphagia [26].

CMS clinical manifestations are summarized in Fig. 20.1.

20.4 Pathophysiology

Since the first reports on cerebellar mutism syndrome, questions have been raised about its pathophysiology [17, 18]. Although cases of transient mutism with behavioral and neurologic problems have been reported also after vascular [35] or traumatic brain injury [36], and in adults, this syndrome is considered peculiar of children after surgery for posterior fossa tumor removal. The specific association of these features, together with the delayed onset, and the association with motor, cognitive and behavioral disorders have provided the basis for many different theories to explain CMS.

A satisfactory understanding of the pathophysiology of cerebellar mutism syndrome may help to better define the prognosis and the risk of developing CMS when informing patients and their families in a pre-operative setting, as well as reducing the incidence of CMS eventually.

Currently, cerebellar mutism syndrome is believed to be caused by interruption of the efferent cerebellar pathway, mainly represented by the dentato-thalamo-cortical (DTC) tract [19, 29, 37–39]. As evidenced by several imaging studies [40–43], the specific site of injury of this pathway that seems to be involved in CMS is the proximal efferent cerebellar pathway (pECP). See Fig. 20.2.

This pathway involves the dentate nuclei, located symmetrically in the white matter adjacent to the vermis. The efferent tracts reach the brainstem through the superior cerebellar peduncles, where they cross the midline and, after passing through the red nucleus, reach the contralateral ventro-lateral thalamus and motor and pre-frontal cortex. According to this theory, damage to the DTC tract along its proximal part leads to a secondary diaschisis of the supratentorial areas connected to the cerebellum.

The term diaschisis refers to a loss of function in one area of the brain following an injury to a distant area connected and normally sending inputs to the former [44].

The first reports referred to supratentorial strokes causing contralateral cerebellar metabolism impairment [45]. In cerebellar mutism syndrome, the injured component is the infratentorial

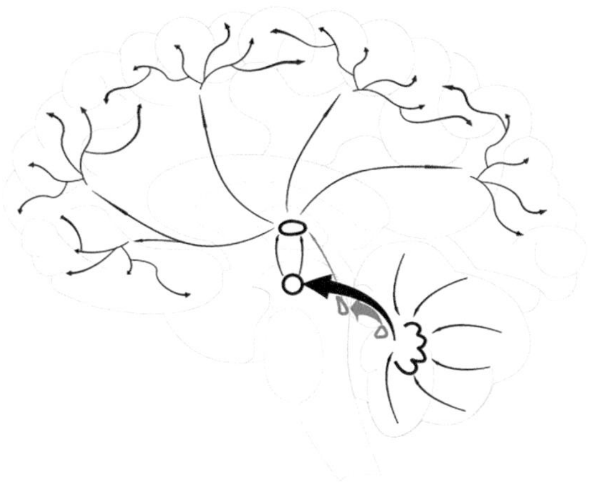

Fig. 20.2 Anatomical pathways whose damage has been involved in the genesis of CMS are illustrated. Cerebellar cortex diffusely projects to deep nuclei, namely, dentate (black) and fastigial (grey). Deep nuclei respectively project to mesencephalic red nucleus (black) and periaqueductal grey matter (grey). Final projection is through the thalamus to contribute to cerebral network modulation. The size of arrows is proportional to functional density of information travelling through white matter bundles and reaches its peak between deep cerebella and mesencephalic nuclei, at superior cerebellar peduncles (large black and grey arrows). (*Graphics by Matteo Barba*)

region, leading to "reversed cerebellocerebral diaschisis," in which cerebellar injury causes a decrease in perfusion and metabolism predominantly of the contralateral frontal cortex [46–48]. Decreased perfusion is believed to be caused by a reduction in metabolic demands; this could explain the improvement in symptoms over time due to neuronal plasticity, particularly in young populations.

Interestingly, the perfusion changes described in cerebro-cerebellar diaschisis in gray matter are not immediate after a supratentorial stroke [49]. Time-to-peak alterations were observed 5 days after the adverse event, while cerebral blood volume changes occurred subacutely, 6–120 days after the stroke [50]. The reasons for this latent period are unknown, although they fit well in the context of cerebellar mutism syndrome, due to its characteristic delayed onset [49].

As evidence from advanced imaging studies accumulates, proofs regarding a pivotal role of cerebellum in modulating virtually any known cerebral network and function are progressively becoming more robust [51, 52]. This theory might explain the symptoms that are not classically related to a purely cerebellar injury, such as the apraxic features of the speech disorder, as well as the cognitive and behavioral impairment [53].

Intriguingly, recent research suggests that there might be phylogenetically more ancient cerebellar projections which might be involved in CMS as well. Periaqueductal grey projections originating at fastigial nuclei have been postulated to participate in gating of vocalization and movement and found to be disrupted in patients developing CMS [51].

Apart from considering direct surgical injury to selected neuroanatomical structures, other attempts to explain this peculiar aspect of CMS have been made since the first reports [18, 24]. Edema of the regions surrounding the surgical cavity has been proposed as an explanation for the timing of CMS onset. Superior and middle cerebellar peduncles have variably been associated with CMS in some studies [20, 43, 54], although there is still a lack of consensus on this subject [53]. Vascular mechanisms have also been reported, and the role of intraoperative and post-operative vasospasm of posterior circulation arteries in contributing to CMS is felt to deserve additional investigations [55].

20.5 Pre-operative Risk Factors

The reported incidence of cerebellar mutism syndrome varies widely across studies [10, 11]. This has raised the question of whether there may be low- and high-risk groups of patients. The ability to stratify a patient's risk of developing CMS is crucial, because of the increasing overall survival of patients with posterior fossa tumors and the impact of CMS on their quality of life.

The well-known risk factors for cerebellar mutism syndrome include medulloblastoma histology, midline tumor location, and brainstem invasion [11, 12, 25, 56].

A recent meta-analysis by Pettersson et al., which included 28 studies with 2276 patients, reviewed CMS risk factors. They found that, in addition to the already clearly associated determinants, fourth ventricle and superior cerebellar peduncle invasion, medulloblastoma size >5 cm, left handedness, and vermis incision were significantly associated with a greater risk of developing CMS [57].

Grønbæk et al. reported similar results in their European multicenter prospective cohort study, which included 376 patients, and they found atypical teratoid rhabdoid tumor histology to be a significant risk factor together with MB histology. They also found that age was an independent risk factor for the development of CMS [56].

Midline location is believed to be a risk factor for CMS due to the lateral displacement of the superior cerebellar peduncles. This exposes the proximal cerebellar efferent pathway to a greater risk of manipulation during tumor resection and therefore to a higher risk of direct damage or post-operative swelling [41].

For similar reasons, brainstem, fourth ventricle, and superior cerebellar peduncles invasion and a tumor size >5 cm might all be considered as expected risk factors, considering the current pathophysiology model of cerebellar mutism syndrome [58].

Left-handedness was associated with cerebellar mutism syndrome in two of the studies included in Petterson meta-analysis [59, 60]. Gronbaek et al. specifically analyzed this risk factor in a prospective study including 250 patients, 20 of whom were left-handed. Among the left-handed patients, 5 (25%) developed post-operative speech impairment (POSI), and 61 out of 230 (27%) right-handed patients developed it. These findings are not consistent with a significant association between handedness and CMS [61].

The association between medulloblastoma histology and CMS has been clear since the first reports [17]. Medulloblastomas are currently divided into four groups (Wingless, Sonic Hedgehog, and groups 3 and 4) which, in fact, represent distinct pathologies. They originate from different cells in the cerebellum and tend to have specific locations. The Wingless (WNT) subgroup is believed to originate from the lower rhombic lip and is located in the lateral recess. The Sonic Hedgehog (SHH) group arises from the external granule layer and is located in the cerebellar hemispheres. Group 3 and 4 arise from Nestin + cells and unipolar brush cells, respectively, and they are typically located in the fourth ventricle [62–64].

Jabarkheel et al. reevaluated CMS risk factors considering the molecular classification of medulloblastoma. They observed a cohort of 370 patients with medulloblastoma from five centers and analyzed age at diagnosis, sex, tumor volume, and CMS development together with molecular subgroup. The results showed a lower risk of developing CMS in the Sonic Hedgehog (SHH) group compared with Wingless (WNT), groups 3 and 4 [65].

Previous studies have shown a lower incidence of CMS in the SHH subgroup [66]. This might be justified by its preferential hemispheric location. Interestingly, Jabarkheel et al. reported that even when arising from the midline, the SHH subgroup have a lower incidence of CMS if compared to the other groups. They observed that midline SHH have a reduced risk of disruption of the pECP compared to other groups arising from the midline [65].

These findings represent a further step toward a better understanding of CMS risk factors, since some might be manifestations of the underlying subgroup. Although subgroup identification is not definitively possible in a pre-operative setting, it is possible to predict with variable grades of probability which subgroup a lesion belongs to, based on its location and enhancement pattern [64, 67, 68]. The reported risk factors for CMS are summarized in Table 20.1.

Recently, some models based on pre-operative MRI findings have been proposed to provide patients and their parents with the most accurate risk stratification in the presence of a posterior fossa tumor [69–71]. After the pioneering work of Liu et al. [69], many efforts have been made to develop reliable preoperative predictive scores. The Rotterdam pediatric cerebellar mutism syndrome prediction model was proposed by Bae et al. based on the previous existing models and has acceptable accuracy, sensitivity, and specificity [71]. More recently, artificial intelligence approaches have been applied to improve performance of preoperative CMS risk scoring, obtain-

Table 20.1 Reported risk factors for CMS are summarized

Risk factor	OR (95% CI)	Statistical significance	Reference
Brainstem invasion	4.28 (2.23–8.23)	$p < 0.0001$	Petterson et al. [57]
IV ventricle invasion	12.84 (4.29–38.44)	$p < 0.00001$	Petterson et al. [57]
SCP invasion	6.77 (2.35–19.48)	$p = 0.0004$	Petterson et al. [57]
MB histology	3.26 (1.93–5.52)	$p < 0.0001$	Petterson et al. [57]
WNT subgroup[a]	4.91 (1.64–16.52)	$p = 0.0063$	Jabarkeel et al. [65]
Group 3[a]	5.56 (1.95–17.94)	$p = 0.0022$	Jabarkeel et al. [65]
Group 4[a]	8.57 (3.11–27.33)	$p = 9.1 \times 10^{-5}$	Jabarkeel et al. [65]
AT/RT histology[b]	10.30 (2.10–54.45)	$p = 0.003$	Grønbæk et al. [56]
MB >50 mm	8.85 (1.3–60.16)	$p = 0.03$	Petterson et al. [57]
Vermis incision	5.44 (2.09–14.16)	$p = 0.0005$	Petterson et al. [57]

SCP superior cerebellar peduncle, *MB* medulloblastoma, *WNT* Wingless, *AT/RT* atypical teratoid rhabdoid tumor
[a]Risk of CMS compared with Sonic Hedgehog molecular subgroup
[b]Risk of CMS compared with pilocytic astrocytoma

ing an accuracy of over 90% [72]. Whatever the described method, a common limitation concerns interobserver variability, especially in respect to predicting tumor histology and ruling out tumor compression from invasion of brainstem and cerebellar peduncles (Table 20.2).

Finally, there is growing evidence that some degree of cerebellar disfunction precedes surgical injury in children with posterior fossa tumors. Although formal neuropsychological and speech assessment might be challenging, especially in children with symptomatic hydrocephalus, a double hit mechanism has been postulated [73, 74].

20.6 Surgical Risk Factors

Whatever the predisposing conditions, there is little discussion about surgery being the substantial offender determining the occurrence of CMS. Lack of a convincing pathophysiological explanation and a general feeling that CMS was a generally transient benign condition prevented for a long time the surgical community from addressing the issue of avoiding it.

For decades, access to fourth ventricle tumors has been achieved through the transvermian approach. Since the first reports of cerebellar mutism syndrome, vermian splitting has been deemed responsible for this disabling condition [18]. This has led to the introduction of the telovelar approach, which allows access to the fourth ventricle through the cerebellomedullary fissure [75, 76] The medial opening of the cerebellomedullary fissure allows the surgeon to use a natural anatomical corridor, avoiding direct damage to the vermis while providing better lateral exposure [77–79].

Since its introduction for the management of fourth ventricle tumors, many studies have analyzed the role of the telovelar approach in CMS. The reported results have been controversial, with a generalized tendency to favor the telovelar approach because of its supposed protective role against CMS [75, 80–82].

In a meta-analysis by Pettersson et al., vermis incision was found to be a risk factor for CMS, while the use of transvermian or telovelar approach was not correlated with CMS [57].

Recently, in a European prospective multicenter cohort study, including 376 patients, the transvermian approach was not found to be a risk factor compared to the telovelar approach [56]. In a retrospective study by Toescu et al. analyzing 167 pediatric patients with fourth ventricle tumors, no significant difference in the incidence of CMS was found between the two approaches [83]. Similar results were observed by Onorini et al. in a retrospective cohort of 92 patients [84]. These are the largest series comparing the telovelar and transvermian approaches for fourth ventricle tumors.

Table 20.2 Comparison between CMS predictive models

	Accuracy	Sensitivity	Specificity	Interobserver variability	Time consuming
Liu et al. [69]	0.88	–	–	+++	–
Bae et al. [71]	0.87	0.97	0.84	+++	–
Sidpra et al. [72]	0.90	0.77	0.99	–	+++

Patient selection for the right approach depends on many factors, and even though in many cases it is possible to approach the same tumor through both approaches, this is not always true. In fact, the telovelar approach allows direct access to the floor of the fourth ventricle and lateral recesses, while the transvermian approach is more suitable for larger tumors invading the vermis and provides more comfortable access to the rostral portion of the fourth ventricle. Moreover, the experience of the surgeon, who might be more comfortable with one approach over another, must be considered. Therefore, randomizing posterior fossa tumor patients for the choice of surgical approach will hardly be possible. However, it cannot be underestimated that the surgeon should abstain from any avoidable cerebellar resection or manipulation during posterior fossa tumor resection. This principle has progressively emerged from multiple surgical experiences.

Incidence of CMS was found to be higher and clinical manifestations more severe in children who were operated in low-volume neurosurgical centers by Khan et al. [27].

Conversely, in experienced hands, refinement of surgical technique with the aim of minimize manipulation of normal tissue has been shown to reduce the incidence of CMS by 70% [85, 86].

Use of intraoperative imaging has been found to be a protective factor against the development of cerebellar mutism syndrome, although there is heterogeneity in the methods utilized (ultrasound vs intraoperative MRI) among different studies [57, 83, 85, 87].

20.7 Prognosis

The natural history of cerebellar mutism syndrome has been described over the years in several papers. The main characteristic of the syndrome, which is mutism, is generally transient. It can last from a few days to up to 2.5 years, although usually it does not last more than 6 months [24, 26, 88]. Recovery of complex movements of the tongue and mouth usually precedes recovery from mutism. The latter usually improves within a few weeks, with gradual regain of speech, although severely dysarthric. Dysarthria can have variable features; some patients experience ataxic dysarthria, with scanning speech and articulatory breakdowns, while others have dysarthria with apraxic characteristics, defined by a slow speech rate [89]. Dysarthria gradually becomes milder or evolves in an almost normal speech [53].

Complete recovery from a speech perspective is not always achieved, as confirmed by long-term follow-up studies [88, 90, 91]. A mutism phase lasting more than 4 weeks has been found to be a predictor of a worse neurological outcome 1 year after diagnosis [23, 25, 43].

Many aspects of recovery must be considered, as CMS affects not only the language area, but also motor, neurobehavioral, and cognitive areas in the long term. In medulloblastoma patients, the neurocognitive sequelae of CMS cannot always be separated by chemotherapy and radiotherapy treatments toxicity.

In a study by De Smet et al., long-term language outcomes were evaluated through auditory perceptual-speech analysis up to 12 years after posterior fossa tumor resection in 14 patients with CMS, and 12 patients exhibited persistent motor speech deficits. Medulloblastoma histology and radiation therapy were found to be correlated with worse long-term speech outcomes [90].

Steinlin et al. reported similar results in terms of persistence of verbal fluency, attention, and behavior problems in patients who underwent surgery for resection of pilocytic astrocytoma without any further treatments 2–18 years after resection [92].

All these aspects of posterior fossa tumor patient recovery have a not negligible influence on quality of life [53].

Currently, there are no standardized pharmacological treatment protocols for cerebellar mutism syndrome.

Rehabilitation of such a complex brain injury requires careful and diversified planning since it needs to cover all the affected domains [58]. Even if considerable experience exists to guide rehabilitation of cerebellar motor impairment, this might not necessarily be readily translated in the exquisite setting of CMS. In fact, for the motor domain, there is a lack of evidence regarding specific CMS rehabilitation programs. From a neuro-behavioral point of view attention, memory, executive functions, and academic achievements should be contextually addressed [93].

Speech rehabilitation has been investigated in multiple studies. First, pre-operative language assessment should be obtained; this usually occurs after the patient has undergone surgery through an accurate interview with the caregivers. Second, the type of speech impairment must be assessed to distinguish whether it is a pure dysarthric disorder, or if it has mostly apraxic features [58].

Recently, an international survey study investigated rehabilitation approaches in children with CMS in different disciplines such as physical and occupational therapy, speech-language pathology, and neuropsychology. Although there is no identified gold standard in rehabilitation practice, many interventions are similar across different geographic regions [94].

20.8 Conclusions

Cerebellar mutism syndrome is a complex, disabling complication of posterior fossa tumor surgery in children, with not negligible long-term negative effects on the quality of life of these patients. The affected population is particularly frail not only because of their young age and developing brain, but also because it is represented by oncological patients, and often needs chemo- and radiotherapy treatments as soon as they recover from the acute post-operative phase.

Currently, the main goal for cerebellar mutism syndrome is to prevent its occurrence. Unfortunately, this is hardly possible due to the known and often unmodifiable, risk factors for CMS. A possible strategy could be the mitigation of known risk factors during surgery.

Although maximal safe resection is the standard of care for medulloblastoma surgery, intentional subtotal resection might become an option in selected patients at high risk for the development of CMS, as more evidence accumulates regarding the effective prognostic impact of residual disease in the molecular era [95–97]. For example, in patients with dentate nucleus or superior cerebellar peduncle infiltration, the decision to leave a small residue might help avoid CMS, without significantly affecting the patient oncological prognosis in terms of overall survival [71, 95, 96]. Neoadjuvant chemotherapy for patients with an MRI diagnosis of medulloblastoma at greater risk of developing CMS has been described to downsize the burden of disease at the time of surgery, but additional investigation is warranted [65].

Unquestionable evidence indicates that high-quality surgery is protective against CMS occurrence, urging the neurosurgical community to seriously address this issue, by promoting investigation on the impact of specific technical nuances, maximizing efforts towards a standardization of surgical quality, and exploring the need to centralize these patients in selected high-volume centers [27, 85, 86].

Further treatment strategies are warranted to allow patients with CMS to achieve a more rapid and complete recovery. Clearly, rehabilitation will play a central role until new treatment protocols are developed, although future intervention-based clinical trials are warranted [94].

Many drugs have been proposed for the treatment of CMS, such as zolpidem, midazolam, fluoxetine, and bromocriptine, although none have shown clear benefits [98].

Transcranial magnetic stimulation together with rehabilitation might be helpful in the future to modulate brain plasticity, as already observed in adults [99].

References

1. Howlader N, Noone AM, Krapcho M, et al. SEER Cancer Statistics Review, 1975–2017, National Cancer Institute. Bethesda, MD, https://seer.cancer.gov/csr/1975_2017/, based on November 2019 SEER data submission, posted to the SEER web site, April 2020.
2. Rickert C, Paulus W. Epidemiology of central nervous system tumors in childhood and adolescence based on the new WHO classification. Childs Nerv Syst. 2001;17:503–11.
3. Formentin C, Joaquim AF, Ghizoni E. Posterior fossa tumors in children: current insights. Eur J Pediatr. 2023;182:4833–50.
4. Brandão LA, Poussaint TY. Pediatric brain tumors. Neuroimaging Clin N Am. 2013;23:499–525.
5. Gudrunardottir T, Lannering B, Remke M, Taylor MD, Wells EM, Keating RF, Packer RJ. Treatment developments and the unfolding of the quality of life discussion in childhood medulloblastoma: a review. Childs Nerv Syst. 2014;30:979–90.
6. Packer RJ. Childhood brain tumors: accomplishments and ongoing challenges. J Child Neurol. 2008;23:1122–7.
7. Bonfield CM, Steinbok P. Pediatric cerebellar astrocytoma: a review. Childs Nerv Syst. 2015;31:1677–85.
8. Michiels EMC, Schouten-Van Meeteren AYN, Doz F, Janssens GO, van Dalen EC. Chemotherapy for children with medulloblastoma. Cochrane Database Syst Rev. 2015;1:CD006678.
9. Zacharoulis S, Moreno L. Ependymoma: an update. J Child Neurol. 2009;24:1431–8.
10. De Smet HJ, Baillieux H, Catsman-Berrevoets C, De Deyn PP, Mariën P, Paquier PF. Postoperative motor speech production in children with the syndrome of 'cerebellar' mutism and subsequent dysarthria: a critical review of the literature. Eur J Paediatr Neurol. 2007;11:193–207.
11. Reed-Berendt R, Phillips B, Picton S, Chumas P, Warren D, Livingston JH, Hughes E, Morrall MCHJ. Cause and outcome of cerebellar mutism: evidence from a systematic review. Childs Nerv Syst. 2014;30:375–85.
12. Catsman-Berrevoets CE, Van Dongen HR, Mulder PG, y Geuze DP, Paquier PF, Lequin MH. Tumour type and size are high risk factors for the syndrome of "cerebellar" mutism and subsequent dysarthria. J Neurol Neurosurg Psychiatry. 1999;67:755–7.
13. Catsman-Berrevoets CE, Aarsen FK. The spectrum of neurobehavioural deficits in the Posterior Fossa Syndrome in children after cerebellar tumour surgery. Cortex. 2010;46:933–46.
14. Bailey P, Buchanan DN, Bucy PC. Intracranial tumors of infancy and childhood. Chicago: The University of Chicago Press; 1939.
15. Cairns H, Oldfield RC, Pennybacker JB, Whitteridge D. Akinetic mutism with an epidermoid cyst of the 3rd ventricle. Brain. 1941;64:273–90.
16. Daly DD, Love JG. Akinetic mutism. Neurology. 1958;8:238–42.
17. Hirsch JF, Renier D, Czernichow P, Benveniste L, Pierre-Kahn A. Medulloblastoma in childhood. Survival and functional results. Acta Neurochir (Wien). 1979;48:1–15.
18. Wisoff JH, Epstein FJ. Pseudobulbar palsy after posterior fossa operation in children. Neurosurgery. 1984;15:707–9.
19. Rekate HL, Grubb RL, Aram DM, Hahn JF, Ratcheson RA. Muteness of cerebellar origin. Arch Neurol. 1985;42:697–8.
20. Pollack IF, Polinko P, Albright AL, Towbin R, Fitz C. Mutism and pseudobulbar symptoms after resection of posterior fossa tumors in children: incidence and pathophysiology. Neurosurgery. 1995;37:885–93.
21. Pollack IF. Posterior fossa syndrome. Int Rev Neurobiol. 1997;41:411–32.
22. Schmahmann JD, Sherman JC. Cerebellar cognitive affective syndrome. Int Rev Neurobiol. 1997;41:433–40.
23. Levisohn L, Cronin-Golomb A, Schmahmann JD. Neuropsychological consequences of cerebellar tumour resection in children. Brain. 2000;123:1041–50.
24. van Dongen HR, Catsman-Berrevoets CE, van Mourik M. The syndrome of "cerebellar" mutism and subsequent dysarthria. Neurology. 1994;44:2040–6.
25. Robertson PL, Muraszko KM, Holmes EJ, Sposto R, Packer RJ, Gajjar A, Dias MS, Allen JC. Incidence and severity of postoperative cerebellar mutism syndrome in children with medulloblastoma: a prospective study by the Children's Oncology Group. J Neurosurg Pediatr. 2006;105:444–51.
26. Gudrunardottir T, Morgan AT, Lux AL, et al. Consensus paper on post-operative pediatric cerebellar mutism syndrome: the Iceland Delphi results. Childs Nerv Syst. 2016;32:1195–203.
27. Khan RB, Patay Z, Klimo P, et al. Clinical features, neurologic recovery, and risk factors of postoperative posterior fossa syndrome and delayed recovery: a prospective study. Neuro-Oncology. 2021;23:1586–96.
28. Siffert J, Poussaint TY, Goumnerova LC, Scott RM, LaValley B, Tarbell NJ, Pomeroy SL. Neurological dysfunction associated with postoperative cerebellar mutism. J Neuro-Oncol. 2000;48:75–81.
29. Riva D, Giorgi C. The cerebellum contributes to higher functions during development: evidence from a series of children surgically treated for posterior fossa tumours. Brain. 2000;123(Pt 5):1051–61.
30. Scott RB, Stoodley CJ, Anslow P, Paul C, Stein JF, Sugden EM, Mitchell CD. Lateralized cognitive deficits in children following cerebellar lesions. Dev Med Child Neurol. 2001;43:685–91.
31. Aarsen FK, Van Dongen HR, Paquier PF, Van Mourik M, Catsman-Berrevoets CE. Long-term sequelae in children after cerebellar astrocytoma surgery. Neurology. 2004;62:1311–6.
32. Ozimek A, Richter S, Hein-Kropp C, Schoch B, Gorissen B, Kaiser O, Gizewski E, Ziegler W,

Timmann D. Cerebellar mutism--report of four cases. J Neurol. 2004;251:963–72.
33. Ricci FS, D'Alessandro R, Somà A, et al. Development and application of a diagnostic and severity scale to grade post-operative pediatric cerebellar mutism syndrome. Eur J Pediatr. 2022;181:941–50.
34. Turkel SB, Shu Chen L, Nelson MD, Hyder D, Gilles FH, Woodall L, Braslow K, Tavaré CJ. Case series: acute mood symptoms associated with posterior fossa lesions in children. J Neuropsychiatry Clin Neurosci. 2004;16:443–5.
35. Baillieux H, Weyns F, Paquier P, De Deyn PP, Mariën P. Posterior fossa syndrome after a vermian stroke: a new case and review of the literature. Pediatr Neurosurg. 2007;43:386–95.
36. Erşahin Y, Mutluer S, Saydam S, Barçin E. Cerebellar mutism: report of two unusual cases and review of the literature. Clin Neurol Neurosurg. 1997;99:130–4.
37. Catsman-Berrevoets CE, van Breemen M, van Veelen ML, Appel IM, Lequin MH. Supratentorial arterial ischemic stroke following cerebellar tumor resection in two children. Pediatr Neurosurg. 2005;41:206–11.
38. Wells EM, Walsh KS, Khademian ZP, Keating RF, Packer RJ. The cerebellar mutism syndrome and its relation to cerebellar cognitive function and the cerebellar cognitive affective disorder. Dev Disabil Res Rev. 2008;14:221–8.
39. Ammirati M, Mirzai S, Samii M. Transient mutism following removal of a cerebellar tumor. A case report and review of the literature. Childs Nerv Syst. 1989;5:12–4.
40. Miller NG, Reddick WE, Kocak M, Glass JO, Löbel U, Morris B, Gajjar A, Patay Z. Cerebellocerebral diaschisis is the likely mechanism of postsurgical posterior fossa syndrome in pediatric patients with midline cerebellar tumors. Am J Neuroradiol. 2010;31:288–94.
41. Morris EB, Phillips NS, Laningham FH, Patay Z, Gajjar A, Wallace D, Boop F, Sanford R, Ness KK, Ogg RJ. Proximal dentatothalamocortical tract involvement in posterior fossa syndrome. Brain. 2009;132:3087–95.
42. Ojemann JG, Partridge SC, Poliakov AV, Niazi TN, Shaw DW, Ishak GE, Lee A, Browd SR, Geyer JR, Ellenbogen RG. Diffusion tensor imaging of the superior cerebellar peduncle identifies patients with posterior fossa syndrome. Childs Nerv Syst. 2013;29:2071–7.
43. Wells EM, Khademian ZP, Walsh KS, Vezina G, Sposto R, Keating RF, Packer RJ. Postoperative cerebellar mutism syndrome following treatment of medulloblastoma: neuroradiographic features and origin. J Neurosurg Pediatr. 2010;5:329–34.
44. Monakow C. Die Lokalization in Grosshirn und de Abbau der Function durch korticale Herde. Wiesbaden: J.F. Bergmann; 1914.
45. Baron JC, Bousser MG, Comar D, Castaigne P. "Crossed cerebellar diaschisis" in human supratentorial brain infarction. Trans Am Neurol Assoc. 1981;105:459–61.
46. Sagiuchi T, Ishii K, Aoki Y, Kan S, Utsuki S, Tanaka R, Fujii K, Hayakawa K. Bilateral crossed cerebello-cerebral diaschisis and mutism after surgery for cerebellar medulloblastoma. Ann Nucl Med. 2001;15:157–60.
47. Patay Z. Postoperative posterior fossa syndrome: unraveling the etiology and underlying pathophysiology by using magnetic resonance imaging. Childs Nerv Syst. 2015;31:1853–8.
48. Kusano Y, Tanaka Y, Takasuna H, Wada N, Tada T, Kakizawa Y, Hongo K. Transient cerebellar mutism caused by bilateral damage to the dentate nuclei after the second posterior fossa surgery. Case report. J Neurosurg. 2006;104:329–31.
49. Patay Z, Parra C, Hawk H, George A, Li Y, Scoggins M, Broniscer A, Ogg RJ. Quantitative longitudinal evaluation of diaschisis-related cerebellar perfusion and diffusion parameters in patients with supratentorial hemispheric high-grade gliomas after surgery. Cerebellum. 2014;13:580–7.
50. Yamada H, Koshimoto Y, Sadato N, Kawashima Y, Tanaka M, Tsuchida C, Maeda M, Yonekura Y, Ishii Y. Crossed cerebellar diaschisis: assessment with dynamic susceptibility contrast MR imaging. Radiology. 1999;210:558–62.
51. McAfee SS, Liu Y, Sillitoe RV, Heck DH. Cerebellar coordination of neuronal communication in cerebral cortex. Front Syst Neurosci. 2022;15:781527. https://doi.org/10.3389/fnsys.2021.781527.
52. Schmahmann JD, Sherman JC. The cerebellar cognitive affective syndrome. Brain. 1998;121(Pt 4):561–79.
53. Catsman-Berrevoets C, Patay Z. Cerebellar mutism syndrome. Handb Clin Neurol. 2018;155:273–88.
54. Toescu SM, Hales PW, Aquilina K, Clark CA. Quantitative MRI in post-operative paediatric cerebellar mutism syndrome. Eur J Radiol. 2018;108:43–51.
55. Deghedy M, Pizer B, Kumar R, Mallucci C, Avula S. Basilar artery vasospasm as a cause of postoperative cerebellar mutism syndrome. Case Rep Pediatr. 2022;2022:1–5.
56. Grønbæk JK, Wibroe M, Toescu S, et al. Postoperative speech impairment and surgical approach to posterior fossa tumours in children: a prospective European multicentre cohort study. Lancet Child Adolesc Health. 2021;5:814–24.
57. Pettersson SD, Kitlinski M, Miękisiak G, Ali S, Krakowiak M, Szmuda T. Risk factors for postoperative cerebellar mutism syndrome in pediatric patients: a systematic review and meta-analysis. J Neurosurg Pediatr. 2022;29:467–75.
58. Fabozzi F, Margoni S, Andreozzi B, Musci MS, Del Baldo G, Boccuto L, Mastronuzzi A, Carai A. Cerebellar mutism syndrome: from pathophysiology to rehabilitation. Front Cell Dev Biol. 2022;10:1082947. https://doi.org/10.3389/fcell.2022.1082947.

59. Law N, Greenberg M, Bouffet E, et al. Clinical and neuroanatomical predictors of cerebellar mutism syndrome. Neuro-Oncology. 2012;14:1294–303.
60. McEvoy SD, Lee A, Poliakov A, Friedman S, Shaw D, Browd SR, Ellenbogen RG, Ojemann JG, Mac Donald CL. Longitudinal cerebellar diffusion tensor imaging changes in posterior fossa syndrome. Neuroimage Clin. 2016;12:582–90.
61. Grønbæk JK, Laustsen AF, Toescu S, et al. Left-handedness should not be overrated as a risk factor for postoperative speech impairment in children after posterior fossa tumour surgery: a prospective European multicentre study. Childs Nerv Syst. 2022;38:1479–85.
62. Vladoiu MC, El-Hamamy I, Donovan LK, et al. Childhood cerebellar tumours mirror conserved fetal transcriptional programs. Nature. 2019;572:67–73.
63. Raybaud C, Ramaswamy V, Taylor MD, Laughlin S. Posterior fossa tumors in children: developmental anatomy and diagnostic imaging. Childs Nerv Syst. 2015;31:1661–76.
64. Wefers AK, Warmuth-Metz M, Pöschl J, et al. Subgroup-specific localization of human medulloblastoma based on pre-operative MRI. Acta Neuropathol. 2014;127:931–3.
65. Jabarkheel R, Amayiri N, Yecies D, et al. Molecular correlates of cerebellar mutism syndrome in medulloblastoma. Neuro Oncol. 2019;22(2):290–7. https://doi.org/10.1093/neuonc/noz158.
66. Moxon-Emre I, Taylor MD, Bouffet E, et al. Intellectual outcome in molecular subgroups of medulloblastoma. J Clin Oncol. 2016;34:4161–70.
67. Perreault S, Ramaswamy V, Achrol AS, et al. MRI surrogates for molecular subgroups of medulloblastoma. Am J Neuroradiol. 2014;35:1263–9.
68. Ismail M, Craig S, Ahmed R, de Blank P, Tiwari P. Opportunities and advances in radiomics and radiogenomics for pediatric medulloblastoma tumors. Diagnostics. 2023;13:2727.
69. Liu J-F, Dineen RA, Avula S, et al. Development of a pre-operative scoring system for predicting risk of post-operative paediatric cerebellar mutism syndrome. Br J Neurosurg. 2018;32:18–27.
70. Zhang H, Liao Z, Hao X, Han Z, Li C, Gong J, Liu W, Tian Y. Establishing reproducible predictors of cerebellar mutism syndrome based on pre-operative imaging. Childs Nerv Syst. 2019;35:795–800.
71. Bae D, Mlc VV, Catsman-Berrevoets C. Preoperative prediction of postoperative cerebellar mutism syndrome. Validation of existing MRI models and proposal of the new Rotterdam pCMS prediction model. Childs Nerv Syst. 2020;36:1471–80.
72. Sidpra J, Marcus AP, Löbel U, et al. Improved prediction of postoperative pediatric cerebellar mutism syndrome using an artificial neural network. Neurooncol Adv. 2022;4(1):vdac003. https://doi.org/10.1093/noajnl/vdac003.
73. Di Rocco C, Chieffo D, Frassanito P, Caldarelli M, Massimi L, Tamburrini G. Heralding cerebellar mutism: evidence for pre-surgical language impairment as primary risk factor in posterior fossa surgery. Cerebellum. 2011;10:551–62.
74. Bianchi F, Chieffo DPR, Frassanito P, Di Rocco C, Tamburrini G. Cerebellar mutism: the predictive role of preoperative language evaluation. Childs Nerv Syst. 2020;36:1153–7.
75. Kellogg JX, Piatt JH Jr. Resection of fourth ventricle tumors without splitting the vermis: the cerebellomedullary fissure approach. Pediatr Neurosurg. 1997;27:28–33.
76. Gok A, Alptekin M, Erkutlu I. Surgical approach to the fourth ventricle cavity through the cerebellomedullary fissure. Neurosurg Rev. 2004;27:50–4.
77. Matsushima T, Rhoton AL, Lenkey C. Microsurgery of the fourth ventricle: part 1. Neurosurgery. 1982;11:631–67.
78. Matsushima T. Microsurgical anatomy of the cerebellomedullary fissure and variations of the transcerebellomedullary fissure approach. In: Microsurgical anatomy and surgery of the posterior cranial fossa. Tokyo: Springer Japan; 2015. p. 73–99.
79. Mussi ACM, Rhoton AL. Telovelar approach to the fourth ventricle: microsurgical anatomy. J Neurosurg. 2000;92:812–23.
80. Qiu B, Wang Y, Wang W, Wang C, Wu P, Bao Y, Ou S, Guo Z, Wang Y. Microsurgical management of pediatric ependymomas of the fourth ventricle via the transcerebellomedullary fissure approach: a review of 26 cases. Oncol Lett. 2016;11:4099–106.
81. Eissa E. The role of telovelar approach in fourth ventricular surgery: a new perspective. Turk Neurosurg. 2017;28(4):523–9. https://doi.org/10.5137/1019-5149.JTN.21209-17.1.
82. Zaheer SN, Wood M. Experiences with the telovelar approach to fourth ventricular tumors in children. Pediatr Neurosurg. 2010;46:340–3.
83. Toescu SM, Samarth G, Layard Horsfall H, Issitt R, Margetts B, Phipps KP, Jeelani N-O, Thompson DNP, Aquilina K. Fourth ventricle tumors in children: complications and influence of surgical approach. J Neurosurg Pediatr. 2021;27:52–61.
84. Onorini N, Spennato P, Orlando V, et al. The clinical and prognostic impact of the choice of surgical approach to fourth ventricular tumors in a single-center, single-surgeon cohort of 92 consecutive pediatric patients. Front Oncol. 2022;12:821738.
85. Cobourn K, Marayati F, Tsering D, Ayers O, Myseros JS, Magge SN, Oluigbo CO, Keating RF. Cerebellar mutism syndrome: current approaches to minimize risk for CMS. Childs Nerv Syst. 2020;36:1171–9.
86. Avula S, Mallucci C, Kumar R, Pizer B. Posterior fossa syndrome following brain tumour resection: review of pathophysiology and a new hypothesis on its pathogenesis. Childs Nerv Syst. 2015;31:1859–67.
87. El Beltagy MA, Atteya MME. The benefits of navigated intraoperative ultrasonography during resection of fourth ventricular tumors in children. Childs Nerv Syst. 2013;29:1079–88.
88. Steinbok P, Cochrane DD, Perrin R, Price A. Mutism after posterior fossa tumour resection in children:

incomplete recovery on long-term follow-up. Pediatr Neurosurg. 2003;39:179–83.
89. Tamburrini G, Frassanito P, Chieffo D, Massimi L, Caldarelli M, Di Rocco C. Cerebellar mutism. Childs Nerv Syst. 2015;31:1841–51.
90. De Smet HJ, Catsman-Berrevoets C, Aarsen F, Verhoeven J, Mariën P, Paquier PF. Auditory-perceptual speech analysis in children with cerebellar tumours: a long-term follow-up study. Eur J Paediatr Neurol. 2012;16:434–42.
91. Morgan AT, Liégeois F, Liederkerke C, Vogel AP, Hayward R, Harkness W, Chong K, Vargha-Khadem F. Role of cerebellum in fine speech control in childhood: persistent dysarthria after surgical treatment for posterior fossa tumour. Brain Lang. 2011;117:69–76.
92. Steinlin M. Neuropsychological long-term sequelae after posterior fossa tumour resection during childhood. Brain. 2003;126:1998–2008.
93. Chieffo DPR, Lino F, Arcangeli V, Moriconi F, Frassanito P, Massimi L, Tamburrini G. Posterior fossa tumor rehabilitation: an up-to-date overview. Children. 2022;9:904.
94. Samargia-Grivette S, Hartley H, Walsh K, Lemiere J, Payne AD, Litke E, Knight A. REhabilitation approaches in CHildren with cerebellar mutism syndrome (REACH): an international cross-disciplinary survey study. J Pediatr Rehabil Med. 2024;17(2):185–97.
95. Thompson EM, Hielscher T, Bouffet E, et al. Prognostic value of medulloblastoma extent of resection after accounting for molecular subgroup: a retrospective integrated clinical and molecular analysis. Lancet Oncol. 2016;17:484–95.
96. Thompson EM, Bramall A, Herndon JE, Taylor MD, Ramaswamy V. The clinical importance of medulloblastoma extent of resection: a systematic review. J Neuro-Oncol. 2018;139:523–39.
97. Keeling C, Davies S, Goddard J, Ramaswamy V, Schwalbe EC, Bailey S, Hicks D, Clifford SC. The clinical significance of sub-total surgical resection in childhood medulloblastoma: a multi-cohort analysis of 1100 patients. EClinicalMedicine. 2024;69:102469.
98. Noris A, Zicca A, Lenge M, Picetti E, Zanaboni C, Rossi S, Giordano F. The medical therapy for cerebellar mutism syndrome: a case report and literature review. Childs Nerv Syst. 2021;37:2727–34.
99. Sathappan AV, Luber BM, Lisanby SH. The dynamic duo: combining noninvasive brain stimulation with cognitive interventions. Prog Neuropsychopharmacol Biol Psychiatry. 2019;89:347–60.

Long-Term Follow-Up and Quality of Life

21

Olga Nigro, Alessandro Cattoni, Francesca Filippi, Marta Podda, Paolo Grampa, Angela Mastronuzzi, Veronica Biassoni, Elisabetta Schiavello, Veronica Capelli, Silvia Molinari, Federica Pallotti, Maura Massimino, and Monica Terenziani

21.1 Introduction

Approximately 35,000 children and adolescents in Europe [1] and 450,000 in the United States [2] are diagnosed with cancer every year. Pediatric central nervous system (CNS) tumors are the most common solid tumors in children and comprise 15–20% of all malignancies in children. Unfortunately, many subtypes continue to have a suboptimal long-term outcome. During the last several years, however, remarkable advances in our understanding of the molecular underpinnings of these tumors have occurred as a result of high-resolution genomic, epigenetic, and transcriptomic profiling, which have provided insights for improved tumor categorization and molecularly directed therapies [3].

The increase in survival rates in those with a brain tumor in childhood has altered the clinical research emphasis from quantity to quality of survival, and in terms of the cost of life prolongation. In its widest sense, the term "quality of survival" encompasses any enduring physical, psychosocial, or socioeconomic problems within the predicament of a person surviving a serious life-threatening illness. The concept of "quality of life" relates to a person's subjective view of their own physical, psychosocial, or

O. Nigro (✉) · M. Podda · P. Grampa · V. Biassoni · E. Schiavello · M. Massimino · M. Terenziani (✉)
Pediatric Oncology Unit, Fondazione IRCCS Istituto Nazionale dei Tumori, Milan, Italy
e-mail: olga.nigro@istitutotumori.mi.it; marta.podda@istitutotumori.mi.it; paolo.grampa@istitutotumoi.mi.it; veronica.biassoni@istitutotumori.mi.it; elisabetta.schiavello@istitutotumori.mi.it; maura.massimino@istitutotumori.mi.it; monica.terenziani@istitutotumori.mi.it

A. Cattoni · S. Molinari
Fondazione IRCCS San Gerardo dei Tintori, Monza, Italy
e-mail: alessandro.cattoni@unimib.it; s.molinari3@campus.unimib.it

F. Filippi
Infertility Unit, Fondazione IRCCS Ca' Granda Ospedale Maggiore Policlinico, Milan, Italy
e-mail: francesca.filippi@policlinico.mi.it

A. Mastronuzzi
Area of Hematology-Oncology, Cell Therapy, Gene Therapies, and Hematopoietic Transplantation Bambino Gesù Children's Hospital, IRCCS, Rome, Italy

Department of Life Sciences and Public Health, Università Cattolica del Sacro Cuore, Rome, Italy
e-mail: angela.mastronuzzi@opbg.net

V. Capelli · F. Pallotti
Nuclear Medicine Department, Fondazione IRCCS Istituto Nazionale dei Tumori, Milan, Italy
e-mail: veronica.capelli@opbg.net; federica.pallotti@istitutotumori.mi.it

A. Mastronuzzi, A. Carai (eds.), *Navigating Pediatric Brain Tumors*,
https://doi.org/10.1007/978-3-032-18992-9_21

socioeconomic functioning in their own environment [4].

More than 95% of childhood cancer survivors (CCSs) will experience a health-related toxicity by 45 years of age, and about 30% will have severe chronic health condition/s (CHC/s) [5, 6]. Elevated risk for morbidity and mortality increases over the years, and this affects the future clinical demands of this population concerning active surveillance and interventions.

The ideal approach to survivors' care involves a risk-based model based on previous treatments, which incorporates routine healthcare, and a personalized plan of surveillance and prevention. Specific professionals are required, and a multidisciplinary team approach should be warranted. Healthcare providers must also educate and follow these survivors to drive them toward a better quality of life and a correct lifestyle.

The screening and surveillance of at-risk treatment groups could facilitate early detection and timely intervention of curable diseases [7].

Many previous studies reported on a long list of CHCs, including endocrinological and cardiovascular events, second malignant neoplasms (SMNs), ototoxicity, pulmonary events, long-term renal function impairment, neurocognitive and psychosocial outcomes, infertility, offspring's health status, and late mortality, specifically in brain tumor survivors.

21.2 Endocrine Late Effects

The remarkable and progressive increase in the population of childhood cancer survivors (CCSs) has led the scientific community to shed light on the growing burden of endocrine late effects experienced following diagnosis and treatment of pediatric brain tumors. In retrospective cohorts of patients with composite histologic backgrounds, the prevalence of endocrine late effects following CNS tumors generally exceeded 60% [8, 9], emphasizing that surveillance programs for the timely detection and treatment of hormonal disorders represent a pivotal part of the long-term care of survivors.

Endocrine *sequelae* can be regarded as the integrated detrimental result of brain cancer and its treatment. First, patients diagnosed with sellar or suprasellar tumors often experience hypopituitarism because of the tumor's "mass-effect" and dedicated surgical resection, resulting in the direct disruption of the hypothalamic–pituitary area (HPA) secreting activity [10]. In addition, neuro-endocrine disorders may arise whenever the HPA lies within the irradiation field of patients exposed to external radiation therapy [11]. In this setting, hormonal HP axes show a differential radiosensitivity, in a spectrum that ranges from the most vulnerable (growth hormone, GH) to the most radioresistant (TSH) axis. Accordingly, increasing exposure thresholds have been set in order to identify patients at risk of developing differential pituitary hormone disorders following a given HPA dosimetry: GH deficiency (>18 Gy), central precocious puberty (18–24 Gy), hypogonadotropic hypogonadism (30–40 Gy), ACTH deficiency (>40–50 Gy), and TSH deficiency (>40–50 Gy) [12]. In addition, cranial/craniospinal scatter irradiation may affect thyroid function, thus resulting in primary thyroid function disorders [13].

Finally, though the HPA shows a well-demonstrated resistance to the detrimental effects of chemotherapy, survivors of both genders often experience primary gonadal insufficiency and impaired residual fertility as a result of the cumulative effect of alkylating agents administered in the setting of polypharmacological protocols.

21.2.1 Growth Hormone Deficiency

Short stature is a frequent finding among childhood brain cancer survivors. Though faltering growth may result from the detrimental effect of spinal radiation on growth plates [14, 15], growth hormone deficiency (GHD) should always be ruled out in the case of impaired height velocity, as it represents the most common pituitary endocrine *sequela* in this subset of patients. The reported incidence achieves 12.5% in cohorts of brain tumor survivors, with an average time of 2.5 years (0.05–8.4) elapsing between tumor treatment and GHD diagnosis. Radiation is the major independent risk factor for iatrogenic GHD [16, 17]. Accordingly, in childhood brain tumor survivors, standing and sitting height should be assessed every 6–12 months [14]. Diagnosis of iatrogenic GHD may be challenging. First, IGF1 and IGFBP3 have been described as not reliable surrogate markers among irradiated patients [14]. Accordingly, standardized provocative tests are mandatory to diagnose GHD also in CCS [18]. Insulin tolerance test is regarded as the gold standard to assess GH secretion in children and adolescents with irradiated brain tumors, while the GHRH-arginine test should be prescribed in this setting, as it is associated with a high occurrence of falsely negative results [19]. The use of arginine (AST) and glucagon stimulation tests (GST) is constrained by the effect of radiotherapy on GH responsiveness to AST [20], the effect of body mass index on GST-induced GH secretion, and the impact of pubertal status on GH peaks. Retesting GH residual reserve in late adolescence and early adulthood is warranted following cranial irradiation, since iatrogenic adult-age GHD is not a rare finding among brain tumor survivors [14, 21, 22]. In the case of GHD, recombinant human GH (rhGH) should be administered by daily subcutaneous injections, with dosage and monitoring schedule superimposable to those undertaken in the general population [23]. The timing for starting rhGH should be discussed within a multidisciplinary team and tailored to the patient's specificities and risk factors. A recent consensus statement suggests that clinicians should wait at least 12 months following the end of antineoplastic treatments before prescribing rhGH in patients with malignant brain tumors. An exception is represented by patients with craniopharyngioma, for whom rhGH can be started as early as 3 months after the end of treatment [24]. In children with co-occurring treatment for central hypothyroidism or adrenal insufficiency, it may be needed to titrate the dose of hydrocortisone or L-thyroxine after starting rhGH [23, 24].

Over the last few years, the scientific community has witnessed an outburst of data about the administration of long-acting rhGH (LAGH) once-weekly formulations in children and adolescents [25]. Nevertheless, information about the safety and effectiveness of LAGH among childhood cancer survivors is still extremely poor, and a larger body of literature should be pursued before proceeding with its routine administration in this subset of fragile individuals.

21.2.2 Hypothyroidism

TSH deficiency (TSHD), also known as *central hypothyroidism*, is one of the most frequent *sequelae* among childhood brain tumor survivors, with a reported incidence of 9.2–47.0% in different study cohorts. HPA radiation doses exceeding 30–40 Gy and surgery are regarded as major risk factors for TSHD. In addition, younger age upon brain tumor diagnosis and suprasellar and infratentorial tumor location play an additional detrimental role [15, 26].

In brain tumor survivors, the co-occurrence of low fT4 and normal or reduced TSH prompts the diagnosis of overt TSHD. Milder pictures may be more insidious, as fT4 may fall into the lower interquartile range. In this setting, the European Thyroid Association guidelines highlight that a 20% or greater decrease in fT4 levels over time not associated with a compensatory increase in TSH should shed light on a potential disruption of the HP-thyroid axis [27, 28]. Lastly, patients with a predominant hypothalamic involvement may present with a slight elevation in TSH levels associated with remarkably low fT4, potentially resembling primary hypothyroidism [28]. Levotiroxine replacement should be started in TSHD after ruling out or correcting co-occurring hypocortisolism. In children and adolescents, the starting daily dose should be set at 2.0 μg/kg, and it should be subsequently titrated, aiming at FT4 levels above the median value of the reference range [28].

The incidence of *primary hypothyroidism* (PH) is remarkably greater among brain tumor survivors compared to the general population, with a reported incidence ranging from 5.8% to 9.4%, mostly due to the well-known radiosensitivity of the thyroid [16, 26]. The overall occurrence of post-radiation PH is related to the extent of the radiation field, the cumulative radiation dose, and the age at radiotherapy. A recent review from the Pediatric Normal Tissue Effects in the Clinic (PENTEC) initiative reports expected rates of subclinical hypothyroidism as high as 12%, 25%, and 44% following 10, 20, and 30 Gy exposure, respectively [29]. Among childhood cancer survivors, hypothyroidism arises as the result of an interplay of direct thyrocyte damage and cell-mediated cytotoxicity due to thyroid antigen exposure following radiation. Medulloblastoma is the brain tumor most frequently associated with PH [26, 30, 31]. The treatment for PH in brain tumor survivors does not differ from that undertaken in the general population.

21.2.3 Central Precocious Puberty

Precocious puberty is defined as the finding of clinical signs consistent with pubertal onset (breast budding in girls, testicular volume $\geq$ 4 mL in boys) before the age of 8 years in females and 9 years in males. Following GH and TSH deficiency, disorders in the timing of onset and progression of puberty represent the third most frequently reported pituitary pathological findings among brain tumor survivors [32]. Central precocious puberty (CPP) can be regarded as either the result of a direct detrimental effect of tumors arising from the hypothalamic area (hypothalamic gliomas, optic pathways gliomas, suprasellar craniopharyngiomas) or as a consequence of the disruptive effect of radiotherapy or neurosurgery [33].

Indeed, the timing of pubertal onset and *tempo* is controlled by a delicate balance of inhibiting (hypothalamic GABA-) and stimulating (glutamate-, kisspeptin-) neural networks exerting their action on the gonadotropin-releasing hormone (GnRH) secreting neurons [34]. Pulsatile release of GnRH has been identified as the pivotal factor triggering pubertal onset and progression, leading to a progressive surge in circulating luteinizing hormone (LH) and follicle-stimulating hormone (FSH) levels. Accordingly, as hypothalamic GABA-secreting neurons are extremely sensitive to iatrogenic damage, radiotherapy and surgery involving the HPA often result in an indirect promotion of pro-activating networks, thus leading to premature pubertal onset [35]. Finally, CPP may occur in patients with brain cancer presenting with hydrocephalus, irrespective of the site of the tumor itself. Indeed, increased intracranial pressure is regarded as an additional factor playing a potentially detrimental role in the hypothalamic inhibitory regulation of GnRH-secreting tumors [36, 37].

Treatment with GnRH analogs is the standard of care in both idiopathic and organic CPP. These compounds show a decreased enzymatic degradation along with an increased affinity for the GnRH pituitary receptor. As the prolonged exposure to GnRH results in desensitization of its receptor and in a downregulation of gonadotropin-secreting activity, GnRH analogs exert their action by inhibiting LH and FSH secretion, thus arresting any further pubertal progression.

21.2.4 Hypogonadism in Female Survivors

Brain cancer survivors may experience either hypo- or hypergonadotropic hypogonadism, mostly depending on the tumor site and treatment burden.

Hypogonadotropic hypogonadism (HH) is defined as an impaired secretion of gonadotropins, leading to pubertal delay, pubertal arrest, or amenorrhea as a result of inadequate circulating sexual hormones. It may arise as either the detrimental mass/infiltrative effect of tumors directly involving the HPA (i.e., craniopharyngiomas, germ cell tumors) or as an outcome of cranial irradiation or neurosurgery. HP dosimetry as high as 30–50 Gy has been reported by different authors as a major risk factor for the onset of HH [12, 38].

Conversely, antineoplastic therapies often affect ovarian secreting reserve, thus leading to *hypergonadotropic hypogonadism*. Gonadal dysfunction can be regarded as one of the most frequently experienced late effects, with reported incidence as high as 8% in mixed cohorts of CCS but achieving 60% among brain cancer survivors [39, 40].

Alkylating agents, widely recognized as the most gonadotoxic medications [41], have been demonstrated to present a dose-dependent toxicity profile. In addition, radiation affects oocyte maturation and function, leading to the depletion of ovarian follicles that eventually results in impaired fertility and hypoestrogenism [42]. Accordingly, among brain cancer survivors, those exposed to craniospinal irradiation may experience impaired ovarian function as a result of scatter irradiation involving the pelvis [43].

The clinical presentation of hypergonadotropic hypogonadism mostly depends on the age at presentation. Pre- and peripubertal girls may display clinical and auxological findings suggestive of pubertal delay or pubertal arrest, with the latter being defined as the failure to progress through pubertal stages over time [44]. In post-pubertal adolescents and women under the age of 40, the co-occurrence of oligo-amenorrhea alongside elevated FSH levels within the menopausal range—confirmed on at least two occasions 4 weeks apart—prompts the diagnosis of primary ovarian insufficiency (POI) [45]. Survivors with POI report a spectrum of symptoms related to hypoestrogenism, including vasomotor phenomena (hot flashes and night sweats), sleep disturbances, fatigue, decreased libido, depression, and vaginal dryness [46].

Childhood cancer survivors diagnosed with either hypo- or hypergonadotropic hypogonadism deserve timely prescription of hormonal replacement therapy (HRT), aiming at restoring age-specific physiological estrogen levels [47]. In pre-peripubertal patients experiencing pubertal delay or arrest, progressively increasing doses of estrogens, mostly delivered by transdermal patches, are prescribed, with the aims of mimicking the physiological course of puberty, inducing secondary sexual features, maximizing height spurt, and promoting bone mass accrual. Conversely, adult-dose combined estro-progestin formulations are prescribed in post-pubertal adolescents and women experiencing hypogonadism, in order to prevent them from experiencing symptoms and clinical signs consistent with hypogonadism [48].

21.2.5 Hypogonadism in Male Survivors

As for females, also among male brain cancer survivors, inadequate circulating testosterone levels may arise as a consequence of either hypo- or hypergonadotropic hypogonadism [49]. The pathophysiology of *hypogonadotropic hypogonadism* (HH) in male brain cancer survivors is complex and multifactorial, involving an interplay of direct tumor invasion, neurosurgery, and cranial radiation, potentially affecting the HP-gonadal axis [12].

Conversely, in patients experiencing primary testicular insufficiency, both Leydig and germ cells can be variably affected. Leydig cells' failure leads to a progressive decline in androgen concentrations. Accordingly, pre- and peripubertal individuals may exhibit pubertal delay or arrest, along with elevated LH and follicle-stimulating hormone (FSH) levels, in the setting of a clinical and biochemical picture suggestive of *hypergonadotropic hypogonadism* [50]. In post-pubertal males, diminished testosterone secretion may precipitate sexual dysfunction and affect libido, alongside complications such as impaired glucose tolerance, insulin resistance, osteopenia, decreased lean mass, fatigue, and an overall decline in quality of life (QoL) [51].

In addition, treatment protocols including alkylating agents, radiotherapy involving the pelvis/groin and/or stem cell transplantation often result in Sertoli/germ cells damage and subsequent impaired spermatogenesis. The extent of chemotherapy-induced germ cell damage is dose-dependent, and cyclophosphamide-equivalent doses below 4000 mg/m^2 do not generally affect residual fertility [52]. On the other hand, the sterilizing dose following testicular radiation exposure is set at 3 Gy [53]. Interestingly, the co-occurrent administration of alkylating agents and radiation exacerbates and intensifies the risk of impaired spermatogenesis. As the reliability of serum FSH and inhibin B levels as surrogates for assessing germ cell function still needs to be confirmed among survivors, semen analysis represents the gold standard following gonadotoxic treatments [54, 55].

All brain tumor survivors exposed to potentially gonadotoxic treatments should receive counseling regarding the risk of testosterone deficiency and impaired fertility. From a clinical perspective, annual follow-up for prepubertal boys should include height monitoring and pubertal assessment, while postpubertal patients should undergo a yearly thorough sexual history review and physical examination, including evaluations of body mass index and early detection of clinical signs potentially consistent with hypogonadism. Early morning testosterone, LH, and FSH levels should be assessed at least yearly, from peripubertal age onward [56].

Peripubertal boys experiencing pubertal delay or arrest, as in the setting of hypergonadotropic hypogonadism, should receive progressively increasing doses of testosterone in order to mimic spontaneous pubertal attainment and to induce secondary sexual characteristics. Conversely, pubertal induction among brain tumor survivors diagnosed with hypogonadotropic hypogonadism can be achieved by offering different potential treatment solutions [57]. On the one hand, testosterone replacement therapy provides adolescents with prompt improvement in circulating sexual hormones and virilization but does not stimulate testicular volume and Sertoli/germ cell maturation. On the other hand, subcutaneous gonadotropins promote both testosterone secretion and sperm production, though this approach involves multiple weekly injections [58].

21.2.6 ACTH Deficiency

Among brain tumor survivors, ACTH deficiency (ACTHD) may arise as a result of neurosurgery or radiation involving the HPA. The theoretical radiation threshold for iatrogenic ACTHD is generally set beyond 30 Gy [12]. The clinical presentation of ACTHD encompasses a spectrum of findings, ranging from insidious pictures (fatigue, weight loss, mild early morning hypoglycemia) to the acute occurrence of a life-threatening critically ill state (adrenal crisis) [59]. As demanding clinical events may trigger an acute presentation, at-risk patients should receive a systematic HP-adrenal axis assessment before undergoing neurosurgery [60]. Early morning serum cortisol levels could be used as a screening tool to timely identify overt deficiency. Nevertheless, in case of more subtle subclinical pictures, despite retained baseline cortisol levels, the HP-adrenal system may fail to achieve a proper secretive response to stressful clinical conditions, thus precipitating an adrenal crisis. Accordingly, a dynamic assessment (ACTH test) is warranted in high-risk patients with clinical complaints consistent with ACTHD, in order to explore adrenal secretory residual reserve. The cornerstone treatment of ACTHD is represented by glucocorticoid replacement therapy. Oral daily hydrocortisone is preferred in children because of its shorter duration, lower potency, and a less detrimental effect on linear growth. The starting dose is 8–10 mg/m^2, and it must be subsequently titrated based on the patient's symptoms and response [61].

Finally, patients and caregivers should always be trained to timely recognize co-occurring clinical conditions exposing patients to a potential risk of adrenal crisis and to double or triple the daily hormonal replacement dose with reference to the magnitude of the stressor ("sick day rule").

21.2.7 Central Diabetes Insipidus

Central diabetes insipidus (CDI) occurs in children with brain malignancy, due to the mass effect of the tumor itself (mainly CNS germ-cell tumors or Langerhans cell histiocytosis) or as a consequence of the surgery involving the pituitary or diencephalon area. Rarely, radiotherapy involving the HPA may result in CDI [62, 63]. Accordingly, CDI is mostly detected upon brain tumor diagnosis or in the early post-surgical period. Though post-surgical CDI may be transient, the 15-year cumulative incidence of permanent CDI is as high as 2.6%. Given this pathogenic background, it is not surprising that the reported prevalence of CDI among patients with suprasellar (SS) tumors is remarkably greater than for non-SS tumors (63.2% versus 0.9%, respectively) [15].

The physiopathology of post-surgical CDI is generally triphasic. Indeed, CDI may initially become overt within the first 2 days following CNS surgery due to local edema. In some cases, between 2 and 14 days following surgery, hypothalamic and pituitary damaged cells can inappropriately secrete ADH, leading to a phase of hyponatremic fluid overload. This phase is generally transient. Thereafter, the irreversible impairment of posterior pituitary cells leads to permanent CDI [63, 64]. The prolonged excretion of hypoosmotic urine, resulting in polyuria, polydipsia, and a trend toward dehydration and hypernatremia, is the consequence of the insufficient secretion of antidiuretic hormone.

Oral, intranasal, or sublingual desmopressin should be promptly started as soon as CDI is confirmed. Subsequently, the dose must be titrated, aiming at identifying the lowest dose effective in maintaining normal blood sodium levels and euvolemia [64, 65].

A limited subset of patients with CDI may also experience direct or secondary damage involving the diencephalic centers that regulate the sense of thirst, with an irreversible impairment of this pivotal physiological compensatory mechanism. Accordingly, adipsic CDI is associated with the highest mortality rates, and its treatment is extremely challenging [66, 67]. It has been reported in 1.3–20% of patients with brain tumors. Di Iorgi et al. hypothesized that the risk of developing adipsic CDI mostly depends on the aggressiveness and extent of the surgical intervention rather than the tumor extension or histotype itself [67].

21.3 Fertility

Impairment in gonadal function and infertility are common treatment-related toxicities among childhood cancer survivors with central nervous system (CNS) and skull base tumors [68].

Several studies have also reported that these patients may be less likely to conceive or even make any attempt during their adult lives due to cognitive damage and lower likelihood of establishing romantic relationships [69, 70].

Successful fertility requires functional testes, ovaries, and genitourinary organs as well as a functional hypothalamic–pituitary–gonadal (HPG) axis, all of which can be affected by the initial cancer involvement, treatment, and the psychogenic effects of therapies. In fact, surgery, chemotherapies, and radiotherapies can all impact future fertility [71].

Female survivors may face ovarian dysfunction due to the direct effects of chemotherapy or radiation and/or the indirect effects from the HPG axis dysfunction [49]. Radiotherapy of the uterus and vagina may also contribute to fertility difficulties as well as compromised sexual health.

Ovaries contain a finite pool of primordial follicles, which represents the ovarian reserve and peaks at 6–7 million follicles during fetal life, at approximately midgestation. In a normal female, the number of ovarian follicles declines with age from >1 million at birth to approximately 1000 at normal menopause (on average 50 years). Chemotherapies and radiotherapies can hasten the natural decline of follicle number that therefore leads to impaired ovarian hormone production, uterine dysfunction due to inadequate estrogen exposure, early menopause, and infertility [72, 73].

Ovarian damage can lead to diminished ovarian reserve (DOR), delayed puberty, primary amenorrhea, or secondary amenorrhea due to premature ovarian insufficiency (POI). DOR is diagnosed when anti-Müllerian hormone (AMH) and antral follicular count (AFC) by ultrasound are below the 5th–10th percentile of the age-related nomograms [74, 75]. POI is characterized by persistent amenorrhea and FSH levels greater than 30–40 IU/L at two random tests at least 1 month apart, before the age of 40 [76].

Gonadal damage from chemotherapy is primarily related to the cumulative doses of chemotherapies received, especially alkylating agents, and the patient's age at the time of treatment [77, 78].

The cyclophosphamide equivalent dose (CED) and alkylating agent dose score (AAD) are the most common methods for calculating the cumulative dose of alkylating agents. Several studies have reported an independent association between POI and CED, showing nearly a threefold increased risk of POI with a CED of ≥8000 mg/m^2 (HR 2.77; 95% CI, 1.18–6.51), which increases to fourfold with a CED of ≥12,000 mg/m^2 (HR 3.9; 95% CI, 1.8–8.43). A CED score of >6000 mg/m^2 is currently considered high risk for POI [52, 78, 79].

Although primordial follicles before puberty are mitotically inactive, they remain vulnerable to the direct effects of radiotherapy. Indeed, radiotherapy has a profound and permanent impact on ovarian function, its extent depending on several factors such as age of the patient (the younger the patient is at the time of radiation, the greater the damage), exposure dose, exposure time, and eventually associated chemotherapy [80, 81]. In the prepubertal age, it's estimated that ≤2 Gy of radiation would destroy half of immature oocytes [73, 82], while 25–50 Gy would produce infertility in a third of young women and in almost all women over 40 years of age.

It is well known that the secretion of GnRH, FSH, LH, estradiol, progesterone, and prolactin follows a pulsatile rhythm, which is responsible for the reproductive hormonal environment [83]. Disturbances of the pulsatile rhythm of FSH/LH production induced by cerebral irradiation can affect fertility and libido and can disrupt the menstrual cycle [84]. Irreversible dysfunction of the HPG axis can be overcome with hormonal therapies for ovarian stimulation.

The uterus could also be affected by radiotherapy, and the consequent damage could be irreversible. In fact, exposure to radiation during childhood leads to altered uterine vascularization, decreased uterine volume and elasticity, myometrial fibrosis and necrosis, and endometrial atrophy and insufficiency. The cervix gets atrophic and loses its elasticity, especially in older patients [85]. Similarly, radiation to the vagina can result in vaginal stenosis/fibrosis, dryness, and soft tissue changes.

Small uterine size after radiation therapy has been associated with adverse obstetrical outcomes, including miscarriage, difficulty with implantation (likely due to endometrial dysfunction), premature birth, and low birthweight offspring. Sufficient evidence is not available to determine a safe uterine dose, although high-quality evidence indicates that cancer survivorship did not increase the risk of congenital abnormalities in births to survivors [86].

Male survivors may have impaired spermatogenesis from gonadotoxic chemotherapy or radiation on testes, as well as gonadotropin deficiency from CNS-direct radiotherapy causing central hypogonadism [87]. Spine or pelvic surgery or radiotherapy may also cause erectile or ejaculatory dysfunction [88]. In men, germ cell failure is commonly reported with a CED score of ≥7500 mg/m^2 [78]. The Childhood Cancer Survivor Study reported a relative risk (RR) of 2.13 (95% CI, 1.69–2.68) for infertility when the AAD was ≥3 in male survivors.

Spermatogenesis can be impaired when the testes are exposed to radiation doses as low as 0.1–0.2 Gy, with doses >4 Gy resulting in permanent azoospermia [89].

Testicular Leydig cells, which produce testosterone, are more resistant to radiation. Hypoandrogenism usually develops in the case of testicular radiation doses of ≥24 Gy in prepubertal patients and ≥30 Gy in postpubertal males, respectively [90]. Due to this variability in radiation dose susceptibility, testicular irradiation often compromises spermatogenesis, while puberty and testosterone levels are unaffected.

Little is known about the effects on gonadal function of the newer treatment protocols, like proton-beam therapy and molecular-matched targeted therapy. Further research is needed.

Ovarian reserve and sperm quality testing represent a cornerstone in counselling and evaluating all patients who underwent gonadotoxic regimens. At present, there is no perfect test, and common methods to assess the ovarian reserve include dosage of follicle-stimulating hormone (FSH) and estradiol (E2) levels at day 3 of the menstrual cycle, dosage of AMH, and an ultrasound-assessed AFC.

In light of the variety of ways that CNS cancers can impact patients' fertility, several international societies have recognized the clinical importance of establishing fertility preservation techniques in those wishing to preserve their future reproductive potential [91] and recommend counselling in all patients of reproductive age.

21.4 Neurocognitive and Psychosocial Late Effects

Long-term neurocognitive and psychosocial effects of treatment for brain tumor CCSs represent important areas of clinical focus and research. Indeed, it is estimated that as many as 40–100% of survivors demonstrate impairment in at least one neurocognitive domain [92] and CCSs report the poorest health-related quality of life among all childhood cancers [93].

21.4.1 Factors Associated with a Less Favorable Neurocognitive Outcome

A vast corpus of studies shows that multiple factors contribute significant risk to cognitive function. We can divide these factors into three clusters of variables: clinical factors, treatment factors, and individual patient characteristics. Clearly, tumor type and size have been associated with poorer neurocognitive outcomes [92, 94, 95]; also, tumor location and histological grade have effects on neuropsychological variables [96]. In addition to these features, longer time since diagnosis and treatment factors like cranial radiation therapy [97], chemotherapy [98], and surgical complications [99] play an important role in neurocognitive development. Lastly, demographic factors, such as low socioeconomic status, correlate with worse outcomes [10, 100], while young age at diagnosis is a positive prognostic factor.

21.4.2 Cognitive and Neuropsychological Outcomes

Historically, the measurement of neurocognitive function has been conducted through the assessment of intellectual quotient (IQ) because the IQ decline can be reasonably interpreted as demonstrating a failure in achieving age-related gains in cognitive function [101]. However, more recently, researchers and clinicians have focused on neuropsychological functions and have identified the ones at greatest risk [101, 102].

The most frequently impaired functions include attention, working memory, processing speed, and executive functions (EFs) [10, 102, 103].

Attention is not a unitary construct, and the subset of skills that falls under the concept of attention includes sustained, focused, selective, divided, alternating, shifting, and resistance to distraction. Attention deficits are commonly found in brain tumor CCSs [102, 104].

Working memory is a temporary workspace in which information is stored and handled for a brief period of time. A working memory deficit can emerge very early with a progressive decline over time [102]; moreover, some authors showed that working memory was the only domain with a continuous decline over time despite a stable IQ score 20–40 years after diagnosis of CNS tumor [105]. Processing speed (the promptness in performing relatively automatic mental tasks) is the first domain to be impaired after treatment and to be specifically correlated with craniospinal irradiation dose [102]. Given the importance of myelin in the conduction speed of neural impulses, it is not surprising that a deficit in this domain is frequent in children with cancer involving the CNS [106].

EFs are different skills, and they are often identified as the ability to control, organize, and manage cognitive, emotional, and behavioral responses. EFs involve inhibition, mental flexibility, planning and decision-making, abstract reasoning, concept formation, problem solving, and awareness [107]. Deficits in this area can manifest in daily life as problems with organization, time management, and emotional and behavioral control and will also negatively impact social development. Studies on EFs in brain tumor CCSs have reported these patients to be particularly susceptible to EF impairments, both in the short and long term. CCSs exhibit similar patterns of impairment in executive functions, in particular in forward-thinking and mental flexibility. Furthermore, language and speech deficits are documented among nearly all survivors after post-surgery posterior fossa syndrome [103, 108].

21.4.3 Psychological and Social Late Effects

Brain tumor CCSs are at increased risk for long-term psychological morbidities, including depression, anxiety, suicidal ideation, and behavior problems when compared to the general population [106, 109–112]. When compared with survivors of other childhood cancers, CCSs experience significantly more depressive symptoms as well as lower self-esteem and quality of life. At last, social deficits like social adjustment problems, isolation, and poor peer relations have also been well documented [113–115].

It should be underlined the fundamental relevance of the early detection of delayed acquisition or decline of neuropsychological functioning. Early psychological and neuropsychological evaluation allows individualized rehabilitative interventions that can reduce subsequent disability and improve quality of life. Therefore, from a clinical point of view, psychological and neuropsychological assessment is recommended, starting with a baseline evaluation at diagnosis and extending long-term neurocognitive follow-up to detect the late effects that manifest years after treatment. Transition to adulthood presents one of the major challenges for brain tumor CCSs: they are at increased risk for a range of adverse late effects that affect broad domains of functioning as neuropsychological, social-emotional, and achievement/vocational.

21.5 Second Malignant Neoplasms (SMNs)

Second malignant neoplasms (SMNs) are the most severe late complications in childhood cancer survivors and are the leading cause of death in long-term survivors. The cumulative incidence of SMNs does not reach a plateau even at 10 years after the treatment of primary cancer; more than 10% of long-term survivors develop SMNs [116].

The risk and histologic type of SMNs are often associated with specific therapies [117]. Brain tumor CCSs represent a high-risk population for developing SMNs due to the intensive therapies administered during childhood. Managing the long-term risks associated with these therapies is crucial to improving the quality of life and overall survival of these patients.

In a retrospective cohort of children and adolescent CCSs treated for CNS malignancies at 26 collaborating institutions in the United States and Canada, 76 subsequent malignant neoplasms were identified among the 1877 survivors evaluated [118]. The overall standardized incidence ratio (SIR) was 4.1 (95% CI = 3.2–5.2); the most common subsequent malignant neoplasms were CNS tumors (15 gliomas, four malignant meningiomas, one medulloblastoma or primitive neuroectodermal tumor; SIR = 25.3, 95% CI = 15.5–39.1), soft tissue sarcomas (SIR = 8.4, 95% CI = 3.6–16.5), and thyroid cancers (SIR = 11.2, 95% CI = 5.8–19.6).

Patients receiving cranial RT of 50 or more Gy had a cumulative incidence of a CNS subsequent neoplasm 25 years after diagnosis of 7.1% (95% CI = 4.5–9.6) compared with 5.2% for those receiving more than 0 but less than 50 Gy (95% CI = 2.1–8.3) and 1.0% for no RT exposure (95% CI = 0–2.3).

Various factors can affect the risk of developing second tumors: the treatment received (radiation therapy, and DNA-damaging agents, most notably alkylating agents), the patient's genetic background, the age of onset of the first cancer, and gender [119, 120].

21.5.1 Genetic Background

Pediatric cancer patients have a high frequency of germline pathogenic variants in cancer-predisposing genes (CPGs) [121].

A comprehensive study of childhood cancer survivors reported that 6.4% of the patients had germline pathogenic variants of CPGs [122].

Overlapping effects of genetic background and primary cancer treatment contribute to the development of SMNs after treatment of pediatric solid tumors [123].

Established familial cancer syndromes that increase brain tumor susceptibility include neurofibromatosis type 1 (NF1), neurofibromatosis type 2 (NF2), tuberous sclerosis (TSC1 or TSC2), Li–Fraumeni (TP53 or CHEK2), nevoid basal cell carcinoma or Gorlin syndrome (PTCH1), Turcot (APC), Cowden (PTEN), hereditary retinoblastoma (RB1), and Rubinstein–Taybi [124].

21.5.2 Treatment Received

Radiotherapy DNA damage induced by radiation in healthy tissues can lead to mutations that increase the risk of malignant tumors, particularly in the CNS. Nearly all of the reported survivors of childhood, adolescent, and young adult cancer who subsequently developed CNS tumors had received treatment with cranial radiation. Cohort studies [125, 126] showed that the dose of radiation exposure to the brain has a linear relationship with the risk of subsequent high-grade gliomas and meningiomas. Age at treatment is another important determinant, with younger children showing greater sensitivity to radiation-induced damage [127]. The risk profile for SMNs following radiation therapy (RT) may have shifted over time, particularly since children under 3 years of age are no longer routinely exposed to radiation. Over the past three decades, advancements in radiation therapy have transitioned treatments from two-dimensional (2D) techniques to three-dimensional (3D) methods, including the more precise three-dimensional conformal radiation therapy (3D-CRT) and, a decade later, intensity-modulated radiation therapy (IMRT). Both techniques aim to focus the radiation dose within the tumor while minimizing exposure to surrounding healthy tissues. However, IMRT may be considered a "double-edged sword" regarding cancer induction compared to 3D-CRT. At lower doses, there is a linear relationship with the development of SMNs, and IMRT exposes a larger volume of normal tissue to these lower doses [128]. As new radiation techniques like proton beam therapy become more widely available, it is crucial to assess their comparative risk of secondary cancers. While some solid SMNs developed in the lower dose region, the most common site was within the highest dose region, suggesting that the benefit of proton therapy, sparing the risk of SMNs compared to IMRT, may not be profound. Further studies conducted with similar analyses are needed to better compare the risk between these two modalities [129]. Proton arc therapy (PAT) is emerging as a promising innovation, with studies indicating potential to minimize the delivered integral dose and thus the risk of SMNs [130].

Chemotherapy Only a few studies examined whether chemotherapy alone is linked to the risk of developing SMNs. In a large cohort of CCSs, it was found that those treated solely with chemotherapy had a higher risk of developing an SMN compared to the general population [119]. Their risk and cumulative incidence were about half of what was seen in survivors who received both radiation and chemotherapy. Additionally, survivors who received higher cumulative doses of alkylating agents and/or platinum-based drugs had increased SMN rates, and there is a linear dose–response relationship between the cumulative dose of alkylating agents and the relative rate of SMNs [119]. In the Childhood Cancer Survivor Study [131], the mortality and morbidity were analyzed among 5-year survivors of medulloblastoma diagnosed between 1970 and 1999. The introduction of adjuvant chemotherapy in the 1980s and risk-stratified therapy in the 1990s significantly improved the 5-year survival rates for children with medulloblastoma. However, these advances have also been linked to a higher risk of late effects, including SMNs. Survivors of standard-risk multimodal therapy have shown a higher 15-year cumulative incidence of SMNs compared to those who received only radiation therapy (RT). For example, a long-term follow-up of the Children's Oncology Group trial A9961 estimated a 10-year cumulative incidence of secondary malignancies at 4.2% [132], while the HIT '91 trial in Germany reported a similar incidence of 4.3% [133]. At St. Jude Children's Research Hospital, the 10-year cumulative incidence rate for SMNs was 5.5%, significantly higher than in historical cohorts treated with RT alone [134].

Interaction between Therapies The combination of radiotherapy and chemotherapy amplifies the risk of SMNs. The concurrent use of alkylating agents and antimetabolites with radiation has shown an increased risk of SMNs [135]. The influence of germline sequence alterations (such as mutations in tumor suppressor genes TP53 and PTEN) in addition to chemo- and radiotherapy in the development of SMNs is gradually being elucidated, but the data are still limited.

21.5.3 Types of SMNs

Second CNS Tumors Survivors are at significantly higher risk (8.1–52.3 times) of developing CNS tumors compared to the general population, especially those who received cranial radiation therapy during treatment [137]. Gliomas, meningiomas, and other CNS neoplasms have a strong correlation between radiation dose and tumor development. The risk does not seem to plateau over time, meaning that survivors may continue to develop CNS tumors many years after treatment [136]. Following cranial radiotherapy, the cumulative incidence of a glioma in CNS tumor survivors is 2.7%, 3.7%, and 5.0% by ages 40, 50, and 60 [137].

High-grade gliomas are among the most aggressive and life-threatening subsequent tumors identified in childhood cancer survivors [127]. Radiation therapy is strongly correlated with the development of high-grade gliomas. Studies, including the British Childhood Cancer Survivor Study (BCCSS) and the North American Childhood Cancer Survivor Study (CCSS), show a linear correlation between radiation dose and the risk of high-grade gliomas [125, 126]. For high-grade gliomas, the risk increases linearly with radiation dose, peaking at exposure levels of 30–44.9 Gy. Odds ratios (OR) for subsequent gliomas are dramatically higher at this dose range, with one study reporting an OR of 21.0, reflecting a 21-fold increased risk. The prognosis for survivors who develop high-grade gliomas is generally poor, with 5-year survival rates ranging from 0% to 19.5%, which is comparable to survival rates of adults with primary gliomas. This grim outlook is a key challenge in the management of these patients, with many studies emphasizing the need for better treatment strategies [138].

Gliomas tend to develop 8–20 years after the initial childhood cancer diagnosis, suggesting that these tumors often manifest long after the initial treatment phase [127].

Meningiomas are the second most common CNS neoplasms in childhood cancer survivors. They are generally considered benign, but malignant forms exist as well. The cumulative incidence of a meningioma after cranial RT in CNS tumor survivors doubled from 5.9% to 12.5% between ages 40 and 60 [139]. Meningiomas have a strong association with prior radiation exposure, particularly high-dose cranial radiation. The BCCSS and CCSS [125, 126] studies showed that meningioma risk increases linearly with radiation dose, with substantial relative risks observed at exposure levels above 20 Gy. For example, at radiation doses of 40 Gy or more, the relative risk of developing meningiomas can rise dramatically, reaching nearly 479 times higher than the general population [125, 126]. Unlike high-grade gliomas, meningiomas generally have better outcomes, with survival rates ranging from 57.3% to 100% depending on the study and tumor grade. For benign meningiomas, 5-year survival can be as high as 84.3%, while malignant forms have lower survival rates, closer to 57.3% [126]. Meningiomas tend to occur after a longer latency period compared to high-grade gliomas. In some studies, meningiomas were diagnosed 10–30 years after the initial cancer diagnosis. The long latency period underscores the need for ongoing vigilance in survivors of childhood cancer.

Primitive Neuroectodermal Tumors (PNETs) are aggressive, high-grade tumors that occur less frequently than gliomas or meningiomas but are still a significant concern among survivors. PNETs are often fatal and challenging to treat [127].

Second Thyroid Tumors The thyroid is particularly sensitive to radiation damage [131]. Thyroid cancer risk increased linearly with radiation dose up to approximately 20 Gy, where the relative risk peaked at 14.6-fold. At thyroid radiation doses >20 Gy, a downturn in the dose–response relationship was observed [136]. Secondary thyroid neoplasms are predominantly differentiated carcinomas. Despite the disease often presenting with lymph node involvement, the prognosis for these patients remains very good [138], similarly to the primary thyroid cancer encouraging a minimalist approach to the treatment of these particular patients wherever possible [139, 140].

21.5.4 Surveillance

The International Late-Effects of Childhood Cancer Guideline Harmonization Group has attempted to provide guidelines regarding the surveillance of CCSs in relation to the development of secondary CNS tumors [141]. They concluded that there is insufficient evidence to determine whether early detection of CNS neoplasms, such as meningiomas or high-grade gliomas, reduces morbidity and mortality, so no recommendation is made for or against routine MRI surveillance. The decision for surveillance should be a shared one between the survivor and the healthcare provider. Children with NF1 are at higher risk for CNS neoplasms, particularly after cranial radiotherapy. Current guidelines recommend considering brain MRIs every 2 years for these patients [141, 142].

21.6 Other Late Effects

Ototoxicity is an adverse effect that has been reported in several brain tumors CCSs, following treatment with platinum-based compounds, head or brain radiotherapy, or both [143, 144]. Children treated with cisplatin at cumulative doses approaching 400 mg/m^2 require long-term surveillance to avoid overlooking hearing deficits. Carboplatin, at a standard dose, does not appear to be a significant risk factor for ototoxicity even in patients who have already been treated with cisplatin [145]. Sensorineural hearing loss is also a common side effect of radiation therapy: a dose–response relationship was observed. Older radiotherapy techniques are more likely to cause serious ototoxic sequelae than available therapies, such as intensity-modulated radiotherapy (IMRT), which reduces exposure to crucial aural structures because of their improved conformality in targeting tumors [144, 146].

Both types of damage, whether from platinum derivatives or radiotherapy, are irreversible. Treatment-induced ototoxicity typically presents as hearing loss of high-frequency sounds, often accompanied by tinnitus.

Moreover, permanent or long-term ventriculoperitoneal derivation also confers risk for hearing loss [144, 146]. One hypothesis is that surgical injury might affect the occurrence of hearing loss for some patients, but the role of the extent of surgery, or the degree of hydrocephalus at diagnosis, in contributing to hearing loss and whether shunting and correction of increased intracranial pressure facilitates healing from surgical injury over time remain unclear.

Based on the evidence and expert consensus [147], the guideline panel agreed that CCSs treated with cisplatin (with or without high-dose carboplatin [>1500 mg/m^2], level C evidence), head or brain radiotherapy of 30 Gy or more (expert opinion), or both, and their healthcare providers should be aware of the potential risks of tinnitus. Referral to an audiologist is recommended for survivors who have symptoms of tinnitus (strong recommendation).

Subclinical, progressive, irreversible, and sometimes fatal treatment-related cardiovascular events may manifest both during and after the end of chemotherapeutic treatment. Among antineoplastic drugs, anthracyclines, widely used in many anticancer treatments, are well known for their cardiotoxicity and have been extensively studied over the past years. Furthermore, screening protocols have been suggested for early detection of anthracycline-induced cardiotoxicity, both in adult and pediatric populations [148–150].

HD-cyclophosphamide, etoposide, thiotepa, and platinum-derived compounds used for high-risk medulloblastoma patients have been associated with increased risk of cardiovascular toxicity (less frequently than anthracyclines, and mostly in adult populations), such as pericardial effusion, left ventricular (LV) dysfunction and heart failure (HF), arrhythmias, thrombotic events, and myocardial infarction [148, 151, 152].

Main late-onset cancer therapy-related cardiovascular toxicities (CTR-CVT) [153] include congestive heart failure (CHF) or cardiomyopathy, valvular abnormalities, coronary artery disease (CAD), and pericardial disease [154].

Cerebro- and cardiovascular diseases represent the third leading cause of death in brain tumor CCSs, following cancer recurrence and secondary malignancies [155]. Stroke is a well-documented issue in CNS tumor survivors treated with radiotherapy [156–159]. Campen et al. showed a 100-fold higher incidence of stroke or transient ischemic attack (TIA) compared to the healthy pediatric population, with a median time from first radiation to first event (stroke or TIA) of 4.9 years, with a median follow-up of 6.3 years. In a report from the Childhood Cancer Survivor Study, nearly 50% of all detected strokes in childhood cancer survivors occurred in CNS tumor survivors, who represented only 13% of the study population. They further showed that the risk of experiencing a stroke is additionally increased by the presence of hypertension or diabetes mellitus [159].

Cardiovascular risk factors increase the risk of cardiovascular disease [154]: a positive significant interaction has been reported between hypertension and the risk of development of CAD and CHF. Bhatia et al. suggested a cardio-screening for all CCSs for whom treatment information is not available: a 5-year interval echocardiogram is suggested for potential CHF and/or radiation related valvulopathies [160].

Long-term survivors of pediatric CNS tumors have a higher incidence of pulmonary diseases such as emphysema, obliterative bronchiolitis, asthma, chronic cough, recurrent pneumonia, and pulmonary fibrosis. Craniospinal radiation, cyclophosphamide, bleomycin, and lomustine (CCNU) have been implicated in the causation of pulmonary dysfunction in children with brain tumors [161, 162]. Pulmonary dysfunction in pediatric cancer survivors tends to be gradual in onset with frequent remission and exacerbation [161].

Baseline pulmonary function testing (including DLCO and spirometry) and chest radiography are recommended before starting treatments and 2 or more years after completion of therapy to document any deficits. Revaluation of pulmonary function should be considered in patients with established deficits who require general anesthesia and for those treated with bleomycin [163, 164]. Different parts of the visual system can be affected by the tumors themselves or the treatment. Additionally, cranial radiotherapy may cause optic neuropathy or cataract. Some manifestations can be transient, resolve completely or partially, or persist as late effects. Chemotherapy-induced peripheral neuropathy (CIPN), manifesting as sensory and/or motor deficits of various degrees, is a common side effect of platinum agents and vinca alkaloids. Neuropathic symptoms often resolve following treatment completion, but in some cases, they persist for years [165].

21.7 New Drugs

Among new drugs, immunotherapeutic therapies can lead to significant long-term toxicities, many of which are likely still unknown. Many side effects have been described in adults. Thus, collaborative studies and long-term follow-ups are necessary to understand the long-term effects of these therapies on children who have survived cancer.

CAR T-cell therapy is associated with acute side effects, but we do not yet have sufficient follow-up to assess chronic effects. Emerging reports indicate that one of the most prominent complications is cytokine release syndrome (CRS), which, while often acute, can lead to prolonged inflammatory responses and organ damage [166].

Among the many immunotherapeutic strategies, immune checkpoint blockade has shown remarkable benefits in treating a range of cancer types. The development of immune checkpoint inhibitors (ICIs), such as anti-CTLA-4 and anti-PD-1/PD-L1 antibodies, has heralded a new era in cancer treatment, enabling the possibility of long-term survival in patients with metastatic disease and providing new therapeutic indications in earlier-stage settings. The relevant time frame of important patient-specific/toxicity-related factors includes acute toxicities, which are largely relevant while patients are on therapy, and chronic toxicities, all known as immune-related adverse events (IRAEs). These probably slowly decline over time, and the potential (theoretical) effects of such toxicities on other immune processes, such as atherosclerosis, could increase over time (Fig. 21.1).

Even if a majority of irAEs occur within the first 5–15 weeks, there are reports of late-onset irAEs both in the setting of ongoing immunotherapy and after treatment cessation. These delayed irAEs have been reported to occur months to years after discontinuation of therapy.

IRAEs most commonly involve the gastrointestinal tract, endocrine glands, skin, and liver. Less often, the central nervous system and cardiovascular, pulmonary, musculoskeletal, and hematologic systems are involved. The effects of ICIs on a diverse range of immune processes, including atherosclerosis, heart failure, neuroinflammation, obesity, and hypertension, have not been characterized but remain an important area of research with potential relevance to cancer survivors. Data on the chronicity of irAEs, especially in real-world settings, are currently limited and often incomplete. Tong et al., in a retrospective chart review of 161 adult patients with melanoma treated with immunotherapy, show that ICI treatment in melanoma is associated with a wide range of toxicities that can be permanent and may have long-lasting impacts on patients [167].

Late IRAEs can be divided by apparatus, in order of incidence [168] (Fig. 21.2).

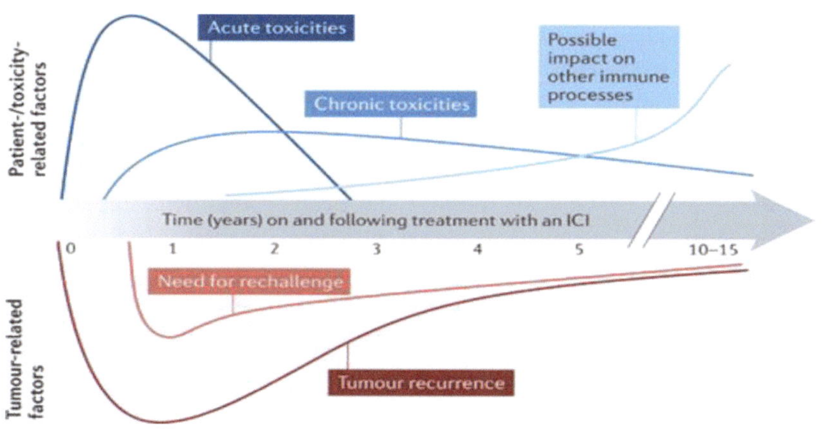

Fig. 21.1 Toxicities over time

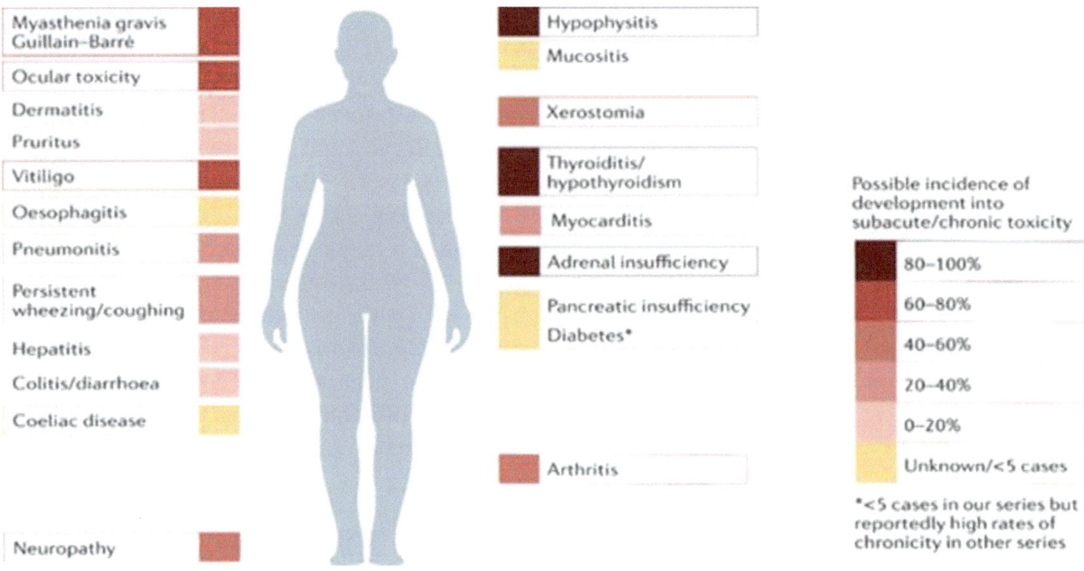

Fig. 21.2 irAEs

Endocrinological complications, such as thyroiditis, type 1 diabetes, and pituitary disfunctions, are of particular concern and often require long-term management [169–178]. In contrast to other adverse ICI effects, hypopituitarism is often permanent. Steroids are mostly not beneficial, and therapeutic strategies should mainly focus on appropriate hormone replacement [173]. Furthermore, there have been rare case reports documenting isolated arginine vasopressin deficiency caused by posterior pituitary/hypothalamus dysfunction in patients undergoing treatment with ICIs [174, 175].

Also, chronic cardiovascular toxicities from ICIs play a relevant role, as cardiovascular disease is the leading cause of non–cancer-related death in cancer survivors, even in the pre-ICI era, due to overlapping risk factors as well as treatment-related effects. Late ICI-associated CAE cases exhibited significantly more left ventricular systolic dysfunction (LVSD) and heart failure (HF) and less frequent supraventricular arrhythmias. Early and late ICI-associated CAE cases had similarly high mortality rates [179]. There is a growing appreciation of late-onset cardiotoxicities, such as atherosclerotic CAD and non-ischemic left ventricular dysfunction. The risk of accelerated CAD with ICIs is biologically plausible due to its proinflammatory mechanisms. Late-onset left ventricular dysfunction could occur as a consequence of subclinical myocarditis during ICI treatment [180].

The critical role of inflammation and adaptive immunity in atherosclerosis has been well characterized in preclinical studies, and several emerging clinical studies indicate a potential role of ICIs in the development and exacerbation of atherosclerosis; immune checkpoint therapy determines the progression of atherosclerosis, due to the role of T-cell immunity in atherogenesis [181].

From a dermatological point of view, IrCARs (immune-related cutaneous adverse reactions) might have a widespread clinical manifestation profile, with the most common ones including eczematous, morbilliform, vitiligo, and lichenoid lesions, but also relatively rarer severe cutaneous adverse reactions (SCARs) and bullous conditions might be seen. Anti-CTLA-4 agents exhibited higher cutaneous toxicity compared to anti-PD-1 and anti-PD-L1 agents [182]. Rare adverse events also extend up to hair conditions, ICI-induced scleroderma, and vasculitis. Oral/mucosal involvement has been reported but is relatively overlooked and requires further elucidation. The onset of presentation of overall

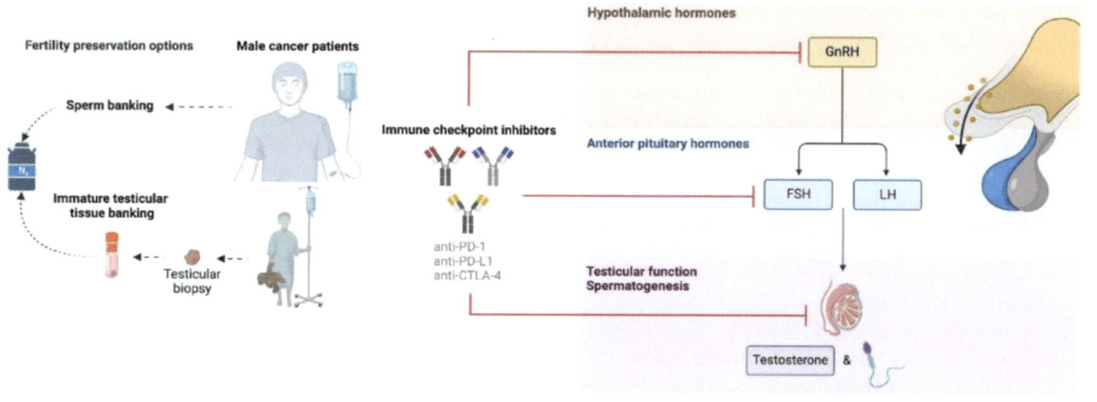

Fig. 21.3 Reproductive dysfunction caused by ICIs

irCAR was delayed as the patient's age increased, which may be attributed to the weakening of the immune system associated with the aging process. Lastly, some cutaneous reactions such as "skin disorders" or "skin toxicities" were ambiguously labeled, highlighting the challenges and lack of awareness in characterizing specific skin lesions [183].

As far as fertility is concerned, while there are several indications for testicular tissue banking, ICI treatment and immunotherapy are not included due to the lack of evidence. Despite the limited data on the impact of ICIs on spermatogenesis and testicular function, the guidelines from the European Society for Medical Oncology and the European Society of Human Reproduction and Embryology emphasize the importance of fertility counseling for all patients [184] (Fig. 21.3).

In conclusion, it can be stated that despite advances in immunotherapy, the long-term effects on pediatric cancer survivors remain largely unknown and of no small importance [181, 184].

Therefore, comprehensive long-term follow-up protocols are crucial, especially for CAR T-cell therapies, including regular monitoring, early intervention, and tailored supportive care. Collaboration among oncologists, primary care physicians, and specialists is essential to optimize health outcomes and quality of life for these patients.

References

1. Childhood Cancer International Europe [Internet]. Available online: https://ccieurope.eu/. Accessed 20 Aug 2024.
2. Cure Search. Available online: https://curesearch.org/. Accessed 20 Aug 2024.
3. Pollack IF, Agnihotri S, Broniscer A. Childhood brain tumors: current management, biological insights, and future directions. J Neurosurg Pediatr. 2019;23(3):261–73. https://doi.org/10.3171/2018.10.PEDS18377.
4. Bull KS, Kennedy CR. Neurocognitive effects of CNS tumors. Handb Clin Neurol. 2013;112:967–72. https://doi.org/10.1016/B978-0-444-52910-7.00017-9.
5. GBD 2017. Childhood Cancer Collaborators. The global burden of childhood and adolescent cancer in 2017: an analysis of the Global Burden of Disease Study 2017. Lancet Oncol. 2019;20(9):1211–25. https://doi.org/10.1016/S1470-2045(19)30339-0.
6. Bhakta N, Force LM, Allemani C. Childhood cancer burden: a review of global estimates. Lancet Oncol. 2019;20(1):e42–53. https://doi.org/10.1016/S1470-2045(18)30761-7.
7. Kremer LCM, Mulder RL, Oeffinger KC, et al. A worldwide collaboration to harmonize guidelines for the long-term follow-up of childhood and young adult cancer survivors: a report from the International Late Effects of Childhood Cancer Guideline Harmonization Group. Pediatr Blood Cancer. 2013;60(4):543–9. https://doi.org/10.1002/pbc.24445.
8. Ramezan NW, Hussain S, Mohamad N, Yaacob NM. Endocrine disorders in childhood brain tumour survivors: a single-centre study. J ASEAN Fed Endocr Soc. 2024;39(1):12–7. https://doi.org/10.15605/jafes.039.01.05. Epub 2023 Dec 22. PMID: 38863912; PMCID: PMC11166355.
9. Jensen MV, Rugbjerg K, de Fine Licht S, et al. Endocrine late effects in survivors of cancer

in adolescence and young adulthood: a Danish population-based cohort study. JAMA Netw Open. 2018;1(2):e180349. https://doi.org/10.1001/jamanetworkopen.2018.0349. Erratum in: JAMA Netw Open. 2018 Jul 6;1(3):e182037. 10.1001/jamanetworkopen.2018.2037. PMID: 30646084; PMCID: PMC6324403.

10. Roddy E, Mueller S. Late effects of treatment of pediatric central nervous system tumors. J Child Neurol. 2016;31(2):237–54. https://doi.org/10.1177/0883073815587944. Epub 2015 Jun 4. PMID: 26045296.
11. Vatner RE, Niemierko A, Misra M, et al. Endocrine deficiency as a function of radiation dose to the hypothalamus and pituitary in pediatric and young adult patients with brain tumors. J Clin Oncol. 2018;36(28):2854–62. https://doi.org/10.1200/JCO.2018.78.1492. Epub 2018 Aug 17. PMID: 30118397; PMCID: PMC6161835.
12. Darzy KH, Shalet SM. Hypopituitarism following radiotherapy. Pituitary. 2009;12:40–50. https://doi.org/10.1007/s11102-008-0088-4.
13. Cattoni A, Molinari S, Gaiero A, et al. Thyroid disorders following hematopoietic stem cell transplantation in childhood: impact of conditioning regimen on thyroid dysfunction, volume changes, and occurrence of nodules. Transplant Cell Ther. 2022;28(8):506.e1–506.e12. https://doi.org/10.1016/j.jtct.2022.05.040. Epub 2022 Jun 1. PMID: 35660063.
14. Sklar CA, Antal Z, Chemaitilly W, et al. Hypothalamic–pituitary and growth disorders in survivors of childhood cancer: an Endocrine Society clinical practice guideline. J Clin Endocrinol Metab. 2018;103:2761–84.
15. González Briceño LG, Kariyawasam D, Samara-Boustani D, et al. High prevalence of early endocrine disorders after childhood brain tumors in a large cohort. J Clin Endocrinol Metab. 2022;107(5):e2156–66. https://doi.org/10.1210/clinem/dgab893. PMID: 34918112.
16. Clement SC, Schouten-van Meeteren AY, Boot AM, et al. Prevalence and risk factors of early endocrine disorders in childhood brain tumor survivors: a Nationwide, Multicenter Study. J Clin Oncol. 2016;34(36):4362–70. https://doi.org/10.1200/JCO.2016.67.5025. Epub 2016 Oct 31. PMID: 27998218.
17. Laughton SJ, Merchant TE, Sklar CA, et al. Endocrine outcomes for children with embryonal brain tumors after risk-adapted craniospinal and conformal primary-site irradiation and high-dose chemotherapy with stem-cell rescue on the SJMB-96 trial. J Clin Oncol. 2008;26:1112–8.
18. Sfeir JG, Kittah NEN, Tamhane S, et al. Diagnosis of GH deficiency as a late effect of radiotherapy in survivors of childhood cancers. J Clin Endocrinol Metab. 2018;103:2785–93.
19. Patti G, Noli S, Capalbo D, et al. Accuracy and limitations of the growth hormone (GH) releasing hormone-arginine retesting in young adults with childhood-onset GH deficiency. Front Endocrinol. 2019;10:525.
20. Lissett CA, Saleem S, Rahim A, et al. The impact of irradiation on growth hormone responsiveness to provocative agents is stimulus dependent: results in 161 individuals with radiation damage to the somatotropic axis. J Clin Endocrinol Metab. 2001;86:663–8.
21. Dichtel LE, Yuen KC, Bredella MA, et al. Overweight/Obese adults with pituitary disorders require lower peak growth hormone cutoff values on glucagon stimulation testing to avoid overdiagnosis of growth hormone deficiency. J Clin Endocrinol Metab. 2014;99:4712–9.
22. Hamrahian AH, Yuen KC, Gordon MB, et al. Revised GH and cortisol cut-points for the glucagon stimulation test in the evaluation of GH and hypothalamic-pituitary- adrenal axes in adults: results from a prospective randomized multicenter study. Pituitary. 2016;19:332–41.
23. Boguszewski MCS, Boguszewski CL, Chemaililly W, et al. Safety of growth hormone replacement in survivors of cancer and intracranial and pituitary tumours: a consensus statement. Eur J Endocrinol. 2022;186:P35–52.
24. Grimberg A, DiVall SA, Polychronakos C, et al. Guidelines for growth hormone and insulin-like growth factor-I treatment in children and adolescents: growth hormone deficiency, idiopathic short stature, and primary insulin-like growth factor-I deficiency. Horm Res Paediatr. 2016;86:361–97.
25. Deal CL, Steelman J, Vlachopapadopoulou E, et al. Efficacy and safety of weekly somatrogon vs daily somatropin in children with growth hormone deficiency: a phase 3 study. J Clin Endocrinol Metab. 2022;107(7):e2717–28. https://doi.org/10.1210/clinem/dgac220. PMID: 35405011; PMCID: PMC9202717.
26. Lawson SA, Horne VE, Golekoh MC, et al. Hypothalamic-pituitary function following childhood brain tumors: analysis of prospective annual endocrine screening. Pediatr Blood Cancer. 2019;66(5):e27631. https://doi.org/10.1002/pbc.27631. Epub 2019 Jan 28. PMID: 30693650.
27. Jostel A, Ryder WD, Shalet SM. The use of thyroid function tests in the diagnosis of hypopituitarism: definition and evaluation of the TSH index. Clin Endocrinol. 2009;71(4):529–34. https://doi.org/10.1111/j.1365-2265.2009.03534.x. Epub 2009 Feb 18. PMID: 19226261.
28. Persani L, Brabant G, Dattani M, et al. 2018 European Thyroid Association (ETA) Guidelines on the diagnosis and Management of Central Hypothyroidism. Eur Thyroid J. 2018;7:225–37.
29. Milano MT, Vargo JA, Yorke ED, et al. Primary hypothyroidism in childhood cancer survivors treated with radiation therapy: a PENTEC comprehensive review. Int J Radiat Oncol Biol Phys.

2024;119(2):482–93. https://doi.org/10.1016/j.ijrobp.2021.02.001.
30. Reiners C, Drozd V, Yamashita S. Hypothyroidism after radiation exposure: brief narrative review. J Neural Transm. 2020;127(11):1455–66.
31. Nagayama Y. Radiation-related thyroid autoimmunity and dysfunction. J Radiat Res. 2018;59(suppl_2):ii98–ii107.
32. Gurney JG, Kadan-Lottick NS, Packer RJ, Childhood Cancer Survivor Study, et al. Endocrine and cardiovascular late effects among adult survivors of childhood brain tumors: Childhood Cancer Survivor Study. Cancer. 2003;97(3):663–73. https://doi.org/10.1002/cncr.11095. PMID: 12548609.
33. Aslan IR, Cheung CC. Early and late endocrine effects in pediatric central nervous system diseases. J Pediatr Rehabil Med. 2014;7(4):281–94. https://doi.org/10.3233/PRM-140299. PMID: 25547881.
34. Ojeda SR, Lomniczi A, Mastronardi C, et al. Minireview: the neuroendocrine regulation of puberty: is the time ripe for a systems biology approach? Endocrinology. 2006;147(3):1166e74.
35. Soriano-Guillén L, Argente J. Central precocious puberty, functional and tumor-related. Best Pract Res Clin Endocrinol Metab. 2019;33(3):101262. https://doi.org/10.1016/j.beem.2019.01.003. Epub 2019 Jan 22. PMID: 30733078.
36. Trivin C, Couto-Silva AC, Sainte-Rose C, et al. Presentation and evolution of organic central precocious puberty according to the type of CNS lesion. Clin Endocrinol. 2006;65(2):239–45. https://doi.org/10.1111/j.1365-2265.2006.02582.x. PMID: 16886967.
37. Dahl M, Proos LA, Arnell K, Gustafsson J. Swedish cohort study found that half of the girls with shunted hydrocephalus had precocious or early puberty. Acta Paediatr. 2024;113(4):827–32. https://doi.org/10.1111/apa.17115. Epub 2024 Jan 17. PMID: 38233740.
38. Armstrong GT, Whitton JA, Gajjar A, et al. Abnormal timing of menarche in survivors of central nervous system tumors: a report from the Childhood Cancer Survivor Study. Cancer. 2009;115(11):2562–70. Epub 2009/03/25.
39. Anderson RA, Mitchell RT, Kelsey TW, et al. Cancer treatment and gonadal function: experimental and established strategies for fertility preservation in children and young adults. Lancet Diabetes Endocrinol. 2015;3(7):556–67.
40. Kuohung W, Ram K, Cheng DM, et al. Laparoscopic oophoropexy prior to radiation for pediatric brain tumor and subsequent ovarian function. Hum Reprod. 2008;23(1):117–21. Epub 2007/11/16.
41. COG guidelines 2023.
42. van Dorp W, Mulder RL, Kremer LC, et al. Recommendations for premature ovarian insufficiency surveillance for female survivors of childhood, adolescent, and young adult cancer: a report from the International Late Effects of Childhood Cancer Guideline Harmonization Group in collaboration with the PanCareSurFup Consortium. J Clin Oncol. 2016;34(28):3440–50. https://doi.org/10.1200/JCO.2015.64.3288. Epub 2016 Jul 25. PMID: 27458300; PMCID: PMC5569686.
43. Chow EJ, Friedman DL, Yasui Y, et al. Timing of menarche among survivors of childhood acute lymphoblastic leukemia: a report from the Childhood Cancer Survivor Study. Pediatr Blood Cancer. 2008;50(4):854–8.
44. McGlacken-Byrne SM, Conway GS. Premature ovarian insufficiency. Best Pract Res Clin Obstet Gynaecol. 2022;81:98–110. https://doi.org/10.1016/j.bpobgyn.2021.09.011. Epub 2021 Nov 16. PMID: 34924261.
45. De Vos M, Devroey P, Fauser BC. Primary ovarian insufficiency. Lancet. 2010;376(9744):911–21. https://doi.org/10.1016/S0140-6736(10)60355-8. Epub 2010 Aug 11. PMID: 20708256.
46. Stuenkel CA, Gompel A. Primary ovarian insufficiency. N Engl J Med. 2023;388(2):154–63. https://doi.org/10.1056/NEJMcp2116488. PMID: 36630623.
47. Sullivan SD, Sarrel PM, Nelson LM. Hormone replacement therapy in young women with primary ovarian insufficiency and early menopause. Fertil Steril. 2016;106(7):1588–99. https://doi.org/10.1016/j.fertnstert.2016.09.046. PMID: 27912889; PMCID: PMC5137796.
48. Cattoni A, Parissone F, Porcari I, et al. Hormonal replacement therapy in adolescents and young women with chemo- or radio-induced premature ovarian insufficiency: practical recommendations. Blood Rev. 2021;45:100730. https://doi.org/10.1016/j.blre.2020.100730. Epub 2020 Jul 4. PMID: 32654893.
49. van Iersel L, Mulder RL, Denzer C, et al. Hypothalamic-pituitary and other endocrine surveillance among childhood cancer survivors. Endocr Rev. 2022;43(5):794–823. https://doi.org/10.1210/endrev/bnab040.
50. Skinner R, Mulder RL, Kremer LC, et al. Recommendations for gonadotoxicity surveillance in male childhood, adolescent, and young adult cancer survivors: a report from the International Late Effects of Childhood Cancer Guideline Harmonization Group in collaboration with the PanCareSurFup Consortium. Lancet Oncol. 2017;18(2):e75–90.
51. Faw CA, Brannigan RE. Hypogonadism and cancer survivorship. Curr Opin Endocrinol Diabetes Obes. 2020;27(6):411–8. https://doi.org/10.1097/MED.0000000000000583. PMID: 33003070.
52. https://www.ighg.org/wp-content/uploads/2023/06/IGHG-Recommendations-June-2023.pdf [2nd Oct 2024].
53. Chemaitilly W, Liu Q, van Iersel L, et al. Leydig cell function in male survivors of childhood cancer: a report from the st jude lifetime cohort study. J Clin Oncol. 2019;37(32):3018–31.

54. Rendtorff R, Beyer M, Müller A, et al. Low inhibin B levels alone are not a reliable marker of dysfunctional spermatogenesis in childhood cancer survivors. Andrologia. 2012;44:219–25.
55. Kelsey TW, McConville L, Edgar AB, et al. Follicle stimulating hormone is an accurate predictor of azoospermia in childhood cancer survivors. PLoS One. 2017;12:e0181377.
56. Han TS, Gleeson HK. Long-term and late treatment consequences: endocrine and metabolic effects. Curr Opin Support Palliat Care. 2017;11(3):205–13. https://doi.org/10.1097/SPC.0000000000000289. PMID: 28661901.
57. Pereira N, Schattman GL. Fertility preservation and sexual health after cancer therapy. J Oncol Pract. 2017;13(10):643–51. https://doi.org/10.1200/JOP.2017.023705. Epub 2017 Aug 15. PMID: 28809602.
58. Alexander EC, Faruqi D, Farquhar R, Unadkat A, Ng Yin K, Hoskyns R, Varughese R, Howard SR. Gonadotropins for pubertal induction in males with hypogonadotropic hypogonadism: systematic review and meta-analysis. Eur J Endocrinol. 2024;190(1):S1–S11. https://doi.org/10.1093/ejendo/lvad166. PMID: 38128110; PMCID: PMC10773669.
59. Bleicken B, Hahner S, Ventz M, Quinkler M. Delayed diagnosis of adrenal insufficiency is common: a cross-sectional study in 216 patients. Am J Med Sci. 2010;339:525–31.
60. Inder WJ, Hunt PJ. Glucocorticoid replacement in pituitary surgery: guidelines for perioperative assessment and management. J Clin Endocrinol Metab. 2002;87(6):2745–50. https://doi.org/10.1210/jcem.87.6.8547. PMID: 12050244.
61. Grossman AB. Clinical review: the diagnosis and management of central hypoadrenalism. J Clin Endocrinol Metab. 2010;95(11):4855–63. https://doi.org/10.1210/jc.2010-0982. Epub 2010 Aug 18. PMID: 20719838.
62. Castle-Kirszbaum M, Kyi M, Wright C, Goldschlager T, Danks RA, Parkin WG. Hyponatraemia and hypernatraemia: disorders of water balance in neurosurgery. Neurosurg Rev. 2021;44:2433–58.
63. Bereket A. Postoperative and long-term endocrinologic complications of craniopharyngioma. Horm Res Paediatr. 2020;93:497–509.
64. Edate S, Albanese A. Management of electrolyte and fluid disorders after brain surgery for pituitary/suprasellar tumours. Horm Res Paediatr. 2015;83:293–301.
65. Claude F, Ubertini G, Szinnai G. Endocrine disorders in children with brain tumors: at diagnosis, after surgery, radiotherapy and chemotherapy. Children (Basel). 2022;9(11):1617. https://doi.org/10.3390/children9111617. PMID: 36360345; PMCID: PMC9688119.
66. Arima H, Wakabayashi T, Nagatani T, et al. Adipsia increases risk of death in patients with central diabetes insipidus. Endocr J. 2014;61:143–8.
67. Di Iorgi N, Morana G, Napoli F, et al. Management of diabetes insipidus and adipsia in the child. Best Pract Res Clin Endocrinol Metab. 2015;29:415–36.
68. Green DM, Kawashima T, Stovall S, et al. Fertility of female survivors of childhood cancer: a report from the childhood cancer survivor study. J Clin Oncol. 2009;27:2677–85.
69. Magelssen H, Melve KK, Skjaerven R, Fossa SD. Parenthood probability and pregnancy outcome in patients with a cancer diagnosis during adolescence and young adulthood. Hum Reprod. 2008;23:178–86.
70. Meirow D, Biederman H, Anderson RA, Wallace WHB. Toxicity of chemotherapy and radiation on female reproduction. Clin Obstet Gynecol. 2010;53(4):727–39.
71. Stern E, Ben-Ami M, Gruber N, et al. Hypothalamic-pituitary-gonadal function, pubertal development, and fertility outcomes in male and female medulloblastoma survivors: a single-center experience. Neuro-Oncology. 2023;25(7):1345–54.
72. Wo JY, Viswanathan AN. The impact of radiotherapy on fertility, pregnancy, and neonatal outcomes in female cancer patients. Int J Radiat Oncol Biol Phys. 2009;73:1304–12.
73. Wallace WHB, Thomson AB, Kelsey TW. The radiosensitivity of the human oocyte. Hum Reprod. 2003;18:117–21.
74. Anderson RA, Mitchell RT, Kelsey TW, et al. Cancer treatment and gonadal function: experimental and established strategies for fertility preservation in children and young adults. Lancet Diabetes Endocrinol. 2015;3:556–67.
75. Anderson RA, Wallace WHB. Antimüllerian hormone, the assessment of the ovarian reserve, and the reproductive outcome of the young patient with cancer. Fertil Steril. 2013;99(6):1469–75.
76. Pastore LM, Christianson MS, Stelling J, et al. Reproductive ovarian testing and the alphabet soup of diagnoses: DOR, POI, POF, POR, and FOR. J Assist Reprod Genet. 2018;35:17–23.
77. Frange P, Alapetite C, Gaboriaud G, et al. From childhood to adulthood: long-term outcome of medulloblastoma patients. The institut curie experience (1980–2000). J Neuro-Oncol. 2009;95(2):271–9.
78. van der Perk MM, van der Kooi AL, Bos AM, et al. Oncofertility perspectives for girls with cancer. J Pediatr Adolesc Gynecol. 2022;35(5):523–6. https://doi.org/10.1016/j.jpag.2022.03.005. Epub 2022 Mar 28.
79. Mulder RL, Font-Gonzales A, Hudson MM, et al. Fertility preservation for female patients with childhood, adolescent, and young adult cancer: recommendations from the PanCareLIFE Consortium and the International Late Effects of Childhood Cancer

Guideline Harmonization Group. Lancet Oncol. 2021;22(2):e45–56. PMID: 33539753 Review.
80. Bath LE, Wallace WH, Critchley HO. Late effects of the treatment of child- hood cancer on the female reproductive system and the potential for fertility preservation. BJOG. 2002;109(2):107–14.
81. Gross E, Champetier C, Pointreau Y, Zaccariotto A, Dubergé T, Guerder C, et al. Normal tissue tolerance to external beam radiation therapy: ovaries. Cancer Radiother. 2010;14:373–5.
82. Wallace WHB, Shalet SM, Hendry JH, Morris-Jones PH, Gattamaneni HR. Ovarian failure following abdominal irradiation in childhood: the radiosensitivity of the human oocyte. Br J Radiol. 1989;62:995–8.
83. Veldhuis JD. The hypothalamic pulse generator: the reproductive core. Clin Obstet Gynecol. 1990;33(3):538–50.
84. Darzy KH, Shalet SM. Hypopituitarism following radiotherapy revisited. Endocr Dev. 2009;15:1–24.
85. Teh WT, Stern C, Chander S, Hickey M. The impact of uterine radiation on subsequent fertility and pregnancy outcomes. Biomed Res Int. 2014;2014:482968.
86. van der Kooi ALF, Mulder RL, Hudson MM, et al. Counseling and surveillance of obstetrical risks for female childhood, adolescent, and young adult cancer survivors: recommendations from the International Late Effects of Childhood Cancer Guideline Harmonization Group. Am J Obstet Gynecol. 2021;224(1):3–15.
87. Romerius P, Stahl O, Moell C, Relander T, Cavallin-Stahl E, Wiebe T, et al. Hypogonadism risk in men treated for childhood cancer. J Clin Endocrinol Metab. 2009;94:4180–6.
88. Kenney LB, Cohen LE, Shnorhavorian M, Metzger MB, Lockart B, Hijiya N, et al. Male reproductive health after childhood, adolescent, and young adult cancers: a report from the Children's Oncology Group. J Clin Oncol. 2012;30:3408–16.
89. Shalet SM, Tsatsoulis A, Whitehead E, Read G. Vulnerability of the human Leydig cell to radiation damage is dependent upon age. J Endocrinol. 1989;120:161–5.
90. Izard MA. Leydig cell function and radiation: a review of the literature. Radiother Oncol. 1995;34:1–8.
91. National Institute for Health and Care Excellence. Fertility problems: assessment and treatment. National Institute for Health and Care Excellence; 2013.
92. Palmer SL, Armstrong C, Onar-Thomas A, Wu S, Wallace D, Bonner MJ, Schreiber J, Swain M, Chapieski L, Mabbott D, Knight S, Boyle R, Gajjar A. Processing speed, attention, and working memory after treatment for medulloblastoma: an international, prospective, and longitudinal study. J Clin Oncol. 2013;31(28):3494–500. https://doi.org/10.1200/JCO.2012.47.4775. Epub 2013 Aug 26. PMID: 23980078; PMCID: PMC3782147.
93. Schreiber JE, Gurney JG, Palmer SL, Bass JK, Wang M, Chen S, Zhang H, Swain M, Chapieski ML, Bonner MJ. Examination of risk factors for intellectual and academic outcomes following treatment for pediatric medulloblastoma. Neuro-Oncology. 2014;16:1129–36.
94. Tonning Olsson I, Perrin S, Lundgren J, Hjorth L, Johanson A. Long-term cognitive sequelae after pediatric brain tumor related to medical risk factors, age, and sex. Pediatr Neurol. 2014;51(4):515–21. https://doi.org/10.1016/j.pediatrneurol.2014.06.011. Epub 2014 Jun 26. PMID: 25266614.
95. Fraley CE, Thigpen JC, Pearson MM, Kuttesch JF Jr, Desjardins L, Hoskinson KR, Alvarado-Gonzalez A, Esbenshade AJ, Pastakia D, Friedman DL, Wellons JC, McNally CM, Siciliano RE, Compas BE. Predictors of cognitive function in pediatric brain tumor patients: pre-surgery through 24-month follow-up. Appl Neuropsychol Child. 2021;10(4):340–7. https://doi.org/10.1080/21622965.2019.1706179. Epub 2019 Dec 30. PMID: 31887256; PMCID: PMC7326643.
96. de Ruiter MA, van Mourik R, Schouten-van Meeteren AY, Grootenhuis MA, Oosterlaan J. Neurocognitive consequences of a paediatric brain tumour and its treatment: a meta-analysis. Dev Med Child Neurol. 2013;55(5):408–17. https://doi.org/10.1111/dmcn.12020. Epub 2012 Nov 15. PMID: 23157447.
97. Riva D, Giorgi C, Nichelli F, Bulgheroni S, Massimino M, Cefalo G, Gandola L, Giannotta M, Bagnasco I, Saletti V, Pantaleoni C. Intrathecal methotrexate affects cognitive function in children with medulloblastoma. Neurology. 2002;59(1):48–53. https://doi.org/10.1212/wnl.59.1.48. PMID: 12105306.
98. Ater JL, Moore BD 3rd, Francis DJ, Castillo R, Slopis J, Copeland DR. Correlation of medical and neurosurgical events with neuropsychological status in children at diagnosis of astrocytoma: utilization of a neurological severity score. J Child Neurol. 1996;11(6):462–9. https://doi.org/10.1177/088307389601100610. PMID: 9120225.
99. Oprandi MC, Oldrati V, Cavatorta C, Gandola L, Massimino M, Bardoni A, Poggi G. The influence of socioeconomic status (SES) and processing speed on the psychological adjustment and well-being of pediatric brain tumor survivors. Cancers (Basel). 2022;14(13):3075. https://doi.org/10.3390/cancers14133075. PMID: 35804846; PMCID: PMC9264789.
100. Patel SK, Fernandez N, Dekel N, Turk A, Meier A, Ross P, Rosenthal J. Socioeconomic status as a possible moderator of neurocognitive outcomes in children with cancer. Psychooncology. 2016;25(1):115–8. https://doi.org/10.1002/pon.3797. Epub 2015 Mar 17. PMID: 25780996.
101. Stavinoha PL, Askins MA, Powell SK, Pillay Smiley N, Robert RS. Neurocognitive and psychosocial outcomes in pediatric brain tumor survi-

vors. Bioengineering (Basel). 2018;5(3):73. https://doi.org/10.3390/bioengineering5030073. PMID: 30208602; PMCID: PMC6164803.
102. Doger de Spéville E, Kieffer V, Dufour C, Grill J, Noulhiane M, Hertz-Pannier L, Chevignard M. Neuropsychological consequences of childhood medulloblastoma and possible interventions: a review. Neurochirurgie. 2021;67(1):90–8. https://doi.org/10.1016/j.neuchi.2018.03.002. Epub 2018 Apr 30. PMID: 29716738.
103. Chevignard M, Câmara-Costa H, Doz F, Dellatolas G. Core deficits and quality of survival after childhood medulloblastoma: a review. Neurooncol Pract. 2017;4(2):82–97. https://doi.org/10.1093/nop/npw013. Epub 2016 Aug 26. PMID: 31385962; PMCID: PMC6655396.
104. Margelisch K, Studer M, Ritter BC, Steinlin M, Leibundgut K, Heinks T. Cognitive dysfunction in children with brain tumors at diagnosis. Pediatr Blood Cancer. 2015;62(10):1805–12. https://doi.org/10.1002/pbc.25596. Epub 2015 Jun 5. PMID: 26053691; PMCID: PMC5054885.
105. Edelstein K, Spiegler BJ, Fung S, Panzarella T, Mabbott DJ, Jewitt N, D'Agostino NM, Mason WP, Bouffet E, Tabori U, Laperriere N, Hodgson DC. Early aging in adult survivors of childhood medulloblastoma: long-term neurocognitive, functional, and physical outcomes. Neuro-Oncology. 2011;13(5):536–45. https://doi.org/10.1093/neuonc/nor015. Epub 2011 Mar 2. PMID: 21367970; PMCID: PMC3093335.
106. Brinkman TM, Krasin MJ, Liu W, Armstrong GT, Ojha RP, Sadighi ZS, Gupta P, Kimberg C, Srivastava D, Merchant TE, Gajjar A, Robison LL, Hudson MM, Krull KR. Long-term neurocognitive functioning and social attainment in adult survivors of pediatric CNS tumors: results from the St Jude lifetime cohort study. J Clin Oncol. 2016;34(12):1358–67. https://doi.org/10.1200/JCO.2015.62.2589. Epub 2016 Feb 1. PMID: 26834063; PMCID: PMC4933131.
107. Anderson PJ, Reidy N. Assessing executive function in preschoolers. Neuropsychol Rev. 2012;22(4):345–60.https://doi.org/10.1007/s11065--012-9220-3. Epub 2012 Oct 30. PMID: 23109046.
108. Murphy C, Upshaw NC, Thomas AS, Fong G, Janss A, Mazewski C, Ingerski LM. Impact of executive functioning on health-related quality of life of pediatric brain tumor survivors. Pediatr Blood Cancer. 2021;68(8):e29130. https://doi.org/10.1002/pbc.29130. Epub 2021 May 27. PMID: 34047487.
109. Baldwin RT, Preston-Martin S. Epidemiology of brain tumors in childhood--a review. Toxicol Appl Pharmacol. 2004;199(2):118–31. https://doi.org/10.1016/j.taap.2003.12.029. PMID: 15313584.
110. Brinkman TM, Liptak CC, Delaney BL, Chordas CA, Muriel AC, Manley PE. Suicide ideation in pediatric and adult survivors of childhood brain tumors. J Neuro-Oncol. 2013;113(3):425–32. https://doi.org/10.1007/s11060-013-1130-6. Epub 2013 Apr 27. PMID: 23624716.
111. Chow C, Liptak C, Chordas C, Manley P, Recklitis C. Adolescent and young adult brain tumor survivors report increased anxiety even years after successful treatment for relapse. J Adolesc Young Adult Oncol. 2019;8(1):90–3. https://doi.org/10.1089/jayao.2018.0053. Epub 2018 Aug 29. PMID: 30156441.
112. Shah SS, Dellarole A, Peterson EC, Bregy A, Komotar R, Harvey PD, Elhammady MS. Long-term psychiatric outcomes in pediatric brain tumor survivors. Childs Nerv Syst. 2015;31(5):653–63. https://doi.org/10.1007/s00381-015-2669-7. Epub 2015 Mar 1. PMID: 25726165.
113. Cheung AT, Li WHC, Ho LLK, Ho KY, Chiu SY, Chan CG, Chung OK. Impact of brain tumor and its treatment on the physical and psychological well-being, and quality of life amongst pediatric brain tumor survivors. Eur J Oncol Nurs. 2019;41:104–9. https://doi.org/10.1016/j.ejon.2019.06.003. Epub 2019 Jun 10. PMID: 31358242.
114. Emond A, Edwards L, Peacock S, Norman C, Evangeli M. Social competence in children and young people treated for a brain tumour. Support Care Cancer. 2016;24(11):4587–95. https://doi.org/10.1007/s00520-016-3301-4. Epub 2016 Jun 16. PMID: 27312844.
115. Schulte F. Social competence in pediatric brain tumor survivors: breadth versus depth. Curr Opin Oncol. 2015;27(4):306–10. https://doi.org/10.1097/CCO.0000000000000193. PMID: 26049269.
116. Effinger KE, Stratton KL, Fisher PG, Ness KK, Krull KR, Oeffinger KC, Armstrong GT, Robison LL, Hudson MM, Leisenring WM, Nathan PC. Long-term health and social function in adult survivors of paediatric astrocytoma: a report from the childhood cancer survivor study. Eur J Cancer. 2019;106:171–80. https://doi.org/10.1016/j.ejca.2018.10.016. Epub 2018 Dec 5. PMID: 30528801; PMCID: PMC6647033.
117. Turcotte LM, Whitton JA, Friedman DL, et al. Risk of subsequent neoplasms during the fifth and sixth decades of life in the childhood cancer survivor study cohort. J Clin Oncol. 2015;33(31):3568–75.
118. Armstrong GT, Liu W, Leisenring W, et al. Occurrence of multiple subsequent neoplasms in long-term survivors of childhood cancer: a report from the Childhood Cancer Survivor Study. J Clin Oncol. 2011;29:3056–64.
119. Armstrong GT. Long-term survivors of childhood central nervous system malignancies: the experience of the Childhood Cancer Survivor Study. Eur J Paediatr Neurol. 2010;14(4):298–303.
120. Turcotte LM, Liu Q, Yasui Y, et al. Chemotherapy and risk of subsequent malignant neoplasms in the childhood cancer survivor study cohort. J Clin Oncol. 2019;37(34):3310–9.
121. Azarova AM, Lyu YL, Lin CP, et al. Roles of DNA topoisomerase II isozymes in chemotherapy and secondary malignancies. Proc Natl Acad Sci USA. 2007;104(26):11014–9.

122. Kim J, Gianferante M, Karyadi DM, et al. Frequency of pathogenic germline variants in cancer-susceptibility genes in the Childhood Cancer Survivor Study. JNCI Cancer Spectr. 2021;5(2):pkab007. https://doi.org/10.1093/jncics/pkab007. eCollection 2021 Apr.
123. Wang Z, Wilson CL, Easton J, et al. Genetic risk for subsequent neoplasms among long-term survivors of childhood cancer. J Clin Oncol. 2018;36(20):2078–87.
124. de Blank PMK, Lange KR, Xing M, et al. Temporal changes in treatment and late mortality and morbidity in adult survivors of childhood glioma: a report from the Childhood Cancer Survivor Study. Nat Cancer. 2024;5(4):590–600. https://doi.org/10.1038/s43018-024-00733-0. Epub 2024 Mar 1. PMID: 38429413.
125. Johnson KJ, Cullen J, Barnholtz-Sloan JS, et al. Childhood brain tumor epidemiology: a brain tumor epidemiology consortium review. Cancer Epidemiol Biomarkers Prev. 2014;23(12):2716–36. https://doi.org/10.1158/1055-9965.EPI-14-0207. Epub 2014 Sep 5.
126. Neglia J, Robison L, Stovall M, et al. New primary neoplasms of the central nervous system in survivors of childhood cancer: a report from the Childhood Cancer Survivor Study. J Nat Cancer Inst. 2006;98:1528–15.
127. Taylor AJ, Little MP, Winter DL, et al. Population-based risks of CNS tumors in survivors of childhood cancer: the British Childhood Cancer Survivor Study. J Clin Oncol. 2010;28:5287–93.
128. Bowers DC, Nathan PC, Constine L, et al. Subsequent neoplasms of the CNS among survivors of childhood cancer: a systematic review. Lancet Oncol. 2013;14(8):e321–8. https://doi.org/10.1016/S1470-2045(13)70107-4.
129. Marks LB, Ma J. Challenges in the clinical application of advanced technologies to reduce radiation-associated normal tissue injury. Int J Radiat Oncol Biol Phys. 2007;69:4–12.
130. Tringale KR, Casey DL, Niyazov G, et al. Second cancer risk in childhood cancer survivors treated with intensity-modulated radiation therapy: an updated analysis of more than 10 years of follow-up. Pediatr Blood Cancer. 2022;69(5):e29600. https://doi.org/10.1002/pbc.29600. Epub 2022 Mar 2.
131. Toussaint L, Indelicato DJ, Muren LP, Stokkevåg CH. Risk of second primary cancer from proton arc therapy of pediatric brain tumors. Phys Imaging Radiat Oncol. 2023;27:100480. https://doi.org/10.1016/j.phro.2023.100480.
132. Salloum R, Chen Y, Yasui Y, et al. Late morbidity and mortality among medulloblastoma survivors diagnosed across three decades: a report from the Childhood Cancer Survivor Study. J Clin Oncol. 2019;37(9):731–40. https://doi.org/10.1200/JCO.18.00969. Epub 2019 Feb 7.
133. Packer RJ, Zhou T, Holmes E, et al. Survival and secondary tumors in children with medulloblastoma receiving radiotherapy and adjuvant chemotherapy: results of Children's Oncology Group Trial A9961. Neuro Oncol. 2013;15:97–103.
134. von Hoff K, Hinkes B, Gerber NU, et al. Long-term outcome and clinical prognostic factors in children with medulloblastoma treated in the prospective randomised multicentre trial HIT'91. Eur J Cancer. 2009;45:1209–17.
135. Tsui K, Gajjar A, Li C, et al. Subsequent neoplasms in survivors of childhood central nervous system tumors: risk after modern multimodal therapy. Neuro Oncol. 2015;17:448–56.
136. Neglia JP, Friedman DL, Yasui Y, et al. Second malignant neoplasms in five-year survivors of childhood cancer: Childhood Cancer Survivor Study. J Natl Cancer Inst. 2001;93(8):618–29.
137. Bhatti P, Veiga L, Ronckers C, et al. Radiotherapy for childhood cancer and risk of thyroid cancer in a large cohort study: an update from the Childhood Cancer Survivor Study. Radiat Res. 2010;174:741–75.
138. Heymer EJ, Hawkins MM, Winter DL, et al. Risk of subsequent gliomas and meningiomas among 69,460 5-year survivors of childhood and adolescent cancer in Europe: the PanCareSurFup study. Br J Cancer. 2024;130(6):976–86. https://doi.org/10.1038/s41416-024-02577-y. Epub 2024 Jan 19.
139. Carret AS, Tabori U, Crooks B, et al. Outcome of secondary high-grade glioma in children previously treated for a malignant condition: a study of the Canadian Pediatric Brain Tumour Consortium. Radiother Oncol. 2006;81:33–8.
140. Shaha MA, Wang LY, Migliacci JC, et al. Previous external beam radiation treatment exposure does not confer worse outcome for patients with differentiated thyroid cancer. Thyroid. 2017;27:412–7.
141. Podda MG, Meazza C, Gattuso G. Treating secondary malignant neoplasms: a burden of childhood cancer survivors. Tumori. 2023;109(5):436–41. https://doi.org/10.1177/03008916231160824. Epub 2023 Mar 24.
142. Bowers DC, Verbruggen LC, Kremer LCM. Surveillance for subsequent neoplasms of the CNS for childhood, adolescent, and young adult cancer survivors: a systematic review and recommendations from the International Late Effects of Childhood Cancer Guideline Harmonization Group. Lancet Oncol. 2021;22(5):e196–206. https://doi.org/10.1016/S1470-2045(20)30688-4. Epub 2021 Apr 9.
143. Knight KR, Kraemer DF, Neuwelt EA. Ototoxicity in children receiving platinum chemotherapy: underestimating a commonly occurring toxicity that may influence academic and social development. J Clin Oncol. 2005;23:8588–96.
144. Bass JK, Hua CH, Huang J, et al. Hearing loss in patients who received cranial radiation therapy for childhood cancer. J Clin Oncol. 2016;34:1248–55.

145. Bertolini P, Lassalle M, Mecier G, et al. Platinum compound-related ototoxicity in children: long-term follow-up reveals continuous worsening of hearing loss. J Pediatr Hematol Oncol. 2004;26(10):649–55.
146. Merchant TE, Gould CJ, Xiong X, et al. Early neuro-otologic effects of three-dimensional irradiation in children with primary brain tumors. Int J Radiat Oncol Biol Phys. 2004;58:1194–207.
147. Clemens E, van den Heuvel-Eibrink MM, Mulder RL, et al. Recommendations for ototoxicity surveillance for childhood, adolescent, and young adult cancer survivors: a report from the International Late Effects of Childhood Cancer Guideline Harmonization Group in collaboration with the PanCare Consortium. Lancet Oncol. 2019;20(1):e29–41.
148. Armenian SH, Lacchetti C, Barac A, et al. Prevention and monitoring of cardiac dysfunction in survivors of adult cancers: american society of clinical oncology clinical practice guideline. J Clin Oncol. 2017;35(8):893–911. https://doi.org/10.1200/JCO.2016.70.5400.
149. Lipshultz SE, Franco VI, Miller TL, Colan SD, Sallan SE. Cardiovas- cular disease in adult survivors of childhood cancer. Annu Rev Med. 2015;66:161–76.
150. Zamorano JL, Lancellotti P, Rodriguez Muñoz D, et al. 2016 ESC position paper on cancer treatments and cardiovascular toxicity developed under the auspices of the ESC committee for practice guidelines: The Task Force for cancer treatments and cardiovascular toxicity of the European Society of Cardiology (ESC). Eur Heart J. 2016;37(36):2768–801. https://doi.org/10.1093/eurheartj/ehw211.
151. Bansal N, Amdani S, Lipshultz ER, Lipshultz SE. Chemotherapy-induced cardiotoxicity in children. Expert Opin Drug Metab Toxicol. 2017;13:817–32.
152. Cuomo A, Mercurio V, Pugliese M, et al. Cardiovascular events and treatment of children with high risk medulloblastoma. ClinicalMedicine. 2021;43:101251. https://doi.org/10.1016/j.eclinm.2021.101251.
153. Howard E, Steingart RM, Armstrong GT, et al. Cardiovascular events in cancer survivors. Semin Oncol. 2019;46(6):426–32. https://doi.org/10.1053/j.seminoncol.2019.01.007.
154. Bisceglia I, Canale ML, Silvestris N, et al. Cancer survivorship at heart: a multidisciplinary cardio-oncology roadmap for healthcare professionals. Front Cardiovasc Med. 2023;10:1223660. https://doi.org/10.3389/fcvm.2023.1223660.
155. Mertens AC, Liu Q, Neglia JP, et al. Cause-specific late mortality among 5-year survivors of childhood cancer: the Childhood Cancer Survivor Study. J Natl Cancer Inst. 2008;100:1368–79.
156. Bowers DC, Mulne AF, Reisch JS, et al. Nonperioperative strokes in children with central nervous system tumors. Cancer. 2002;94:1094–101.
157. Bowers DC, Liu Y, Leisenring W, et al. Late-occurring stroke among long-term survivors of childhood leukemia and brain tumors: a report from the Childhood Cancer Survivor Study. J Clin Oncol Off J Am Soc Clin Oncol. 2006;24:5277–82.
158. Haddy N, Mousannif A, Tukenova M, et al. Relationship between the brain radiation dose for the treatment of childhood cancer and the risk of long-term cerebrovascular mortality. Brain. 2011;134:1362–72.
159. Mueller S, Fullerton H, Stratton K, et al. Radiation, atherosclerotic risk factors, and stroke risk in survivors of pediatric cancer: a report from the Childhood Cancer Survivor Study. Int J Radiat Oncol Biol Phys. 2013;86:649–55.
160. Bhatia S, Tonorezos ES, Landier W. Clinical care for people who survive childhood cancer: a review. JAMA. 2023;330(12):1175–86. https://doi.org/10.1001/jama.2023.16875.
161. Mertens AC, Yasui Y, Liu Y, et al. Pulmonary complications in survivors of childhood and adolescent cancer. A report from the Childhood Cancer Survivor Study. Cancer. 2002;95:2431–41.
162. Huang TT, Chen Y, Dietz AC, Yasui Y, Donaldson SS, Stokes DC, et al. Pulmonary outcomes in survivors of childhood central nervous system malignancies: a report from the Childhood Cancer Survivor Study. Pediatr Blood Cancer. 2014;61:319–25.
163. Liles A, Blatt J, Morris D, et al. Monitoring pulmonary complications in long-term childhood cancer survivors: guidelines for the primary care physician. Cleve Clin J Med. 2008;75(7):531–9. https://doi.org/10.3949/ccjm.75.7.531.
164. Çetingül N, Demir E, Sayiner A, et al. Evaluation of long term respiratory complications in childhood and adolescent cancer surrvivors. J Pediatr Res. 2023;10(1):13–8. https://doi.org/10.4274/jpr.galenos.2022.98216.
165. Streckmann F, Balke M, Cavaletti G, Toscanelli A, et al. Exercise and neuropathy: systematic review with meta-analysis. Sports Med. 2021;52:1–23.
166. Shalabi H, Gust J, Taraseviciute A, et al. Beyond the storm — Subacute toxicities and late effects in children receiving CAR T cells. Nat Rev Clin Oncol. 2021;18(6):363–78.
167. Tong J, Kartolo A, Yeung C, et al. Long-term toxicities of immune checkpoint inhibitor (ICI) in melanoma patients. Curr Oncol. 2022;29(10):7953–63.
168. Ghisoni E, Wicky A, Bouchaab H, et al. Late-onset and long-lasting immune-related adverse events from immune checkpoint-inhibitors: an overlooked aspect in immunotherapy. Eur J Cancer. 2021;149:153–64.
169. Basek A, Jakubiak GK, Cieślar G, Stanek A. Life-threatening endocrinological immune-related adverse events of immune checkpoint inhibitor therapy. Cancers (Basel). 2023;15(24):5786.
170. Barroso-Sousa R, Barry WT, Garrido-Castro AC, et al. Incidence of endocrine dysfunction following the use of different immune checkpoint inhibitor

regimens: a systematic review and meta-analysis. JAMA Oncol. 2018;4:173–82.
171. Chamorro-Pareja N, Faje AT, Miller KK. Pituitary complications of checkpoint inhibitor use. Endocrinology. 2024;165(9):bqae084.
172. Suijkerbuijk KP, Valk GD, Dankbaar JW, et al. Differences in checkpoint-inhibitor-induced hypophysitis: mono- versus combination therapy induced hypophysitis. Front Endocrinol. 2024;15:1400841.
173. Husebye ES, Castinetti F, Criseno S, et al. Endocrine-related adverse conditions in patients receiving immune checkpoint inhibition: an ESE clinical practice guideline. Eur J Endocrinol. 2022;187:G1–G21.
174. Angelousi A, Papalexis P, Karampela A, et al. Diabetes insipidus: a rare endocrine complication of immune check point inhibitors: a case report and literature review. Exp Ther Med. 2022;25(1):10.
175. Caturegli P, Di Dalmazi G, Lombardi M, et al. Hypophysitis secondary to cytotoxic T lymphocyte-associated protein 4 blockade: insights into pathogenesis from an autopsy series. Am J Pathol. 2016;186(12):3225–35.
176. Kanie K, Iguchi G, Bando H, et al. Mechanistic insights into immune checkpoint inhibitor-related hypophysitis: a form of paraneoplastic syndrome. Cancer Immunol Immunother. 2021;70(12):3669–77.
177. Özdemir BC. Immune checkpoint inhibitor-related hypogonadism and infertility: a neglected issue in immuno-oncology. J Immunother Cancer. 2021;9(2):e002220.
178. Chera A, Stancu AL, Bucur O. Thyroid-related adverse events induced by immune checkpoint inhibitors. Front Endocrinol. 2022;13:1010279.
179. Dolladille C, Ederhy S, Allouche S, et al. Late cardiac adverse events in patients with cancer treated with immune checkpoint inhibitors. J Immunother Cancer. 2020;8(1):e000261.
180. Tan S, Day D, Nicholls SJ, Segelov E. Immune checkpoint inhibitor therapy in oncology: current uses and future directions: JACC: CardioOncology state-of-the-art review. JACC CardioOncol. 2022;4(5):579–97.
181. Tan S, Spear E, Sane N, et al. Blood pressure surveillance in cancer patients treated with immune checkpoint inhibitors. J Hum Hypertens. 2023;37(11):1043–6.
182. Esen BH, Özbek L, Oğuz S, Selçukbiricik F. Characterizing immune checkpoint inhibitor-related cutaneous adverse reactions: a comprehensive analysis of FDA adverse event reporting system (FAERS) database. Heliyon. 2024;10(13):e33765.
183. Khoja L, Day D, Wei-Wu Chen T, et al. Tumour- and class-specific patterns of immune-related adverse events of immune checkpoint inhibitors: a systematic review. Ann Oncol. 2017;28(10):2377–85.
184. Ntemou E, Delgouffe E, Goossens E. Immune checkpoint inhibitors and male fertility: should fertility preservation options be considered before treatment? Cancers (Basel). 2024;16(6):1176.

Supportive Care and Rehabilitation

22

Antonella Cacchione and Susanna Staccioli

22.1 Introduction

The new WHO classification of Central Nervous System (CNS) tumors (2021) [1], as a new diagnostic tool, with new neurosurgical techniques and therapeutic trials have led to an extraordinary improvement in the survival of children with brain tumors. This success is accompanied by new challenges arising from the morbidity experienced by those surviving. In particular, physical, psychological, and social/emotional sequelae are the weight that follows from improved recovery rate, and the goal of supportive care and rehabilitation has the aim to minimize the impact of the tumor itself and/or of the treatments received on the patient and relative quality of life. Pediatric supportive care and rehabilitation comprise minimizing the impairment and maximizing activities in routine life using a multidisciplinary team. A multidisciplinary approach provides major success in terms of outcome and for prevention or limitation of short- and long-term morbidity [2]. An interdisciplinary group usually includes an oncologist, nurse, physiatrist, motor physical therapist, occupational therapist, speech pathologist, psychologist, educator and teacher, orthotist, therapeutic recreation specialist, and dietician. The importance of these concepts and their clinical evidence are supported by the literature [3]. This chapter describes supportive care requirements during treatment and rehabilitation, specifically focused on pediatric brain tumor patients.

A. Cacchione (✉)
Area of Hematology-Oncology, Cell Therapy, Gene Therapies, and Hematopoietic Transplantation, Bambino Gesù Children's Hospital, IRCCS, Rome, Italy
e-mail: antonella.cacchione@opbg.net

S. Staccioli
Neurorehabilitation Unit, Neurological Science and Neurorehabilitation Area, "Bambino Gesù" Children's Hospital – IRCCS, Rome, Italy

22.2 Supportive Care

22.2.1 Diagnosis Communication, Psychosocial Assessment, and Takeover

Children and adolescents diagnosed with brain tumors encounter distinct challenges, and their healthcare needs are unique, as are those of the families and caregivers supporting them. The diagnosis often overwhelms families with a large amount of information at a time when emotions are high and clear communication from the healthcare team is critical during this period. Offering the opportunity to ask questions, providing written materials, and ensuring a thorough exchange of information are key steps in supporting families during the diagnostic pro-

A. Mastronuzzi, A. Carai (eds.), *Navigating Pediatric Brain Tumors*,
https://doi.org/10.1007/978-3-032-18992-9_22

cess [4]. The mental health, relationships, and employment of parents can be deeply affected, and siblings may feel sidelined due to the time and attention required for caring for a child with brain cancer. Parents frequently require guidance from mental health professionals on how and when to discuss the diagnosis with their child in a way that is appropriate for their age. The goal is to strengthen the child's trust in the healthcare team and in the treatment plan. A pediatric patient's reaction to illness and treatment is shaped by the preexisting developmental and psychological stage, prior life experiences, family dynamics, and, importantly, how the diagnosis is conveyed. The way information is communicated is crucial in influencing the patient's response and coping strategies throughout the course of treatment [5]. Children and adolescents may consequently exhibit a diminished interest in previously enjoyed activities, withdraw from social interactions, and experience a depressive affect [6]. The psychosocial support team plays a critical role in bolstering the children and alleviating parental concerns by affirming that such behavioral manifestations are not atypical. Facilitating the normalization of activities to the greatest extent feasible, implementing consistent behavioral management strategies, and refraining from excessive indulgence or overprotection can mitigate long-term behavioral issues and enhance the child's self-esteem. Reintegration into the educational environment is a crucial component for reinstating normative developmental trajectories in the context of illness [7].

The presence of brain neoplasm, in pediatric and adolescent oncological populations, further complicates the pathway due to significant physical and cognitive advancements (e.g., acquisition of speech and locomotion) alongside psychosocial maturation (e.g., the development of sexual identity) typical of this age. Due to alterations in cerebral architecture induced either by the tumor or therapeutic interventions, these patients often experience deficits in memory functioning and diminished mental health, adversely affecting social interactions and overall quality of life both during treatment and in subsequent follow-up [8]. The physiological transformations and treatment-related side effects can significantly influence the child's self-concept and body image, thereby affecting peer interactions and autonomy. Children at heightened risk for social integration challenges include those with conspicuous alterations in physical appearance and those experiencing central nervous system involvement [9]. It is imperative to prioritize the evaluation and enhancement of social relationships and functional capabilities in these young patients.

The resources available to families may enter a crisis phase, complicating their ability to navigate the challenges associated with a new cancer diagnosis and to provide appropriate support to their child. It is essential and beneficial to conduct a comprehensive assessment of the family unit, encompassing its composition, specific medical history, and unique concerns. A documented written evaluation outlining the strengths and vulnerabilities of the familial structure should be communicated to the treatment team to enhance support for both the family and the patient. Indeed, failure to convey the family's specific needs and sociocultural characteristics among the healthcare team may adversely impact overall treatment outcomes and care provision [10].

22.2.2 Posterior Fossa Syndrome (PFS)

Medulloblastoma (MD), the most prevalent malignant brain tumor in the pediatric population [11], along with other malignant brain tumors such as ependymomas and low-grade gliomas, occurs within the posterior fossa—the region of the intracranial cavity that houses the cerebellum and brainstem. Surgical intervention for these childhood brain tumors causes not only the resection of malignant tissues but also significantly affects adjacent neural structures

[12]. The cerebellum plays a crucial role in various complex behavioral and functional processes in humans; hence, disruption or damage to this area can result in pronounced sequelae in pediatric patients afflicted with posterior fossa tumors. Approximately 25% of children who undergo surgical excision of posterior fossa tumors develop a range of impairing and distressing symptoms, including mutism, ataxia, hypotonia, and emotional lability [13]. These complications may obstruct subsequent treatment strategies and often necessitate further therapeutic interventions. Accompanying speech difficulties, significant behavioral alterations manifest, including personality regression and apathy. Notably, another defining characteristic of the syndrome is emotional lability, characterized by rapid fluctuations in emotional expression, ranging from inconsolable crying and agitation to episodes of giggling and heightened distractibility [14–16].

Currently, there are no evidence-based pharmacological protocols established for the treatment of PFS, and clinical management primarily concentrates on functional recovery through targeted behavioral, physical, occupational, and speech therapies. Pharmacological treatment attempts [17] may include: (a) aripiprazole, a partial dopamine agonist; (b) zolpidem, a benzodiazepine-like agent that may produce a paradoxical effect on the cortico-striatopallidal-thalamocortical pathway potentially reversing the impact of intraoperative damage to this region; and (c) risperidone, utilized for the management of agitation and behavioral dysregulation. The duration of pharmacotherapy is contingent upon the severity of the child's symptoms and their influence on overall quality of life and medical management.

Awareness of the potential onset of PFS facilitates timely recognition and individualized pharmacological management to address acute mood symptoms. Psychosocial interventions are vital for assessing family dynamics and supporting both the patients and their families in mitigating the subsequent sequelae [18, 19].

22.2.3 Chemotherapy Side Affects

22.2.3.1 Nausea and Vomiting

Chemotherapy-induced nausea and vomiting (CINV) represents the prevalent adverse effect of oncological treatments, persisting despite substantial advancements in antiemetic strategies, which now include a diverse array of pharmacological interventions [20]. Approximately 60% of pediatric cancer patients experience nausea or vomiting at some stage during their chemotherapy and radiotherapy regimens [21].

The emetogenic potential of various antineoplastic agents used in pediatric oncology has been systematically evaluated, leading to the categorization of these medications in a classification framework established in 2011. This specific classification was designed to optimize antiemetic therapy by aligning treatment protocols with the identified emetogenic risk associated with different drugs [22] (Table 22.1).

A classification of CINV has been defined [23], with important implications for both prevention and management.

Table 22.1 Emetogenic potential of antineoplastic medication

Emetogenic potential	Chemotherapy drugs
High level (>90% in the absence of prophylaxis)	Carboplatin, methotrexate, cisplatin, procarbazine, cyclophosphamide, thiotepa
Moderate level (30–90% in the absence of prophylaxis)	Etoposide, ifosfamide, intrathecal therapy (methotrexate and cytarabine), busulfan, irinotecan, lomustine, melphalan, cyclophosphamide <1 g/m^2, oxaliplatin, cytarabine, temozolomide, vinorelbine, doxorubicin
Low level (10 to <30% in the absence of prophylaxis)	Methotrexate >50 to <250 mg/m^2, docetaxel, 5-fluorouracil, topotecan, gemcitabine
Minimal (<10% in the absence of prophylaxis)	Bevacizumab, vinblastine, vincristine, vinorelbine

(a) Anticipatory nausea and vomiting: prior to administration of chemotherapy. It is thought to be a conditioned response linked to visual, gustatory, olfactory, and environmental factors related to previously administered chemotherapy. It is relatively common among adolescent patients.
(b) Acute nausea and vomiting: within 24 h after chemotherapy administration. It is most commonly observed within 1–2 h of chemotherapy administration. It is worth noting that delayed emesis is often observed following the administration of cisplatin, carboplatin, cyclophosphamide, or doxorubicin.
(c) Breakthrough: this term is used to describe instances of nausea or vomiting that occur despite the use of antiemetic prophylaxis and are refractory to treatment.

It is important to be aware that the consequences of CINV can be wide-ranging, affecting both physical and psychological well-being. These can include dehydration, malnutrition, stress, poor functional status, and anxiety state before each cycle of chemotherapy. It would be beneficial for all patients receiving emetogenic chemotherapy to have access to good antiemetic therapy.

It is thought that the pathophysiology of CINV has a central mechanism [24], which appears to activate the chemoreceptor trigger zone located in the area postrema in the floor of the fourth ventricle. This is exposed directly to emetogenic substances, such as chemotherapy, through the blood system or cerebrospinal fluid. It is thought that the trigger zone releases neurotransmitters such as serotonin and dopamine, which may activate the brain stem vomiting center. There is also a further way of causing vomiting, with a peripheral mechanism, whereby chemotherapeutic drugs may cause local gastrointestinal irritation and damage to the gastric mucosa, which could lead to the production and release of serotonin that interacts with 5-HT3 receptors on the vagal afferent terminals in the wall [25].

The amygdala may be involved in anticipatory vomiting. It seems plausible to suggest that memory, fear, anticipation, and sensory input, such as smell, are all generated in the higher cortical center and directly stimulate the vomiting center, which could result in emesis. It seems that, regardless of the source of afferent input, the vomiting center, located in the lateral reticular formation of the medulla oblongata, serves as the final pathway along with efferent impulses to induce emesis [26].

The development of 5-hydroxytryptamine (5-HT3) receptor antagonists has greatly improved the control of chemotherapy-induced emesis, and these agents are considered to be the gold standard of treatment among the available options. Dexamethasone may not be the best option as an antiemetic for children with brain tumors, due to the concern that corticosteroids, by repairing damage to the blood–brain barrier (BBB), may cause a reduction in the uptake of cytotoxic agents into the brain tissue, which could potentially impact the efficacy of chemotherapy in the treatment of a child with a brain tumor [27]. In light of the abovementioned considerations, it may be advisable to exercise caution when considering the use of dexamethasone as an antiemetic in children undergoing treatment for a brain tumor. Ondansetron, the most studied 5-HT3 antagonist, is generally well tolerated in children with minimal toxicity and is considered an effective first-line antiemetic in children undergoing chemotherapy, radiotherapy, and surgery [28].

A similarity in the efficacy of ondansetron, granisetron, dolasetron, and tropisetron as first-generation 5-HT3 antagonists has been highlighted, as evidenced by various studies [29]. It would appear that the efficacy of the intravenous and oral routes of ondansetron is equivalent. The recommended dose of ondansetron for children receiving moderately or highly emetogenic chemotherapy should be 5 mg/m^2/dose (0.15 mg/kg/dose) intravenous (IV)/oral pretherapy, followed by one dose and then every 8 h for highly emetogenic chemotherapy and every 12 h for moderately emetogenic chemotherapy. It may be beneficial to consider conversion to an alternate 5-HT3 antagonist as a potential intervention for patients who do not respond to the initial 5-HT3 antagonist. In such cases, there is a possibility of observing benefit in 40–50% of patients [30]. In the event of an inadequate response to a 5-HT3 receptor antagonist as a standalone treatment, the addition of chlorpromazine may be a potential avenue for consideration in the management of CINV [29]. Metoclopramide is another antiemetic acting as a 5-HT3 receptor antagonist [31].

Regarding anticipatory signs in children who experience breakthrough nausea and vomiting, benzodiazepines can be prescribed for their action on the vomiting center [29].

A new agent, aprepitant, an NK-1 receptor antagonist that is thought to block NK-1 receptors in the brain and gut, showed efficacy when administered with 5HT3 antagonists in the management of acute and delayed onset of vomiting in highly emetogenic protocols, particularly those containing cisplatin [32]. It may be helpful to consider a range of nonpharmacological interventions that could potentially contribute to the management of CINV in children receiving antineoplastic agents of any emetic risk: acupuncture, music therapy, progressive muscle relaxation, and psychoeducational support and information, for children receiving antineoplastic agents [33].

22.2.3.2 Peripheral Neuropathy

Pediatric chemotherapy-induced peripheral neuropathy (CIPN) is a common, debilitating side effect of chemotherapy and the actual incidence in pediatric populations is between 50% and 90% (respectively, with platinum-derived compounds and with vinca alkaloids), depending on the type of drug and relative cumulative dosage [34]. Some specific agents used in the treatment of pediatric brain tumors (the vinca alkaloid vincristine, platinum-based antineoplastic as cisplatin, carboplatin, and oxaliplatin) affect the function of the sensory, motor, and/or autonomic peripheral nervous systems, leading to the development of debilitating and untreatable symptoms [35]. Paraesthesia, dysesthesia, hyperalgesia, allodynia, numbness, pain, and loss of proprioception are typical sensory symptoms, developing first in the feet and hands. Motor symptoms are less common and include gait abnormalities, balance deficits, fine motor, and muscle weakness [36]. Similarly, autonomic symptoms are not as common as sensory symptoms and consist of diarrhea, constipation, urinary retention, incontinence, paralytic ileus, and orthostatic hypotension [37]. The severity of CIPN symptoms is related to the cumulative dose of chemotherapy administered. As a result, specifically, these manifestations can lead to pain, functional impairment, reduced patient quality of life, and increased healthcare costs.

The assessment and diagnosis of CIPN in pediatric cancer patients can be challenging. Children are generally unable or find it difficult to recognize and describe symptoms associated with CIPN. In addition, the signs and symptoms of CIPN experienced by individuals can be highly variable and often change over the course of treatment. Quality of life (QoL) questionnaires and pain/neuropathy scales represent subjective assessments. Electrophysiological tests are objective assessments used for diagnosis or assessment of CIPN. These tests are routinely used to assess the electrophysiological abnormalities associated with patients with CIPN and consist of nerve conduction studies, electromyography (EMG) [38]. Combined subjective and objective assessments are tests that utilize questionnaires and combine these with functional, neurological, or electrophysiological assessments. They include tests such as the pediatric–modified Total Neuropathy Scale (ped-m TNS) and the Total Neuropathy Scale–Pediatric Version (TNS-PV). The questionnaire assesses sensory, motor, and autonomic neuropathy symptoms and clinical examinations test for light touch, pain and vibration sensation, muscle function, and deep tendon reflexes [39].

Management of VIPN encompasses micronutrient supplementation—particularly antioxidants—as well as pharmacological interventions aimed at alleviating pain and allodynia, utilizing agents such as gabapentin, pregabalin, amitriptyline, lidocaine, or cannabinoids. Additionally, nonpharmacological modalities, such as acupuncture and neurofeedback, play a significant role in the management of this clinical condition. Rehabilitation strategies focused on motor function are crucial for the restoration of muscle strength and overall physical capabilities.

22.2.3.3 Endocrinological Deficits

Midline tumors (craniopharyngioma, optic pathway glioma, hamartoma, germ cell tumor, low-grade gliomas) count for 20–30% of all pediatric brain tumors [40]. Onset presentation symptoms, due to mass effect of the tumor, usually include neurological, visual complaints and various endocrine abnormalities [41]. Endocrinopathies related to midline neoplasms are diabetes insipidus (DI), changes in weight, height and growth velocity, and precocious or delayed puberty [42, 43]. These endocrine disturbances (above all DI) can manifest long before radiological diagnosis of the tumor. Central precocious puberty is defined as the onset of secondary sexual development arriving before the age of 8 years in girls and 9 years in boy and it is associated with a neoplasm of the CNS. Etiology of CPP has a direct relationship to the location and type of lesions, resulting from the secretion of stimulatory substances [42].

DI is usually the first, earlier manifestation of suprasellar tumors; its mechanism of appearance is the interruption of the transport of the vasopressin neurosecretory granules along the hypothalamic–neurohypophysis pathway [43]. Growth hormone deficiency has been found in almost 50% of cases, and delayed growth can be an early sign in suprasellar region's tumors. Mass effect or infiltrative lesions exerted by sellar/suprasellar neoplasms cause decreased hormone production or secretion, leading to either increased or decreased levels of cortisol, sexual hormones, TSH, and thyroxin.

Mandatory therapeutic approaches, including surgery and radiotherapy, can damage hypothalamic/pituitary cells, and preexisting hypopituitarism can get worse [44].

During chemotherapy treatment, the presence of DI is a risk factor for chemotherapy-related complications when platins of ifosfamide/cyclophosphamide-based protocols are used. Despite vigilant monitoring of electrolytes and desmopressin dose adjustment, significant variations in sodium level have been documented, leading to adverse clinical manifestations [45].

Endocrinopathies are not only neoplastic disease's manifestation but also a common iatrogenic complication of multimodality treatment, with either surgical or radiotherapy approach [46]. In fact, hormonal disturbances are markedly increased after gross total resection compared with partial resection, with or without radiation, with over 50% of patients experiencing at least one endocrinopathy and over 10% developing panhypopituitarism [47]. Therefore, a sparing surgery is the preferred choice when chemo or radiotherapy are feasible thereafter [48]. Hypothalamic obesity is common at diagnosis and augments post-treatment. It is important to recognize endocrine symptoms and clinical signs as they can occur long before the diagnosis of hypothalamic pituitary lesions is made. Height, weight, and BMI plotting may be helpful in shortening the time taken to diagnose. Careful history and clinical examination, as well as timely reevaluation, need to be done in patients with abnormal BMI or BMI progression, as the presence of other neurological, ophthalmologic, and endocrine signs and symptoms may be indicative of the presence of an underlying hypothalamic–pituitary lesion.

22.2.4 Nutritional Aspects

Malnutrition may be experienced by patients undergoing childhood cancer treatment as a consequence of their underlying malignancy and also as a result of treatment-related factors. Malnutrition results in a reduction in muscle mass, which affects an individual's capacity to engage in physical activity. Furthermore, nearly 40% of children with brain tumors experience difficulties with swallowing [49], which serves to exacerbate anorexia and fatigue. Despite the frequent utilization of nutritional support, the prevalence of malnutrition ranges from 5% to 90% across different cohorts of pediatric brain tumor patients [50]. Malnutrition has been demonstrated to impact a number of important clinical outcomes, including wound healing, infection risk, tolerance to chemotherapy, response to treatment, and quality of life. It is also associated with an increased risk of mortality [51]. The nutritional decline observed in children diagnosed with brain tumors is frequently influenced by additional factors, including the location of the tumor and the specific treatment administered. Tumors in the posterior fossa, which account for approximately 60–70% of all pediatric brain tumors [11], can be associated with suboptimal nutrition due to prolonged nausea and vomiting and neurological impairment, resulting in swallowing difficulties and an increased risk of aspiration. Chemotherapy and radiation therapy, whether localized or including the craniospinal axis, may cause emesis, somnolence, or mucositis [52]. It is imperative that infants be observed closely, as their nutritional status may decline rapidly at the outset of treatment [53]. The involvement of a dietician and a speech-language pathologist is crucial in the management of this aspect of patient care. A variety of nutritional intervention strategies are available, including the use of commercial supplemental drinks or caloric additives, which are beneficial in low-risk patients. It is of the utmost importance for all patients to control nausea and vomiting as well as to provide appropriate analgesia for mucositis and esophagitis. Enteral feedings via nasogastric tube or gastrostomy tube should be initiated as soon as possible for those patients who are unable to maintain their weight by the aforementioned strategies.

22.3 Rehabilitation

22.3.1 Rehabilitation Approach Modality

Rehabilitation is the process aimed at enabling children with disabilities due to the neoplasm and related treatments to reach and maintain optimal physical, sensory, intellectual, psychological, and social function. It includes providing the tools children need to gain and maintain independence and self-determination [54]. Using the framework of International Classification of Functioning and Disabilities, and Health [55] to describe the domains of functioning and disability, the focus of rehabilitation may encompass body structures and function (e.g., strength, muscle tone, and swallowing) activities and participation (mobility, play, learning, and communication), environmental factors (physical, attitudinal, and resource barriers), and quality of life.

The basis of the treatment is to consider the child in all dimensions and domains of his life (multidimensional holistic rehabilitation) without neglecting family engagement.

From a rehabilitative point of view, CNS tumors can be considered an acquired brain injury (ABI). Plasticity mechanism in the developing brain consists of a variety of processes essential for synaptic formation and rewiring of neuronal networks. These mechanisms optimize the propagation time and processing of stimuli and critical to learning and memory [56].

The goal of rehabilitation treatment after ABI is to stimulate the natural reorganization of connections to offset damaged pathways. Teamwork is a crucial strategy, usually including many disciplines and healthcare workers, such as pediatric physiatrist and neurologist, speech therapist, psychomotor therapist, dysphagia therapist, occupational therapist, and cognitive therapist [57].

In pediatric CNS tumors, rehabilitative treatment implementation is necessary in the post-surgical phase or in between oncological treatments, to plan a short- and long-term management, providing not only an outpatient program but also an inpatient rehabilitation to maximize the mechanisms of recovery [58].

22.3.1.1 Early-Term Morbidity and Rehabilitative Care

Clinical manifestations of pediatric brain tumors depend on several conditions, such as age, site location, tumor's grade of infiltration/compression, and type of treatment (radiotherapy vs. chemotherapy). Typical onset signs and symptoms suggestive of CNS lesions are: cranial nerve palsy, seizures, motor palsy, ataxia, visual deficit, endocrine dysfunctions, abnormal posture of the head (due to local compression), headache, and vomiting (secondary to increased intracranial pressure). Early-delayed reactions occur from a few weeks to 3 months after radiation treatment and are thought to be due to a combination of tumor response, peritumoral edema, and demyelination. Findings include transient focal neurologic deficits, somnolence syndrome (characterized by extreme sleepiness and signs of increased intracranial pressure [ICP], such as headache, nausea, vomiting, anorexia, and irritability). Brain tumors in children under the age of one are a special clinical situation. Their diagnosis is often delayed because of the mobility of the skull bone. It is also possible to recognize prenatal signs such as polyhydramnios and macrocephaly [59]. Cranial ultrasound and magnetic resonance imaging (MRI) must be ordered promptly to prevent secondary neurological complications. Spinal cord tumors present mainly with urinary dysfunction, weakness, back and abdominal pain, abnormal head posture or respiratory problems, and bladder and bowel dysfunction. Following diagnosis and an integrated report, a multidisciplinary assessment is carried out, including a neurosurgeon, pediatric oncologist, and radiotherapist. Treatment of hydrocephalus usually precedes tumor resection or biopsy. In some types of CNS tumors, radical resection is essential, but in relation to the functionally critical area, in some cases complete resection is generally limited by the inability to remove the tumor with surrounding clear margins of normal tissue because of the risk of producing permanent neurological deficits [60]. Intraoperative neurophysiological monitoring is important to minimize this risk. Early rehabilitation programs usually start in the intensive care unit (ICU) with passive mobilization, prevention of secondary complications (placement of orthosis, skin care), botulinum toxin injection, and respiratory rehabilitation. Intensive rehabilitation is usually provided in an inpatient setting (Rehabilitative Unit), where it is also possible to manage in a multidisciplinary team, neurological complications, endocrinological problems, and respiratory failure in a close way [58]. Weaning from mechanical ventilation and tracheostomy is an important goal of this phase of treatment, favored by motor and respiratory passive and active exercises.

22.3.1.2 Feeding and Swallowing Problems

In a recent consensus statement [61], the importance of examining and managing nutritional issues in pediatric oncology, both for overnutrition and undernutrition, has been stressed. Rehabilitation is primarily involved when the child is unable to take food by mouth, detected and treated by a speech therapist and through medical exams. Dysphagia is defined as a disorder affecting any phase of swallowing (oral, oral propulsive, pharyngeal, esophageal, or gastric) involving the intake of food and liquids. Anamnesis and clinical assessment could reveal signs of dysphagia, such as: aspiration, laryngeal penetration, coughing during meals, history of aspiration pneumonia, or respiratory morbidity. Respectively, video fluoroscopy swallow study (VFSS) and fiberoptic endoscopic evaluation (FESS) radiographically and anatomically examine the progression of bolus from the mouth to the stomach [62]. It can be requested to confirm clinical suspects, using different viscosities for fluids. Mentioning some issues well summarized from Dodrill et al. 2016 [63], the technique of treatment depends on dysphagic disorders, mainly consistent in using thickening agents, chopping the solid meal, offering different bottles or cups, modifying posture (seating equipment), and trailing swallowing maneuvers (e.g., chin tuck) to assist swallow safety [64]. In patients whose motor oral rehabilitation is not a short-term solution, to guarantee a complete daily nutritional intake, surgical indication of percutaneous gastrostomy is mandatory.

In childhood brain tumors, the dysphagia presentation is dependent on the location and tumor type as well as treatment options, including surgery, radiotherapy, and chemotherapy. It may appear as a symptom of the above-mentioned “Cerebellar mutism syndrome” or as a direct insult of cranial nerve, after surgical treatment of posterior fossa tumors. Given the many complex factors influencing the child’s dysphagia and eating and drinking management, a multidisciplinary team approach is essential to provide comprehensive assessment and management of their difficulties [65]. Drooling problems are frequently associated with dysphagia. Drugs commonly used to treat sialorrhea are glycopyrrolate, trihexyphenidyl, chloralhydrate, and scopolamine patch. Surgical treatment is sometimes necessary in cases of pharmacological ineffectiveness. Saliva gram is the gold standard examination indicated to verify the suspicion of chronic inhalation.

22.3.1.3 Respiratory Problems

Posterior fossa and cervico-medullary tumors are associated with a high risk of developing respiratory problems, mainly due to muscle weakness, injury to the respiratory centers, and loss of brainstem reflexes. These evidences are consequences of tumor location, compression effect, surgical treatment, or intracranial hypertension. In acute or post-acute phase, some patients need tracheostomy, mechanical ventilation, or noninvasive ventilation. Early respiratory and motor rehabilitation treatment in the intensive care unit has the goal to facilitate extubating. In post-acute inpatient rehabilitation, respiratory rehabilitation is important for managing secretions, applying positive expiratory pressure (PEP) therapy, ensuring effective cough (e.g., mechanical cough assistance), providing inhalation therapy, and supporting lung expansion using an Ambu bag. These procedures, united with feed recovery by mouth, are preparatory for a possible weaning from mechanical ventilation or tracheostomy.

22.3.1.4 Long-Term Morbidity

Late effects of cancer therapy are treatment-related complications that include secondary malignancies, organ-system dysfunction, psychosocial difficulties, cognitive disabilities, and death [66]. Networking is essential to reduce morbidity and to ensure the best possible quality of life. Whole brain irradiation may induce a wide spectrum of cognitive deficits that can emerge over time, including long-term effects on learning and memory, as well as global cognitive decline. In rare cases, severe leukoencephalopathy may occur. These are among the major radiotherapy-related complications in pediatric patients [67]. Several pharmacologic interventions have been tested to improve cognitive function in patients treated with focal or whole-brain radiation. Lacking better options, drugs such as methylphenidate, donepezil, and memantine are generally well tolerated and may be beneficial in a subset of patients, along with neurocognitive rehabilitation aimed at compensatory strategies [68]. Over the last two decades, proton radiation therapy has emerged as a treatment of choice in some brain tumors. Proton irradiation decreases dose radiation exposure for patients as well as its long-term cognitive effects [69, 70].

22.3.2 Rehabilitative Care

22.3.2.1 Neurological and Cognitive Dysfunctions

Lumsden et al. [71] provided evidence that pediatric patients may exhibit a higher rate of neuropsychiatric and neurodevelopmental disorders even prior to the diagnosis of a brain tumor. In their study, 4.6% of the 131 patients had a diagnosis of autism spectrum disorder. Neuropsychiatric presentations, as well as general cognitive and behavioral impairments (not limited to supratentorial tumor locations) are common in children with brain tumors [72, 73].

Long-term follow-up studies of children with brain tumors have demonstrated a range of cognitive deficits, affecting intelligence, memory, attention, executive function, and academic performance, depending on tumor location (critical areas), age, comorbidity (epilepsy), hydrocephalus at onset and/or shunt dysfunctions, post-surgical complications, and oncological treatment (as mentioned above) with volume and dose of irradiation [74–76].

Cognitive assessment includes a standardized cognitive battery and questionnaires:

General intelligence:

- Griffiths III (scales for psychomotor development, for children less than 48 months) includes five domains: Foundation of

Learning; Language and Communication; Eye and Head Coordination; Personal–Social–Emotional; Gross Motor).
- Wechsler Intelligence Scale for Children (WISC-IV).
- Leiter for nonverbal IQ.
- NEPSY II test for neuropsychological screening (from 3 to 16 years old).

Margelish et al. have shown [77] how to analyze all the subscales to detect specific skills (visuo-perceptual abilities, verbal comprehension, verbal learning, memory, attention, processing speed, verbal fluency, executive functions) or integrate with other tests of measurement:

- Corsi test (visuo-spatial memory).
- BVN for short-term memory.
- Conners Continuous Performance Test for sustained attention.
- Visual memory: Rey figure.
- Wisconsin card sorting tests for cognitive flexibility.
- London of tower test for executive functions.
- Bell's test: visuo-spatial attention.
- PedsQL questionnaire for quality of life.
- Self-management skills scale.
- Vineland Adaptive Behavior Scale (semi-structured interview for adaptive behavior).

22.3.2.2 Neuropsychological Outcomes and Cognitive–Emotional Rehabilitation

Cognitive behavioral interventions are widely used in children with brain tumors post-treatment, aiming to stimulate and to reinforce compensatory attention and memory, improving neurocognitive functions. Cognitive remediation programs could be distinguished in two main approaches: the face-to-face remediation approach oriented to single cognitive domains and the computerized approach [78].

The goal of the training may concern visuo-spatial abilities, memory, executive functions, and language.

Interventions may involve function-specific training and cognitive processing.

Evidence-based rehabilitative programs have brought to light the possibility of using telerehabilitation using virtual reality and applications on the computer. In pediatric oncological patients, it is usually more effective in terms of motivation and comfort.

It is well established that rehabilitation should adopt an ecological approach; therefore, in addition to cognitive and motor interventions, networking with schools, healthcare providers, families, and other elements of the child's living environment is fundamental to improving outcomes and quality of life.

The diagnosis of malignancy in a child is one of the most stressful life events. It is helpful to conduct an assessment of the family, including family composition, history, strengths, vulnerabilities, and preexisting problems, including psychosocial and practical resources, socioeconomic status, and marital, parental, and sibling relationships [2–5].

Emotional support and cognitive behavioral intervention take part in a more global restorative and supportive therapies, with the aim of social integration.

Psychosocial support and a parent's training are strongly recommended.

22.3.2.3 Motor Deficit Treatment

The earliest timing of intervention on motor deficits and spasticity in children with acquired brain injury is crucial to obtain better results [79].

Functional measures of postural control, self-care, and motor skills, as well as gait analysis, widely used in cerebral palsy, can be extended to acquired brain injury (GMFM, Ashworth, Wee-Fim). These tools are also effective for outcome assessment [80, 81].

In cases of spasticity (e.g., hypertonia, clonus), pharmacological treatment may be beneficial and is also indicated in pediatric patients. This includes the use of muscle relaxant medications—most commonly baclofen—as well as botulinum toxin injections [82].

The botulinum toxin injection seems to interact with intrafusal and extrafusal fibers, producing a reduction of hypertonia both through synaptic blockade and inhibition of the stretch reflex loop, and these changes may influence not only the spinal cord but also the CNS. These findings suggest that spasticity itself can be considered as a factor affecting the cortical sensitive potentials [83].

To prevent secondary complications from prolonged immobilization or to sustain the limbs in sitting position or during gait, it is necessary to pack early orthoses (static or dynamic orthoses) [84, 85].

Summarizing the totality of rehabilitation approaches in the case of pediatric patients with brain tumors and motor deficits due to disease or related treatments, we can highlight several interventions in ABI, based on clinical practice [81, 86]:

- Constraint-induced movement therapy: the aim is to stimulate the functional use of the affected limb through the physical constraint of the unaffected limb, to stimulate brain reorganization.
- Bimanual therapy: improving functional integration, for children with hemiparesis.
- Strength training: repetitive muscle contraction, and may include electrical stimulation.
- Treadmill training: may include partial-weight body support, not for severely affected children.
- Virtual reality: used advanced technology to stimulate experiences, also in-home setting.
- Motor imagery: through mental stimulation and cognitive motor process.
- Mirror Therapy: takes advantage of the mirror reflection of the less impaired limb, in bimanual activities.
- Robot-assisted rehabilitation, also effective on cognitive processes related to sensory-motor deficits. Lokomat is a robotic tool for gait training, motivated by virtual reality [87]. Results appear promising also in upper limb rehabilitation.

22.3.2.4 Speech Problems

Children with brain injury, above all for posterior fossa location, frequently suffer from speech problems with or without feeding difficulties. It is related to tumor location (posterior fossa, brain stem, and midline localization) or secondary to a cognitive dysfunction (aphasia, dysphasia, verbal fluency) and may regard several aspects of language: lexical-semantics, phonological, learning, and fluency. In addition to patient observation in a therapeutic setting, an assessment battery is usually administered. Among the various standardized tests [88] can be mentioned:

- Peabody picture verbal test for lexical comprehension.
- Metaphor comprehension and metasemantic ability (MCT test).
- Rey auditory verbal learning test for verbal memory.
- Visual motor integration per visual perception.
- Test for learning problems (Conner's).

22.3.2.5 Occupational Therapy

Children with CNS tumors have a high likelihood of experiencing a variety of disabilities related to their tumor and the effects of the aforementioned various treatment modalities. Rehabilitative services such as occupational and physical therapy are needed by many children for weakness ranging from a hemiplegia of the arm and leg to a subtle change in fine motor skills. Occupational and speech therapists can assist the child to recover full function in older children and adolescents with acquired brain injury. In older children and adolescents with acquired brain injury, occupational therapy is indicated to work on self-care abilities, dressing, bathing, and self-feeding [89]. Independence supports a higher mood in a holistic rehabilitation concept.

22.3.2.6 Visual Functions in Children with Brain Tumors

Brain tumors can alter the normal anatomy of structures involved in both the afferent and efferent visual system, leading to dysfunction of these systems, vision loss, and ocular motility disturbances [90]. Damage to visual function can be secondary to tumor location (hemispheres, optic pathways), surgical and oncological treatment, and can involve parenchymal zones, lateral geniculate ganglion, optic nerve, and optic pathways. Also, chronic papilledema could lead to loss of vision and visual field defects. Visual field defects are common in hemispheric, sellar/suprasellar, or temporo-parietal visual function assessment, and ophthalmological examination mainly assesses reaction to light, pupillary reaction, eye fundus examination, visual acuity, refractive error, computerized visual field, visual evoked potential, and optic coherence tomography. Orthoptic examination is possible to assess ocular motility, manual visual field, and visual acuity in younger children. In preverbal or cooperative children, visual quantitative acuity can be assessed by the visual acuity cards (Teller) procedure. Mainly in vision loss and low vision problems, integrated rehabilitation with an orthoptic and occupational therapist is crucial to stimulate residual vision, using an optical device (prisms, software) and recent strategies based on virtual reality [91, 92, 93].

22.4 Conclusions

Brain tumors are the most common solid tumors in children, and an increased survival rate is accompanied by increased need for neurorehabilitation because many subtypes continue to have a suboptimal long-term outcome. During the last several years, however, remarkable advances in understanding the molecular underpinnings of these tumors and the most personalized treatment have been made. A part of this category of patients continues to have motor behavioral and cognitive problems, the severity of which seems to be related to the malignancy and also to the severity of treatment. An optimal supportive care approach—encompassing attention to the collateral effects of therapies, psychological assessment, nutritional support, and comprehensive speech, motor, and neurocognitive rehabilitation—may lead to meaningful improvements in outcomes and quality of life.

References

1. Louis DN, Perry A, Wesseling P, Brat DJ, Cree IA, Figarella-Branger D, Hawkins C, Ng HK, Pfister SM, Reifenberger G, Soffietti R, von Deimling A, Ellison DW. The 2021 WHO classification of tumors of the central nervous system: a summary. Neuro-Oncology. 2021;23(8):1231–51. https://doi.org/10.1093/neuonc/noab106. PMID: 34185076; PMCID: PMC8328013.
2. Pruitt DW, Ayyangar R, Craig K, White A, Neufeld JA. Pediatric brain tumor rehabilitation. J Pediatr Rehabil Med. 2011;4(1):59–70. https://doi.org/10.3233/PRM-2011-0154. PMID: 21757811.
3. Fountain DM, Burke GA. Multidisciplinary rehabilitation for children with brain tumors: a systematic review. Dev Neurorehabil. 2017;20(2):68–75. https://doi.org/10.3109/17518423.2015.1065017. Epub 2015 Jul 29. PMID: 26222675.
4. Park M, Choi EK, Lyu CJ, Han JW, Hahn SM. Family resilience factors affecting family adaptation of children with cancer: a cross-sectional study. Eur J Oncol Nurs. 2022;56:102078. https://doi.org/10.1016/j.ejon.2021.102078. Epub 2021 Nov 24. PMID: 34847403.
5. Yamaji N, Suzuki D, Suto M, Sasayama K, Ota E. Communication tools used in cancer communication with children: a scoping review protocol. BMJ Open. 2022;12(2):e056403. https://doi.org/10.1136/bmjopen-2021-056403. PMID: 35197351; PMCID: PMC8867319.
6. Desjardins L, Barrera M, Schulte F, Chung J, Cataudella D, Janzen L, Bartels U, Downie A. Predicting social withdrawal, anxiety and depression symptoms in pediatric brain tumor survivors. J Psychosoc Oncol. 2019;37(1):22–36. https://doi.org/10.1080/07347332.2018.1535531. Epub 2019 Jan 7. PMID: 30614410.
7. Kearney JA, Salley CG, Muriel AC. Standards of psychosocial care for parents of children with cancer. Pediatr Blood Cancer. 2015;62(Suppl 5):S632–83. https://doi.org/10.1002/pbc.25761. PMID: 26700921; PMCID: PMC5066591.
8. Young K, Bowers A, Bradford N. Families' experiences of child and adolescent brain tumor: a systematic review and synthesis of qualitative research. Psychooncology. 2021;30(10):1643–62. https://doi.org/10.1002/pon.5745. Epub 2021 Jun 14. PMID: 34124814.
9. Szabados M, Kolumbán E, Agócs G, Kiss-Dala S, Engh MA, Hernádfői M, Takács K, Tuboly E, Párniczky A, Hegyi P, Garami M. Association of tumor location with anxiety and depression in childhood brain cancer survivors: a systematic review and meta-analysis. Child Adolesc Psychiatry Ment Health. 2023;17(1):124. https://doi.org/10.1186/s13034-023-00665-0. PMID: 37891679; PMCID: PMC10612250.

10. Levesque A, Ogez D, Gravel V, Marcil V, Curnier D, Rondeau É, Sinnett D, Péloquin K, Sultan S. Feasibility study of taking back control together, an intervention to support parents of children with cancer. J Clin Psychol Med Settings. 2024;31(2):444–54. https://doi.org/10.1007/s10880-023-09998-6. Epub 2023 Dec 21. PMID: 38127090.
11. Jackson K, Packer RJ. Recent advances in pediatric medulloblastoma. Curr Neurol Neurosci Rep. 2023;23(12):841–8. https://doi.org/10.1007/s11910-023-01316-9. Epub 2023 Nov 9. PMID: 37943476; PMCID: PMC10724301.
12. Lanier JC, Abrams AN. Posterior fossa syndrome: review of the behavioral and emotional aspects in pediatric cancer patients. Cancer. 2017;123(4):551–9. https://doi.org/10.1002/cncr.30238. Epub 2016 Oct 27. PMID: 27787875.
13. Thacker N, Bouffet E. Posterior fossa syndrome-time to unmute the silence on cerebellar mutism. Neuro-oncol. 2021;23(9):1427–8. https://doi.org/10.1093/neuonc/noab147. PMID: 34139019; PMCID: PMC8408842.
14. Bakhshi SK, Mitha R, Mushtaq N, Shamim MS. Cerebellar mutism syndrome after surgical resection of posterior fossa neoplastic lesions. J Pak Med Assoc. 2020;70(9):1667–8. PMID: 33040137.
15. De Smet HJ, Catsman-Berrevoets C, Aarsen F, Verhoeven J, Marien P, Paquier PF. Auditory-perceptual speech analysis in children with cerebellar tumours: a long-term follow-up study. Eur J Paediatr Neurol. 2012;16:434–442.24.
16. Di Rocco C, Chieffo D, Pettorini BL, Massimi L, Caldarelli M, Tamburrini G. Preoperative and postoperative neurological, neuropsychological and behavioral impairment in children with posterior cranial fossa astrocytomas and medulloblastomas: the role of the tumor and the impact of the surgical treatment. Childs Nerv Syst. 2010;26(9):1173–88. https://doi.org/10.1007/s00381-010-1166-2. Epub 2010 Jun 16. PMID: 20552208.
17. Yap JL, Wachtel LE, Ahn ES, et al. Treatment of cerebellar cognitive affective syndrome with aripiprazole. J Pediatr Rehabil Med. 2012;5:233–8.
18. Gordon AL, di Maggio A. Rehabilitation for children after acquired brain injury: current and emerging approaches. Pediatr Neurol. 2012;46(6):339–44. https://doi.org/10.1016/j.pediatrneurol.2012.02.029. PMID: 22633627.
19. Li N, Yang Y, Glover DP, Zhang J, Saraswati M, Robertson C, Pelled G. Evidence for impaired plasticity after traumatic brain injury in the developing brain. J Neurotrauma. 2014;31(4):395–403. https://doi.org/10.1089/neu.2013.3059. Epub 2013 Dec 10. PMID: 24050267; PMCID: PMC3922417.
20. Patel P, Robinson PD, Wahib N, Cheung P, Wong T, Cabral S, Parker A, Cohen M, Devine K, Gibson P, Holdsworth MT, Neumann E, Orsey A, Phillips R, Spinelli D, Thackray J, van de Wetering M, Woods D, Sung L, Dupuis LL. Interventions for the prevention of acute phase chemotherapy-induced nausea and vomiting in adult and pediatric patients: a systematic review and meta-analysis. Support Care Cancer. 2022;30(11):8855–69. https://doi.org/10.1007/s00520-022-07287-w. Epub 2022 Aug 12. PMID: 35953731; PMCID: PMC10153509.
21. Ganguly S, Sasi A, Nagaraju SKK, Bakhshi S. Anti-emetics in children receiving chemotherapy for solid tumors and leukemia: pharmacology and optimization of therapy for nausea and vomiting. Pharmaceuticals (Basel). 2024;17(5):616. https://doi.org/10.3390/ph17050616. PMID: 38794186; PMCID: PMC11124061.
22. Dupuis LL, Boodhan S, Sung L, Portwine C, Hain R, McCarthy P, Holdsworth M, Pediatric Oncology Group of Ontario. Guideline for the classification of the acute emetogenic potential of antineoplastic medication in pediatric cancer patients. Pediatr Blood Cancer. 2011;57(2):191–8. https://doi.org/10.1002/pbc.23114. Epub 2011 Apr 4. PMID: 21465637; PMCID: PMC6554029.
23. Sherani F, Boston C, Mba N. Latest update on prevention of acute chemotherapy-induced nausea and vomiting in pediatric cancer patients. Curr Oncol Rep. 2019;21(10):89. https://doi.org/10.1007/s11912-019-0840-0. PMID: 31418119; PMCID: PMC6695477.
24. Meena JP, Gupta AK, Jat KR, Anandani G, Sasidharan A, Tanwar P. Efficacy and safety of olanzapine for the prevention of chemotherapy-induced nausea and vomiting in children: a systematic review and meta-analysis of randomized controlled trials. J Pediatr Hematol Oncol. 2023;45(7):361–9. https://doi.org/10.1097/MPH.0000000000002737. Epub 2023 Aug 3. PMID: 37539996.
25. Hesketh PJ. Chemotherapy-induced nausea and vomiting. N Engl J Med. 2008;358(23):2482–94. https://doi.org/10.1056/NEJMra0706547. PMID: 18525044
26. Gupta K, Walton R, Kataria SP. Chemotherapy-induced nausea and vomiting: pathogenesis, recommendations, and new trends. Cancer Treat Res Commun. 2021;26:100278. https://doi.org/10.1016/j.ctarc.2020.100278. Epub 2020 Dec 11. PMID: 33360668.
27. Agre S, Agre M, Pol P, Tonse M, Mohanty M, Shaikh A. Retrospective evaluation of a dexamethasone sparing antiemetic regimen: an antiemetic prophylaxis study on NEPA (Netupitant plus Palonosetron) for preventing chemotherapy-induced nausea and vomiting (CINV) in cancer patients. Cureus. 2023;15(11):e49763. https://doi.org/10.7759/cureus.49763. PMID: 38161895; PMCID: PMC10757726.
28. Ruktrirong J, Traivaree C, Monsereenusorn C, Photia A, Lertvivatpong N, Rujkijyanont P. Single daily dosing versus divided dosing intravenous ondansetron to prevent chemotherapy-induced nausea and vomiting among children: a comparative randomized double-blind controlled trial. Pediatr Blood Cancer. 2021;68(6):e29002. https://doi.org/10.1002/pbc.29002. Epub 2021 Mar 23. PMID: 33754455.

29. Dupuis LL, Nathan PC. Options for the prevention and management of acute chemotherapy-induced nausea and vomiting in children. Paediatr Drugs. 2003;5(9):597–613. https://doi.org/10.2165/00148581-200305090-00003. PMID: 12956617.
30. Tran K, Loshak H. Palonosetron for patients undergoing high or moderate Emetogenic chemotherapy [internet]. Ottawa (ON): Canadian Agency for Drugs and Technologies in Health; 2021. PMID: 36191121.
31. Lau Moon Lin M, Robinson PD, Flank J, Sung L, Dupuis LL. The safety of metoclopramide in children: a systematic review and meta-analysis. Drug Saf. 2016;39(7):675–87. https://doi.org/10.1007/s40264-016-0418-9. PMID: 27003816.
32. Bauters TG, Verlooy J, Robays H, Benoit Y, Laureys G. Emesis control by aprepitant in children and adolescents with chemotherapy. Int J Clin Pharm. 2013;35(6):1021–4. https://doi.org/10.1007/s11096-013-9842-4. Epub 2013 Sep 4. PMID: 24002338.
33. Dupuis LL, Nathan PC. Optimizing emetic control in children receiving antineoplastic therapy: beyond the guidelines. Paediatr Drugs. 2010;12(1):51–61. https://doi.org/10.2165/11316190-000000000-00000. PMID: 20034341.
34. Kandula T, Park SB, Cohn RJ, Krishnan AV, Farrar MA. Pediatric chemotherapy induced peripheral neuropathy: a systematic review of current knowledge. Cancer Treat Rev. 2016;50:118–28. https://doi.org/10.1016/j.ctrv.2016.09.005.
35. Starobova H, Vetter I. Pathophysiology of chemotherapy-induced peripheral neuropathy. Front Mol Neurosci. 2017;10:174. https://doi.org/10.3389/fnmol.2017.00174.
36. Kandula T, Farrar MA, Cohn RJ, Mizrahi D, Carey K, Johnston K, et al. Chemotherapy-induced peripheral neuropathy in long-term survivors of childhood cancer: clinical, neurophysiological, functional, and patient-reported outcomes. JAMA Neurol. 2018;75(8):980–8. https://doi.org/10.1001/jamaneurol.2018.0963.
37. Courtemanche H, Magot A, Ollivier Y, Rialland F, Leclair-Visonneau L, Fayet G, et al. Vincristine-induced neuropathy: atypical electrophysiological patterns in children. Muscle Nerve. 2015;52(6):981–5. https://doi.org/10.1002/mus.24647.
38. Tay N, Laakso EL, Schweitzer D, Endersby R, Vetter I, Starobova H. Chemotherapy-induced peripheral neuropathy in children and adolescent cancer patients. Front Mol Biosci. 2022;9:1015746. https://doi.org/10.3389/fmolb.2022.1015746. PMID: 36310587; PMCID: PMC9614173.
39. Gilchrist LS, Tanner L. The pediatric-modified total neuropathy score: a reliable and valid measure of chemotherapy-induced peripheral neuropathy in children with non-CNS cancers. Support Care Cancer. 2013;21(3):847–56. https://doi.org/10.1007/s00520-012-1591-8.
40. Lim EA, Alves CAPF, Picariello S, Aquilina K, Bisdas S, Loebel U, Mankad K, D'Arco F. Neuroimaging of paediatric pineal, sellar and suprasellar tumours: a guide to differential diagnosis. Childs Nerv Syst. 2022;38(1):33–50. https://doi.org/10.1007/s00381-021-05359-6. Epub 2021 Sep 16. PMID: 34529090.
41. McCrea HJ, George E, Settler A, Schwartz TH, Greenfield JP. Pediatric suprasellar tumors. J Child Neurol. 2016;31(12):1367–76. https://doi.org/10.1177/0883073815620671. Epub 2015 Dec 15. PMID: 26676303.
42. Khadilkar V, Karguppikar M. Endocrinological management of sellar and supra-sellar tumors in children. Neurol India. 2020;68(Supplement):S28–32. https://doi.org/10.4103/0028-3886.287676. PMID: 32611889.
43. Alter CA, Shekdar KV, Cohen LE. Pituitary tumors in children. Adv Pediatr Infect Dis. 2021;68:211–25. https://doi.org/10.1016/j.yapd.2021.05.007. PMID: 34243854.
44. Müller HL, Zhou J, Peng J. Editorial: recent advances in pediatric craniopharyngioma. Front Endocrinol (Lausanne). 2024;15:1413744. https://doi.org/10.3389/fendo.2024.1413744. PMID: 38706703; PMCID: PMC11066279.
45. Devaraja J, Sloan S, Lee V, Dimitri P. Arginine-vasopressin infusion in a child with cranial diabetes insipidus during hyperhydration therapy with chemotherapy: a therapeutic challenge. Endocrinol Diabetes Metab Case Rep. 2021;2021:20–0122. https://doi.org/10.1530/EDM-20-0122. Epub ahead of print. PMID: 33597311; PMCID: PMC7923125.
46. Gabay S, Merchant TE, Boop FA, Roth J, Constantini S. Shifting strategies in the treatment of pediatric Craniopharyngioma. Curr Oncol Rep. 2023;25(12):1497–513. https://doi.org/10.1007/s11912-023-01471-9. Epub 2023 Nov 28. PMID: 38015373.
47. Claude F, Ubertini G, Szinnai G. Endocrine disorders in children with brain tumors: at diagnosis, after surgery, radiotherapy and chemotherapy. Children (Basel). 2022;9(11):1617. https://doi.org/10.3390/children9111617. PMID: 36360345; PMCID: PMC9688119.
48. Del Baldo G, Vennarini S, Cacchione A, Amelio D, De Ioris MA, Fabozzi F, Colafati GS, Mastronuzzi A, Carai A. Multidisciplinary management of craniopharyngiomas in children: a single center experience. Diagnostics (Basel). 2022;12(11):2745. https://doi.org/10.3390/diagnostics12112745. PMID: 36359587; PMCID: PMC9689811.
49. Brinksma A, Sanderman R, Roodbol PF, et al. Malnutrition is associated with worse health-related quality of life in children with cancer. Support Care Cancer. 2015;23(10):3043–52.
50. Zimmermann K, Ammann RA, Kuehni CE, et al. Malnutrition in pediatric patients with cancer at diagnosis and throughout therapy: a multicenter cohort study. Pediatr Blood Cancer. 2013;60(4):642–9.
51. Sung L, Zaoutis T, Ullrich NJ, et al. Children's Oncology Group's 2013 blueprint for research: can-

cer control and supportive care. Pediatr Blood Cancer. 2013;60(6):1027–30.
52. Grabenbauer GG, Holger G. Management of radiation and chemotherapy related acute toxicity in gastrointestinal cancer. Best Pract Res Clin Gastroenterol. 2016;30(4):655–64. https://doi.org/10.1016/j.bpg.2016.06.001. Epub 2016 Jun 25. PMID: 27644912.
53. Otmani N, Hattad S. Clinical outcome in children with chemotherapy-induced Mucositis. Semin Oncol Nurs. 2021;37(3):151160. https://doi.org/10.1016/j.soncn.2021.151160. Epub 2021 Jun 1. PMID: 34088558.
54. World Health Organisation. Rehabilitation: health topics 2011. Available at: http://www.who.int/topics/rehabilitation/en/. Accessed 21 Jan 2011.
55. World Health Organization. International classification of functioning, disability and health (ICF). Geneva: World Health Organisation; 2001.
56. Gmelig Meyling C, Verschuren O, Rentinck IR, Engelbert RHH, Gorter JW. Physical rehabilitation interventions in children with acquired brain injury: a scoping review. Dev Med Child Neurol. 2022;64(1):40–8. https://doi.org/10.1111/dmcn.14997. Epub 2021 Jul 26. PMID: 34309829; PMCID: PMC9292549.
57. Perkins A, Gracey F, Kelly G, Jim J. A new model to guide identity-focused multidisciplinary rehabilitation for children and young people following acquired brain injury: I-FoRM. Neuropsychol Rehabil. 2022;32(8):1928–69. https://doi.org/10.1080/09602011.2022.2100794. Epub 2022 Jul 27. PMID: 35895321.
58. Rossi F, Ricci F, Botti S, Bertin D, Breggiè S, Casalaz R, Cervo M, Ciullini P, Coppo M, Cornelli A, Esposito M, Ferrarese M, Ghetti M, Longo L, Morri M, Naretto G, Orsini N, Fagioli F, AIEOP Rehabilitation Working Group Members. The Italian consensus conference on the role of rehabilitation for children and adolescents with leukemia, central nervous system, and bone tumors, part 1: review of the conference and presentation of consensus statements on rehabilitative evaluation of motor aspects. Pediatr Blood Cancer. 2020;67(12):e28681. https://doi.org/10.1002/pbc.28681. Epub 2020 Sep 17. PMID: 32940000.
59. Simone V, Rizzo D, Cocciolo A, Caroleo AM, Carai A, Mastronuzzi A, Tornesello A. Infantile brain tumors: a review of literature and future perspectives. Diagnostics (Basel). 2021;11(4):670. https://doi.org/10.3390/diagnostics11040670. PMID: 33917833; PMCID: PMC8068230.
60. Blaney SM, Hass-Kogan D, Poussaint TY, et al. Gliomas, ependymomas, and other nonembryonal tumors of the central nervous system. In: Pizzo P, Poplack D, editors. Principles and practice of pediatric oncology. 6th ed. Philadelphia: Lippincott Williams & Wilkins; 2011. p. 717.
61. Fabozzi F, Trovato CM, Diamanti A, Mastronuzzi A, Zecca M, Tripodi SI, Masetti R, Leardini D, Muratore E, Barat V, Lezo A, De Lorenzo F, Caccialanza R, Pedrazzoli P. Management of nutritional needs in pediatric oncology: a consensus statement. Cancers (Basel). 2022;14(14):3378. https://doi.org/10.3390/cancers14143378. PMID: 35884438; PMCID: PMC9319266.
62. Lefton-Greif MA, Okelo SO, Wright JM, Collaco JM, McGrath-Morrow SA, Eakin MN. Impact of children's feeding/swallowing problems: validation of a new caregiver instrument. Dysphagia. 2014;29(6):671–7. https://doi.org/10.1007/s00455-014-9560-7. Epub 2014 Aug 27. PMID: 25159316; PMCID: PMC4359894.
63. Dodrill P, Gosa MM. Pediatric dysphagia: physiology, assessment, and management. Feeding disorders in infants and children. Ann Nutr Metab. 2015;66(suppl 5):24–31.
64. Kilcommons A, Rawlinson D. Dysphagia and long-term feeding difficulties in the pediatric brain tumor population. Perspect ASHA Spec Interest Groups. 2016;1(13):143–8.
65. Plimpton SR, Stence N, Hemenway M, Hankinson TC, Foreman N, Liu AK. Cerebral radiation necrosis in pediatric patients. Pediatr Hematol Oncol. 2015;32(1):78–83. https://doi.org/10.3109/08880018.2013.791738. Epub 2013 May 7. PMID: 23647507.
66. Richard NM, Bernstein LJ, Mason WP, Laperriere N, Maurice C, Millar BA, Shultz DB, Berlin A, Edelstein K. Cognitive rehabilitation for executive dysfunction in brain tumor patients: a pilot randomized controlled trial. J Neuro-Oncol. 2019;142(3):565–75. https://doi.org/10.1007/s11060-019-03130-1. Epub 2019 Mar 7. PMID: 30847839.
67. Lassaletta Á, Morales JS, Valenzuela PL, Esteso B, Kahalley LS, Mabbott DJ, Unnikrishnan S, Panizo E, Calvo F. Neurocognitive outcomes in pediatric brain tumors after treatment with proton versus photon radiation: a systematic review and meta-analysis. World J Pediatr. 2023;19(8):727–40. https://doi.org/10.1007/s12519-023-00726-6. Epub 2023 May 8. PMID: 37154861; PMCID: PMC10348930.
68. Kirkman MA, Ekert JO, Hunn BHM, Thomas MSC, Tolmie AK. A systematic review of cognitive interventions for adult patients with brain tumours. Cancer Med. 2023;12(10):11191–210. https://doi.org/10.1002/cam4.5760. Epub 2023 Mar 7. PMID: 36880363; PMCID: PMC10242361.
69. Yahya N, Manan HA. Neurocognitive impairment following proton therapy for paediatric brain tumour: a systematic review of post-therapy assessments. Support Care Cancer. 2021;29(6):3035–47. https://doi.org/10.1007/s00520-020-05808-z. Epub 2020 Oct 11. PMID: 33040284.
70. Mahajan A, Stavinoha PL, Rongthong W, Brodin NP, McGovern SL, El Naqa I, Palmer JD, Vennarini S, Indelicato DJ, Aridgides P, Bowers DC, Kremer L, Ronckers C, Constine L, Avanzo M. Neurocognitive effects and necrosis in childhood cancer survivors treated with radiation therapy: a PENTEC com-

prehensive review. Int J Radiat Oncol Biol Phys. 2024;119(2):401–16. https://doi.org/10.1016/j.ijrobp.2020.11.073. Epub 2021 Mar 30. PMID: 33810950.
71. Lumsden DE, Woodthorpe C, Hargrave D, Hedderly TJ. Pre-existing neurodevelopmental and neuropsychiatric difficulties in children with brain tumours: implications for future outcome studies. Dev Med Child Neurol. 2011;53(1):93. https://doi.org/10.1111/j.1469-8749.2010.03822.x. Epub 2010 Nov 18. PMID: 21087234.
72. Zyrianova Y, Alexander L, Faruqui R. Neuropsychiatric presentations and outcomes in children and adolescents with primary brain tumours: systematic review. Brain Inj. 2016;30(1):1–9. https://doi.org/10.3109/02699052.2015.1075590. Epub 2015 Nov 5. PMID: 26536821.
73. Iuvone L, Peruzzi L, Colosimo C, Tamburrini G, Caldarelli M, Di Rocco C, Battaglia D, Guzzetta F, Misciagna S, Di Giannatale A, Ruggiero A, Riccardi R. Pretreatment neuropsychological deficits in children with brain tumors. Neuro-Oncology. 2011;13(5):517–24. https://doi.org/10.1093/neuonc/nor013. Epub 2011 Mar 3. PMID: 21372071; PMCID: PMC3093333.
74. George AP, Kuehn SM, Vassilyadi M, Richards PM, Parlow SE, Keene DL, Ventureira EC. Cognitive sequelae in children with posterior fossa tumors. Pediatr Neurol. 2003;28:42–7.
75. Poggi G, Liscio M, Galbiati S, Adduci A, Massimino M, Gandola L, Spreafico F, Clerici CA, Fossati-Bellani F, Sommovigo M, Castelli E. Brain tumors in children and adolescents: cognitive andpsychological disorders at different ages. Psychooncology. 2005;14:386–95.
76. Knab B, Connell PP. Radiotherapy for pediatric brain tumors: when and how. Expert Rev Anticancer Ther. 2007;7(12 Suppl):S69–77. https://doi.org/10.1586/14737140.7.12s.S69. PMID: 18076312.
77. Margelisch K, Studer M, Ritter BC, Steinlin M, Leibundgut K, Heinks T. Cognitive dysfunction in children with brain tumors at diagnosis. Pediatr Blood Cancer. 2015;62(10):1805–12. https://doi.org/10.1002/pbc.25596. Epub 2015 Jun 5. PMID: 26053691; PMCID: PMC5054885.
78. Butler RW, Copeland DR. Attentional processes and their remediation in children treated for cancer: a literature review and the development of a therapeutic approach. J Int Neuropsychol Soc. 2002;8(1):115–24. PMID: 11843068.
79. Day AM, Slomine BS, Salama C, Quinton TL, Suskauer SJ, Salorio CF. Functional gains in children receiving inpatient rehabilitation after brain tumor resection. Arch Phys Med Rehabil. 2021;102(11):2134–40. https://doi.org/10.1016/j.apmr.2021.05.001. Epub 2021 May 25. PMID: 34044002; PMCID: PMC8572161.
80. Gavazzi F, Patel V, Charsar B, Glanzman A, Erler J, Sevagamoorthy A, McKenzie E, Kornafel T, Ballance E, Pierce SR, Teng M, Formanowski B, Woidill S, Shults J, Wassmer E, Tonduti D, Magrinelli F, Bernard G, Van Der Knaap M, Wolf N, Adang L, Vanderver A. Gross motor function in pediatric onset *TUBB4A*-related leukodystrophy: GMFM-88 performance and validation of GMFC-MLD in *TUBB4A*. J Child Neurol. 2023;38(8–9):498–504. https://doi.org/10.1177/08830738231188159. Epub 2023 Jul 17. PMID: 37461315; PMCID: PMC10527384.
81. Chieffo DPR, Lino F, Arcangeli V, Moriconi F, Frassanito P, Massimi L, Tamburrini G. Posterior fossa tumor rehabilitation: an up-to-date overview. Children (Basel). 2022;9(6):904. https://doi.org/10.3390/children9060904. PMID: 35740841; PMCID: PMC9221689.
82. Brandenburg JE, Rabatin AE, Driscoll SW. Spasticity interventions: decision-making and management. Pediatr Clin N Am. 2023;70(3):483–500. https://doi.org/10.1016/j.pcl.2023.01.005. Epub 2023 Mar 21. PMID: 37121638.
83. Frascarelli F, Di Rosa G, Bisozzi E, Castelli E, Santilli V. Neurophysiological changes induced by the botulinum toxin type a injection in children with cerebral palsy. Eur J Paediatr Neurol. 2011;15(1):59–64. https://doi.org/10.1016/j.ejpn.2010.04.002. Epub 2010 May 20. PMID: 20493744.
84. Morgan C, Fetters L, Adde L, Badawi N, Bancale A, Boyd RN, Chorna O, Cioni G, Damiano DL, Darrah J, de Vries LS, Dusing S, Einspieler C, Eliasson AC, Ferriero D, Fehlings D, Forssberg H, Gordon AM, Greaves S, Guzzetta A, Hadders-Algra M, Harbourne R, Karlsson P, Krumlinde-Sundholm L, Latal B, Loughran-Fowlds A, Mak C, Maitre N, McIntyre S, Mei C, Morgan A, Kakooza-Mwesige A, Romeo DM, Sanchez K, Spittle A, Shepherd R, Thornton M, Valentine J, Ward R, Whittingham K, Zamany A, Novak I. Early intervention for children aged 0 to 2 years with or at high risk of cerebral palsy: international clinical practice guideline based on systematic reviews. JAMA Pediatr. 2021;175(8):846–58. https://doi.org/10.1001/jamapediatrics.2021.0878. PMID: 33999106; PMCID: PMC9677545.
85. Bleyenheuft Y, Ebner-Karestinos D, Surana B, Paradis J, Sidiropoulos A, Renders A, Friel KM, Brandao M, Rameckers E, Gordon AM. Intensive upper- and lower-extremity training for children with bilateral cerebral palsy: a quasi-randomized trial. Dev Med Child Neurol. 2017;59(6):625–33. https://doi.org/10.1111/dmcn.13379. Epub 2017 Jan 30. PMID: 28133725.
86. Castelli E. Robotic rehabilitation in children. Psychiatr Danub. 2023;35(Suppl 3):93–4. PMID: 37994072.
87. Van Kammen K, Reinders-Messelink HA, Elsinghorst AL, Wesselink CF, Meeuwisse-de Vries B, van der Woude LHV, Boonstra AM, den Otter R. Amplitude and stride-to-stride variability of muscle activity during Lokomat guided walking and treadmill walking in children with cerebral palsy. Eur J Paediatr Neurol. 2020;29:108–17. https://doi.org/10.1016/j.ejpn.2020.08.003. Epub 2020 Aug 21. PMID: 32900595.

88. Broome K, McCabe P, Docking K, Doble M. A systematic review of speech assessments for children with autism Spectrum disorder: recommendations for best practice. Am J Speech Lang Pathol. 2017;26(3):1011–29. https://doi.org/10.1044/2017_AJSLP-16-0014. PMID: 28772287.
89. Fischer C, Petriccione M, Donzelli M, Pottenger E. Improving care in pediatric neuro-oncology patients: an overview of the unique needs of children with brain tumors. J Child Neurol. 2016;31(4):488–505. https://doi.org/10.1177/0883073815597756. Epub 2015 Aug 5. PMID: 26245798; PMCID: PMC5032907.
90. Peragallo JH. Effects of brain tumors on vision in children. Int Ophthalmol Clin. 2018;58(4):83–95. https://doi.org/10.1097/IIO.0000000000000237. PMID: 30239365; PMCID: PMC6152840.
91. Ricci D, Lucibello S, Orazi L, Gallini F, Staccioli S, Serrao F, Olivieri G, Quintiliani M, Sivo S, Rossi V, Leone D, Ferrantini G, Romeo DM, Frezza S, Amorelli GM, Molle F, Vento G, Lepore D, Mercuri E. Early visual and neuro-development in preterm infants with and without retinopathy. Early Hum Dev. 2020;148:105134. https://doi.org/10.1016/j.earlhumdev.2020.105134. Epub 2020 Jul 11. PMID: 32688300.
92. Leat SJ. A proposed model for integrated low-vision rehabilitation services in Canada. Optom Vis Sci. 2016;93(1):77–84. https://doi.org/10.1097/OPX.0000000000000750. PMID: 26583792.
93. De Luca R, Portaro S, Le Cause M, De Domenico C, Maggio MG, Cristina Ferrera M, Giuffrè G, Bramanti A, Calabrò RS. Cognitive rehabilitation using immersive virtual reality at young age: a case report on traumatic brain injury. Appl Neuropsychol Child. 2020;9(3):282–7. https://doi.org/10.1080/21622965.2019.1576525. Epub 2019 Mar 6. PMID: 30838889.

Palliative Care and End-of-Life Considerations

23

Antonella Cacchione, Michele Salata and Valentina Di Ruscio

23.1 Introduction

Brain tumors (BTs) represent the second most common malignancy of children and adolescents, with an incidence of approximately 5000 children affected per year [1], and have the highest disease-related mortality rate of all pediatric cancers [2].

As the disease progresses, children suffering from BT experience significant physical, psychosocial, and spiritual challenges as well as progressive loss of functions. High symptom burden throughout the disease trajectory, particularly at the end of life, is disproportionately different from other childhood malignancies [3]. In order to face quality of life obstacles throughout their illness journey, it is crucial to have expert guidance with a team specialized and skilled to manage symptoms, optimize quality of life, access supportive services, strive for comfort and dignity at the end of life, and provide bereavement support to the child and overall to caregivers. Underlining and emphasizing these needs, the World Health Organization (WHO) released a document titled Cancer Pain Relief and Palliative Care (PC) in Children, in which PC is recommended in all cases of pediatric oncology patients, at diagnosis, irrespective of prognosis [4].

BTs are categorized as either high- or low-grade. High-grade tumors have a poorer prognosis, but patients with either high- or low-grade tumors experience the adverse effects of chemotherapy, radiation, surgery, and direct disease sequelae, which may be alleviated with supportive/palliative care [2].

PC is a key facet of high-quality pediatric neuro-oncology care as it addresses physical symptom burden, goals of care, advanced care planning, medical decision-making, and end-of-life (EOL) care, optimizing quality of life and minimizing distress [5]. Some specific pediatric BTs (high-grade gliomas, diffuse midline gliomas) are characterized from a particularly dismal prognosis, and the median survival is generally less than 16–24 months [6] independently from the treatment received. In these cases, from the time of diagnosis, a PC may be the chosen approach for treatment by the families.

This chapter will review the fundamentals of providing primary pediatric palliative care in pediatric patients with a diagnosis of a brain tumor.

A. Cacchione · V. D. Ruscio
Area of Hematology-Oncology, Cell Therapy, Gene Therapies, and Hematopoietic Transplantation, IRCCS, Bambino Gesù Children's Hospital IRCCS, Rome, Italy

M. Salata (✉)
Pediatric Palliative Care Center, IRCCS "Bambino Gesù Children's Hospital", Passoscuro, Fiumicino, Italy
e-mail: michele.salata@opbg.net

A. Mastronuzzi, A. Carai (eds.), *Navigating Pediatric Brain Tumors*,
https://doi.org/10.1007/978-3-032-18992-9_23

23.2 The Distinctive Nature of Pediatric Neuro-Oncology Palliative Care

The specific and peculiar nature of pediatric neuro-oncology, due to specific neurological/neuropsychiatric/psychological issues starting from the onset of illness and that become worse during treatments, makes the inclusion of palliative care in the patient care pathway even more important to incorporate in the right way and timing compared to other branches of pediatric oncology [7].

The optimal timing for the introduction of palliative care for children with BT remains unclear. The association of palliative care with death and the discontinuation of treatment often creates obstacles to meeting the needs of children living with brain tumors. PC is viewed as representing failure, a persistent legacy that must be dismantled. Furthermore, the perceived sharp division between curative cancer therapy and palliative care among health professionals and parents represents a further complication. In the context of prognostic uncertainty, PC may not be introduced late in the illness trajectory, conceptualizing that PC is a part of the care paradigm and not synonymous with end-of-life care [8]. In this perspective, the transition to predominantly comfort care can occur gradually. A fundamental and relevant aspect of palliative care management in the pediatric brain tumor patient is the continuity of communication and shared management with the primary oncology team to allow continuity of care well perceived by patients and families [9]. Unique to pediatrics is the concept of "concurrent care," which allows children to receive curative therapies and to stay in hospice [10–12].

23.3 Timing and Location

In recent years, the incorporation of specialized pediatric PC into the management of childhood cancers has significantly advanced, tailored to address the unique challenges faced by children with progressive malignancies. Traditionally, palliative care was only introduced after all curative treatment options had been exhausted (Fig. 23.1), while now the inclusion of PC in the care pathway has a different place and time, with overlapping of the two medical care media (Fig. 23.2) [13].

Palliative care, sometimes referred to as supportive care, currently prioritizes symptom management and relief, as well as the enhancement of quality of life (QoL) at any stage of the illness. Specialty pediatric palliative care is defined by a holistic approach, encompassing medical, psychosocial, and spiritual support facilitated by an interdisciplinary team of trained professionals; notably, this care begins at the point of diagnosis and persists irrespective of whether disease-directed therapies are being administered.

Central to effective pediatric PC is a multidisciplinary team approach that assists patients and their families in establishing individualized goals of care. The American Academy of Pediatrics provides foundational principles for guiding palliative care practices [14], which include (1) the ethical obligation of healthcare providers to pursue interventions only when the anticipated benefits exceed associated risks; (2) the primary aim of palliative care to improve quality of life, irre-

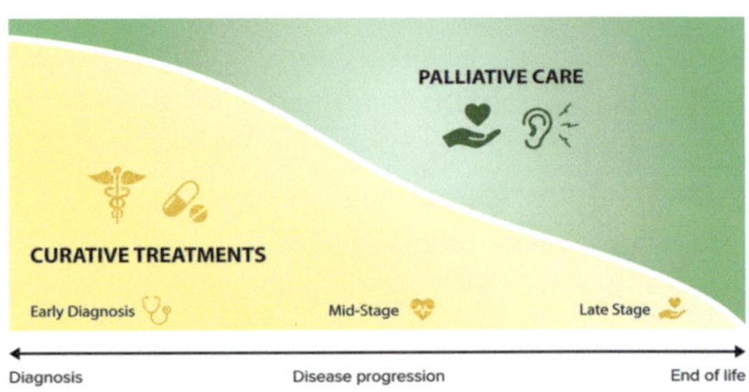

Fig. 23.1 Sequential succession of curative treatments and palliative care

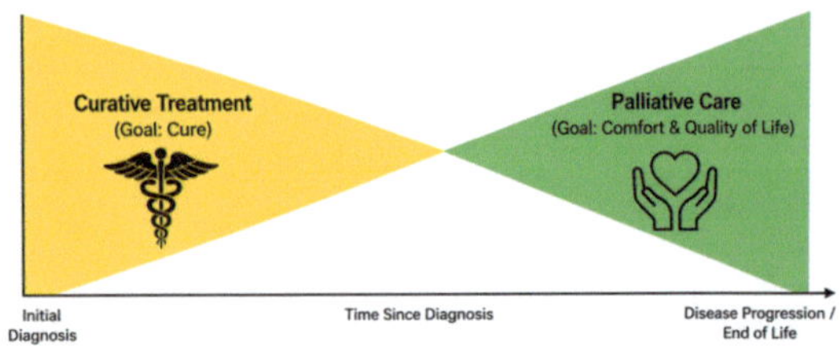

Fig. 23.2 Overlapping of curative treatments and palliative care

spective of the disease trajectory; (3) a strong focus on alleviating symptoms and managing comorbidities; and (4) a commitment to fostering healthy bereavement processes for the families of patients.

This comprehensive model of pediatric palliative care underscores the importance of addressing both immediate and long-term needs, thereby enhancing the overall well-being of affected children and their families throughout the illness experience [15].

In addition to the imbrication of the time of the PC intake, the reflection on the place where their child will be taken in charge is fundamental. The mainstay decision put to families is whether and when to enroll in hospice.

Home care program or recovery in residential formula (hospice) is a comprehensive care program that provides on-call nurse visits, regular medical evaluations, some medication delivery, and bereavement support. In order to be eligible for hospice care, a reasonable possibility of death within the next six months and a shared awareness about the patient's wishes regarding resuscitation should exist [16]. Hospice employs a multidisciplinary approach, with a primary focus on ensuring comfort and enhancing quality of life. It is of the utmost importance to engage in advanced care planning for those nearing the end of their lives. This encompasses the patient's or their family's preference regarding the location of their death. In their examination of hospice referral patterns among pediatric oncologists with a survey, Fowler et al. [17] identified two key barriers to referral: the inability of hospice to administer palliative chemotherapy and the inability to provide blood transfusions. Improved psychological outcomes for families have been associated with household management and the ability to die at home, when possible [18].

23.4 Symptoms

The symptoms experienced by children with BT, in addition to the most common symptoms of other childhood cancers (fatigue, pain, dyspnea), may have a significant impact from the time of diagnosis through to the end of life. These symptoms often include neurological signs that significantly reduce the child's autonomy and QoL. Tumor location can predict the type of associated problems: supratentorial tumors present with seizures and cognitive or behavioral changes; infratentorial tumors are associated with ataxia; and brainstem tumors are associated with speech problems, cranial nerve palsies (including dysphagia and dysarthria), hearing and vision loss, neurological motor deficits, difficulties with secretion management, and headache [15]. It is therefore important to consider the use of alternative and/or augmentative communication to aid communication at the end of life [19].

23.4.1 Headache

Headache occurs in around 30–40% of patients with brain tumors [20], usually due to increased intracranial pressure. The main treatment pharmacological modality includes paracetamol, opioids, and steroids (dexamethasone). Pharmacological agents that target neuropathic pain may offer benefits, although their efficacy often manifests after at least one week. Low-dose methadone (0.04 mg/kg/dose two times a day) is an opioid with N-methyl-D-aspartic acid (NMDA) receptor antagonist properties and is particularly efficacious in the treatment of cancer-related headaches [21]. Nonsteroidal anti-inflammatory drugs are usually contraindicated due to the potential for bleeding at the tumor site and the risk of developing gastric ulcers. In cases of neuropathic neck and back pain related to leptomeningeal irritation, the administration of gabapentin, methadone, or ketamine may be indicated [22].

23.4.2 Dysphagia and Nutritional Support

In patients affected by BT, dysphagia secondary to posterior fossa and brainstem tumors may impair the child's ability to swallow fluids and food orally. In such cases, the insertion of a nasogastric tube for feeding may become necessary. Parents of children with bulbar dysfunctions and specifically with eating capability experience significant distress about the starvation and the inability to eat [23]. Oromotor dysfunctions arising from bulbar impairment cause loss of the ability to control oral muscles and reduce mental alertness in managing secretions. The objective of treatment is to reduce respiratory distress, the aesthetic distress caused by secretions, and to achieve maximum patient comfort. The pharmacological agents employed are muscarinic anticholinergics, including glycopyrrolate, scopolamine, and atropine [24]. Glycopyrrolate does not cross the blood–brain barrier, thereby avoiding the potential for central nervous system side effects. Scopolamine patches provide a convenient transdermal delivery system. Atropine ophthalmic 1% solution can be administered sublingually, with one drop every four hours, providing 0.5 mg of atropine per dose [25]. It may be beneficial to consider alternative treatment strategies, such as regular oral care and suction, in addition to lateral positioning of the patient. Families may find it reassuring to be informed that the rattling noise is not painful and that deep suction is generally not beneficial, while conversely regular oral care and lateral positions are simple but useful tricks. As oromotor dysfunction progresses to dysphagia, it is crucial to consider the fundamental nature of care through feeding and to pay particular attention to nutrition and hydration. It is important to consider nutrition and hydration within the context of the patient's prognosis, the risks of an exacerbation of symptoms (dyspnea, edema, pain) in comparison to mild dehydration, the risk of aspiration pneumonia, and the benefits to the child of enjoying their favorite foods [26]. In specific cases, it may be reasonable to consider more invasive solutions (such as surgically placed feeding tubes or total parenteral nutrition) if these procedures align with the values of the family and the patient's short-term prognosis. In the event that the prognosis is shorter, a nasogastric feeding tube is a more appropriate option, with a reduced risk profile. Withholding/withdrawing artificial nutrition and hydration is a deeply personal decision for patients and parents, often influenced by geographical provenience, religion, culture, and tradition. For healthcare professionals, the ethical issue of withholding or withdrawing nutrition is complex. It is important to inform parents that providing nutrition to an unresponsive child who is dying will not improve the quality of life or alter the outcome [27, 28].

23.4.3 Seizures

Seizures are not uncommon during the entire illness trajectory and can be a very distressing symptom overall in the terminal phase [29]. The goals of treatment are control of seizures and optimization of periods of wakefulness, avoiding worsening cognitive and behavioral functioning [30]. There is no evidence to support routine prophylactic antiepileptic use in the absence of a documented seizure history, and these agents may cause sedation or agitation [31], but when indicated, due to dysphagia, the administration of concentrated sublingual compounds and rectally administered antiepileptic medications is often necessary. The benzodiazepines are most useful in the acute treatment of seizures [32]. Diazepam and lorazepam can be given rectally, and lorazepam and midazolam are both absorbed intranasally. For the long-term management of seizures, levetiracetam, a broad-acting agent, has few adverse effects, is well tolerated, and is often effective [33, 34]. A significant proportion of patients experience a brief, initial period of aggression on levetiracetam, reversible with vitamin B6 supplementation [35].

23.4.4 Nausea and Vomiting

Nausea and vomiting in the context of pediatric neural tumors are common symptoms and may be attributed to either treatment or direct effects of the tumor [36]. The objective of treatment is to reduce nausea and vomiting to a level that allows patients to interact with their families, consume foods they enjoy by mouth, and maintain adequate nutrition and hydration. It is crucial to consider the potential causes of nausea, including direct pressure from the tumor, chemotherapy, hepatic failure, or gastrointestinal pathology (obstruction, ulcers, mucositis, constipation), to address the pharmacological management in a specific way [37]. In the case of increased intracranial pressure, steroids represent the first-line treatment option. In the event of chemotherapy or radiation-induced nausea and vomiting, prophylaxis with a serotonin-3 receptor antagonist (5HT3RA) is recommended, with several published guidelines for children already in existence [38]. In order to achieve the most effective control of nausea and vomiting, it is recommended that both a scheduled medication and an as-needed medication be utilized. It is also advisable to select medications from different classes. Nonmedical therapies may include hypnosis and acupuncture [39].

23.4.5 Agitation, Alteration of Mental Status/ Psychological Symptoms

In the palliative phase, sadness, difficulties in talking about their feelings, fear about illness and death, fear of being alone, and loss of perspective are the most common and typical psychological symptoms [40, 41]. Mood disorders, particularly anxiety, depression, and agitation, are also not uncommon, even among children. Agitation is a common phenomenon at the end of life and presents as restlessness, moaning, and grimacing [42], and it can be a significant source of distress for family members, necessitating timely and aggressive symptom management. Treatment may include benzodiazepines, neuroleptics (haloperidol), reduction of steroid dosage, or administration of opioids if agitation is associated with pain. Moreover, patients with BT are at high risk for skin breakdown related to functional deficits, immobility, and weight gain secondary to steroid use [9]. Patients may present with delayed wound healing and/or wound infection as a result of steroid treatment. With disease progression, leptomeningeal disease, or spinal metastases, patients may develop a neurogenic bowel and bladder and become incontinent of urine and stool. Corticosteroids are frequently employed for the alleviation of progressive neurological symptoms. Initially, they provide a marked improvement; however, this efficacy is generally transient. The dilemma often arises as to whether to further increase the dose of corticosteroids for symptom relief, which often results in a concomitant increase in the side effects of steroids, which are often burdensome in themselves. These adverse effects include hyperphagia, weight gain, body transformation, glucose intolerance, hypertension, mood disturbance, gastrointestinal bleeding and ulcers, and obstructive sleep apnea [43]. Hyperphagia in itself can be of particular concern in those children with swallowing disturbances, as they are permanently hungry and are at risk of choking.

23.5 End-of-Life Care and Palliative Sedation

Although a set of quality measures exists for adults with advanced cancer, these did not directly translate to the pediatric context owing to the delicate balance of parent and child, delegated decision-making, and families' values about advanced childhood cancer care. Hence, to optimize care value, there is an imminent need to establish end-of-life care quality measures that attend to the preferences and priorities of children with cancer and their families, but also coordinated and regulated by a skilled multidisciplinary team [44].

Approximately 80% of pediatric patients with cancer in the terminal phase experience pain that is refractory to traditional analgesia; respiratory symptoms with irregular breathing patterns (hypoventilation, apnea, Cheyne–Stokes respirations, and agonal breathing) are greatly impacted by neurological decline and progressive somnolence. The pharmacological analgesia based on opioids and benzodiazepines allows pain to be kept under control in approximately 30% of cases [45, 46].

Palliative sedation therapy is defined as the intentional reduction of the patient's alert state, using pharmacological tools, up to the point of loss of consciousness, with the aim of decreasing or eliminating a symptom perception or a psychological mood that is otherwise intolerable for the patient. Palliative sedation therapy may be employed in pediatric cancer patients at the end of life when experiencing intractable pain, restlessness, agitation, and psychological suffering, refractory to standard management [47]. The primary objective is to induce a state of deep sleep, which can be achieved through the administration of sedative drugs. Midazolam, neuroleptics, and barbiturates are the drugs most commonly used in this context [48].

The initiation of palliative sedation occurs once the medical team and parents have determined that the child has true refractory symptoms causing unbearable suffering. It is of the utmost importance that the intention of palliative sedation be clearly communicated to parents before its initiation; in order to reach a unified approach to end-of-life, it is essential to engage parents and the multidisciplinary team early.

23.6 Pharmacological Requirements

The pharmacological support of PC in pediatric BT patients makes use of numerous drugs, the main purpose of which is to contain symptoms, alleviate discomfort, contain fear and anxiety, and try to maintain (at least in the initial stages) a good contact of the child with his or her family [23] (Table 23.1).

23.7 Bioethical Aspects

Effective and direct communication is a fundamental aspect of quality pediatric PC, facilitating decision-making and reducing parental distress [49]. The precocious formulation of end-of-life decisions, including Do Not Attempt Resuscitation (DNAR) directives [50, 51], serves to mitigate the potential for a crisis to arise during the progressive deterioration. End-of-life decisions for children with BT include ending treatment, withholding artificial nutrition, determining the location of care, and assessing the need for palliative sedation [52]. The complexity of such decisions requires a skilled and supportive multidisciplinary team.

Table 23.1 Most common drugs used in pediatric neurooncological palliative care

Class		Form	Dose	
Antiemetics				
Ondansetron		Oral, IV	0.15 mg/kg Q8h	
Aprepitant (emend)				
		Oral	Day 1: 3 mg/kg PO (max 125 mg) day 2, 3: 2 mg/kg PO (max 80 mg)	
Metoclopramide		Oral, IV	0.1–0.5 mg/kg q6 hours (max 10 mg)	
Dexamethasone		Oral, IV	10 mg/m2 Daily	
Anti edema				
Dexamethasone		IV, OS	0.25–0.5 mg/kg/dose Q 8–12 h	
Analgesia				
Morphine		OS, SC IV Continuous infusion (IV)	0.1–0.3 mg/kg/dose Q3–4 h 0.05–0.15 mg/kg/dose Q4 h 0.01–0.06 mg/kg/h	Also for dyspnea

(continued)

Table 23.1 (continued)

Class		Form	Dose	
Fentanest		IV Continuous IV Transdermal patch	0.5–2 μg/kg/dose Q30 min–1 h 0.5–2 μg/kg/h Q72 h: 12.5, 25, 50, 75, 100 μg/kg/h	
Gabapentin		IV OS	0.04 mg/kg 10 mg/kg/day to 50 mg/kg/day Q8h	Also for neuropathic pain
Tramadol		OS	1–2 mg/kg/dose Maximum daily Dose 400 mg Every 4–6 hours	
Seizures				
Midazolam		OS Intranasal SC, IV	0.3 mg/kg Q 5 min) to Q4 h 0.1 mg/kg/dose 0.025–0.05 mg/kg/dose	Also for dyspnea, seizures, agitation
Agitation				
Lorazepam		Oral	0.002–0.01 mg/kg/dose Q4–6–12 h	
Haloperidol				
Respiratory secretions				
Glycopyrrolate		IV SC	0–100 μg/kg Q6 h 4–10 μg/kg Q3–4 h	
Anticholinergic scopolamine	Cutaneous patch 1.5 mg		1.5 Mg. Every 72 hours	Over 45 kg

IV intravenous, *SC* subcutaneous, *Q* interval, *h* hours

Another main aspect is represented by involvement and awareness that children and adolescents possess and their wish to be involved in decisions affecting their future healthcare. Parents usually prefer strongly to protect their children from the reality of the disease, and clinicians are also reluctant to routinely include them in sharing medical updates and in making decisions [53]. The legal aspects regulate this much-discussed and articulated field, keeping the age of 14 as the watershed for sharing and communicating the disease status to pediatric patients [54, 55].

23.8 Conclusions

Children with BT have distinct PC needs and unique symptom management compared with children suffering from other malignancies. Patient's progressive cognitive impairment and decline in neurological functions are the major issues that impact communication, decision-making, and safety. The early initiation and take-over of a palliative care approach with the management of symptoms from a skilled multidisciplinary team is essential to alleviate the burden of the peculiar aspect of pediatric BT because the neurologic deterioration that characterizes the dying trajectory of children with brain tumors may create significant challenges for healthcare professionals and the children's parents.

References

1. Ostrom Quinn CBTRUS Statistical report. Primary brain and other central nervous system tumors diagnosed in the US 2010–2014. Neuro-oncol. 2017;19:1–88.
2. Ward E, DeSantis C, Robbins A, Kohler B, Jemal A. Childhood and adolescent cancer statistics, 2014. CA Cancer J Clin. 2014;64:83–103.
3. Baenziger PH, Moody K. Palliative care for children with central nervous system malignancies. Bioengineering (Basel). 2018;5(4):85. https://doi.org/10.3390/bioengineering5040085. PMID: 30322131; PMCID: PMC6315897
4. WHO. Cancer pain relief and palliative care in children. Geneva: World Health Organization; 1998.
5. Committee on Approaching Death: Addressing Key End of Life Issues; Institute of Medicine. Dying in

America: improving quality and honoring individual preferences near the end of life. Washington, DC: National Academies Press (US); 2015.
6. Koschmann C, et al. A road map for the treatment of pediatric diffuse midline glioma. Cancer Cell. 2024;42(1):1–5.
7. Zelcer S, Cataudella D, Cairney AE, Bannister SL. Palliative care of children with brain tumors: a parental perspective. Arch Pediatr Adolesc Med. 2010;164(3):225–30. https://doi.org/10.1001/archpediatrics.2009.284.
8. Brock KE, DeGroote NP, Allen KE. Behind the scenes: care coordination time in an outpatient pediatric palliative oncology clinic. J Palliat Med. 2021;24(3):413–7. https://doi.org/10.1089/jpm.2020.0197. Epub 2020 Jun 23. PMID: 32584641
9. Pérez-Torres Lobato M. Palliative care for children with central nervous system tumors: results of a Spanish multicenter study. Clin Transl Oncol. 2024;26(3):786–95.
10. Lamki AI, et al. Improving cancer Care for children in the developing world: challenges and strategies. Curr Pediatr Rev. 2017;13(1)
11. Levine DR, et al. Does phase 1 trial enrollment preclude quality end-of-life care? Phase 1 trial enrollment and end-of-life care characteristics in children with cancer. Cancer. 2015;121:1508–12.
12. Andre N, Pasquier E. Metronomics during palliative care in paediatric oncology? For sure! But handle me with care. Acta Paediatr. 2016;105(8):874–5. https://doi.org/10.1111/apa.13365. PMID: 27383517
13. Pyke-Grimm KA, Fisher B, Haskamp A, Bell CJ, Newman AR. Providing palliative and hospice care to children, adolescents and young adults with cancer. Semin Oncol Nurs. 2021;37(3):151166. https://doi.org/10.1016/j.soncn.2021.151166. Epub 2021 Jun 24. PMID: 34175165; PMCID: PMC9683514
14. Abdel-Baki MS, Hanzlik E, Kieran MW. Multidisciplinary pediatric brain tumor clinics: the key to successful treatment? CNS Oncol. 2015;4:147–55.
15. Fischer C, Petriccione M, Donzelli M, Pottenger E. Improving care in pediatric neuro-oncology patients: an overview of the unique needs of children with brain tumors. J Child Neurol. 2016;31:488–505.
16. Cuviello A, Raisanen JC, Donohue PK, Wiener L, Boss RD. Initiating palliative care referrals in pediatric oncology. J Pain Symptom Manag. 2021;61(1):81–9.e1
17. Fowler K, Poehlin K, Billheimer D, et al. Hospice referral practice for children with cancer: a survey of pediatric oncologists. J Clin Oncol. 2006;24(7):1099–104.
18. Lotstein D, Klein MJ, Lindley LC, Wolfe J. From hospital to home: referrals to pediatric hospice and home-based palliative care. J Pain Symptom Manag. 2023;65(6):570–9. https://doi.org/10.1016/j.jpainsymman.2023.02.009. Epub 2023 Feb 23. PMID: 36828291
19. Epelman CL. End of life management in pediatric cancer. Curr Oncol Rep. 2012;14(2):191–6.
20. Pace A, Di Lorenzo C, Guariglia L, Jandolo B, Carapella CM, Pompili A. End of life issues in brain tumor patients. J Neuro-Oncol. 2009;91:39–43.
21. Madden K, Bruera E. Very-low-dose methadone to treat refractory neuropathic pain in children with cancer. J Palliat Med. 2017;20(11):1280–3. https://doi.org/10.1089/jpm.2017.0098. Epub 2017 Jun 13. PMID: 28609177
22. Mazandi VM, Lang SS, Rahman RK, Nishisaki A, Beaulieu F, Zhang B, Griffis H, Tucker AM, Storm PB, Heuer GG, Gajjar AA, Ampah SB, Kirschen MP, Topjian AA, Yuan I, Francoeur C, Kilbaugh TJ, Huh JW. Co-administration of ketamine in pediatric patients with neurologic conditions at risk for intracranial hypertension. Neurocrit Care. 2023;38(2):242–53. https://doi.org/10.1007/s12028-022-01611-2. Epub 2022 Oct 8. PMID: 36207491; PMCID: PMC10267668
23. Kuhlen M, Hoell J, Balzer S, Borkhardt A, Janssen G. Symptoms and management of pediatric patients with incurable brain tumors in palliative home care. Eur J Paediatr Neurol. 2016;20:261–9. https://doi.org/10.1016/j.ejpn.2015.12.004. Epub 2015 Dec 22. PMID: 26753538
24. Diekeman DS, Botkin JR. Clinical report-forgoing medically provided nutrition and hydration in children. Pediatrics. 2009;124:813–22.
25. Protus BM, Grauer PA, Kimbrel JM. Evaluation of atropine 1% ophthalmic solution administered sublingually for the management of terminal respiratory secretions. Am J Hosp Palliat Care. 2013;30(4):388–92.
26. Anderson AK, Burke K, Bendle L, Koh M, McCulloch R, Breen M. Artificial nutrition and hydration for children and young people towards end of life: consensus guidelines across four specialist paediatric palliative care centres. BMJ Support Palliat Care. 2021;11(1):92–100. https://doi.org/10.1136/bmjspcare-2019-001909. Epub 2019 Oct 19. PMID: 31630111
27. Druml C, Ballmer PE, Druml W, Oehmichen F, Shenkin A, Singer P, Soeters P, Weimann A, Bischoff SC. ESPEN guideline on ethical aspects of artificial nutrition and hydration. Clin Nutr. 2016;35(3):545–56. https://doi.org/10.1016/j.clnu.2016.02.006. Epub 2016 Feb 16. PMID: 26923519
28. Tsai E. Withholding and withdrawing artificial nutrition and hydration. Paediatr Child Health. 2011;16(4):241–4. https://doi.org/10.1093/pch/16.4.241. PMID: 22468129; PMCID: PMC3076180
29. Wusthoff CJ, Shellhaas RA, Licht DJ. Management of common neurologic symptoms in pediatric palliative care: seizures, agitation, and spasticity. Pediatr Clin N Am. 2007;54:709–33.
30. Barrett L, Fraser L, Noyes J, Taylor J, Hackett J. Understanding parent experiences of end-of-life care for children: a systematic review and qualitative evidence synthesis. Palliat Med. 2023;37(2):178–202. https://doi.org/10.1177/02692163221144084.

31. Harris N, Baba M, Mellor C, Rogers R, Taylor K, Beringer A, Sharples P. Seizure management in children requiring palliative care: a review of current practice. BMJ Support Palliat Care. 2020;10(3):e22. https://doi.org/10.1136/bmjspcare-2017-001366. Epub 2017 Jul 7. PMID: 28687558
32. Krouwer HG, Pallagi JL, Graves NM. Management of seizures in brain tumor patients at the end of life. J Palliat Med. 2000;3:465–75.
33. Sutherland AE, Curtin J, Bradley V, Bush O, Presswood M, Hedges V, Naessens K. Subcutaneous levetiracetam for the management of seizures at the end of life. BMJ Support Palliat Care. 2018;8(2):129–35. https://doi.org/10.1136/bmjspcare-2016-001261. Epub 2017 Jul 22. PMID: 28735270
34. Pace A, Villani V, Di Lorenzo C, Guariglia L, Maschio M, Pompili A, Carapella CM. Epilepsy in the end-of-life phase in patients with high-grade gliomas. J Neuro-Oncol. 2013;111(1):83–6.
35. Romoli M, Perucca E, Sen A. Pyridoxine supplementation for levetiracetam-related neuropsychiatric adverse events: A systematic review. Epilepsy Behav. 2020;103(Pt A):106861. https://doi.org/10.1016/j.yebeh.2019.106861. Epub 2020 Jan 6. PMID: 31917143
36. Vern-Gross TZ, Lam CG, et al. Patterns of end-of-life care in children with advanced solid tumor malignancies enrolled on a palliative care service. J Pain Symptom Manag. 2015;50(3):305–12. ISSN 0885-3924
37. Marcus KL, Kao PC, Ma C, Wolfe J, DeCourcey DD. Symptoms and suffering at end of life for children with complex chronic conditions. J Pain Symptom Manag. 2022;63(1):88–97. https://doi.org/10.1016/j.jpainsymman.2021.07.010. Epub 2021 Jul 24. PMID: 34311060
38. Patel P, Robinson PD, Cohen M, Devine K, Gibson P, Holdsworth MT, Neumann E, Orsey A, Phillips R, Spinelli D, Thackray J, van de Wetering M, Woods D, Cabral S, Sung L, Dupuis LL. Prevention of acute and delayed chemotherapy-induced nausea and vomiting in pediatric cancer patients: a clinical practice guideline. Pediatr Blood Cancer. 2022;69(12):e30001. https://doi.org/10.1002/pbc.30001. Epub 2022 Oct 11. PMID: 36221901
39. Bettini E, Idiokitas R, Mahmood L, Jacobs S, Steinhorn D. Safety and acceptance of acupuncture and acupressure in children, adolescents, and young adults undergoing hematopoietic stem cell transplant. Cancer Nurs. 2023;46(3):E204–7. https://doi.org/10.1097/NCC.0000000000001135. Epub 2022 Dec 1. PMID: 35679148
40. Massie MC, Ebelhar J, Allen KE, DeGroote NP, Wasilewski-Masker K, Brock KE. Defining and timing of palliative opportunities in children with central nervous system tumors. Neuro-Oncology Practice. 2021;8(4):451–9.
41. Theunissen JM, Hoogerbrugge PM, van Achterberg T, Prins JB, Vernooij-Dassen MJ, van den Ende CH. Symptoms in the palliative phase of children with cancer. Pediatr Blood Cancer. 2007;49(2):160–5. https://doi.org/10.1002/pbc.21042. PMID: 16972239
42. Weaver MS, Heinze KE, Bell CJ, Wiener L, Garee AM, Kelly KP, Casey RL, Watson A, Hinds PS. Pediatric palliative care special interest group at Children's National Health System. Establishing psychosocial palliative care standards for children and adolescents with cancer and their families: an integrative review. Palliat Med. 2016;30:212–23.
43. Jaward LR, O'Neil TA, Marks A, Smith MA. Differences in adverse effect profiles of corticosteroids in palliative care patients. Am J Hosp Palliat Care. 2019;36(2):158–68. https://doi.org/10.1177/1049909118797283. Epub 2018 Aug 30. PMID: 30165748
44. Ananth P, Mun S, Reffat N, et al. A stakeholder-driven qualitative study to define high quality end of-life care for children with cancer. J Pain Symptom Manage. 2021;62(3):492–502. https://doi.org/10.1016/j.jpainsymman.2021.01.134. PubMed: 33556497
45. Miele E, Mastronuzzi A, et al. Propofol-based palliative sedation in terminally ill children with solid tumors: a case series. Medicine (Baltimore). 2019;98(21):e15615.
46. Vallero SG, Lijoi S, Bertin D, Pittana LS, Bellini S, Rossi F, Peretta P, Basso ME, Fagioli F. End-of-life care in pediatric neuro-oncology. Pediatr Blood Cancer. 2014;61:2004–2011.
47. Harris MB. Palliative care in children with cancer: which child and when? JNCI Monographs. 2004;2004(32):144–9.
48. Postovsky S, Moaed B, Krivoy E, et al. Practice and palliative sedation in children with brain tumors and sarcomas at end of life. Pediatr Hematol Oncol. 2007;24(6):409–15.
49. Hendricks-Ferguson VL, Pradhan K, Shih CS, Gauvain KM, Kane JR, Liu J, Haase JE. Pilot evaluation of a palliative and end-of-life communication intervention for parents of children with a brain tumor. J Pediatr Oncol Nurs. 2017;34:203–13.
50. Cuviello A, Pasli M, Hurley C, Bhatia S, Anghelescu DL, Baker JN. Compassionate de-escalation of life-sustaining treatments in pediatric oncology: an opportunity for palliative care and intensive care collaboration. Front Oncol. 2022;12(13):1017272. https://doi.org/10.3389/fonc.2022.1017272. PMID: 36313632; PMCID: PMC9606590
51. Park HS, DeGroote NP, Lange A, Kavalieratos D, Brock KE. The scope of practice of an embedded pediatric palliative oncology clinic. J Pain Symptom Manag. 2024;67(3):250–259.e5. https://doi.org/10.1016/j.jpainsymman.2023.11.030. Epub 2023 Dec 6. PMID: 38065424
52. Lee A, DeGroote NP, Brock KE. Early versus late outpatient pediatric palliative care consultation and its association with end-of-life outcomes in children with cancer. J Palliat Med. 2023;26(11):1466–73. https://doi.org/10.1089/jpm.2023.0063. Epub 2023 May 24. PMID: 37222727
53. Brouwer M, Maeckelberghe E, Brincke HT, Meulenbeek-Ten Brincke M, Verhagen E. Pediatric

brain tumors: narrating suffering and end-of-life decision-making. Camb Q Healthc Ethics. 2020;29(3):338–45. https://doi.org/10.1017/S0963180120000055. PMID: 32484136
54. Miller EG, Feudtner C. Health reform law allows children in hospice to be treated for their disease. AAP News. 2013;34:14.
55. Clelland D, van Steijn D, Macdonald ME, et al. Global development of children's palliative care: an international survey of in-nation expert perceptions in 2017. Wellcome Open Res. 2020;5:99.

Patient Organisations and Advocacy: Championing Voices, Changing Lives

24

Anita Granero, Yuko Moue, Christine Mungoshi, Kathy Oliver, Roberto Premuselli, and Chris Tse

24.1 Volunteering, Advocacy, and Lobbying: Essential Vocabulary for Patients' Organizations

When we think of words like "giving", "supporting", "helping", and "being of service", another word usually comes immediately to mind: volunteering.

Though its meaning has never changed, it is now often associated with others like "advocacy" and "lobbying" because the realm of "volunteering" is perpetually in flux, prompting the need for fresh terminology to articulate its relevance and role in today's society.

24.1.1 Advocacy

The word advocacy comes from the Latin word "advocatus" and encompasses any action aimed at pleading, supporting, defending, or speaking on behalf of other individuals or a cause.

Advocacy lacks a specific start date because fundamentally, it entails the act of standing up for others, and in various forms, humans have been engaged in this practice throughout history.

Advocacy activities have had a particularly significant impact in healthcare, starting from the 1950s when Sidney Farber, a Harvard physician and cancer researcher, devised the idea of "Total Care" for paediatric cancer patients and launched the notion of "patient and family advocacy", changing forever the dynamics between patients, families, and healthcare professionals in care and communication.

The earliest tangible example of hospital-based advocacy likely emerged through the efforts of nurses, largely due to the work of Florence Nightingale. Although she never explicitly addressed the concept of advocacy, Nightingale demonstrated its significance in a practical manner throughout her lifetime [1].

A. Granero (✉)
Oscar's Angels France, Blagnac, France

Oscar's Angels Italia, Monza, MB, Italy

Y. Moue
Pediatric Brain Tumor Network of Japan, c/o Rare Cancers Japan, Kudan-Minami, Chiyoda-ku, Japan
e-mail: contact@pbtnjapan.com

C. Mungoshi
Zimbabwe Brain Tumour Association, Belvedere, Harare, Zimbabwe

K. Oliver
International Brain Tumour Alliance (IBTA), Tadworth, Surrey, UK
e-mail: kathy@theibta.org

R. Premuselli
Oncology Research Unit, IRCCS Ospedale Pediatrico Bambino Gesù, Piazza Sant'Onofrio, Rome, Italy
e-mail: roberto.premuselli@opbg.net

C. Tse
Brain Tumour Support NZ, Enderley, Hamilton, New Zealand
e-mail: chris.tse@braintumoursupport.org.nz

A. Mastronuzzi, A. Carai (eds.), *Navigating Pediatric Brain Tumors*,
https://doi.org/10.1007/978-3-032-18992-9_24

In the early days, especially in areas like mental health or chronic illness, patients were typically expected to accept treatments without question or input. Those who tried to advocate for themselves often encountered resistance or were labelled as non-compliant.

As time passed, the necessity for patients to voice their needs gave rise to the patient advocacy movement.

Patient advocacy groups initially began as support and self-help groups, uniting individuals with a shared illness or disease to aid those who have been diagnosed and have survived.

These were the foundation stones of modern patient advocacy that finds its roots in the activism surrounding HIV/AIDS in the 1980s, along with the advocacy movements related to breast cancer in the 1990s [2].

Since then, patients' organisations have significantly evolved to encompass families and caregivers who are therefore recognised as essential partners by health authorities.

The European Medicines Agency (EMA) has developed a definition of patients' organisations which is now widely used:

"Patients' organisations are defined as not-for profit organisations which are patient focused, and whereby patients *and/or carers* (the latter when patients are unable to represent themselves because of their illness or their age) represent a majority of members in governing bodies" [3] (Fig. 24.1).

24.1.2 Volunteering

The word "volunteering" comes from the Latin "voluntas", which means "will" or "desire". It was first used in the military world, describing those who offer themselves to military service.

The non-military sense of the term was initially documented in the 1630s and over time became increasingly associated with the idea of community service and engagement [4] whose defining feature remains, to this day, free will.

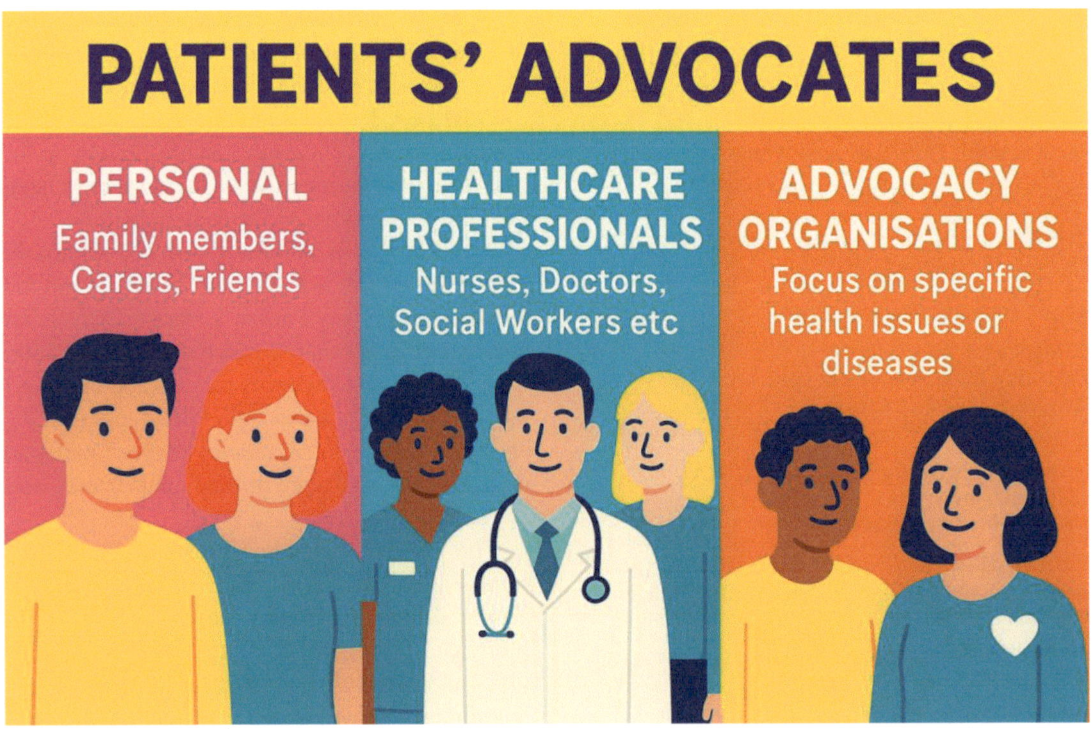
PATIENTS' ADVOCATES
PERSONAL
Family members, Carers, Friends
HEALTHCARE PROFESSIONALS
Nurses, Doctors, Social Workers etc
ADVOCACY ORGANISATIONS
Focus on specific health issues or diseases

Fig. 24.1 Types of patients' advocates

But if you think of volunteering simply as people helping other people, its origin is then probably as old as humanity.

Throughout the ages, communities of various cultures have demonstrated forms of mutual help and solidarity. During the ancient Egyptian, Greek, and Roman civilizations, the practice of assistance to the less fortunate was widespread, often guided by moral and religious principles.

The first "organised" volunteering institutions, as we know them today, were still closely associated with religion and came from the monastic orders of the early Christian church, such as the Franciscans, and their equivalents in other religions. Their mission was mainly to care for the poor and the sick.

The nineteenth century was a pivotal period in the development of volunteering organisations due to various social, economic, and humanitarian needs of the time. Institutions like the Red Cross and the Salvation Army laid the groundwork for the development of organised volunteering on a larger scale, setting the stage for the proliferation of volunteer organizations in the twentieth and twenty-first centuries, reflecting changes in society, technology, and global challenges.

"Modern" volunteering still has its roots in altruistic, charitable, and campaigning behaviours, but the number of "beneficiaries" and "causes" has certainly dramatically increased over the years, and organizations now use volunteers in many different roles.

Despite the evolution of society, one constant remains true over the years: volunteering originated from necessity and compassion, and these principles continue to embody its essence.

Even among experts, the definition of "volunteering" remains very wide and sometimes controversial.

Since 2011, every three years, the United Nations Volunteers program produces the "State of the World's Volunteerism Report", "a flagship UN publication designed to strengthen understanding on volunteerism and demonstrate its universality, scope and reach in the twenty-first century" [5].

One of the aims of their first publication was to promote a better understanding of volunteerism, trying also to define what the term "volunteer" meant. Despite its simplicity, the question revealed a multitude of definitions influenced by social-cultural context and national legal frameworks [6].

In some measure, this is still valid to this day, even if the official definition used worldwide is the one adopted by the United Nations General Assembly in 2001: *"Volunteering is a wide range of activities undertaken of free will, for the general public good, for which monetary reward is not the principal motivating factor"* [7, 8].

24.1.3 Lobbying

Along with influencing, campaigning, demonstrations, and boycotts, lobbying is considered an advocacy tactic [9].

Healthcare lobbying frequently involves collaborating with legislators, regulatory agencies, and policymakers to convey patients' needs and concerns.

It has become a crucial tool for healthcare advocacy organizations, allowing them to shape policies, funding decisions, and regulations that directly affect patient care and access to healthcare.

The once very clear line between the activities of volunteering, advocacy, and lobbying is now more difficult to draw, and, especially in healthcare, the distinctions have become increasingly blurred.

This overlap highlights a growing trend in healthcare, where meeting patient needs increasingly calls for a multi-dimensional approach.

Nowadays, patient organisations rooted in volunteerism and operating in healthcare systems not only actively "roll up their sleeves" by engaging in hands-on, ground-level activities, but also play a crucial role in advocacy by raising awareness of patients' rights and engaging in lobbying efforts to promote policy change.

Their advocacy role has often become an essential part of their work [10].

For the nonprofit organisations working in this sector, advocacy and active volunteerism at the patient's bedside have become two activities very difficult to separate because of the patients' and families' need to feel heard and represented on a more grassroots level during hospitalisations. Like all things, volunteering and advocacy must change with the times, adapting to the needs and problems of society.

This was even more apparent during the COVID pandemic when volunteers demonstrated how absolutely necessary they were. In a very short period of time, the Coronavirus crisis managed to cripple the health systems of the wealthiest countries in the world, proving to us all the existential vulnerability of the human condition. In this mayhem, a sure example of human strength was shown by the extraordinary response of volunteers all around the world.

At present health systems grapple with increasing pressures. Navigating a growing population, shifting health requirements, and intricate socioeconomic factors, volunteers emerge as an invaluable resource, providing a diverse support network that goes beyond conventional medical assistance.

24.2 Brain Tumor Advocacy

The history of brain tumor advocacy shows a gradual rise in awareness and action surrounding a condition that has often been overlooked. Over the decades, this movement has been driven by the dedication of patients, caregivers, healthcare professionals, and advocacy organizations, all committed to increasing awareness, securing research funding, and improving care for those impacted by brain tumors.

Before the 1970s, brain tumors were largely unknown to the public, primarily due to limited diagnostic tools and minimal public awareness; therefore, few resources existed to support patients. Unlike more common cancers, brain tumors received little attention or advocacy.

In the following decade, specific support groups were established by families affected by the disease, with the goal of connecting patients and raising funds for research. Their reach was very limited because of a lack of resources and interconnections with other groups.

Dedicated brain tumor organisations began to emerge in the 1970s, and with time, in addition to providing patient resources and funding research, they expanded their focus to include launching public awareness campaigns and advocating for improved healthcare policies.

In the 2000s, patient-driven advocacy gained momentum as social media and online communities allowed patients and families to share experiences and amplify their voices. National organisations set up large-scale campaigns, virtual support groups, and educational events, with patients actively pushing for research funding and policy changes. National awareness campaigns, such as brain tumor awareness weeks and months in various countries, raised public awareness and funding.

In the 2010s, advocacy efforts increased research funding, although brain tumors remained underfunded compared to other cancers. High-profile cases brought attention to brain tumors, strengthening calls for research and new treatments. Advocacy groups prioritized clinical trials and access to innovative therapies.

More recently, brain tumor advocacy has focused on public awareness, research funding, and patient-centred policies, including reimbursement for advanced treatments and support for mental health, rehabilitation, and social services. International collaboration has grown, with groups like the International Brain Tumor Alliance (IBTA) coordinating global efforts.

Many advocates now promote precision medicine to provide targeted, personalized treatments for complex brain tumors.

As brain tumor advocacy progressed, making significant advancements in raising awareness and securing funding for adult brain tumor research, attention slowly began to shift towards the unique challenges faced by paediatric patients. This shift has sparked dedicated efforts to address the specific needs of children with brain tumors, with advocacy campaigns now placing greater emphasis on not only raising awareness but also advocating for research breakthroughs and better treatment options tailored to younger patients, all while highlighting the emotional and physical toll these tumors take on young patients and their families.

Through a variety of efforts, from grassroots movements to large-scale partnerships, advocates have worked tirelessly to address the critical gaps in research and care for children battling brain tumors. Advocates have worked relentlessly through a variety of efforts, from grassroots initiatives to large-scale collaborations, to bridge the crucial gaps in research and care for children fighting brain tumors, often prioritising not only their survival but also their quality of life.

Here are some *international examples* of paediatric brain tumor advocacy efforts that emphasize raising awareness, funding research, and improving the quality of life for young patients.

24.3 Case History 1: In-House Paediatric Brain Tumors Advocates in France and Italy

24.3.1 Challenges

From the moment of diagnosis and throughout treatment, a paediatric brain tumor profoundly affects the child and their family in numerous ways.

Paediatric brain tumors follow a complex care pathway that includes visits to different units (neurology, neurosurgery, intensive care, neuro-oncology, etc.), where families have difficulty finding their way, often in emergency situations and face often-long stages of care including the following:

- The announcement of the diagnosis.
- The therapies involving complex management (neurosurgery, radiotherapy, chemotherapy, etc.), the long-term follow-up.
- The management of sequelae.

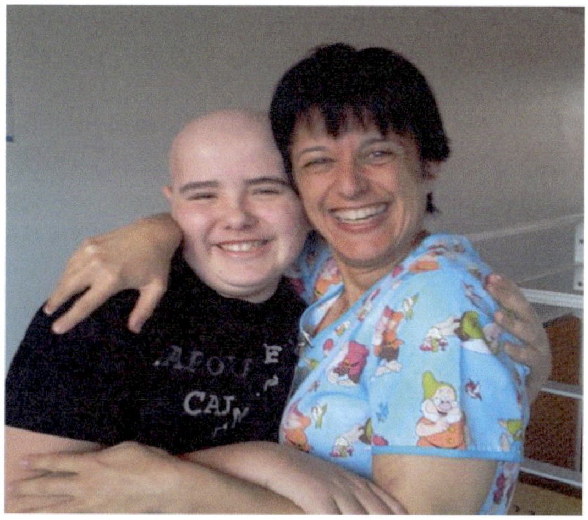

Fig. 24.2 Anita Granero, Founder of Oscar's Angels Italy and Oscar's Angels France, with Jojo, a young brain tumor patient who sadly passed away

- Transition to adult follow-up.
- The end-of-life care.

Emotional support for parents and families is paramount to help them navigate such a challenging and life-altering experience (Fig. 24.2).

24.3.2 Solutions

In this context, since 2001 at the Paediatric Hospital in Toulouse, France, a partnership was established between the healthcare staff and the advocacy organization Oscar's Angels.

It became evident to the advocacy organization that a comprehensive daily support project should be developed in collaboration with healthcare teams. This initiative, involving trained advocates, aimed to enhance the quality of care for all family members within this complex care pathway, focusing on two primary objectives:

1. Promote health mediation by allowing a strong link between the daily reality of patients and their families, with that of the hospital rhythm. This mediation involves daily and active support for the families by a patient/family advocate all along the care pathway, allowing unique exchanges between them and the medical and para-medical teams.

2. To support the evolution of the healthcare system and influence effective changes in public health policies.

The Oscar's Angels volunteers, based within the hospital, undergo specialized training to learn how to collaborate effectively with healthcare professionals.

Beyond direct support, these volunteers also offer unique insights into the needs of patients and their families, enriching the understanding of the hospital's medical teams.

Recognizing the patient's central role within the healthcare system, fostering effective communication between healthcare staff and patients/families enhances health outcomes and patient satisfaction while minimizing the likelihood of errors, misunderstandings, distress, and negligence [11].

The volunteers' presence promotes a friendlier environment and can help prevent or defuse tensions between parents and caregivers and thus maintain a favourable environment [12].

24.3.3 What Has Been Achieved

The Oscar's Angels patient/family advocates have been specifically trained to help neuro-oncology patients and their families during the different stages of care with some innovative support practices:

- A dedicated phone line is available for hospital staff to notify the patient/family advocate about new arrivals and emergency admissions, enabling them to arrange family support as quickly as possible.
- The volunteers' support is systematically offered to all families. The advocate/volunteer is considered a member of the multidisciplinary team.
- At the request of families, the volunteers can be present during diagnostic announcements or therapeutic stages. With the medical team's approval, the volunteers can assist families in better understanding medical or care-related information.

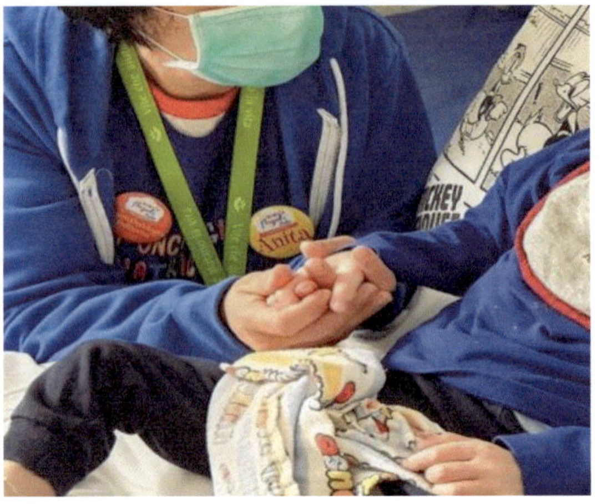

Fig. 24.3 An Oscar's Angels Italia's volunteer bringing comfort and support to a young patient

- Specific family support programs involving the patient/family advocates have been institutionalised/formalised on:
  1. Surgery day.
  2. Transition consultation to adult follow-up.
  3. Palliative care/end-of-life (Fig. 24.3).

This innovative partnership between healthcare professionals and advocates has been presented at various scientific congresses and meetings, and this has led, in 2018, to the use of the organisation in Italy at the request of the neuro-oncology team of the Paediatric Hospital Bambino Gesù in Rome, Italy.

24.3.4 Next Steps

In 2025, Oscar's Angels will lead the evaluation of an advocates/volunteers training project in support of the patients' families for the Adult Emergency Department of the Pierre Paul Riquet Hospital in Toulouse, France.

Two surveys will be conducted between 2026 and 2028 to evaluate the implementation of the "Paediatric Neurosurgery Support Program" and assess its effectiveness and impact. They will be addressed to both families and healthcare professionals.

24.4 Case History 2: Brain Tumor Patient Advocacy in Zimbabwe

Brain tumor care in the sub-Saharan Africa region, particularly in Zimbabwe, reveals a significant gap in patient advocacy and involvement. There is limited patient representation in decision-making, which is rooted in the hierarchical structure of the healthcare system and cultural perceptions of healthcare professionals. For many poor brain tumor patients, challenging the authority of powerful professionals is especially difficult, leaving them with limited ability to influence their own care.

When discussing the silencing of patient voices in sub-Saharan Africa, it is essential to examine the power dynamics within healthcare systems, particularly in specialised fields like brain tumor care. Neurosurgical specialists were often regarded with a near "demigod" status and challenging their recommendations was unthinkable; they were the experts, and patients and caregivers were expected to follow their advice. This reverence for specialists fostered a deferential relationship where patients were expected to comply with recommendations rather than engage in a dialogue about their care. The specialist's word was seen as final, and patients, treated as passive recipients, typically accepted treatment decisions without voicing concerns or preferences.

In Zimbabwe, the notion of seeking a second opinion or challenging a doctor's recommendation was virtually unheard of, and this issue was compounded by the scarcity of neurosurgical specialists. In 2005, when the Zimbabwe Brain Tumor Association (ZBTA) was founded, there were only three neurosurgeons serving a population of around 13 million. Limited access to information about brain tumors and treatment options further restricted patients' ability to make informed decisions or influence their treatment pathways, leaving them in a passive role, heavily reliant on professional judgments.

Although there are some changes, shifting this position requires not only the establishment of more robust patient advocacy networks but also the promotion of a healthcare culture that values patient input as essential to effective brain tumor treatment. Efforts to empower patients must address both the hierarchical structure of healthcare and the importance of patient-centred care as central to improving outcomes for brain tumor patients. A patient-centred approach ensures that treatment is respectful, inclusive, and responsive to each individual's needs.

Brain tumor advocacy in Zimbabwe continues to work towards meeting the unique needs of patients and their caregivers. Despite substantial challenges such as limited funding opportunities in this area, with limited resources, the ZBTA has persistently worked to drive change. These efforts include supporting patients and caregivers, and advocating for enhanced diagnosis, treatment, and post-treatment care for brain tumor patients.

Today, brain tumor advocacy in Zimbabwe remains a grassroots movement, relying heavily on the dedication of committed advocates. Volunteer-led initiatives at ZBTA have helped reduce the gap between patient needs and available support. Partnerships with international organisations like the International Brain Tumor Alliance (IBTA) and involvement with regional organisations such as the Society for Neuro-Oncology Sub-Saharan Africa (SNOSSA) highlight the progress being made to align Zimbabwe's efforts with global standards.

Policy limitations, such as insufficient government prioritisation of neurological health, hinder the development of comprehensive national strategies. Access to medical resources, including advanced imaging equipment and specialists, is limited, forcing many patients to seek costly treatment abroad.

24.4.1 Early Efforts and Challenges

The earliest brain tumor advocacy efforts in Zimbabwe were driven by a small but dedicated group of individuals, friends and families of those affected by brain tumors who recognised the urgent need for patient support. These pioneers faced significant challenges, including widespread ignorance about brain tumors and the stigma surrounding neurological conditions. The establishment of the Zimbabwe Brain Tumor Association (ZBTA) marked a critical turning point in advocacy. Founded with a mission to support patients and their families, ZBTA has spearheaded various initiatives, from providing educational resources on brain tumors to organising support groups and advocating for better medical care. Participation in regional collaborations, such as the Society for Neuro-Oncology Sub-Saharan Africa (SNOSSA), demonstrates Zimbabwe's commitment to aligning with broader African and global advocacy strategies.

Current support systems for brain tumor patients in Zimbabwe include counselling services, caregiver training programs, and limited financial assistance, though funding availability remains restricted. These initiatives aim to address the medical, emotional, and practical needs of patients and their families. International partnerships offer supplementary resources, such as educational materials and funding for essential medical supplies. However, these support systems are often overstretched due to high demand and limited resources.

24.4.2 Challenges

Brain tumor patient advocacy remains underdeveloped not only in Zimbabwe but across the wider Sub-Saharan Africa region. In Zimbabwe, the voices of patients are still small, with advocacy efforts striving to achieve broader recognition and impact. The work of the ZBTA is crucial in advocating for a stronger focus on patient-centred care, yet substantial challenges persist.

Limited funding constrains the development of brain tumor patient advocacy groups, which, in other regions, play a pivotal role in elevating the voices of individuals affected by brain tumors and offering a platform for patients to actively participate in shaping their care.

Expanding advocacy efforts is crucial to empower patients and ensure that their perspectives become an essential part of the care process.

24.4.3 Future Initiatives and Aims

The ZBTA aims to become a cornerstone of brain tumor advocacy in Zimbabwe, to offer essential support to patients and their families.

Public education and awareness programs are crucial to advocacy efforts in Zimbabwe. The ZBTA, through funding from its partners, regularly hosts awareness campaigns through social media, community workshops, and public events, such as commemorating the International Brain Tumor Awareness Week, held annually each autumn to raise awareness about the challenges of brain tumors. These initiatives focus on educating the public about early signs of brain tumors and available diagnostic and treatment options available in Zimbabwe. Workshops for caregivers provide practical advice on how to support patients effectively during their recovery.

The future of brain tumor advocacy in Zimbabwe is promising, as it increasingly prioritises sustainable support systems and innovative approaches to training and policy development.

Future strategies include robust caregiver training and support systems.

Brain tumor patient advocacy organisations in Sub-Saharan Africa have a role to ensure that the patient's voice is heard and they are equipped to be involved in decision-making about things that matter to them and their health.

24.5 Case History 3: Patient Advocacy in New Zealand

New Zealand prioritises access to paediatric cancer medicines by a rule in its Pharmaceutical Schedule, which is cited as a putative reason for its high survival rates for childhood cancers. In 2022, a government review was announced in the face of rising drug costs and a perception of unfairness to other disease groups, which threatened to change this rule. The review instigated a campaign by the paediatric cancer community, including patient organisations involved in brain tumor advocacy, in support of continued prioritised medicines access.

24.5.1 Paediatric Brain Tumors in New Zealand

Each year, approximately 150 children in New Zealand, aged 0 to 14 years, are diagnosed with cancer. The most common childhood cancers diagnosed are leukaemia (29%), brain tumors (23%), and lymphomas (15%) [13].

Childhood cancer survival is comparable with that of other high-income countries. New Zealand's five-year overall survival of 85.6% across all tumor types is slightly higher than Australia and the USA (both 85%) and the UK and Canada (both 84%) [14].

Paediatric brain cancer survival statistics are more challenging. Despite being the second most common cancer diagnosed, paediatric brain tumors account for 42% of all childhood cancer deaths in New Zealand, the most of any cancer type. The UK and Australia have five-year survival rates for brain tumors of 76% compared with New Zealand's 73.5% and Canada's 72%.

24.5.2 Treatment

New Zealand citizens are entitled to free or subsidised healthcare provided by the government and funded through general taxation. The vast majority of cancer patients are treated under the public health system.

Treatment for paediatric cancer patients is provided at two specialist centres: Starship's Blood and Cancer Centre in Auckland and the Children's Haematology/Oncology Centre (CHOC) in Christchurch, in conjunction with 14 shared care centres located across the country [15] (Fig. 24.4).

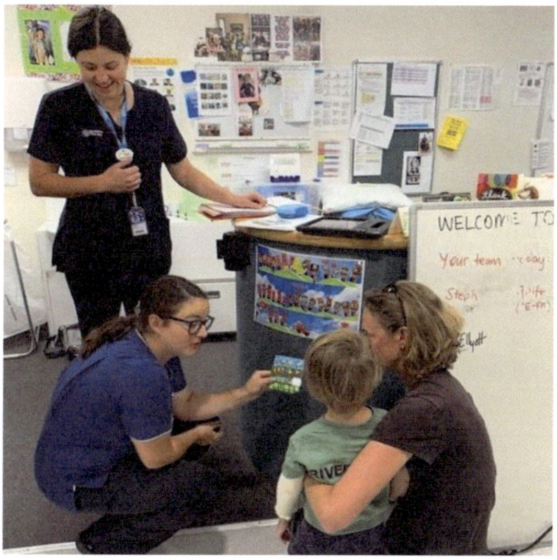

Fig. 24.4 Frankie, his mum Michelle, and healthcare staff at Auckland City Hospital

Oversight and governance are provided by the National Child Cancer Network (NCCN) [16]. The NCCN also manages the New Zealand Child Cancer Registry (NZCCR), which reports on childhood cancer incidence, treatment, and outcomes.

Clinical trials are an essential part of the treatment paradigm for paediatric brain tumors. Access to clinical trials is mainly provided through the Australian and New Zealand Children's Haematology/Oncology Group (ANZCHOG). ANZCHOG actively collaborates with international cooperative groups, such as the Children's Oncology Group, the International Society of Paediatric Oncology (SIOP), and various clinical trial groups [17].

24.5.3 Patient Advocacy

Cancer advocacy in New Zealand is provided through the charitable (not-for-profit) sector; however, there is no single organisation dedicated to paediatric brain tumor advocacy.

The Child Cancer Foundation provides wraparound support, care coordination, counselling, and a range of other support services to paediatric cancer patients and their families [18].

Brain Tumor Support NZ is a support, information, and advocacy organisation primarily for adult brain tumor patients; however, its Brain Tumor Support Kids division offers support and resources to children and families dealing with paediatric brain tumors, including peer-to-peer support [19].

Rare Disorders New Zealand is an umbrella organisation representing over 150 charities and support groups operating in the rare disorders space, including brain tumors [20].

24.5.4 The Problem—Prioritised Medicines Access Under Threat

Access to publicly funded medicines is controlled by Pharmac, the New Zealand government drug procurement agency. Pharmac rigorously evaluates and procures medicines for the Pharmaceutical Schedule, which it manages within a fixed annual budget.

Paediatric cancer medicines are prioritised by rule 8.1b of the Pharmaceutical Schedule. In essence, rule 8.1b provides clinicians with the full decision-making authority to prescribe medicines that are not publicly funded to children who are diagnosed with cancer and are treated in a paediatric setting.

This means that children with cancer can access treatments that aren't on the Pharmaceutical Schedule, or treatments for which they don't meet the usual access criteria, with full reimbursement. This includes access to experimental medicines that are currently under development in clinical trials or not yet registered in New Zealand.

Rule 8.1b is universally supported by New Zealand's paediatric cancer community, including paediatric oncologists, patient organisations, and, most importantly, families affected by childhood cancer. It has been cited as one of the reasons why New Zealand's childhood cancer survival rates are among the highest in the world.

In November 2022, Pharmac announced a review of rule 8.1b following concerns raised around fairness when compared with other conditions and the growing costs of new cancer medicines [21].

Possible outcomes of this review were changes to rule 8.1b or its removal altogether.

24.5.5 The Solution—Power of Patient Advocacy

The announcement galvanised the paediatric cancer community to express their strong and unequivocal support of rule 8.1b.

Brain Tumor Support NZ submitted comprehensive feedback arguing that changes to rule 8.1b have the potential to cause:

(a) A reduction in access to clinical trials by restricting the availability of standard of care or experimental treatments.
(b) Significant financial distress to families by forcing people to purchase medicines privately.
(c) Premature death, increased suffering, and poorer health outcomes by reducing access to essential treatments.
(d) Increased inequity among population groups.

In presenting these issues, Brain Tumor Support NZ highlighted the devastating impact that childhood brain tumors had on the patient and their entire family [22]. Children with highly aggressive tumors were faced with a short-term prognosis and poor quality of life. Others with slower-growing tumors were faced with a lifetime of difficulties such as cognitive and physical deficits, emotional or psychosocial distress.

All submitters argued that changes to rule 8.1b would undermine the whole children's cancer treatment system of care and threaten New Zealand's ability to benchmark international survival outcomes.

Following a lengthy period of public consultation, Pharmac announced in March 2024 that rule 8.1b would remain unchanged [23]. They acknowledged that the rule has a real impact on treatment and health outcomes of children with cancer [24].

The decision to maintain New Zealand's prioritised access to paediatric cancer medicines was an example of patient advocacy at work. Advocacy for less common disorders, such as childhood brain tumors, assumes even greater importance due to the rare nature of the disease.

Patient organisations such as Brain Tumor Support NZ play a vital role in representing the patient perspective and supporting and advocating for their community in situations where individual patients and families may not have the resources or capability.

24.6 Case History 4: Brain Tumor Patients' Rights and Patient Advocacy

Patients' rights are at the forefront of much of the advocacy work that many patient organisations undertake. The International Brain Tumor Alliance (IBTA, www.theibta.org) is no exception, spearheading a global project to create The Brain Tumor Patients' Charter of Rights between 2017 and 2020 [25]. The Charter is intended to address inequalities across countries with regard to diagnosis, treatment, and support of both adult and paediatric patients. It is an aspirational framework for improving healthcare systems, shared decision-making, doctor/patient communication, quality standards, policies, and practices. The Charter is also meant to stimulate debate and discussion while recognising the significant hurdles that exist in some countries regarding the rights of patients.

The Charter is the result of international collaboration between many brain tumor patient advocacy organisations around the world, who contributed to its structure and content. To date, the Charter is supported by nearly 100 patient groups, societies, and others. It is available in 15 languages [25].

The Charter can be used by families of paediatric neuro-oncology patients to underpin the things that matter most to them on their brain tumor journeys. It can also be used by healthcare professionals to highlight elements of services and opportunities for young patients within their own institutions that may be missing or not efficiently or equitably provided.

24.6.1 Challenges

Brain tumors are the most common solid tumor in childhood (representing nearly 25% of all childhood cancers), and they are among the deadliest [26].

In various regions around the world, there are significant unmet needs and challenges for children with brain tumors. In some countries, these include, for example, late/incorrect diagnosis, lack of access to multidisciplinary teams, the dearth of sophisticated neurosurgical care and other treatments, the absence of rehabilitation services, and poor management of late effects of treatment (long-term, health-related complications), which can have a devastating consequence on quality of life.

The influences of culture, religion, and even geography in different parts of the world can also affect how young patients and their families access good quality, effective, and safe treatment for a brain tumor.

A paper written by a group of 28 co-authors representing major brain tumor patient advocacy organisations around the world focusses on many of these issues. The paper, published in *Neuro-Oncology Practice* and titled "Brain tumor patients' rights and the power of patient advocacy: the current international landscape" paints a picture of met and unmet needs of brain tumor patients in 18 countries in the Asia Pacific, Sub-Saharan Africa, North America, Eastern Europe, and Western Europe. The paper states: "Acknowledging that some rights in The Brain Tumor Patients' Charter of Rights are aspirational, there still remain many areas of the world where even basic patient rights are not yet attainable. Patient advocacy organisations stand ready to help change this to achieve the best possible health and quality of life outcomes for adults and children living with brain tumors" [27].

Unmet needs for paediatric brain tumor patients are particularly acute in low- and middle-income countries (LMIC). Care in paediatric neuro-oncology is highly complex, requiring numerous healthcare professionals and others to deliver specialised care at various stages of the patient's brain tumor journey. These specialists include neurosurgeons, oncologists, physiotherapists, ophthalmologists (if a child's vision is affected by a tumor on the optic nerve), epileptologists (to help with seizures), radiation oncologists, oncological nurses, speech and language specialists, care coordinators, play therapists, and others [28].

Therefore, it is crucial that paediatric brain tumor patients have the right to a multidisciplinary team who can deliver optimal care throughout the treatment pathway for these young and very vulnerable people.

Access to a second opinion is also an important right for these patients. Brain tumors are a rare disease in children and as such should be treated in a centre of excellence where there are healthcare professionals with significant experience of paediatric neuro-oncology.

Paediatric patients should have the right to access appropriate support and rehabilitation to ensure that their survivorship includes the best quality of life possible. With the aim of long-term survivorship for some paediatric brain tumor patients, new therapy regimens are being developed, which lessen late effects of the disease and its treatment while still, hopefully, providing extended survival.

Childhood brain tumor patients who survive into adulthood should have the right to robust, structured transition programmes from paediatric to adult care, which is also developmentally appropriate.

The co-authors of the above-mentioned paper in *Neuro-Oncology Practice* say that: "The Brain Tumor Patients' Charter of Rights, if achieved in practice, would potentially meet many of the unmet needs of the [adult and paediatric] brain tumor patient and caregiver community, thus improving patient and caregiver quality of life" [27].

24.6.2 Some Solutions for Gaps in Treatment, Care, and Support

A brain tumor diagnosis is devastating, especially when children and their families are faced with the realities of this relentless disease. But there are steps that can be taken to improve gaps in treatment and care.

For example, there should be a greater focus of attention on healthcare inequalities regarding access to new therapies and to quality care and support. These disparities must be addressed as a matter of urgency. There should be increased clinical trial availability for paediatric brain tumor patients and more funding for research into the causes of paediatric brain tumors. There should also be better, kinder treatments for this young population of patients.

A greater emphasis on the creation of paediatric brain tumor registries is also needed. Creating collaborations between government, researchers, healthcare professionals, neuro-oncology societies, and others to establish and maintain such registries is crucial [27]. Accurate, good quality paediatric brain tumor registries also help policymakers with resource allocation, thus hopefully optimising patient care [29].

Brain tumor patient advocacy organisations can also effectively raise awareness of the multitude of unmet needs facing children with neuro-oncological disease. These organisations provide a powerful and valuable stimulus for meaningful change in healthcare policy and delivery.

Finally, it is hoped that The Brain Tumor Patients' Charter of Rights will have worldwide relevance to adult and paediatric patients with the goal of reducing disparities, improving access to treatments and support, and also instilling a greater measure of hope in the international brain tumor community.

24.7 Case History 5: Adolescent and Young Adult Cancer Patients in Italy

In the complex landscape of paediatric oncology, Adolescents and Young Adults (AYA) represent a distinct yet often overlooked group—patients aged 15–39 who confront a cancer diagnosis. Within this population, brain tumors stand out as one of the most clinically significant neoplasms and a leading cause of morbidity and mortality. Their treatment frequently requires multifaceted, prolonged approaches that can deeply affect neurocognitive development, health-related quality of life, and the educational and vocational paths of young patients.

This stage of life is marked by pivotal transitions—completing school or entering the workforce, forming emotional relationships, and striving for independence. A cancer diagnosis during such a formative period can profoundly reshape not only daily life but also fundamental aspects of identity, social connection, and the pursuit of future aspirations.

In a paediatric oncology setting, the AYA population faces particular challenges. Being in the transition phase between childhood and adulthood, these patients do not identify with either children or adults. Their needs, both medically and psychosocially, may differ greatly from those of younger paediatric patients or older adults. Sometimes, they wish to actively participate in decisions regarding their treatment, seeking more targeted support and sharing their experiences with peers in similar situations. Furthermore, they must address delicate issues such as fertility and sexuality, aspects that are often overlooked in paediatric or adult settings [30].

On the social side, young adults with cancer can face isolation during treatment, difficulty maintaining relationships, and a sense of disconnection from their peers without such a diagnosis. Moreover, financial hardship, arising from both medical expenses and loss of income during treatment, represents a further challenge these patients may encounter.

In this complex context, understanding the specificities and challenges that the AYA population faces becomes essential to provide them with adequate and targeted support, both from a medical and social point of view [31].

In the 1990s, there was increased awareness of the unique needs of AYA patients, driven in part by increasing paediatric cancer survival and increased attention to quality of life (QoL) for survivors. However, it was in the 2000s that the AYA patient association movement began to take shape in a more organised and widespread manner [32]. In the delicate context of oncology treatments, these associative initiatives provide comprehensive support, including individual and family assistance, research promotion, patient education, and public awareness. They act as important points of reference for those who find themselves facing the complexity of life with cancer at a young age. These associations provide not only emotional comfort but also practical information and effective advocacy for patient rights.

The roots of these initiatives often lie in the personal experiences of patients, caregivers, and health workers who, aware of the need for targeted support for the AYA population, have given rise to movements capable of transforming the landscape of cancer care for young adults. Thanks to their unwavering dedication, these organisations have established themselves as irreplaceable reference points for those who find themselves navigating the difficult waters of cancer at a young age.

In the evolutionary context of Bambino Gesù Children's Hospital (OPBG, Rome, Italy), 2017 marked a significant transition in the management of AYA patients. Every year, the hospital welcomes around 70 adolescent patients, paying special attention to their needs and aspirations. In collaboration with psychologists, a questionnaire was developed to better understand the specific needs of this population and evaluate the level of communication, reception, assistance, and intra-hospital socialisation. The analysis of the results gave rise to an innovative organisational model called "4You Progetto Adolescenti", designed to improve the quality of care and the attention to the specific needs of AYAs [33]. This model has various objectives, including improving the activities suggested in the hospital environment, promoting socialisation among young patients, supporting growth and autonomy typical of adolescence, and encouraging collaborations with peers outside the hospital. The "4You" project actively involves the patients themselves, allowing them to be active protagonists of their treatment and growth path. Through monthly meetings, young people have the opportunity to propose and implement initiatives and events tailored to their needs, ranging from sports to entertainment, from fashion to social activities. This model promotes the creativity and planning of adolescents, offering them a space to express their ideas and actively contribute to the improvement of hospital care.

The psychosocial impact of the "4You" project is significant. Psychologists actively participate in group meetings, sharing the needs of the children, helping them express their emotions and experiences, and encouraging them to be active heroes in their own recovery. Thanks to this participatory and patient-centred approach, OPBG confirms itself as a reference point in the care and support of AYA patients suffering from cancer.

In 2018, OPBG further consolidated its focus on AYA patients with haematology-oncology diseases by implementing an innovative, participatory model through the establishment of the "Associazione 4You—Associazione di Promozione Sociale". The 4You Association, the only association in Italy founded by adolescent cancer patients, aims to guarantee, through a peer-to-peer approach, a good quality of life during the treatment process of AYA patients and offers support to families through awareness-raising and psychological and social support activities (Fig. 24.5).

The 4You activities are divided into aspects that include: encouraging communication by encouraging a regular exchange of experiences and sharing of projects; informing the needs of adolescents with cancer and their families; promoting the dissemination of information through social campaigns on the mass media and having demonstrations and meetings; organising seminars and conferences to make all interested parties aware of the psychological and social problems of children affected by cancer and their families; and raising awareness among the public on tumors and leukaemia in adolescents and the psychological and social consequences. The 4You Association operates on a national level, aware of the fact that medical care alone, however indispensable, needs to be integrated with broader support activities such as departments suitable for teenagers, in addition to social spaces, and dedicated activities and projects. The very nature of this association, created and run by patients and former adolescent cancer patients, is a guarantee of a deep commitment to the cause for which they work. For this reason, the heart of the 4You Association is them: the adolescents and young adults.

> "We strive to enhance the quality of life of children with cancer, so that treatment becomes a journey of living rather than of illness."
> The members of 4You

We can say that experiences like these can help AYAs find the resources necessary to face the diagnostic process. Over the years, we have witnessed a 40% increase in requests to meet with 4You volunteers directly from the patients themselves, which in the past rarely occurred.

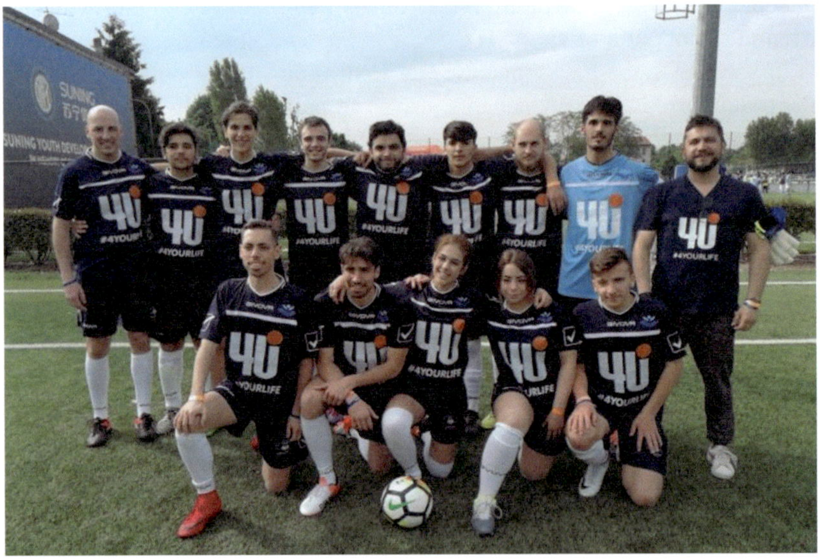

Fig. 24.5 The 4You team took part in the Winner's Cup—a football event for young people in cancer treatment organised by Inter, CSI Milano, and AIEOP (Associazione Italiana Ematologia Oncologia Pediatrica)

As the AYA paradigm continues to evolve, the importance of a holistic approach to patient care becomes increasingly evident. It is through collective efforts such as the 4You Adolescent Project and the 4You Association that the transformative potential of healthcare innovation can be fully achieved, ushering in an era in which patients emerge as active collaborators in the search for healing and hope [34].

These exceptional examples of advocacy programs within the global brain tumor community, while not entirely comprehensive, reflect a shared dedication to enhancing the lives of patients, caregivers, and their families. They underscore the impact of collaboration among healthcare providers, nonprofit organisations, policymakers, and patient advocates in bridging critical gaps in care, advancing early diagnosis, securing greater research funding, and improving access to cutting-edge treatments. Moreover, these initiatives act as symbols of hope, nurturing a sense of solidarity and strength within the brain tumor community and promoting wider public awareness and support.

24.8 Case History 6: Paediatric Brain Tumor Networks in Japan

Around the year 2000, with the widespread use of the internet, children with brain tumors and their families in Japan began to communicate through social media and support one another. Simultaneously with other families' groups for children with cancer, they established groups and organizations based on specific diagnoses or regions, engaging in mutual support and social activities aimed at raising awareness of paediatric cancers and improving quality of life. These activities include promoting awareness of paediatric brain tumors, lobbying efforts, and advancing hospice projects.

Through these efforts, networks of paediatric cancer organizations (including those focused on brain tumors) were established, enabling collaboration towards developing treatments and improving the quality of life of the patients [35] (Fig. 24.6).

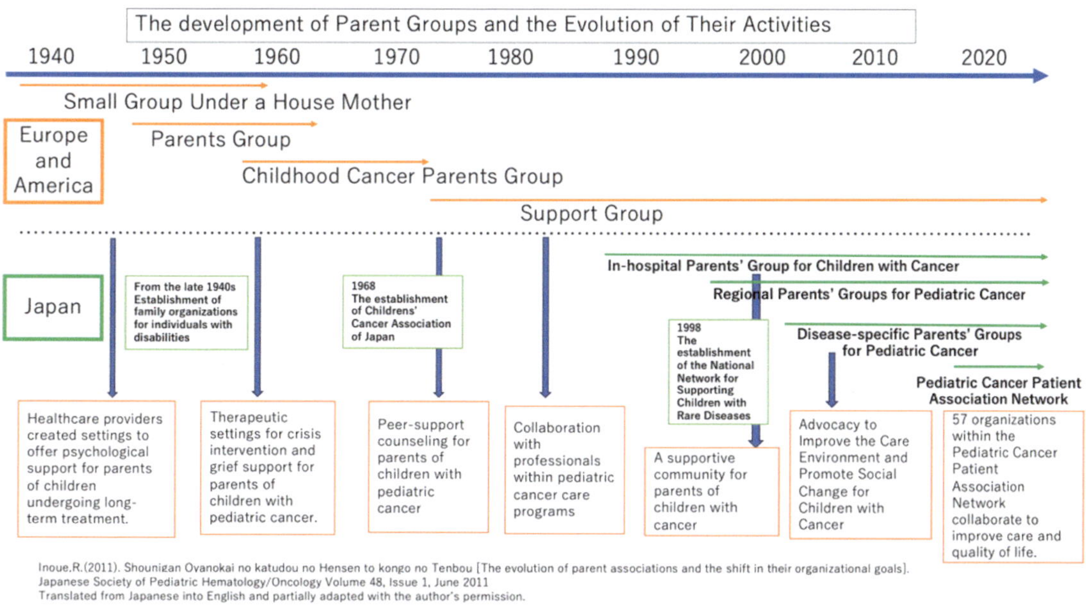

Fig. 24.6 Shounigan Oyanokai no katudou no Hensen to kongo no Tenbou [The evolution of parent associations and the shift in their organizational goals] [35]

24.8.1 Challenges and Responses

Japan has a universal health insurance system, giving everyone access to hospital care. However, for rare diseases such as paediatric brain tumors, it has been extremely difficult for the patients to collect information about treatment options and to identify appropriate hospitals. In 2012, 15 paediatric cancer hub hospitals were designated, but patients' access to specialized medical care still remains insufficient.

In Europe and the United States, regulatory frameworks exist to encourage the development of paediatric cancer treatments, but Japan lacks such a framework. This has been a significant obstacle to the development and implementation of treatments for paediatric brain tumors.

Moreover, there is insufficient understanding in preschools, schools, and society at large regarding the nature of paediatric brain tumors and their late-onset complications. This lack of understanding makes life even more difficult for patients and their families.

To address these challenges, family organizations have been actively sharing and disseminating information about treatment methods and late-onset complications through social media, symposiums, and study meetings. They have also published various guidebooks and promoted the construction of paediatric hospices and the formation of peer support groups. In recent years, notable progress has been made in the following two areas:

24.8.2 Progress in Paediatric Hospices in Japan

Children with severe illnesses or disabilities have the right to live as fulfilling a life as possible, surrounded by the love of their families and friends. Hospices are places where children can spend meaningful and joyful time with their families.

24.8.3 Challenges

According to government statistics, there are 115,012 children in Japan with designated chronic paediatric diseases, of which about 20,000 live with life-threatening conditions (LTCs) such as paediatric cancers. However, as of 2020, only two paediatric hospices existed in Japan.

24.8.4 Solutions

- In autumn 2021, families who had lost a child to a brain tumor opened the third paediatric hospice in Yokohama.
- Exchanges between paediatric hospices in Japan and abroad began, and several nonprofit organizations were established with the aim of building new hospices across the country.
- In 2022, following strong requests from many families, a Parliamentary League for Paediatric Hospice Support was established, along with the National Association for the Support of Children's Hospices.
- In 2024, this association evolved into a general incorporated association, the Japan Children's Hospice Association. Increasingly, local governments are also supporting the establishment of hospices in their regions.

24.8.5 Outlook

Parent organizations will continue to provide support for hospice activities in the years ahead.

24.8.6 The Current Situation and Outlook on Drug Lag and Drug Loss

24.8.6.1 Challenges

Many anticancer drugs are developed in Europe and the United States but require approval before being used in Japan. The Japanese approval process is complex, and domestic regulations may hinder drug development. This poses a major challenge for overseas emerging biotech companies (EBPs) with limited financial resources when entering the Japanese market. For patients with rare or paediatric diseases, the delay before medicines approved overseas become available in Japan is a serious issue.

24.8.6.2 Solutions

1. Patient group activities

Support groups for children with brain tumors have joined forces with other rare disease and paediatric cancer organizations to advocate actively for improvements in drug regulation through petitions and lobbying. As a result, in July 2023, the Ministry of Health, Labour and Welfare (MHLW) established a review committee on pharmaceutical regulation.

2. Ongoing regulatory reforms

This committee has proposed multiple reforms to the current pharmaceutical regulations. In fact, from December 2023 through 2024, the MHLW issued a series of notifications, and reforms are now underway.

24.8.6.3 Outlook

Regulatory reform in Japan has only just begun, but families of children with paediatric cancers, including brain tumors, strongly hope that new drugs developed worldwide will become available in Japan as quickly as possible. They also believe that proactive participation in international joint clinical trials from Phase I is the most effective way to deliver urgently needed new treatments to children without delay.

24.9 Conclusions

In today's evolving healthcare landscape, the role of advocates continues to develop. With a heightened recognition of the significance of a positive patient experience, numerous improvement initiatives are underway in hospitals within healthcare policy and elsewhere. The role of patient advocates is crucial in driving these efforts forward [36].

Amidst the complex fabric of global healthcare institutions, advocates and volunteers constitute an essential cohort. Their relentless devotion, altruistic resolve, and steadfast compassion introduce a catalytic factor that surpasses conventional clinical approaches, profoundly influencing the well-being of patients, their loved ones, and the broader community.

In healthcare, advocacy organisations are instrumental in championing various aspects of public health, patient rights, healthcare access, research funding, and healthcare policy reforms.

Patient organisations, which are a subset of advocacy organisations, primarily concentrate on offering assistance, resources, and services to individuals impacted by particular medical conditions or illnesses, as well as to their families. Their main objective is to empower patients, increase awareness about the condition, and enhance the quality of life of patients and their families.

Despite the significant advancements made by patient advocacy organisations over the last century, challenges persist, particularly for those dedicated to addressing rare diseases like paediatric and adult brain tumors.

Although there are well-established and well-known brain tumor patient organisations around the world, not every country has such a group. Therefore, people affected by brain tumors may need to rely on broader cancer support organisations or general patient advocacy groups for assistance and resources. This situation is not ideal as it may not address the unique needs of brain tumor patients that stem from the complexity of their disease and the effects of treatment on neurological function.

Addressing the unique needs of brain tumor patients requires a comprehensive and multidisciplinary approach that prioritizes personalized care, holistic support, and ongoing communication between patients, caregivers, and healthcare providers.

By addressing these needs, healthcare systems can better meet the diverse challenges faced by individuals affected by brain tumors and improve outcomes and quality of life for patients and their families [37].

Patient advocacy in paediatric neuro-oncology presents a unique complexity compared to the realm of adult brain tumors. This complexity arises from the varying levels of cognitive maturity among young patients, their potential neurological sequels, and the indispensable involvement of a third party in the decision-making process: the parents and family at large.

Carter et al. say that although a clear definition of child-centred care (CCC) and clarity around this concept have yet to be achieved, it has already evolved into family centred care (FCC), as it is now widely recognised that children need to be cared for in the context of their family, that families are the constant in the child's life and the family's values and priorities should be central in the plan of care for the child [38, 39].

Family involvement plays a vital role in improving the quality of life for paediatric brain tumor patients by providing emotional support, facilitating shared decision-making, advocating for their needs, promoting education and empowerment, ensuring continuity of care, fostering social connection, and supporting end-of-life care and bereavement.

Paediatric brain tumor advocacy organisations work to ensure that families are actively involved in decision-making, care planning, and psychosocial support throughout the treatment journey and strive to ensure that children with brain tumors have access to specialized medical care from multidisciplinary teams with expertise in paediatric neuro-oncology.

Therefore, a collaborative partnership between healthcare providers and patient advocacy organisations is essential for optimizing outcomes and enhancing the well-being of paediatric brain tumor patients.

Despite these challenges, the successful history of brain tumor advocacy demonstrates the significant impact that the voices of patients and caregivers can have on healthcare when given the opportunity. By sharing their personal experiences, needs, and perspectives, patients and their families have been able to influence changes in the healthcare system. Their advocacy has not only raised awareness but also led to improvements in research funding, treatment accessibility, and healthcare policies. This grassroots movement has drawn much-needed attention to brain tumors as a critical health issue, resulting in increased resources and support for those affected. Brain tumor advocacy shows that empowering those directly impacted by their disease can drive meaningful progress and transform healthcare outcomes [40].

Websites of Brain Tumor Patient and Caregiver: Advocacy Organizations Highlighted in This Chapter

Associazione 4You, Rome, Italy: https://www.4youaps.org/

Brain Tumour Support NZ: (New Zealand) https://www.braintumoursupport.org.nz/

International Brain Tumour Alliance (IBTA): https://www.theibta.org

Oscar's Angels France: https://www.oscarsangels.com

Oscar's Angels Italia: https://www.oscarsangelsitalia.com

Pediatric Brain Tumor Network of Japan: https://pbtnjapan.com/en/pbtn

Rare Disorders New Zealand: https://raredisorders.org.nz/

The Child Cancer Foundation (New Zealand): https://childcancer.org.nz/

Zimbabwe Brain Tumour Association, Harare, Zimbabwe https://www.ztbazw.org/

References

1. Selanders LC, Crane PC. The voice of Florence Nightingale on advocacy. OJIN. 2012;17:1. https://doi.org/10.3912/OJIN.Vol17No01Man01.
2. Wong-Rieger D. Moving from patient advocacy to partnership; a long and bumpy road. The Patient. 2017;10:271.
3. European Medicines Agency, Stakeholders and Communications Division, (June 2014). Available at: http://www.ema.europa.eu/docs/en_GB/document_library/Regulatory_and_procedural_guideline/2009/12/WC500018099.pdf
4. Online Etymology Dictionary: https://www.etymonline.com/word/volunteerism
5. UN Volunteers: https://www.unv.org/swvr
6. UN Volunteers.: https://www.unv.org/swvr/wellbeing
7. UN Volunteers.: https://www.unv.org/sites/default/files/A%20RES%2056%2038.pdf. Accessed: 17 Apr 2024.
8. UN Volunteers.: https://swvr2022.unv.org/ The fourth State of the World's Volunteerism Report (SWVR) report, titled Building Equal and Inclusive Societies.
9. Chapman J. Monitoring and evaluating advocacy. PLA Notes. 2002;43:48–52.
10. MSG Management Study Guide.: https://managementstudyguide.com/advocacy-and-volunteerism.htm
11. Levinson W, Chaumeton N. Communication between surgeons and patients in routine office visits. Surgery. 1999;125:127–34.
12. Marchal C, Vuillaume C, Plançon ML, Hubert P. Les bénévoles ont-ils une place dans un service de réanimation ? Volunteers in intensive care unit: do they have a place? Reanimation. 2003;12:173–7.
13. National Child Cancer Network, "Childhood Cancer Incidence in Aotearoa, New Zealand 2015–2019": https://childcancernetwork.org.nz/
14. National Child Cancer Network 2022, "Childhood cancer survival in Aotearoa, New Zealand 2010: 2019": https://childcancernetwork.org.nz/
15. Te Aho o Te Kahu. He Pūrongo mate Pukupuku o Aotearoa 2020, the state of cancer in New Zealand 2020. Wellington: Te Aho o Te Kahu, Cancer Control Agency; 2021.
16. Child Cancer Network: https://childcancernetwork.org.nz/
17. Hansford J, et al. "If you build it, they will come": the convergence of funding, research and collaboration in paediatric brain cancer clinical trials. Med J Aust. 2024;221:520–3. https://doi.org/10.5694/mja2.52506.
18. Child Cancer Foundation: https://childcancer.org.nz/
19. Brain Tumor Support NZ: https://www.braintumour-support.org.nz/
20. Rare Disorders NZ: https://raredisorders.org.nz/
21. Pharmac: https://pharmac.govt.nz/news-and-resources/consultations-and-decisions/2022-11-02-consultation-on-funding-medicines-for-paediatric-cancers
22. Brain Tumour Support NZ. December 2022. "Submission to Pharmac's review of rule 8.1b of the Pharmaceutical Schedule". https://static1.squarespace.com/static/5c0062f3e17ba398a2a5aaf4/t/63a0f0b028cfe264b65c6336/1671491761395/BTSNZ+Submission+on+Pharmac+Rule+8.1b_Final.pdf.
23. Pharmac: https://pharmac.govt.nz/news-and-resources/news/funding-process-for-child-cancer-medicines-to-remain
24. Pharmac: March 2024. "Summary of submissions to the review of rule 8.1b of the pharmaceutical schedule". https://pharmac.govt.nz/assets/Uploads/Update-on-Rule-8.1b-Summary-of-submissions-to-the-review.pdf
25. The International Brain Tumour Alliance (IBTA)., https://theibta.org/charter/ [Accessed 25 Jan 2025].
26. Brain Tumour Research, https://braintumourresearch.org/blogs/campaigning/stark-facts?_gl=1*hhmt1h*_up*MQ..*_ga*MTYwNjc1Nzc4OC4xNzM4MTkyNzI3*_ga_FRXYK27L9B*MTczODE5MjcyNi4xLjAuMTczODE5MjcyNi42MC4wLjEwMDAzODQ1Mg [Accessed 26 Jan 2025].
27. Oliver K, et al. Brain tumour patients' rights and the power of patient advocacy: the current international landscape. Neuro-oncol Pract. 2024; https://doi.org/10.1093/nop/npae079. [Accessed 25 Jan 2025]
28. Chan MH, Boop F and Qaddoumi I, Challenges and opportunities to advance paediatric neuro-oncology care in the developing world, Childs Nerv Syst, August 2015, https://doi.org/10.1007/s00381-015-2771-x [Accessed 26 Jan 2025].
29. Moreira DC, Bouffet E Qaddoumi, I, The greatest challenge for pediatric low-grade glioma, Neuro-Oncol, February 2024, https://doi.org/10.1093/neuonc/noae004 [Accessed 27 Jan 2025].
30. Zebrack B. Information and service needs for young adult cancer survivors. Support Care Cancer. 2009;17(4):349–57.
31. Salsman JM, Bingen K, Barr RD. Understanding, measuring, and addressing the financial impact of cancer on adolescents and young adults. Pediatr Blood Cancer. 2016;63(2):219–25.
32. Ferrari A, Thomas D, Franklin AR, Hayes-Lattin BM, Mascarin M, van der Graaf W, Albritton KH. Starting

an adolescent and young adult program: some success stories and some obstacles to overcome. J Clin Oncol. 2010;28(32):4850–7.
33. De Salvo A, De Ioris MA, Secco DE, Bevilacqua F, Premuselli R, Amicucci M, Ciaralli I, Santato F, Mastronuzzi A, Milano GM. The 4YouLab model: a dedicated-program for adolescents and young adults with cancer in a children's hospital. Front Oncol. 2021;
34. Associazione 4 You: https://www.4youaps.org/
35. Inoue R. Shounigan Oyanokai no katudou no Hensen to Kongo no Tenbou [the evolution of parent associations and the shift in their organizational goals]. Japn Soc Pediatric Hematol/Oncol. 2011;48(1)
36. Gonzalez AR. Patient advocacy history, evolution and impact on health. JOJ Pub Health. 2018;3(3):555615. https://doi.org/10.19080/JOJPH.2018.03.555615.
37. Parvataneni R, Polley MY, Freeman T, Lamborn K, Prados M, Butowski N, Liu R, Clarke J, Page M, Rabbitt J, Fedoroff A, Clow E, Hsieh E, Kivett V, Deboer R, Chang S. Identifying the needs of brain tumor patients and their caregivers. J Neuro-Oncol. 2011;104(3):737–44. https://doi.org/10.1007/s11060-011-0534-4. Epub 2011 Feb 11. PMID: 21311950; PMCID: PMC3170122
38. Carter B, Young S, Ford K, Campbell S. The concept of child-centred care in healthcare: a scoping review. Pediatr Rep. 2024;16(1):114–34. https://doi.org/10.3390/pediatric16010012. PMID: 38391000; PMCID: PMC10885088
39. Ahmann E. Family-centered care: shifting orientation. Pediatr Nurs. 1994;20:113–7.
40. Rhee M, Mui P, Cadogan C, Imerman J, Lindsell S, Samant LT. The role of brain tumor advocacy groups. Curr Neurol Neurosci Rep. 2014;14(4):442. https://doi.org/10.1007/s11910-014-0442-z. PMID: 24604060

FSC
www.fsc.org

MIX
Papier aus verantwortungsvollen Quellen
Paper from responsible sources
FSC® C105338

If you have any concerns about our products,
you can contact us on
ProductSafety@springernature.com

In case Publisher is established outside the EU,
the EU authorized representative is:
Springer Nature Customer Service Center GmbH
Europaplatz 3, 69115 Heidelberg, Germany

Printed by Libri Plureos GmbH
in Hamburg, Germany